Gonadotropins and Gonadal Function

ACADEMIC PRESS RAPID MANUSCRIPT REPRODUCTION

Proceedings of a Conference
held at Bangalore, India
in October, 1973
under the joint sponsorship of
the International Union of Biochemistry,
Federation of Asian and Oceanian Biochemists,
and the University Grants Commission, India

Gonadotropins and Gonadal Function

EDITED BY

N. R. Moudgal

Department of Biochemistry
Indian Institute of Science
Bangalore, India

With a Foreword by

C. H. Li

ACADEMIC PRESS, INC. New York San Francisco London 1974

A Subsidiary of Harcourt Brace Jovanovich, Publishers

ACADEMIC PRESS, INC.
111 Fifth Avenue, New York, New York 10003

United Kingdom Edition published by
ACADEMIC PRESS, INC. (LONDON) LTD.
24/28 Oval Road, London NW1

Library of Congress Cataloging in Publication Data
Main entry under title:

Gonadotropins and gonadal functions.

Proceedings of an international symposium, "Advances in chemistry, biology, and immunology of gonadotropins," held in October 1973 at the Indian Institute of Science, Bangalore, India under the joint sponsorship of the International Union of Biochemistry, the Federation of Asian and Oceanian Biochemists, and the University Grants Commission, India.

1. Gonadotropin–Congresses. I. Moudgal, N. R., ed. II. International Union of Biochemistry. III. Federation of Asian and Oceanian Biochemists. IV. India (Republic). University Grants Commission. [DNLM: 1. Gonadotropins–Congresses–Gonads–Physiology–Congresses. WK900 G6353]
QP572.G6G67 596'.01'66 74-16108
ISBN 0–12–508850–7

PRINTED IN THE UNITED STATES OF AMERICA

Contents

List of Contributors ix
Foreword xvii
Preface xix
List of Abbreviations xxi

SECTION I. CHEMISTRY OF GONADOTROPINS

On the Chemistry of Pituitary Interstitial Cell Stimulating Hormone 1
M. R. Sairam, David Chung, Thomas A. Bewley, and Choh Hao Li

Structural Study of Luteinizing Hormone 16
Y. Combarnous, J. Closset, G. Maghuin-Rogister, and G. Hennen

Chemistry of Follicle Stimulating Hormone 23
P. Rathnam and B. B. Saxena

Chemical Aspects of Highly Purified Human Pituitary Follicle Stimulating Hormone 42
J. F. Kennedy

Characterization of Ovine Pituitary Glycoprotein with Dual Gonadotropic Activity 54
G. Sreemathi and S. Duraiswami

Purification and Characterization of Urinary hCG 66
H. Van Hell

Chemistry of Human Chorionic Gonadotropin 79
F. J. Morgan, S. Birken, and R. E. Canfield

Purification and Characterization of Human Chorionic Gonadotropin in Hydatidiform Mole 93
P. K. Chan, C. Y. Lee, and L. Ma

Identification and Chemical Characterization of the Pituitary Gonadotropins in Reptiles and Amphibians 101
Paul Licht and Harold Papkoff

Some Aspects of Chemistry and Biology of Piscine Gonadotropins 118
B. I. Sundararaj and T. S. A. Samy

Studies on Hypothalamic Gonadotropin-Releasing Factors 128
Raghavan M. G. Nair and John A. Colwell

Recent Advances in the Physiology and Chemistry of Gonadotropin-Releasing Factors 149
S. M. McCann, P. G. Harms, C. Libertun, S. R. Ojeda, R. Orias, R. L. Moss, C. P. Fawcett, and L. Krulich

SECTION II. BIOLOGY AND IMMUNOLOGY OF GONADOTROPINS

Gonadotropins: A Correlation of Biological and Immunological Activities 161
Shanta S. Rao, B. Dattatreya Murthy, and Anil R. Sheth

Immunosorbents of Gonadotropins and Their Antibodies 169
K. Muralidhar, T. S. A. Samy, and N. R. Moudgal

The Use of Granulosa Cell Cultures and Short-Term Incubations in the Assay for Gonadotropins 185
Cornelia P. Channing

Gonadotropic Control of the Development of Testes and Accessory Organs 199
M. R. N. Prasad

Gonadotropin Regulation of Follicular Development in the Hamster 205
Gilbert S. Greenwald

Studies on Follicular Maturation — Effects of FSH- and LH Antisera in Hamsters 213
A. Jagannadha Rao, C. S. Sheela Rani, and N. R. Moudgal

Gonadotropins and Functions of Granulosal and Thecal Cells *In Vivo* and *In Vitro* 220
Sardul S. Guraya

Role of Gonadotropins in Ovulation 237
Neena B. Schwartz and Charles A. Ely

Effect of Anti-Gonadotropin Serum on Ovulation in Mice 253
Shuji Sasamoto

Luteotropic Complex in Lactating Rats 260
K. Yoshinaga and J. J. Ford

Role of Luteinizing Hormone and Prolactin in the Luteotropic Process 271
H. G. Madhwa Raj, G. J. MacDonald, and Roy O. Greep

Ultrastructural Changes in the Corpus Luteum of Pregnancy in the Golden Hamster following LH Deprival 281
Mukku Venkatramaiah, T. C. Anand Kumar, Kamala Kumar A. Jagannadha Rao, and N. R. Moudgal

SECTION III. BIOCHEMISTRY OF GONADOTROPINS

Mechanism of Action of Luteinizing Hormone – Releasing Hormone 292
Fernand Labrie, Georges Pelletier, Pierre Borgeat, Jacques Drouin, Muriel Savary, Jean Côté, and Louise Ferland

Hypothalamic Content of Luteinizing Hormone Releasing Factor and Its Mechanism of Action on the Rat Anterior Pituitary 305
Tsunehisa Makino, Michio Takahashi, Koji Yoshinaga, and Roy O. Greep

Biosynthesis of Gonadotropins and Their Releasing Factors 312
Katsumi Wakabayashi, Tadashi Asai, Takashi Higuchi, Bun-Ichi Tamaoki, and Samuel M. McCann

Chorionic Gonadotropin Produced from the Cultivated Trophoblast 321
Shimpei Tojo, Matsuto Mochizuki, and Takeshi Maruo

Interactions between Prostaglandins and Gonadotropins on Corpus Luteum Function 332
Harold R. Behrman, T. S. NG, and Gayle R. Orczyk

Evidence for the Role of Ovarian Prostaglandins in Ovulation 345
D. T. Armstrong, Y. S. Moon, and J. Zamecnik

Possible Role of Prostaglandins in the Secretion of Gonadotropins 357
A. P. Labhsetwar, H. S. Joshi, and A. Zolovick

Gonadotropins and Cyclic AMP in Various Compartments of Rat Ovary 364
K. Ahrén, H. Herlitz, L. Nilsson, J. Perklev, S. Rosberg, and G. Selstam

The Role of Cyclic AMP and Prostaglandins in the Actions of Luteinizing Hormone 376
John M. Marsh and William J. LeMaire

Studies on the Mechanism of Action of LH 391
C. Das, G. L. Kumari, and G. P. Talwar

The Role of Cytochrome P.450 in the Side-Chain Cleavage of Cholesterol 403
Peter F. Hall and Mikio Shikita

Gonadotropin-Receptor Activity and Granulosa Luteal Cell Differentiation 416
A. R. Midgley, Jr., A. J. Zeleznik, H. J. Rajaniemi, J. S. Richards, and L. E. Reichert, Jr.

Studies on Action of Luteinizing Hormone in the Rat 430
N. R. Moudgal and K. Muralidhar

Purification of LH-HCG Receptor from Luteinized Rat Ovaries 444
C. Y. Lee and R. J. Ryan

The Role of Carbohydrate in the Biological Function of Human Chorionic Gonadotropin 460
Om P. Bahl and Leopold Marz

Biochemical Aspects of the Interaction of the Human Chorionic Gonadotropin with Rat Gonads 474
Yoshihiko Ashitaka and Samuel S. Koide

Some Effects of FSH on the Seminiferous Epithelium of Mammalian Testis 485
Anthony R. Means

Cell-Types Influenced by FSH in the Rat Testis 500
Jennifer H. Dorrington and Irving B. Fritz

SECTION IV. GONADOTROPINS IN CLINICAL MEDICINE

Induction of Ovulation with Gonadotropins: Prevention of Ovarian Hyperstimulation 512
Melvin L. Taymor, Merle J. Berger, and Irwin E. Thompson

Use of Urinary Estrone and Other Parameters in Monitoring Gonadotropin Therapy 522
Shanti M. Shahani, P. G. Natrajan, and P. C. Merchant

Regulation of Gonadal Function in the Male by Gonadotropins 531
H. G. Burger, H. W. G. Baker, D. M. DeKretser, B. Hudson, P. Franchimont, and R. J. Pepperell

Serum Gonadotropins in Men with Hypogonadism: Mesterolone in the Treatment of Oligozoospermia 545
G. K. Rastogi, B. N. Datta, R. J. Dash, and M. K. Sinha

Concluding Remarks 551
A. V. Nalbandov

Subject Index 555

List of Contributors

Numbers in parentheses indicate pages on which authors' contributions begin

AHRÉN, K. (364), Department of Physiology, University of Göteberg, Göteborg, & Research Laboratories AB Leo, Helsingbörg, Sweden

ANAND KUMAR, T. C. (281), Neuroendocrine Laboratory, Department of Anatomy, All India Institute of Medical Sciences, New Delhi, India

ARMSTRONG, D. T. (345), Department of Physiology & Obstetrics & Gynecology, University of Western Ontario, London, Ontario, Canada

ASAI, TADASHI (313), Gunma University, Institute of Endocrinology, Maebashi, Japan

ASHITAKA, YOSHIHIKO (474), Department of Obstetrics & Gynecology, Kobe University School of Medicine, Kobe, Japan

BAHL, OM. P. (460), Department of Biochemistry, State University of New New York at Buffalo, Buffalo, New York

BAKER, H. W. G. (531), Department of Medicine, Prince Henry's Hospital Medical Research Center, Monash University, Melbourne, Australia

BEHRMAN, HAROLD, R. (332), Department of Reproductive Biology, Merck Institute of Therapeutic Research, Rahway, New Jersey

BERGER, MERLE, J. (512), Peter Bent Brigham Hospital & Harvard Medical School, Boston, Massachusetts

BEWLEY, THOMAS, A. (1), Hormone Research Laboratory, University of California Medical Center, San Francisco, California

BIRKEN, S. (79), Department of Medicine, College of Physicians & Surgeons, Columbia University, New York, New York

BORGEAT, PIERRE (292), MRC Group in Molecular Endocrinology, Centre Hôpital de L'Universite Laval, Quebec, Canada

BURGER, H. G. (531), Department of Medicine, Prince Henry's Hospital Medical Research Center, Monash University, Melbourne, Australia

CANFIELD, R. E.,(79), Department of Medicine, College of Physicians & Surgeons, Columbia University, New York, New York

CHAN, P. K. (93), Department of Biochemistry, The Chinese University of Hong Kong, Shatin, Hong Kong

CHANNING, CORNELIA, P. (185), Department of Physiology, University of Pittsburgh, Pittsburgh, Pennsylvania

CHUNG, DAVID (1), Hormone Research Laboratory, University of California Medical Center, San Francisco, California

CLOSSET, J. (16), Section d'Endocrinologie, Department de Clinique et de Semeiologie Medicales, Institut de Medecine, Universite de Leige, Belgium

COLWELL, JOHN, A. (128), Department of Medicine, Medical University of South Carolina & V. A. Hospital, Charleston, South Carolina

COMBARNOUS, Y. (16), Section d'Endocrinologie, Department de Clinique et de Semeiologie Medicales, Institut de Medecine, Universite de Liege, Belgium

CÔTÉ, JEAN (292), **MRC** Group in Molecular Endocrinology, Centre Hôpital de L'Universite Laval, Quebec, Canada

DAS. C. (391), Department of Biochemistry, All India Institute of Medical Sciences, New Delhi, India

DASH, R. J. (545), Department of Endocrinology, Post-graduate Institute of Medical Education & Research, Chandigarh, India

DATTA, B. N. (545), Department of Endocrinology, Post-graduate Institute of Medical, Research & Education, Chandigarh, India

DATTATREYA MURTHY, B. (161), Institute for Research in Reproduction, Parel, Bombay, India

DE KRETSER, D. M. (531), Department of Medicine, Prince Henry's Hospital Medical Research Center, Monash University, Melbourne, Australia

DORRINGTON, JENNIFER (500), Banting & Best Department of Medical Research, University of Toronto, Toronto, Ontario, Canada

DROUIN, JACQUES (292), MRC Group in Molecular Endocrinology, Centre Hôpital de L'Universite Laval, Quebec, Canada

DURAISWAMY, S. (54), Department of Zoology, University of Delhi, Delhi, India

ELY, CHARLES, A. (237), Department of Anatomy, Columbia University, College of Physicians & Surgeons, New York, New York

FAWCETT, C. P. (149), Department of Physiology, University of Texas Health Sciences, Southwestern Medical School, Dallas, Texas

FERLAND, LOUISE (292), MRC Group in Molecular Endocrinology, Centre Hôpital de L'Universite Laval, Quebec, Canada

FORD, J. J. (260), Laboratory of Human Reproduction & Reproductive Biology, Harvard Medical School, Boston, Massachusetts

FRANCHIMONT, P. (531), Institut de Medicine, University de Liege, Liege, Belgium

FRITZ, IRVING, B. (500), Banting & Best Department of Medical Research, University of Toronto, Toronto, Ontario, Canada

GREENWALD, GILBERT, S. (205), Department of Obstetrics & Gynecology & Anatomy, University of Kansas Medical Center, Kansas City, Kansas

GREEP, ROY, O. (271, 305), Laboratory of Human Reproduction & Reproductive Biology, Harvard Medical School, Boston, Massachusetts

GURAYA, SARDUL, S. (220), Department of Zoology, Punjab Agricultural University, Ludhiana, Punjab, India

HALL, PETER, F. (403), Department of Physiology, College of Medicine, University of California, Irvine, California

HARMS, P. G., (149), Department of Physiology, University of Texas Health Sciences, Southwestern Medical School, Dallas, Texas

HENNEN, G. (16), Section d'Endocrinologie, Department de clinique et de Semeiologie Medicales, Institut de Medecine, Universite de Liege, Belgium

HERLITZ, H. (364), Department of Physiology, University of Goteborg, Goteborg, & Research Laboratories, AB Leo, Helsingborg, Sweden

HIGUCHI TAKASHI (313), Yokohama City University School of Medicine, Yokohama, Japan

HUDSON, B. (531), Department of Medicine, Prince Henry's Hospital Medical Research Center, Monash University, Melbourne, Australia

JOSHI, H. S. (357), Worcestor Foundation for Experimental Biology, Shrewsbury, Massachusetts

KAMALA KUMAR (281), Neuroendocrine Laboratory, Department of Anatomy, All India Institute of Medical Sciences, New Delhi, India

KENNEDY, J. F. (42), Department of Chemistry, University of Birmingham, Edgbaston, Birmingham, England

KOIDE, SAMUEL, S. (474), The Population Council, The Rockefeller University, New York, New York

KRULICH, L. (149), Department of Physiology, University of Texas Health Sciences, Southwestern Medical School, Dallas, Texas

KUMARI, G. L. (391), National Institute of Family Planning, New Delhi, India

LABHSETWAR, A. P. (357), Worcester Foundation for Experimental Biology, Shrewsbury, Massachusetts

LABRIE, FERNAND (292), MRC Group in Molecular Endocrinology, Centre Hôpital de L'Universite Laval, Quebec, Canada

LEE, C. Y. (93), Department of Biochemistry, The Chinese University of Hong Kong, Shatin, Hong Kong

LEE, C. Y. (444), Department of Endocrine Research, Mayo Medical School, Rochester, Minnesota

LEMAIRE WILLIAM, J. (376), Departments of Biochemistry & Obstetrics & Gynecology, University of Miami School of Medicine, Miami, Florida

LI, CHOH HAO (1), Hormone Research Laboratory, University of California Medical Center, San Francisco, California

LIBERTUN, C. (149), Department of Physiology, University of Texas Health Sciences, Southwestern Medical School, Dallas, Texas

LICHT, PAUL (101), Department of Zoology, University of California, Berkeley, California

MA LIN (93), Department of Biochemistry, The Chinese University of Hong Kong, Shatin, Hong Kong

MacDONALD, G. J. (271), Laboratory of Human Reproduction & Reproductive Biology, Harvard Medical School, Boston, Massachusetts

MADHWA RAJ, H. G. (271), Laboratory for Human Reproduction and Reproductive Biology, Harvard Medical School, Boston, Massachusetts

MAGHUIN-ROGISTER, G. (16), Section d'Endocrinologie, Department de Clinique et de Semeiologie Medicales, Institut de Medicine, Universite de Liege, Belgium

MAKINO, TSUNEHISA (305), Laboratory for Human Reproduction and Reproductive Biology, Harvard Medical School, Boston, Massachusetts (Department of Obstetrics & Gynecology Keio University, School of Medicine Tokyo, Japan)

MARSH, JOHN, M. (376), Departments of Biochemistry & Obstetrics & Gynecology, University of Miami School of Medicine, Miami, Florida

MARUO TAKESHI (321), Department of Obstetrics & Gynecology, Kobe University School of Medicine, Ikuta Ku, Kobe, Japan

MARZ, LEOPOLD (460), Department of Biochemistry, State University of New York at Buffalo, Buffalo, New York, New York

McCANN, S. M. (313), Department of Physiology, University of Texas Health Sciences, Southwestern Medical School, Dallas, Texas

MEANS, ANTHONY, R. (485), Department of Cell Biology, Baylor College of Medicine, Houston, Texas

MERCHANT, P. C. (522), Department of Endocrinology, T. N. Medical College & Nair Hospital, Bombay, India

MIDGLEY, A. R., Jr. (416), Department of Pathology, University of Michigan, Ann Arbor, Michigan

MOCHIZUKI MATSUTO (321), Department of Obstetrics & Gynecology, Kobe University, School of Medicine, Ikuta Ku, Kobe, Japan

MOON, Y. S. (345), Department of Physiology & Obstetrics & Gynecology, University of Western Ontario, London, Ontario, Canada

MORGAN, F. J. (79), Department of Medicine, College of Physicians & Surgeons, Columbia University, New York, New York (St. Vincent's School of Medical Research, Melbourne, Victoria 3065, Australia)

MOSS, R. L. (149), Department of Physiology, University of Texas Health Sciences, Southwestern Medical School, Dallas, Texas

MOUDGAL, N. R. (169, 213, 281, 430), Department of Biochemistry, Indian Institute of Science, Bangalore, India

MUKKU VENKATRAMAIAH (281), Department of Biochemistry, Indian Institute of Science, Bangalore, India

MURALIDHAR, K. (169, 430), Department of Biochemistry, Indian Institute of Science, Bangalore, India

NAIR, RAGHAVAN, M. G. (128), Department of Medicine, Medical University of South Carolina & V. A. Hospital, Charleston, South Carolina

NALBANDOV, A. V. (551), University of Illinois, Urbana, Illinois

NATRAJAN, P. G. (522), Department of Endocrinology, T. N. Medical College & Nair Hospital, Bombay, India

NG, T. S. (332), Department of Reproductive Biology, Merck Institute of Therapeutic Research, Rahway, New Jersey

NILSSON, L. (364), Department of Physiology, University of Göteborg, Göteborg, & Research Laboratories, AB Leo, Helsingborg, Sweden

OJEDA, S. R. (149), Department of Physiology, University of Texas Health Sciences, Southwestern Medical School, Dallas, Texas

ORCZYK, GAYLE, R. (332), Department of Reproductive Biology, Merck Institute of Therapeutic Research, Rahway, New Jersey

ORIAS, R. (149), Department of Physiology, University of Texas Health Sciences, Southwestern Medical School, Dallas, Texas

PAPKOFF, HAROLD (101), Hormone Research Laboratory, University of California Medical Center, San Francisco, California

PELLETIER, GEORGES (292), MRC Group in Molecular Endocrinology, Centre Hospital de L' Universite Laval, Quebec, Canada

PEPPERELL, R. J. (531), Institut de Medicine, University de Liege, Liege, Belgium

PERKLEV, J. (364), Department of Physiology, University of Göteborg, Göteborg, & Research Laboratories, AB Leo, Helsingborg, Sweden

PRASAD, M. R. N. (199), Department of Zoology, University of Delhi, Delhi, India

RAJANIEMI, H. J. (416), Department of Pathology, University of Michigan, Ann Arbor, Michigan

RAO, A. JAGANNADHA (213, 281), Department of Biochemistry, Indian Institute of Science, Bangalore, India (Hormone Research Laboratory University of California Medical Center, San Francisco, California)

RAO, S. SHANTA (161), Institute for Research in Reproduction, Parel, Bombay, India

RASTOGI, G. K. (545), Department of Endocrinology, Post-graduate Institute of Medical, Education & Research, Chandigarh, India

RATHNAM, P. (23), Cornell University Medical College, 1300 York Avenue, New York, New York

REICHERT, L. E., Jr. (416), Department of Biochemistry, Emory University, Atlanta, Georgia

ROSBERG, S. (364), Department of Physiology, University of Göteborg, Göteborg, & Research Laboratories, AB Leo, Helsingborg, Sweden

RICHARDS, J. S. (416), Department of Pathology, University of Michigan, Ann Arbor, Michigan

RYAN, R. J. (444), Department of Endocrine Research, Mayo Medical School, Rochester, Minnesota

SAIRAM, M. R. (1), Hormone Research Laboratory, University of California Medical Center, San Francisco, California

SAMY, T. S. A. (118, 169), Department of Biochemistry, Indian Institute of Science, Bangalore, India (Children's Cancer Research Foundation, Boston, Massachusetts)

SASAMOTO, SHUJI (253), Laboratory of Veterinary Physiology, Tokyo University of Agriculture & Technology, Fuchu, Tokyo, Japan

SAVARY MURIEL (292), MRC Group in Molecular Endocrinology, Centre Hôpital de L'Universite Laval, Quebec, Canada

SAXENA, B. B. (23), Cornell University Medical College, 1300 York Avenue, New York, New York

SCHWARTZ, NEENA, B. (237), Department of Physiology, Northwestern University Medical School, Chicago, Illinois

SELSTAM, G. (364), Department of Physiology, University of Göteborg, Göteborg, & Research Laboratories, AB Leo, Helsingborg, Sweden

SHAHANI, SHANTI, M. (522), Department of Endocrinology, T. N. Medical College & Nair Hospital, Bombay, India

SHEELA RANI, C. S. (213), Department of Biochemistry, Indian Institute of Science, Bangalore, India

SHETH, ANIL, R. (161), Institute for Research in Reproduction, Parel, Bombay, India

SHIKITA MIKIO (403), National Institute of Radiological Sciences, Chiba-Shi, Japan

SINHA, M. K. (545), Department of Endocrinology, Post-graduate Institute of Medical Education & Research, Chandigarh, India

SREEMATHI, G. (54), Department of Zoology, University of Delhi, Delhi, India

SUNDARARAJ, B. I. (118), Department of Zoology, University of Delhi, Delhi, India

TAKAHASHI MICHIO (305), Laboratory of Human Reproduction and Reproductive Biology, Harvard Medical School, Boston, Massachusetts

TALWAR, G. P. (391), Department of Biochemistry, All India Institute of Medical Sciences, New Delhi, India

TAMAOKI, BUN-ICHI (313), National Institute of Radiological Sciences, Chiba, Japan

TAYMOR, MELVIN, L. (512), Peter Bent Brigham Hospital & Harvard Medical School, Boston, Massachusetts

THOMPSON, IRWIN, E. (512), Peter Bent Brigham Hospital & Harvard Medical School, Boston, Massachusetts

TOJO SHIMPEI (321), Department of Obstetrics & Gynecology, Kobe University, School of Medicine, Ikuta-Ku, Kobe, Japan

VAN HELL, H. (66), Research & Development Laboratories of Organon, Oss, Holland

WAKABAYASHI KATSUMI (312), Gunma University, Institute of Endocrinology, Maebashi, Japan,

YOSHINAGA, K. (260, 305), Laboratory of Human Reproduction and Reproductive Biology, Harvard Medical School, Boston, Massachusetts

ZAMECNIK, J. (345), Department of Physiology & Obstetrics & Gynecology, University of Western Ontario, London, Ontario, Canada

ZELEZNIK, A. J. (416), Department of Pathology, University of Michigan, Ann Arbor, Michigan

ZOLOVICK, A. (357), Worcester Foundation for Experimental Biology, Shrewsbury, Massachusetts

Foreword

The first indication of the relationship between the pituitary gland and gonad function was made in 1909 by S. J. Crowe, H. Cushing, and J. Homan during their investigations on the hypophysectomy of the dog. It was not until 1926 that the evidence for gonadotropic activity in the anterior lobe of the pituitary was conclusively demonstrated in the rat by P. E. Smith. This was followed by the observations of S. Ascheim and B. Zondek in 1927 for the existence of human chorionic gonadotropin in the urine of pregnant women, and H. H. Cole and G. H. Hart in 1930 for the presence of gonadotropic activity in the serum of pregnant mares. In 1931, H. L. Fevold, F. L. Hisaw, and S. L. Leonard demonstrated that "the anterior lobe of the hypophysis secretes two hormones which act on the ovary: a gonad stimulating factor which stimulates follicular growth and a luteinizing factor which causes lutenic growth." The latter factor is also known as interstitial cell stimulating hormone.

The four gonadotropins (follicle stimulating hormone, interstitial cell stimulating hormone, human chorionic gonadotropin and pregnant mare serum gonadotropin) have now been completely purified and isolated in their pure form. They are glycoproteins consisting of two chemically different subunits. The amino acid sequence of the two subunits in human chorionic gonadotropin and human pituitary interstitial cell stimulating hormone have only recently been elucidated. It is therefore timely to review the present knowledge on the chemistry and biology of these gonadotropins. We are indebted to Professor N. R. Moudgal for his skillful efforts in organizing the symposium and for editing the proceedings for those who were not able to attend.

Choh Hao Li

Preface

The present volume represents the proceedings of an International Symposium, "Advances in Chemistry, Biology and Immunology of Gonadotropins," held in October 1973 at the Indian Institute of Science, Bangalore, India. The Symposium was sponsored by the International Union of Biochemistry (its 54th symposium), the Federation of Asian and Oceanian Biochemists (1st symposium), and the Society of Biological Chemists, India.

The subject of gonadotropins—the chemistry, physiological and biochemical mechanism of action, mechanisms involved in their release from the pituitary, etc.—has, during the last decade, received keen attention from scientists of different disciplines. This has necessitated periodic reviews and critical evaluations of the vast amount of newer information thus gathered. The proceedings of the present symposium are grouped under four sections—I. Chemistry of Gonadotropins; II. Biology and Immunology of Gonadotropins; III. Biochemistry of Gonadotropins, and IV. Gonadotropins in Clinical Medicine. It is my sincere hope that this volume will serve as a valuable reference work on the current thinking in the rapidly advancing field of gonadotropins.

I am thankful to all the participants and discussants of the symposium, and in particular, to the following distinguished scientists who chaired the various sessions: Drs. C. H. Li, R. K. Meyer, A. R. Midgley, Shanta S. Rao, M. R. N. Prasad, A. V. Nalbandov, J. Marsh, R. J. Ryan, G. P. Talwar, H. G. Burger, and P. N. Shah. Further, I am grateful to Prof. C. H. Li for kindly agreeing to act as the Honorary President of the symposium and also for writing a Foreword for this volume. To Prof. A. V. Nalbandov, my thanks for kindly writing the Concluding Remarks on this symposium.

The following agencies—The University Grants Commission, India, the Indian Council of Medical Research, New Delhi, The Council of Scientific and Industrial Research, India, the Family Planning Foundation, India, the Indian Institute of Science, Bangalore, the Ford Foundation, New Delhi, and the Population Council, New York, kindly made available grants-in-aid. The organizers are grateful to all these agencies for their timely help, without which this symposium would not have materialized.

It is a pleasure to record here my warm appreciation of the excellent editorial and general assistance given to me by my colleague Miss. C. S. Sheela Rani throughout the preparation of this volume. My grateful thanks are to my colleague Mr. K. Muralidhar for helping me in editing some of the manuscripts.

PREFACE

The photo-offset process has been used in the preparation of this volume, with the hope that an early publication of this will benefit the readers. My grateful thanks are due to my secretary, Mr. P. Pasupathy for a patient and excellent job of retyping the manuscripts in a camera-ready form, and to Academic Press for facilitating the publication of this volume.

N. R. Moudgal

List of Abbreviations

adenosine $3',5'$ monophosphate	cyclic AMP or cAMP
adrenocorticotropic hormone	ACTH
antiserum	a/s
centigrade (temp)	t°
follicle stimulating hormone	FSH
follicle stimulating hormone releasing—hormone	FSH-RH
gram (s)	g or gm
gravity	g
growth hormone	GH
hour (s)	hr
human chorionic gonadotropin	hCG
human menopausal gonadotropin	HMG
human placental lactogen	HPL
international unit	IU
intramuscular(ly)	im
intraperitoneal(ly)	ip
intravenous(ly)	iv
interstitial cell stimulating hormone	ICSH, (LH)
luteinizing hormone	LH
luteinizing hormone releasing hormone or factor	LHRF, LHRH, LRF
minute (s)	min
N-acetyl neuraminic acid	NANA
ovarian ascorbic acid depletion	OAAD
pregnant mare serum gonadotropin	PMSG or PMS
prolactin release inhibiting factor	PIF
prostaglandin (s)	PG (s)
probability	p
standard deviation	S. D.
standard error of mean	S. E. M
subcutaneous(ly)	sc
thyroid stimulating hormone	TSH

prefixes o, h, b, r indicate the species ovine, human, bovine and rat, respectively.

ON THE CHEMISTRY OF PITUITARY INTERSTITIAL CELL STIMULATING HORMONE

M.R. Sairam, David Chung, Thomas A. Bewley, and Choh Hao Li

Significant progress has been made in recent years on the isolation and physicochemical characterization of the glycoprotein hormones ICSH, FSH, TSH of the anterior pituitary, and hCG of the placenta. In this paper, we wish to discuss three aspects of the chemistry of ICSH: the comparative chemistry of ovine and human ICSH, the -S-S- bridges in the α subunit of oICSH, and the quaternary structure of oICSH. It is not our intention to review the literature, but rather to present recent data obtained from our laboratory.

THE COMPARATIVE CHEMISTRY OF OVINE AND HUMAN ICSH

As a result of extensive studies carried out independently in two laboratories, the linear amino acid sequence of the two subunits of oICSH has been recently disclosed (1-4). All the amide or acid forms of Asx or Glx residues in ICSH-α (Fig. 1) have been determined (3,5); this information was not provided in the report of Liu et al (1). In addition, there is an inversion of residues at positions 88 and 89. The amino acid sequence of the 119 residues of the β subunit as shown in Fig. 1 are in agreement with report of Liu et al (2), excepting that in the latter, the assignment of Asn/Asp and Gln/Glu are not complete. After the preliminary reports of the completion of the amino acid sequence of oICSH appeared, a number of laboratories began the task of unravelling the structure of the human hormone.

In our investigations, hICSH was isolated either from a side fraction during the isolation of hGH, or from frozen or acetone-dried glands by the procedure described by Hartree (6) with minor modifications. By this procedure, an average of 50 mg of ICSH was obtained from 1000 acetone preserved glands (4 x NIH-LH-S14 - by OAAD assay). For the separation of α and β subunits the method of Closset et al. (7) was employed with an additional purification step by gel filtration on Sephadex G-100; the final yields of the subunits were in the order of 65 %.

Table 1 presents the amino acid and carbohydrate compositions of hICSH and its subunits. It should be pointed out that these values are in good agreement with those reported by other investigators (7-9).

At the begining of our investigation on the amino acid sequence of hICSH-α, we relied on the information already available for the whole molecule (without subunit separation) of the ovine hormone (1,3). This data was later confirmed by isolation and

H-Phe-Pro-Asp-Gly-Glu-Phe-Thr-Met-Gln-Gly-Cys-Pro-Glu-Cys-Lys-Leu-Lys-Glu-Asn-Lys-
10 20

Tyr-Phe-Ser-Lys-Pro-Asp-Ala-Pro-Ile-Tyr-Gln-Cys-Met-Gly-Cys-Cys-Phe-Ser-Arg-Ala-
30 40

CHO
Tyr-Pro-Thr-Pro-Ala-Arg-Ser-Lys-Lys-Thr-Met-Leu-Val-Pro-Lys-Asn-Ile-Thr-Ser-Glu-
50 60

Ala-Thr-Cys-Cys-Val-Ala-Lys-Ala-Phe-Thr-Lys-Ala-Thr-Val-Met-Gly-Asn-Val-Arg-Val-
70 80

CHO
Glu-Asn-His Thr-Glu-Cys-His-Ser-Cys-Thr-Cys-Tyr-Tyr-His-Lys-Ser-OH
90 96

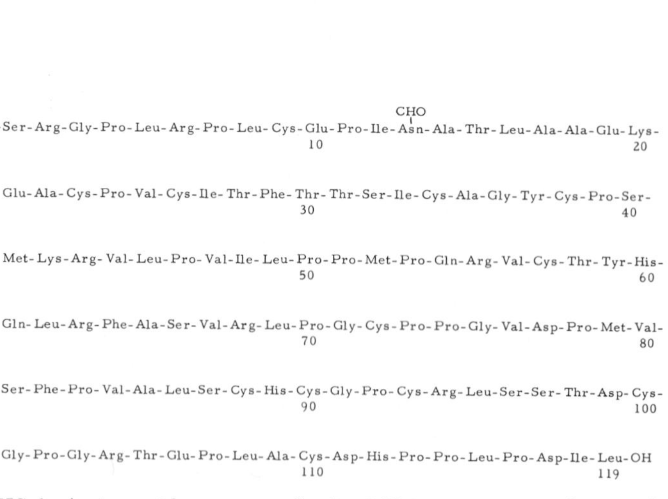

FIG 1. Amino acid sequence of ovine ICSH: upper-α, lower-β.

sequence analysis of tryptic peptides obtained from the isolated α subunit. The complete amino acid sequence of hICSH- α (10) is shown in Fig 2. It may be noted that the α subunit of hCG (11) has an almost identical sequence except for the presence of three more residues, Ala - Pro - Asx, at the NH_2-terminus. Figure 3 presents a comparison of the amino acid sequence of ICSH-α from human, ovine (1,3) and porcine (12) species. A total of 63 amino acid residues have been fully conserved. Locations of the two carbohydrate moieties are in identical positions. The amino acid sequence of bovine (13) ICSH-α has also been reported. The structures of ovine and bovine ICSH- α are almost identical, whereas the porcine subunit differs from the other two species.

Table 1. Amino acid and carbohydrate* composition of human ICSH and its subunits

Composition	ICSH-α Expt.	ICSH-α Sequence	ICSH-β Expt.	ICSH-β Sequence	Human ICSH Expt.	Human ICSH Sequence
Tryptophan**			0.7	1	1.54	1
Lysine	5.7	6	2.1	2	8.3	8
Histidine	3.0	3	2.5	3	6.0	6
Arginine	3.4	3	9.0	10	13.3	13
Aspartic acid	6.1	5	7.0	7	12.0	12
Threonine	7.9	8	6.2	7	15.0	15
Serine	7.7	8	6.1	7	13.2	15
Glutamic acid	9.0	9	7.0	7	15.8	16
Proline	7.0	6	16.9	16	20.2	22
Glycine	4.5	4	8.4	8	11.5	12
Alanine	4.3	4	5.0	5	8.5	9
Half-cystine	10.0	10	11.5	12	20.5	22
Valine	6.6	7	10.1	11	16.5	18
Methionine	2.4	3	1.8	2	4.5	5
Isoleucine	1.0	1	4.4	5	5.5	6
Leucine	4.0	4	8.0	8	12.0	12
Tyrosine	3.8	4	1.8	2	5.6	6
Phenylalanine	4.0	4	2.1	2	5.8	6
Fucose	0.5		1.2		1.64	
Mannose	6.6		3.4		10.40	
Galactose	2.8		1.9		5.0	
N-acetylglucosamine	8.0		4.5		10.8	
N-acetylgalactosamine	2.5		1.1		3.5	
Sialic acid	2.2		1.36		3.1	

*We thank Dr. J. S. Dixon for these values. ** By p-toluene sulfonic acid hydrolysis of the β-subunit and spectrophotometric estimation of the native ICSH.

H-Val-Gln-Asp-Cys-Pro-Glu-Cys-Thr-Leu-Gln- (10)

Glu-Asn-Pro-Phe-Phe-Ser-Gln-Pro-Gly-Ala- (20)

Pro-Ile-Leu-Gln-Cys-Met-Gly-Cys-Cys-Phe- (30)

Ser-Arg-Ala-Tyr-Pro-Thr-Pro-Leu-Arg-Ser- (40)

Lys-Lys-Thr-Met-Leu-Val-Gln-Lys-Asn(CHO)-Val- (50)

Thr-Ser-Glu-Ser-Thr-Cys-Cys-Val-Ala-Lys- (60)

Ser-Tyr-Asn-Arg-Val-Thr-Val-Met-Gly-Gly- (70)

Phe-Lys-Val-Glu-Asn(CHO)-His-Thr-Ala-Cys-His- (80)

Ser-Cys-Thr-Cys-Tyr-Tyr-His-Lys-Ser-OH (89)

FIG 2 Amino Acid Sequence of Human ICSH-α

	5	10	15	20
Ovine/Bovine:	Phe-Pro-Asp-Gly-Glu-	Phe-Thr-Met-Gln-Gly-	Cys-Pro-Glu-Cys-Lys-	Leu-Lys-Glu-Asn-Lys-
Human:		Val-Gln-Asp-	Cys-Pro-Glu-Cys-Thr-	Leu-Gln-Glu-Asn-Pro-
Porcine:		Thr-Met-Glx-Gly-	Cys-Pro-Glx-Cys-Lys-	Leu-Lys-Glx-Asx-Lys-

	25	30	35	40
	Tyr-Phe-Ser-Lys-Pro-	Asp-Ala-Pro-Ile-Tyr-	Gln-Cys-Met-Gly-Cys-	Cys-Phe-Ser-Arg-Ala-
	Phe-Phe-Ser-Gln-Pro-	Gly-Ala-Pro-Ile-Leu-	Gln-Cys-Met-Gly-Cys-	Cys-Phe-Ser-Arg-Ala-
	Tyr-Phe-Ser-Lys-Leu-	Gly-Ala-Pro-Ile-Tyr-	Glx-Cys-Met-Gly-Cys-	Cys-Phe-Ser-Arg-Ala-

	45	50	55	60
	Tyr-Pro-Thr-Pro-Ala-	Arg-Ser-Lys-Lys-Thr-	Met-Leu-Val-Pro-Lys-	Asn(CHO)-Ile-Thr-Ser-Glu-
	Tyr-Pro-Thr-Pro-Leu-	Arg-Ser-Lys-Lys-Thr-	Met-Leu-Val-Gln-Lys-	Asn(CHO)-Val-Thr-Ser-Glu-
	Tyr-Pro-Thr-Pro-Ala-	Arg-Ser-Lys-Lys-Thr-	Met-Leu-Val-Pro-Lys-	Asn(CHO)-Ile-Thr-Ser-Glx-

	65	70	75	80
	Ala-Thr-Cys-Cys-Val-	Ala-Lys-Ala-Phe-Thr-	Lys-Ala-Thr-Val-Met-	Gly-Asn-Val-Arg-Val
	Ser-Thr-Cys-Cys-Val-	Ala-Lys-Ser-Tyr-Asn-	Arg-Val-Thr-Val-Met-	Gly-Gly-Phe-Lys-Val
	Ala-(Thr, Cys, Cys)-Val-	Ala-Lys-Ala-Phe-Thr-	Lys-Ala-Thr-Val-Met-	Gly-Asx-Ala-Arg-Val

	85	90	95
	Glu-Asn(CHO)-His-Thr-Glu-	Cys-His-Ser-Cys-Thr-	Cys-Tyr-Tyr-His-Lys-Ser
	Glu-Asn(CHO)-His-Thr-Ala-	Cys-His-Ser-Cys-Thr-	Cys-Tyr-Tyr-His-Lys-Ser
	Glx-Asn(CHO)-Ser-Thr-Glx-	(Cys-His, His, Cys, Thr, Cys)-	Tyr-Tyr-His-Lys-Ser

FIG 3. Structure comparison of ovine, porcine, and human ICSH-α

By the time of the 1972 Laurentian Hormone Conference, there were at least three other groups independently working on the amino acid sequence of the β subunit. While our own investigations were in progress, Ward et al. (9) presented the sequence of the first 28 amino acid residues. This was soon followed by the presentation of sequence by Closset et al (14), and Shome and Parlow (15). An examination of these proposals revealed significant differences. This prompted us to continue our interest in the problem in order to clarify the discrepancies between published reports. The two dimentional paper chromatography-electrophoretic technique proved very useful in the task of isolating all the tryptic and chymotryptic peptides required for complete sequence analysis. The amino acid composition of the tryptic peptides is recorded in Table 2. The chymotryptic peptides from

Table 2. Amino acid composition (molar ratio) of tryptic peptides of oxidized human ICSH-β

Peptide	Composition	No. of residues
T1	$Arg_{1.0}$ $Ser_{0.7}$	2
T2	$Lys_{1.0}$ $His_{0.9}$ $Arg_{1.0}$ $Cya_{0.8}$ $Asp_{0.9}$ $Glu_{1.7}$ $Pro_{2.9}$ $Ala_{1.8}$ $Val_{1.2}$ $Ile_{2.0}$ $Leu_{2.3}$	18*
T3**	$Arg_{0.9}$ $Cya_{3.5}$ $Asp_{1.3}$ $Met_{1.6}$ $Thr_{3.5}$ $Glu_{1.3}$ $Pro_{2.2}$ $Gly_{2.0}$ $Ala_{1.3}$ $Val_{2.2}$ $Ile_{1.9}$ $Tyr_{0.8}$	23
T4	$Arg_{0.8}$ $Cya_{1.0}$ $Thr_{1.0}$ $Glu_{2.0}$ $Pro_{3.4}$ $Ala_{1.0}$ $Val_{3.3}$ $Leu_{3.1}$ $Tyr_{0.6}$	16
T5	$Arg_{1.0}$ $Asp_{1.0}$ $Val_{1.2}$	3
T6	$Arg_{0.9}$ $Ser_{1.0}$ $Glu_{1.1}$ $Ile_{1.0}$ $Phe_{1.0}$	5
T7	$Arg_{0.9}$ $Cya_{0.9}$ $Pro_{2.3}$ $Gly_{1.0}$ $Leu_{1.0}$	6
T8	$Arg_{0.9}$ $Cya_{1.0}$ $Asp_{1.0}$ $Ser_{2.0}$ $Pro_{2.2}$ $Gly_{0.8}$ $Ala_{1.1}$ $Val_{3.6}$ $Leu_{1.3}$ $Phe_{1.0}$	15
T9	$Arg_{1.0}$ $Cya_{1.7}$ $Pro_{1.1}$ $Gly_{1.4}$	5
T11	$Lys_{0.9}$ $Cya_{1.0}$ $Asp_{1.0}$ $Thr_{0.9}$ $Ser_{1.8}$ $Pro_{1.0}$ $Gly_{2.0}$	9
T12	$His_{1.6}$ $Cya_{1.4}$ $Asp_{2.2}$ $Thr_{1.2}$ $Ser_{0.8}$ $Glu_{1.0}$ $Pro_{1.9}$ $Gly_{1.0}$ $Leu_{1.2}$	12

T10 is free arginine

*This includes Trp which is in the oxidized form. **Glycopeptide.

the reduced and carbamidomethylated subunit provided the necessary overlaps to completely align all the tryptic peptides. The complete amino acid sequence (16) is shown in Fig 4. This formulation is much closer to that proposed by Shome and Parlow (17), but differs considerably from that of Closset et al. (14). The position of all the amide residues have been completely determined (16). The important features to be noted as shown in our proposal are : the presence of free amino terminal serine, the single tryptophan residue at position 8, an extra residue of methionine at position 42, and the absence of lysine near the COOH-terminal. It is likely that because of heterogeneity at this end, we have not been able to isolate a C-terminal lysine containing peptide. If lysine is indeed present, this would be positioned at 116 in our sequence. Shome and Parlow (17) were unable to fix the order of the last three residues (Ser, Gly, Lys) in their proposal. Further, the positioning of two residues, Pro_{111} and Gln_{112}, is reversed in their sequence. In addition to the high degree of heterogeneity noted at the COOH-terminus during the sequence work, evidence for a peculiar internal break along the peptide chain itself was also noted in the region 44-49; this had been observed earlier by Shome and Parlow (17). Such an internal

H-Ser-Arg-Glu-Pro-Leu-Arg-Pro-Trp-Cys-His-Pro-Ile-Asn-Ala-Ile- (5, 10, 15)

Leu-Ala-Val-Gln-Lys-Glu-Gly-Cys-Pro-Val-Cys-Ile-Thr-Val-Asn(CHO)- (20, 25, 30)

Thr-Thr-Ile-Cys-Ala-Gly-Tyr-Cys-Pro-Thr-Met-Met-Arg-Val-Leu- (35, 40, 45)

Gln-Ala-Val-Leu-Pro-Pro-Leu-Pro-Gln-Val-Cys-Thr-Tyr-Arg-Asp- (50, 55, 60)

Val-Arg-Phe-Glu-Ser-Ile-Arg-Leu-Pro-Gly-Cys-Pro-Arg-Gly-Val- (65, 70, 75)

Asp-Pro-Val-Val-Ser-Phe-Pro-Val-Ala-Leu-Ser-Cys-Arg-Cys-Gly- (80, 85, 90)

Pro-Cys-Arg-Arg-Ser-Thr-Ser-Asp-Cys-Gly-Gly-Pro-Lys-Asp-His- (95, 100, 105)

Pro-Leu-Thr-Cys-Asp-Pro-Gln-His-Ser-Gly-OH (110, 115)

FIG 4. The Amino Acid Sequence of Human ICSH-β

break has not been reported in the sequence work on the subunits of ICSH and TSH from other species.

Comparison of hICSH-β with the amino acid sequence of hTSH-β recently reported by us (18) shows a high degree of similarity: a total of 43 residues are identical. Such a structural resemblance had also been noted between oICSH-β (2,4) and bTSH-β subunits (19). Thus, the studies on the human hormones provide additional evidence to the supposition that areas of sequence which are identical in the two β subunits for ICSH and TSH are the points on non-covalent binding with their respective α counterparts. Similarly, areas of non-identity contribute to interaction with target sites (receptors) and therefore must be the principal areas that confer hormonal specificity.

Comparison of human ICSH-β with the structures of ovine (2,4), bovine (20), porcine (21) ICSH-β, and hCG-β (22) shows that as in the case of the α subunit, structural conservation is apparent (Fig. 5). It may also be noted that unlike non-human ICSH, the hICSH-β subunit has the single oligosaccharide moiety linked to asparagine at position 30 instead of 13. The hCG-β, in addition to possessing four more carbohydrate chains, does have a

					5					10					15						20
Human:	H-Ser-	Arg-	Glu-	Pro-	Leu-	Arg-	Pro-	Trp-	Cys-	His-	Pro-	Ile-	Asn-	Ala-	Ile-	Leu-		-Ala-	Val-	Gln-	Lys-
HCG:		Lys	Gln					Arg		Arg			Asn		Thr					Glu	
Ovine/Bovine:			Gly					Leu		Glu			Asn		Thr				Ala	Glu	
Porcine:			Gly					Leu		Glx			Asn		Thr		Arg		Ala	Glx	Asx
													CHO								

					25					30					35					40
Human:	Glu-	Gly-	Cys-	Pro-	Val-	Cys-	Ile-	Thr-	Val-	Asn- CHO	Thr-	Thr-	Ile-	Cys-	Ala-	Gly-	Tyr-	Cys-	Pro-	Thr-
HCG:																				
Ovine/Bovine:									Phe	Thr		Ser								Ser
Porcine:	Glx	Ala							Phe	Thr		Ser								Ser

					45					50					55					60
Human:	Met-	Met-	Arg-	Val-	Leu-	Gln-	Ala-	Val-	Leu-	Pro-	Pro-	Leu-	Pro-	Gln-		-Val-	Cys-	Thr-	Tyr-	Arg-	Asp-
HCG:		Thr					Gly				Ala			Glx	Leu			Asn			
Ovine/Bovine:		Lys				Pro	Val	Ile				Met			Arg					His	Gln
Porcine:		Arg				Pro		Ala				Val		Glx	Pro						Glx

					65					70					75					80
Human:	Val-	Arg-	Phe-	Glu-	Ser-	Ile-	Arg-	Leu-	Pro-	Gly-	Cys-	Pro-	Arg-	Gly-	Val-	Asp-	Pro-	Val-	Val-	Ser-
HCG:																Asn				
Ovine/Bovine:	Leu			Ala		Val							Pro					Met		
Porcine:	Leu	Ile		Ala		Ser							Pro					Thr		

					85					90					95					100
Human:	Phe-	Pro-	Val-	Ala-	Leu-	Ser-	Cys-	Arg-	Cys-	Gly-	Pro-	Cys-	Arg-	Arg-	Ser-	Thr-	Ser-	Asp-	Cys-	Gly-
HCG:	Tyr	Ala						Gln		Ala	Leu						Thr			
Ovine/Bovine:								His						Leu		Ser	Thr			
Porcine:								His						Leu		Ser		Asx		

					105					110					115					147
Human:	Gly-	Pro-	Lys-	Asp-	His-	Pro-	Leu-	Thr-	Cys-	Asp-	Pro-	Gln-	His-	Ser-	Gly-OH		CHO			
HCG:											Asp	Pro	Arg	Phe	Gln	Asp-	Ser-	Ser	. . .	Pro
Ovine/Bovine:	Pro	Gly	Arg	Thr	Glu			Ala			His	Pro	Pro	Leu	Pro	Asp-	Ile -	Leu-OH		
Porcine:	Pro	Gly	Arg	Ala	Glx			Ala		Asx	Arg	Pro	Pro	Leu	Pro	Gly-	Leu	Leu-OH		

FIG 5. Structure comparison of human, ovine and porcine ICSH-β with HCG-β

unit linked to Asn_{30}. The resemblance of hICSH-β to hCG-β is greater than its similarity to non-primate β subunits. In all, a total of 69 amino acid residue positions have been conserved. Tryptophan is present only in human ICSH-β.

THE DISULFIDE BRIDGES IN THE α SUBUNIT OF OVINE ICSH

The ICSH and TSH molecule each has a total of 11 disulfide bonds (five in the α and six in the β) as compared to two in growth hormone and three in lactogenic hormone. The disulfide bonds are the covalent linkages between half-cystine residues located at different parts of the molecule and serve as part of the stabilizing forces that hold the molecule in its native conformation. Although the entire amino acid sequence of the subunits of ICSH have been determined, the knowledge on the primary structure of the molecule is not complete without the identification of all the constituent -S-S bonds.

The ovine ICSH-α subunit has four of its ten half-cystine residues located adjacent to one another (positions 35-36 and 63-64) and as such, the assignment of the -S-S- bonds would obviously be a difficult task. As the amino acid sequence of the α subunits are the same in ICSH and TSH (and possibly FSH), a determination of one of them would provide a solution for the other two.

In preliminary trials with a variety of enzymes such as trypsin, chymotrypsin, pronase, nagarase, subtilisin, thermolysin, acid protease, or collagenase either alone or in combination, we found that no smaller fragment amenable for meaningful evaluation was liberated. Diagonal peptide mapping of these digests yielded a large ninhydrin-positive area which moved slightly off the diagonal, indicating the possibility of the presence of a core material. Further, treatment of ICSH-α with cyanogen bromide which cleaves the peptide chain at accessible methionyl bonds, or urea treatment to make the molecule more susceptible to enzymic attack were both unsuccessful. We have finally resorted to partial acid hydrolysis as a means to obtain information to link the -S-S- bridges.

No single experiment was sufficient in itself to provide information on all the -S-S- bonds. Separate experiments were required to generate peptide fragments that were useful to assign each pairing. Further, each peptide had to be purified by many tedious purification steps. The analytical data obtained on peptides

Table 3. Composition of -S-S peptides of ovine ICSH-α

Peptide	Composition	-S-S- bridge (residues)
P-B-5-2	$Glu_{0.8}$ $Cya_{1.0}$	14-86
P-B-5-3	$Thr_{0.8}$ $Glu_{1.0}$ $Cya_{1.0}$	
2 A-3	$Cya_{2.0}$ $MetSO_{2\,1.3}$ $Thr_{1.0}$ $Glu_{1.0}$ $Gly_{0.8}$ $Ala_{0.6}$ $Val_{1.1}$	11-64
2 B-1-2	$Cya_{2.0}$ $Thr_{0.9}$ $Glu_{0.8}$ $Gly_{0.5}$ $Ala_{0.5}$	35-63
3-2	$Cya_{2.0}$ $Thr_{0.6}$ $Ser_{0.7}$ $Glu_{0.7}$	32-89

enabled us to fix four of the five disulfide bridges as summarized in Table 3. The fifth one linking residues 36 and 91, however, has been suggested by difference. In any particular experiment the yield of usable cystine-containing peptide was low, because of the large number of purification steps involved. The primary structure of the α subunit is seen in Fig 6 (5). The five disulfide bridges are formed by residues 11-64, 14-86, 32-89, 35-63 and 36-91. We propose that -S-S- bonds in ICSH-α from other species and also TSH-α of bovine and human, will have disulfide bridges in the same positions.

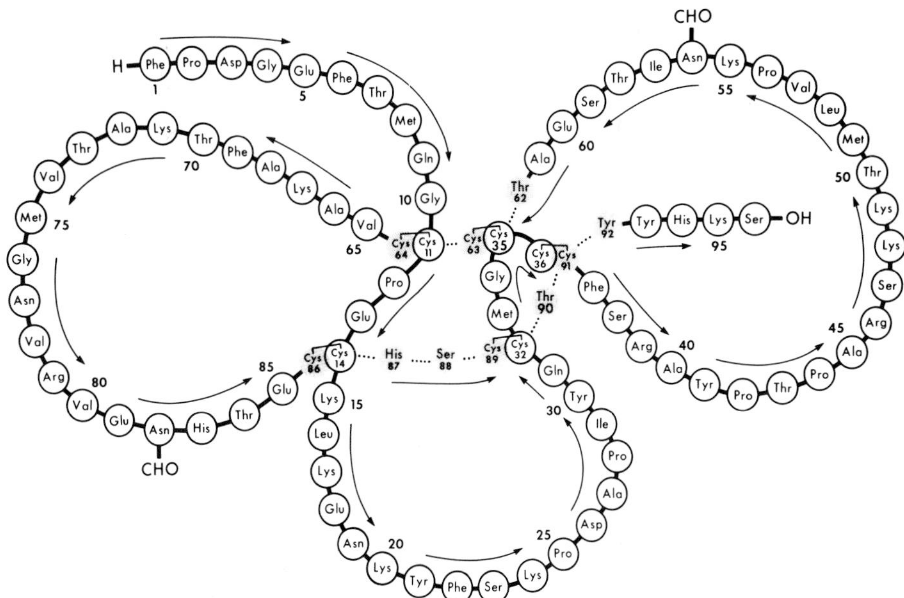

FIG 6. The primary structure of ovine ICSH- α

THE QUARTERNARY STRUCTURE OF OVINE ICSH

Very little direct experimental information is available concerning the kinetics of the dissociation and reassociation of pituitary gonadotropins. However, oICSH provides a unique opportunity for such studies in view of the extensive knowledge available regarding its structure. The circular dichroic (CD) spectra of native and reassociated ICSH, and the isolated α and β subunits, have been previously published (23). Below 240 nm, CD spectra indicate that none of these molecules contain any appreciable amount of ordered secondary structure. In the region of side-chain absorption (Fig. 7) the CD spectra of the native and reassociated hormone are indistinguishable. It may be seen from Fig 7 that the spectrum of native ICSH is not equal to the algebraic sum of the spectra of the α and β subunits. These observations have led us to conclude that definite structural changes occur upon dissociation of the native molecule giving rise to alterations in

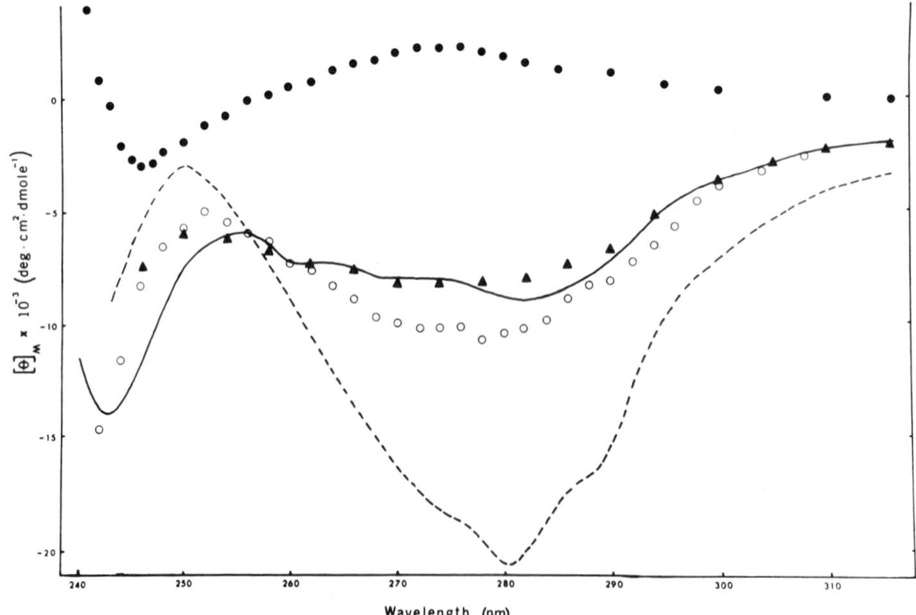

FIG 7. CD spectrum of ovine ICSH and its subunits: ------ native ICSH; oooo, β subunit; ●●●●●, α subunit, ________, algebric sum of α and β ; ▲▲▲▲, native ICSH in 5 M guanidine HCl or pH 3.6.

the environment of the aromatic residues. Further, it is apparent that all CD changes occurring during dissociation, are completely reversed upon reassociation. We have proposed that the negative maxima at 278-279 nm and the shoulder at 289 nm arise in large part from one or more buried tyrosyl residues (23). A study of the reactivity of ovine ICSH toward tetranitromethane has demonstrated that two tyrosines are indeed unreactive, with one buried residue being present in each subunit (24). However, all tyrosyl groups in the isolated subunits are fully reactive. Figure 7 also shows that the CD spectrum of ICSH treated with either guanidine hydrochloride or acidic media is equivalent to the algebraic sum of the CD spectra of the isolated subunits. Accordingly, the 289 nm CD band exhibited by the native protein has been assigned to buried tyrosyl residues. These data clearly indicate that the disappearance or appearance of the 289 and 278-279 nm bands in the CD spectrum can be conveniently used to study the dissociation - reassociation reactions, and is the most direct approach currently available.

In the present study, dissociation was followed by adjusting a solution of the intact hormone to pH 2.2 - 3.6 and continuously monitoring the CD at 280 nm as a function of time. Complete dissociation was confirmed by sedimentation velocity measurements. Reassociation was followed by readjusting the solution of dissociated subunits to pH 7.5, and monitoring the repair of mass by sedimentation velocity and the repair of the native conformation by means of CD spectra.

At pH 2.2, the dissociation is extremely fast and difficult to follow. As shown in Figure 8, the reaction is fairly rapid even at pH 3.6, reaching a stable state in approximately two hours. During this time the $S_{20,w}$ dropped from an original value of 2.54 to a stable value of 1.54, clearly indicating complete dissociation. The kinetics of the dissociation, as followed by changes in the CD spectrum, are essentially of the first order.

As shown in Fig. 8, reassociation begins as soon as the pH has been readjusted to 7.5. It is evident from the rapid increase in $S_{20,w}$ that the increase in mass occurs at a faster rate than the return to the native conformation. An analysis of the $S_{20,w}$ and CD data reveals that the mass repair is approximately of second order, while the conformational repair is approximately of first order. The final $S_{20,w}$ and CD of the reaction mixture reached values indicating 80 % reassociation. The mixture was

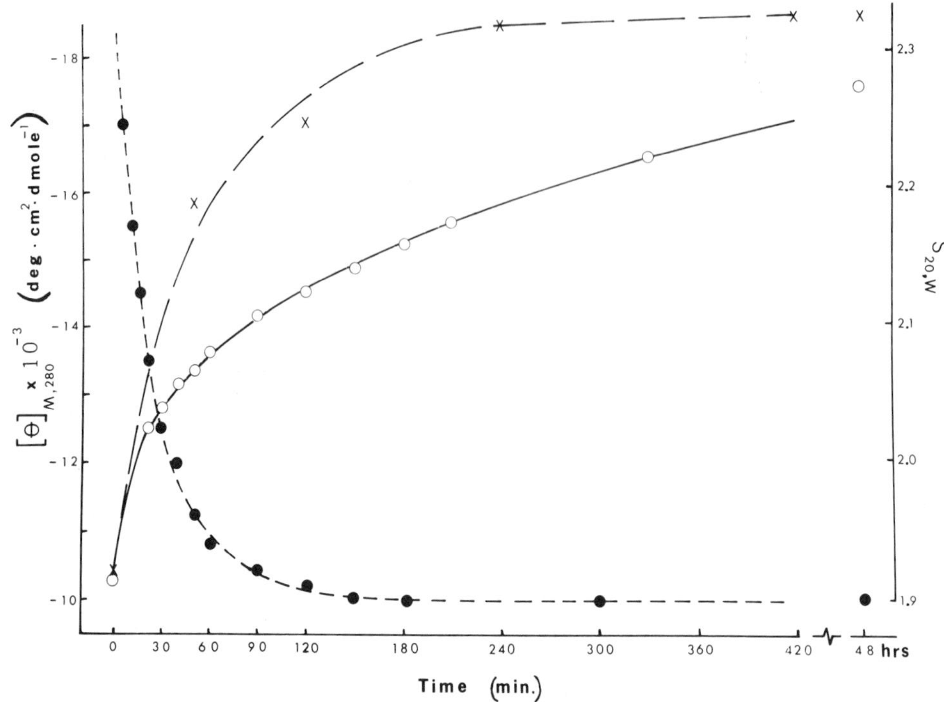

FIG 8. Mass and CD repair during association of ICSH-α and ICSH-β ; ●-----●, dissociation; x———x , repair of S value; o———o , repair of CD.

then purified by exclusion chromatography on Sephadex G-100. The elution pattern showed three distinct peaks with the major component eluting at a position equivalent to native ICSH (≈ 80 % yield by optical density). This product was isolated and found to exhibit both an $S_{20,\,w}$ value and CD spectrum identical to those of the native hormone. The second small peak appeared in the void volume of the column, while the third peak emerged at a position more retarded than native ICSH.

The formation of the reassociated molecule, based on these results, is shown in Fig. 9. The initial step is a rapid second order association producing a 30, 000 dalton intermolecular complex. After this initial "dimer" formation, the 1:1 complex undergoes a slower intramolecular rearrangement in which one of

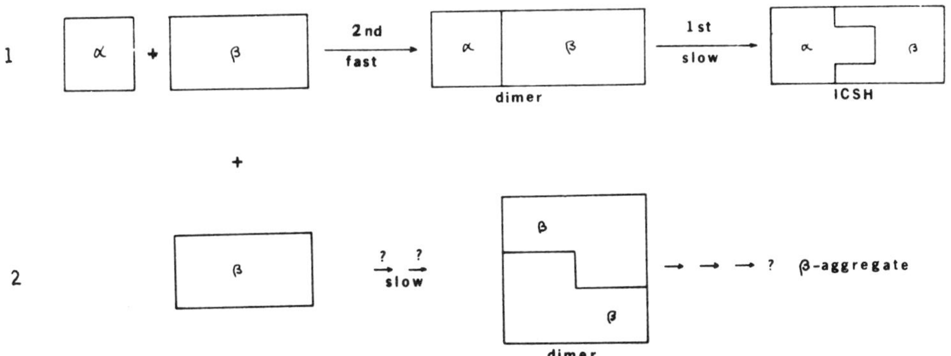

FIG 9. Diagrammatic representation of the reassociation of ICSH-α and ICSH-β

the tyrosine residues in each subunit becomes buried, developing the same local environment characteristic of the native protein. In addition, there is evidence for the presence of a slower, competing reaction which appears to involve the formation of highly aggregated β subunit. This aggregation reaction does not occur as long as the β subunit is kept under acidic conditions. Other investigators, utilizing the binding of a fluorescent dye, have reached similar conclusions regarding the dissociation and reassociation of human ICSH (25).

ACKNOWLEDGEMENTS

We take this opportunity to thank Dan Gordon, Jean Knorr, Peter Geffen, and Richard Wilcox for expert technical assistance. This work was supported in part from grants from the National Institutes of Arthritis, Metabolic and Digestive Diseases (AM 6097). The human pituitary glands were generously supplied by the National Pituitary Agency in Baltimore, Maryland.

REFERENCES

1. Liu, W.K., Nahm, H.S., Sweeney, C.M., Lamkin, W.M., Baker, H.N. and Ward, D.N. (1972). J. Biol. Chem. 247, 4351.
2. Liu, W.K., Nahm, H.S., Sweeney, C.M., Holcomb, G.N., and Ward, D.N. (1972). J. Biol. Chem. 247, 4365.
3. Sairam, M.R., Papkoff, H. and Li, C.H. (1972). Arch. Biochem. Biophys. 153, 554.
4. Sairam, M.R., Papkoff, H., Samy, T.S.A. and Li, C.H. (1972). Arch. Biochem. Biophys. 153, 572.
5. Chung, D., Sairam, M.R. and Li, C.H. (1973). Arch. Biochem. Biophys. 159, 678.
6. Hartree, A.S. (1966). Biochem. J. 100, 754.
7. Closset, J., Hennen, G. and Lequin, R.M. (1972). FEBS Letters 21, 325.
8. Hartree, A.S., Thomas, M., Braikevitch, M., Bell, E.T., Christie, D.W., Spaull, G.V., Taylor, R. and Pierce, J.G. (1971). J. Endocr. 51, 169.
9. Ward, D.N., Reichert, L.E., Jr., Liu, W.K., Nahm, H.S., Hsia, J., Lamkin, W.M. and Jones, N.S. (1973). Rec. Prog. Horm. Res. 29, 533.
10. Sairam, M.R., Papkoff, H. and Li, C.H. (1972). Biochem. Biophys. Res. Comm. 48, 530.
11. Bellisario, R., Carlsen, R.B. and Bahl, O.P. (1973). J. Biol. Chem. 248, 6796.
12. Rogister, G.M., Combarnous, Y. and Hennen, G. (1972). FEBS Letters 25, 57.
13. Pierce, J.G., Liao, T.H., Carlsen, R.B. and Reimo, T. (1971). J. Biol. Chem. 246, 866.
14. Closset, J., Hennen, G. and Lequin, R.M. (1973) FEBS Letters 29, 97.
15. Shome, B. and Parlow, A.F. (1972). Abstr. Intl. Cong. Endocrinol. 4th. 176.
16. Sairam, M.R. and Li, C.H. (1973). J. Int. Res. Comm, 1 No. 9, 14.
17. Shome, B. and Parlow, A.F. (1973). J. Clin. Endo. Metab. 36, 618.
18. Sairam, M.R. and Li, C.H. (1973). Biochem. Biophys. Res. Comm. 54, 426.

19. Liao, T.H. and Pierce, J.G. (1971). J. Biol. Chem. 246, 850.
20. Rogister, G.M. and Dockier, A. (1971). FEBS Letters 19, 209.
21. Rogister, G.M. and Hennen, G. (1972). FEBS Letters 23, 225.
22. Carlson, R.B., Bahl, O.P. and Swaminathan, N. (1973). J. Biol. Chem. 248, 6810.
23. Bewley, T.A., Sairam, M.R. and Li, C.H. (1972). Biochemistry 11, 930.
24. Sairam, M.R., Papkoff, H. and Li, C.H. (1972). Biochem. Biophys. Acta. 278, 421.
25. Aloj, S.M., Ingham, K.C. and Edelhoch (1973). Arch. Biochem. Biophys. 155, 478.

STRUCTURAL STUDY OF LUTEINIZING HORMONE

Y. Combarnous, J. Closset, G. Maghuin-Rogister
and G. Hennen

INTRODUCTION

Our group has determined the amino acid sequence of both the α and β subunits of human and porcine LH as well as that of the β subunit of bovine LH (1-3). As LH has now been studied in several species, preliminary conclusions about its molecular evolution can be drawn. These findings add weight to Liao and Pierce's hypothesis concerning the significance of the structural similarity between pituitary LH and TSH (4). We have also studied the accessibility of the tyrosyl residues in both porcine and bovine LH as well as in their subunits. Our studies on their sequence and conformation show that certain portions in the primary structure of LH (and TSH) have remained relatively constant throughout the course of evolution, and that certain of these invariant portions are probably involved in the binding of the α and β subunits to one another.

PRIMARY STRUCTURE OF LH IN SEVERAL SPECIES

A. LH β subunit

Amino acid sequences of LH β subunits from ovine, bovine, porcine and human species are compared in Table 1. The extent of homology varies from total, as seen between the ovine and bovine chain, to 68 % between the human and bovine subunit. Seventy five positions are common to the four species studied. The ovine and bovine chains exhibit identical amino acid sequences (except for position 54, which is a glutamine in the ovine chain and glutamic acid in the bovine chain); however, they differ in their polysaccharide side chain, attached in both cases to asparagine 13.

Table I. SEQUENCES OF THE β SUBUNIT OF BOVINE, OVINE, PORCINE AND HUMAN LH AND OF BOVINE AND HUMAN TSH.

Positions common to human and bovine TSH β subunits.	F C I P T E Y M H E R E C A Y C L T I N T T C A G Y C M T R B B G K L F L P K Y A L S Q D V C T Y R D F Y T E I P G C P H V P Y F S Y P V A S C K C G K C B T B Y S B C I H E A I K T N Y C T K P Q K S Y
	1 2 3 4 5 6 7 8 9 10 1 2 3 4 5 6 7 8 9 20 1 2 3 4 5 6 7 8 9 30 1 2 3 4 5 6 7 8 9 40 1 2 3 4 5 6 7 8 9 50 1 2 3 4 5 6 7 8 9 60 1 2 3 4 5 6 7 8 9 70 1 2 3 4 5 6 7 8 9 80 1 2 3 4 5 6 7 8 9 90 1 2 3 4 5 6 7 8 9 100 1 2 3 4 5 6 7 8 9 110 1 2 3
TSH β, human [Sairam & Li (7, 8)]	F C I P T E Y M T H I E R R E C A Y C L T I N T T I C A G Y C M T R R I B G K L F L P K Y A L S Q D V C T Y R D F I Y R T V E I P G C P L H V A P Y F S Y P V A L S C K C G K C B T B Y S B C I H E A I K T N Y C T K P Q K S Y
TSH β, bovine [Liao & Pierce (4)]	F C I P T E Y M M H V E R K E C A Y C L T I N T T V C A G Y C M T R B V B G K L F L P K Y Z L S Q D V C T Y R D F M Y K T A E I P G C P R H V T P Y F S Y P V A I S C K C G K C B T B Y S B C I H E A I K T N Y C T K P Q K S Y M
Positions common to bovine LH and TSH β subunits.	C P E C C T T C A G Y C L P V C T Y P G C P V P S P V A S C C G C D C C P
	1 2 3 4 5 6 7 8 9 10 1 2 3 4 5 6 7 8 9 20 1 2 3 4 5 6 7 8 9 30 1 2 3 4 5 6 7 8 9 40 1 2 3 4 5 6 7 8 9 50 1 2 3 4 5 6 7 8 9 60 1 2 3 4 5 6 7 8 9 70 1 2 3 4 5 6 7 8 9 80 1 2 3 4 5 6 7 8 9 90 1 2 3 4 5 6 7 8 9 100 1 2 3 4 5 6 7 8 9 110 1 2 3 4 5 6 7 8 9
LH β, bovine [Maghuin-Rogister et Dockier (9).]	S R G P L R P L C Q P I N A T L A A E K E A C P V C I T F T T S I C A G Y C P S M K R V L P V I L P P M P E R V C T Y H E L R F A S V R L P G C P P G V D P M V S F P V A L S C H C G P C R L S S T D C G P G R T Q P L A C D H P P L P D I L
LH β, ovine [Liu et al (10); Sairam et al (11).]	S R G P L R P L C Q P I N A T L A A E K E A C P V C I T F T T S I C A G Y C P S M K R V L P V I L P P M P Q P V C T Y H E L R F A S V R L P G C P P G V D P M V S F P V A L S C H C G P C R L S S T D C G P G R T Q P L A C D H P P L P D I L
LH β, porcine [Maghuin Rogister & Hennen (12).]	S R G P L R P L C R/Z P I N A T L A A E K E A C P V C I T F T T S I C A G Y C P S M R R V L P A A L P P V P Q P V C T Y R E L I F A S S F L P G C P P G V D P T V S F P V A L S C H C G P C R L S S S D C G P G R A Q P L A C D R P P L P G L L
LH β, human [(Closset et al (3).]	S R Z P L R P W C Z P I N A T L A V Z K Z G C P V C I T V N T T I C A G Y C P T M R M L L Z A V L P P V P Z P V C T Y R B V R F Z S I/G R L P G C P R G V B P V V S F P V A L S C R C G P C R R S T S B C G G P K B H P L T C Z B S K G
Positions common to bovine, ovine, porcine and human LH β subunits.	S R P L R P C P I N A T L A V E E C P V C I T T I C A G Y C P M L L P P P V C T Y F S R L P G C P G V D P V S F P V A L S C C G P C R S D C G P L C

B. LH α subunit

Table 2 shows the comparison of the amino acid sequence of ovine, porcine and human LH-α. According to partial data on the primary structure of the bovine LH α subunit (1,5,6), it appears that once again there is total homology between the ovine and the bovine chains. No more than four amino acid replacements are observed between the porcine and the ovine primary sequence. The human chain differs by 23 positions when compared to the ovine α subunit. Obviously, the primary structure of the LH α subunit exhibits less variability during evolution than the primary structure of the β subunit.

C. Possible allelic forms

From both the LH α and β subunits, we have isolated peptides exhibiting identical sequences, except in one position. In the bovine LH α subunit, position 56 can be occupied by either isoleucine or threonine and position 83 by serine or histidine. In the porcine LH β subunit, position 10 can be occupied by glutamic acid or arginine. In the case of the human LH β subunit, position 67 can be occupied by isoleucine or glycine.

D. Invariant portions in the primary structure of LH and homology with TSH

As seen in Table 2, considerable portions in the amino acid sequence of the LH β subunit remain constant among the various species. Some of these constant regions (26-29, 31-38, 47-50, 56-59, 69-73, 80-91 and 98-100) exhibit a high degree of homology with the TSH β subunit. The invariability of these structural parts in both LH and TSH, whose biological function and specificity are quite distinct, suggests that they might be responsible for the binding of the β subunit with an α subunit common to both LH and TSH within the same species. The hypothesis is further supported by the physicochemical studies described below.

Table II. SEQUENCES OF THE α SUBUNIT OF BOVINE, OVINE, PORCINE AND HUMAN LH AND OF BOVINE AND HUMAN TSH.

Alignement and comparison.

```
                                                  1         2         3         4         5         6         7         8         9
                                         123456789012345678901234567890123456789012345678901234567890123456789012345678901234567890123456

TSH α, human [Sairam & Li (7).]                 VZBCPZCTLZZBPFFSZPGAPILZCMGCCFSRAYPTPLRSKKTMLVZKNVTSZSTCCVAKSYBRVTVMGGFKVZNHTACHCSTCYYHKS

TSH α, bovine [Liao & Pierce (4).]       FPDGEFTMZGCPZCKLKENKYFSKPBAPIYQCMGCCFSRAYPTPARSKKTMLVPKNITSZATCCVAKAFTKATVMGNVRVZNHTECHCSTCYYHKS

Positions common to bovine and human             Z CPZC L EN  FS P API QCMGCCFSRAYPTP RSKKTMLV KN TSZ TCCVAK     TVMG   VZNHT CHCSTCYYHKS
TSH α subunit.

                                                  1         2         3         4         5         6         7         8         9
                                         123456789012345678901234567890123456789012345678901234567890123456789012345678901234567890123456

LH α, ovine [Liu et al (13); Sairam      FPNGZFTMQGCPZCKLKZBKYFSKPBAPIYZCMGCCFSRAYPTPARSKKTMLVPKNITSZATCCVAKAFTKATVMGNVRVZNHTZCHCSTCYYHKS
et al. (14) or bovine.]                             T                                            T                         S

LH α, porcine [Maghuin Rogister,               TMQGCPECKLKENKYFSKLGAPIYQCMGCCFSRAYPTPARSKKTMLVPKNITSEATCCVAKAFTKATVMGNARVENHTECHCSTCYYHKS
Combarnous & Hennen, (2)]

LH α, human [Sairam et al. (15).]               VZBCPZCTLZZBPFFSZPGAPILZCMGCCFSRAYPTPLRSKKTMLVZKNVTSZSTCCVAKSYBRVTVMGGFKVZNHTACHCSTCYYHKS

Positions common to ovine, bovine                Q CPEC L EN  FS   API QCMGCCFSRAYPTP RSKKTMLV KN TSE TCCVAK     TVMG   VENHT CHCSTCYYHKS
porcine and human LHα subunits.
```

ACCESSIBILITY OF TYROSYL RESIDUES OF LH

A. Spectrophotometric titration

Phenolic groups in native porcine, and bovine LH and their isolated subunits have been classified into three groups according to their apparent pK (Table 3) as determined from spectrophotometric titration curves.

It is worth noting that the native hormone is unique in having two tyrosines not ionized below pH 11.5.

Table 3. Apparent pK values of tyrosyl residues of porcine and bovine LH in the native hormones and in the isolated subunits. *

	Class 1		Class 2		Class 3	
	245 nm	295 nm	245 nm	295 nm	245 nm	295 nm
p LHβ	9.8 (0.8)	9.8 (0.7)	10.5 (1.0)	10.5 (1.1)		
b LHβ	9.9 (1.1)	9.9 (1.1)	10.6 (0.9)	10.6 (0.9)		
p LHα	9.4 (0.9)	9.3 (1.3)	10.4 (2.6)	10.4 (2.9)	10.9 (1.0)	10.8 (0.9)
b LHα	9.2 (0.9)	9.1 (1.1)	10.1 (2.0)	10.2 (2.3)	10.9 (1.4)	11.0 (1.5)
p LH	10.4 (2.7)	10.4 (2.9)	11.5 (2.0)	11.5 (2.3)	untitrated (2)**	
b LH	9.9 (2.5) 10.3 (1.0)	10.0 (3.1) 10.4 (1.2)	11.3 (1.5)	11.3 (1.4)	untitrated (2)**	

* pK_{app} values were calculated from the tangent slopes of the plots $[\Delta\varepsilon_M] \times [H^+]$ versus $[\Delta\varepsilon_M]$. The number of tyrosyl residues with similar pK_{app} was determined from $\Delta\varepsilon_M$ max given by the intercept of each tangent with the abscissa.

** The total number of tyrosyl residues per molecule of porcine (or bovine) LH is 7.

B. Catalytic iodination

We noted that when LH is substituted with more than seven iodine atoms, its conformation is markedly affected. Therefore, preparations substituted by two and seven iodine atoms per molecule were used to understand the reactivity of tyrosyl residues towards iodination.

In I_7-porcine LH, we found that all the labels are linked to tyrosines of the α subunit. They were identified after trypsin hydrolysis of the reduced and S-carboxymethylated substituted hormone. Isolation and characterization of the radioactive peptides showed that Tyr α-21, α-92 and α-93 were diiodinated, while Tyr α-41 was monosubstituted and Tyr α-30 was not labeled. In I_2-porcine LH, Tyr α-21 was the only tyrosyl substituted. In addition, the tetrapeptide 21-24 (Tyr-Phe-Ser-Lys) was readily split off by digestion of native LH with trypsin, confirming the exposure of this region to the solvent medium.

Though the two tyrosyls of the LH β subunit were non-reactive towards iodination when the native hormone was substituted, they were easily iodinated when the reaction was performed with the isolated LH β subunit.

As it turns out, these two residues, Tyr β-37 and Tyr β-59, are located precisely in those constant-sequence portions of the LH β chain which are structurally homologous with the TSH β chain.

Our data thus strongly support the hypothesis, suggested by Liao and Pierce (4) that the similarities in the sequences of the LH β and TSH β subunits reflect their interaction with a common α subunit.

REFERENCES

1. Maghuin-Rogister, G. and Hennen, G. (1971). Eur. J. Biochem. 21, 489.
2. Maghuin-Rogister, G., Combarnous, Y. and Hennen, G. (1973). Eur. J. Biochem. 39, 235.
3. Closset, J., Hennen, G. and Lequin, R.M. (1973). FEBS Letters, 29, 97.
4. Liao, T.H. and Pierce, J.G. (1971). J. Biol. Chem. 246, 850.
5. Pierce, J.G., Liao, T.H., Carlsen, R.B. and Reimo, T. (1971). J. Biol. Chem. 246, 866.
6. Hennen, G., Kluh, Y., and Maghuin-Rogister, G. (1971). FEBS Letters, 19, 207.
7. Sairam, M.R., and Li, C.H. (1973). Biochem. Biophys. Res. Comm. 51, 336.
8. Sairam, M.R. and Li, C.H. (1973). Biochem. Biophys. Res. Comm. 54, 426.
9. Maghuin-Rogister, G. and Dockier, A. (1971). FEBS Letters, 19, 209.
10. Liu, W.K., Nahm, H.S., Sweeney, C.M., Holcomb, G.N. and Ward, D.N. (1972). J. Biol. Chem. 247, 4365.

11. Sairam, M.R., Samy, T.S.A. and Papkoff, H. (1972). Arch. Biochem. Biophys. 153, 572.
12. Maghuin-Rogister, G. and Hennen, G. (1973). Eur. J. Biochem. 39, 255.
13. Liu, W.K., Nahm, H.S., Sweeney, C.M., Lamkin, W.M., Baker, H.N. and Ward, D.N. (1972). J. Biol. Chem. 247, 4351.
14. Sairam, M.R., Papkoff, H. and Li, C.H. (1972). Arch. Biochem. Biophys. 153, 554.
15. Sairam, M.R., Papkoff, H. and Li, C.H. (1972). Biochem. Biophys. Res. Comm. 48, 530.

CHEMISTRY OF FOLLICLE STIMULATING HORMONE

P. Rathnam and B. B. Saxena

Highly purified FSH from human pituitary glands, suitable for structural studies, has been prepared by various investigators (1-3). The insufficient yields of FSH, and particularly of its subunits have, however, handicapped the determination of its primary structure. The availability of human pituitary glands, from The National Pituitary Agency, Baltimore, Md., has permitted the development of procedures for the isolation of anterior pituitary hormones of high physicochemical purity in quantities sufficient for structural studies (4).

ISOLATION OF FSH

The pituitary acetone powder from 15,000 glands was extracted with 35 % ethanol containing 10 % ammonium acetate. The extract was made 87 % with respect to ethanol to obtain a precipitate designated as 'crude glycoprotein'. The details of the procedures are described elsewhere (5).

Batches of 7 g of glycoprotein fraction were fractionated by ascending exclusion chromatography on five 10 x 100 cm columns of Sephadex G-100 equilibrated with 0.1 M ammonium bicarbonate, pH 8.0 (Fig 1). The protein in the eluate from this and subsequent columns were monitored by recording absorption at 280 nm. Hormone fractions obtained during various purification steps were characterized by polyacrylamide disc gel electrophoresis, pH 8.6 (Diagram 1) (6), by bioassay (7) and by radioimmunoassay of FSH, and LH (8). Gel filtration on Sephadex G-100 columns removed approximately 70 % of inert material from the crude glycoprotein fraction. A total of 10 g of glycoprotein containing FSH, LH, and TSH were obtained. This was fractionated by ion-exchange chromatography on a 10 x 100 cm column of carboxymethyl Sephadex C-50 (Fig 2). The column was equilibrated with, the material was applied in, and eluted with 0.004 M ammonium acetate buffer with an initial pH of 5.5.

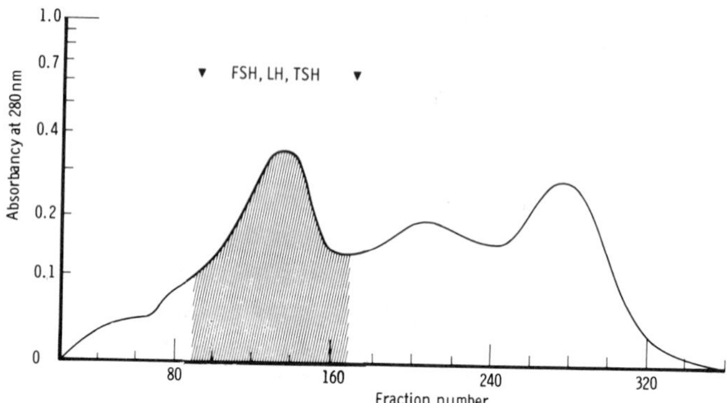

FIG 1. Gel filtration of crude glycoprotein on Sephadex G-100. The hatched area represents the FSH, LH and TSH fraction. Flow rate : 100 ml/hr.

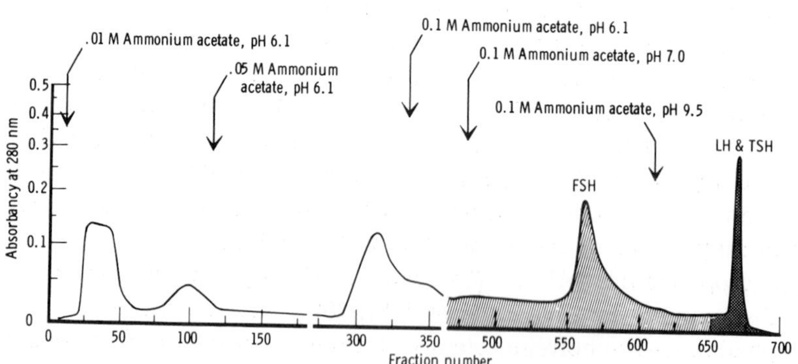

FIG 2. Preparative ion-exchange chromatography of the glycoprotein fraction from the Sephadex G-100 column.

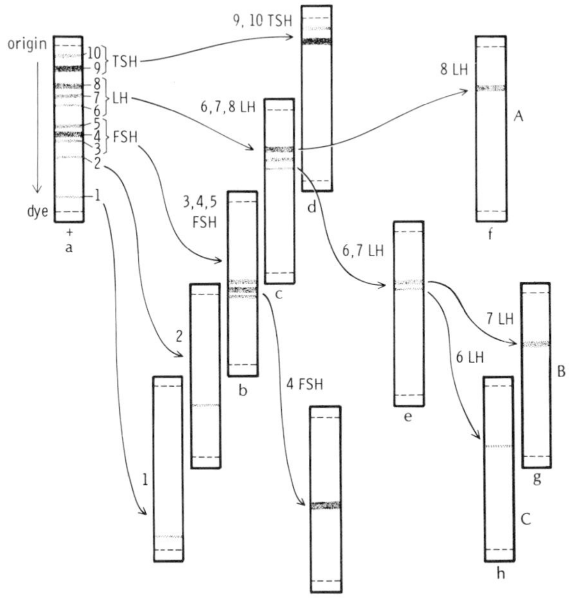

Diagram 1. Disc electrophoretic patterns of : (a) crude FSH, LH and TSH fractions; (b) FSH, (c) LH and (d) TSH fractions obtained after first isoelectric focusing; and (e, f, g, h) LH fractions-A, -B and -C obtained after second isoelectric focusing.

A batch of 0. 8 g of the FSH fraction obtained from CM-Sephadex C-50 column was further purified by preparative zone electrophoresis (Fig 3a) on cellulose column. The active fraction obtained (0. 5 g) was re-electrophoresed on the same column under similar conditions to isolate FSH (Fig 3b). The residual FSH present in the LH and TSH fraction from CM-Sephadex C-50 (Fig 2) was also recovered during the isolation of LH and TSH by isoelectric focusing (9).

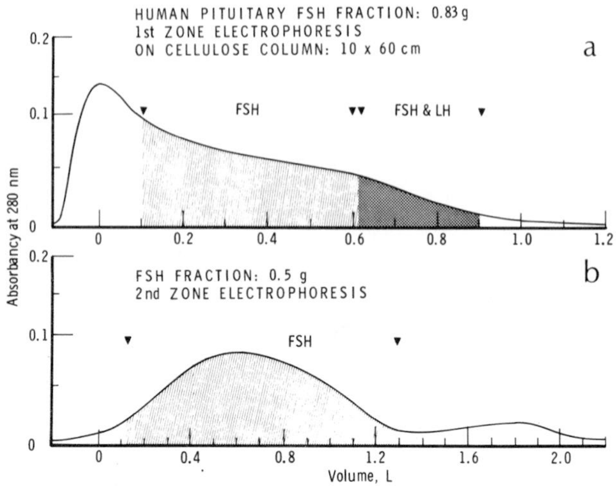

FIG 3. (a) Preparative zone electrophoresis on a cellulose column in 0.05 M tris-HCl buffer, pH 8.2, at 250 volts for 96 hr; a flow rate of eluate 28 ml/hr and 20 ml fractions were collected. (b) Re-electrophoresis of the FSH fraction from the first zone electrophoresis, under similar conditions.

CHARACTERIZATION OF FSH

The FSH isolated by the zone electrophoresis exhibits a high degree of physicochemical purity as demonstrated by disc electrophoresis (Fig 4) and immunoelectrophoresis (Fig 5). Bioassay revealed that this preparation is virtually free of LH (10), GH (11), ACTH (12), TSH (13) and prolactin (PRL) activity (14) (Table 1).

Highly purified preparations of FSH exhibited microheterogeneity as demonstrated by minor differences in electrophoretic mobility, in amino acid and carbohydrate analyses and during ultracentrifugal studies as described hereunder. The isoelectric point of FSH (pI 4.25), $S_{20,W}$ (1.98 and 2.89), and the

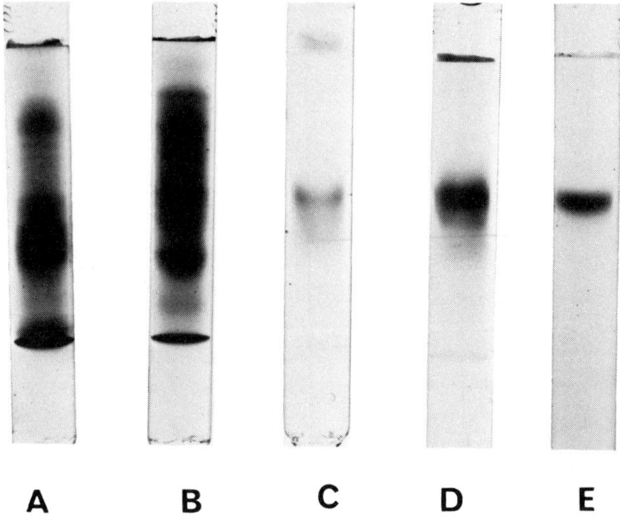

FIG 4. Disc electrophoretic patterns at pH 8.6, of (A) 'Crude glycoprotein'; (B) 'FSH, LH, TSH' fraction from Sephadex G-100 columns; (C) 'FSH' fraction from CM-Sephadex C-50 column; (D) 'FSH' fraction from first zone electrophoretic column; and (E) FSH, after second zone electrophoresis.

Table 1. Yield and specific activity of FSH

Fraction	Yield (g)	Specific activity (units*/mg)					
		FSH	LH	TSH	GH	PRL	ACTH
Glycoprotein**	35	1.05 (0.91-1.21)¶	0.48	0.16	0.034	trace	0.07
FSH	0.3	300 (185-330) §	0.02	none	none	none	none
FSH-α	0.07	none	--	--	--	--	--
FSH-β	0.12	trace	--	--	--	--	--

* FSH-S3; LH-S1; TSH-S4; BGH-10; PRL (NIH standards); ACTH-(Parke Davis).
** Obtained from 15,000 human pituitary glands. ¶ 95 % confidence limits. § Range.

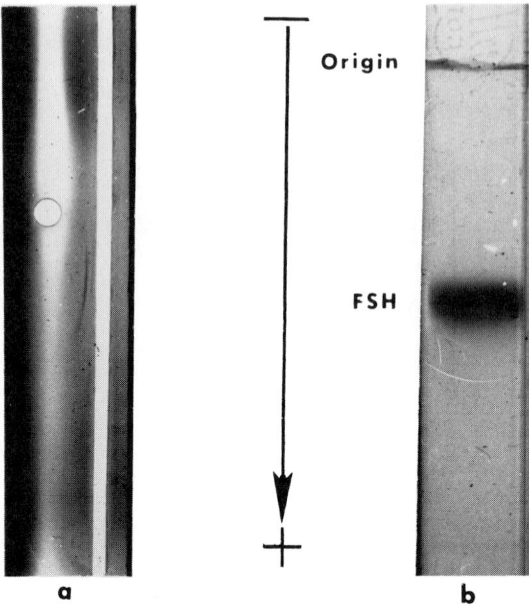

FIG 5. (a) Immunoelectrophoresis of FSH in agar gel at 80 volts for 90 min in the cold, against anti-FSH sera. (b) Disc electrophoretic pattern of FSH at pH 8.6.

effect of various treatments on the biological activity of FSH have been reported earlier (8, 15).

ISOLATION OF THE SUBUNITS OF FSH

A batch of 300 mg FSH isolated from 15,000 pituitary glands was dissolved in 10 ml of 0.04 M tris-phosphate buffer, pH 7.5 containing 8 M cyanate-free urea (Sequenal grade; Pierce Chemical Co., Rockford, Illinois) and incubated for 1 hr at 40°. This material was applied to a column of DEAE-Sephadex A-25 equilibrated with 0.04 M tris-phosphate buffer, pH 7.5, and was eluted with the same buffer followed by a gradient of 0 to 0.2 M

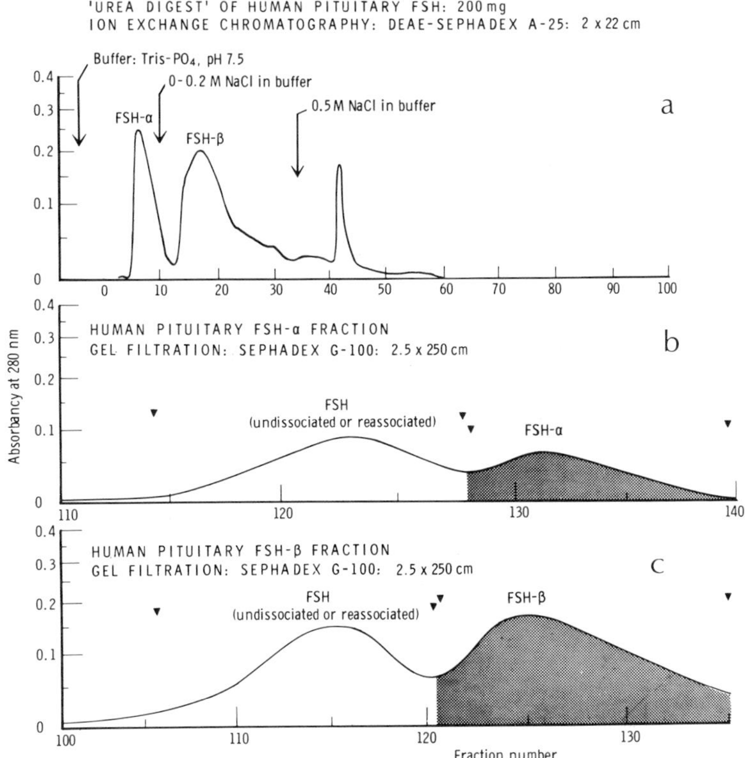

FIG 6. (a) Separation of fractions containing the subunits of FSH, from a 'urea digest' of FSH. Flow rate : 120 ml/hr.
(b) & (c) Purification of the α and β subunits by gel filtration on a column of Sephadex G-100 respectively.

sodium chloride to obtain the α subunit (Fig 6a). The β subunit was eluted with tris-phosphate buffer containing 0.5 M sodium chloride. The α and β subunits were contaminated with 'undissociated or reassociated' FSH and were purified by repeated gel filtration on a column of Sephadex G-100 equilibrated with 0.1 M ammonium bicarbonate buffer (Figs 6b and c).

The yield and activity of FSH and its subunits are summarized in Table 1. Isolation of 300 mg of the FSH represented a 116-fold purification from the crude glycoprotein or a 25,000-fold purification from the fresh pituitary tissue. The FSH contained upto 300 NIH-FSH-S3 units representing approximately a 285-fold purification of the crude glycoprotein and a 6000-fold purification of the fresh pituitary tissue. The yield of the FSH was approximately 25 % of the total present in the gland. It is estimated that each gland may contain 80-100 μg FSH. The yields of α and β subunits are 70 and 120 mg, respectively.

CHARACTERIZATION OF THE SUBUNITS OF FSH

A. Disc electrophoresis

The disc electrophoresis in polyacrylamide gel revealed microheterogeneity of α and β subunits of FSH (Fig 7) as has been demonstrated for the subunits of other glycoprotein hormones (16-18); the subunits were devoid of any biological activity.

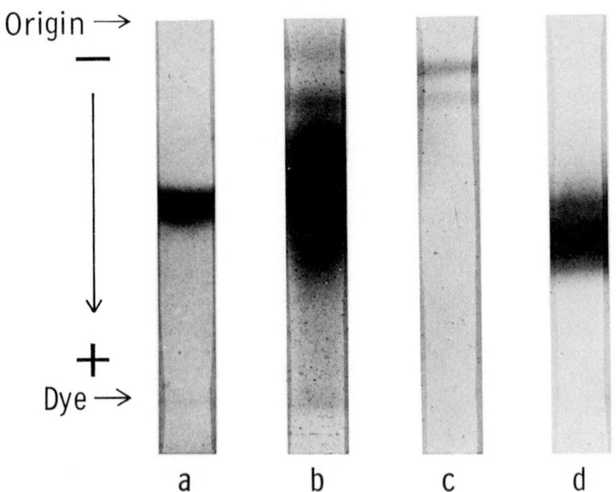

FIG 7. Disc electrophoretic patterns at pH 8.6, of (a) FSH; (b) 'urea digest' of FSH; (c) FSH-α ; and (d) FSH-β .

B. Recombination of the subunits

Partial recombination of α and β subunits to form the native molecule has been reported earlier for FSH (19) and other hormones (20,21). Using α and β subunits in ratio of 1:1.5, at a protein concentration of 1 % in 0.2 M phosphate buffer pH 6.8 and incubation for 16 hr at 37° resulted in a maximum recombination achieving 30 % recovery of the biological activity of the native hormone. The inability to attain a higher recovery suggested incomplete recombination, probably due to irreversible conformational changes in the α and β subunits following urea dissociation, or random recombination of α and β subunits to form modified forms of FSH. These suggestions are further supported by the following experiments. The hormone was treated with 8 M urea for 1 hr at 40°; one aliquot was taken for bioassay, and another was dialyzed against several changes of 0.2 M phosphate buffer, pH 6.8 at 37° to remove the urea, and permit the recombination of the subunits. Aliquots were taken for bioassay, disc electrophoresis and circular dichroism. As shown in Table 2, as much as 30-60 % of the activity was recovered following dialysis, which is significantly greater than the maximum activity recovered under the optimum conditions for recombination. Gel filtration of recombined α and β subunits confirmed the presence of a fraction of recombined subunits and a retarded fraction containing free subunits. The recombined FSH showed poor binding to the gonadotropin receptor of the granulosa cells.

Table 2. Recombination of FSH-α and β

Material	FSH activity * % range	Number of experiments
FSH	100	
FSH : 8M urea	0 - 10	3
FSH : 8M urea (dialyzed)	30 - 60	3
FSH- α & β : recombined	0 - 30	10

* assayed by Steelman & Pohley method (7).

FIG 8

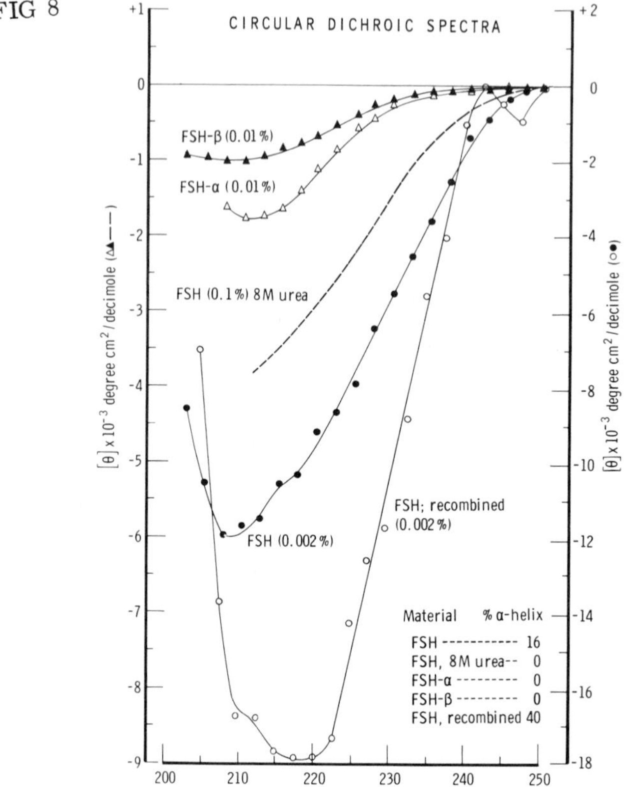

The circular dichroic spectra (Fig 8) of the native FSH shows a maximum of 208 mμ and 16 % α-helix, which is lost following urea treatment. The α and β subunits show little α-helicity. The recombined FSH exhibits a maximum at 217 mμ and an α-helical content of 40 %. This shift indicates a greater percent of the β form and confirms a change of conformation created during recombination of the subunits. These findings strongly suggest that α and β subunits may recombine in other than native conformation, and this may explain the poor recovery of biological activity following reassociation.

C. Ultracentrifugal studies with human FSH and its β -subunit

1. Sedimentation velocity of FSH : We have previously demonstrated the dependence of sedimentation rate of FSH on concentration and the existence of FSH in a monomer-dimer system with extrapolated $S_{20, w}$ values of 1.98 and 2.89 (19). Further, a 1 % solution of FSH during a velocity run at 52,000 rpm for 192 min showed an initial optical density at the meniscus of 0.8, as measured by continuous absorption spectrum at 280 nm. The rate of sedimentation was calculated to be 2.9 $\pm$ 0.1 S. This estimate is in agreement with the sedimentation value of 2.89 S determined previously by extrapolation and represents the dimer of FSH.

2. Equilibrium centrifugation of FSH : Figure 9 shows the results of two equilibrium centrifugation runs on FSH. At each speed, the results from the channels having different initial concentrations are shown. The plot shows local weight average molecular weights $[M_W (r)]$ as a function of the local concentration at given points in the channel. At each speed, the curves do not overlap, and as the initial concentration decreases, the apparent molecular weight at a given local concentration increases. This is the classical behaviour of a disperse solute. By taking the value of the number average molecular weight at the base of the cell, the overall weight average molecular weight (M) of the entire sample, Z average and overall Z + 1 average gave the values: $\overline{M}_W = 31,200 \pm 600$, $\overline{M}_Z = 39,600 \pm 900$, $\overline{M}_{Z+1} = 52,400 \pm 2,000$. The disparity among these values is a further index of the degree of dispersity of the sample. These observations suggest that a monomer of FSH and more than one of its stable polymers coexist in equilibrium.

3. Sedimentation velocity of FSH-β : The rates of sedimentation of FSH-β at various protein concentrations were determined in a Beckman Model E analytical ultracentrifuge. The temperature was maintained at 20 $\pm$ 0.02^{o} with Rotor Temperature Indicator Control (RTIC). For concentrations of 1.7 to

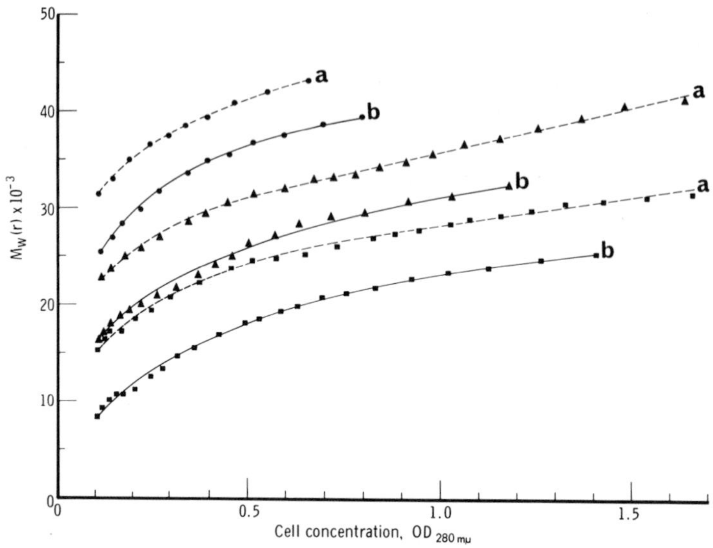

FIG 9. Sedimentation equilibrium of FSH: ● 0.01 %; ▲ 0.03 %; ■ 0.10 %; (a) 32,000 rpm; (b) 44,000 rpm.

0.5 %, aliquots of 0.40 ml of a solution of FSH-β in 0.01 M phosphate buffer, pH 7.0 was used in one sector of a 12 mm double sector cell; the other sector of the cell was filled with 0.42 ml of the buffer alone. The cell was counterbalanced and mounted on a previously cooled AN-D rotor and centrifuged at 60,000 rpm. For solutions of concentrations of 0.35 to 0.2 %, aliquots of 1 ml of FSH-β were centrifuged against 1.1 ml of the solvent in a 30 mm double sector cell, using an AN-E rotor, at 48,000 rpm. The photographs of the sedimentation boundary for each concentration between 2.0 to 0.2 % were taken at 8 min intervals with the Schlieren optics. The sedimentation rate was calculated from the measurements of distances moved by the maximum ordinate or σ made by the aid of a Nikon two-dimensional Micro-comparator (Stangert Corpn., Long Island, New York). The results of these studies are compared with that of native FSH.

As shown in Fig. 10 between 1.7 and 0.2 % concentrations, the FSH- β sedimented as a single symmetrical boundary, suggesting a high degree of homogeneity of FSH- β in the ultracentrifuge. As the concentration decreases the boundary appeared to disperse, a phenomenon characteristic of glycoproteins in general. Between 1.7 to 0.5 % concentrations, a mean $S_{20,w}$ of 1.8 was calculated. Similar to the behaviour of FSH below 0.5 % concentration, the sedimentation rate of FSH- β decreased with concentration, suggesting a dissociation of the protein into smaller molecular weight moieties.

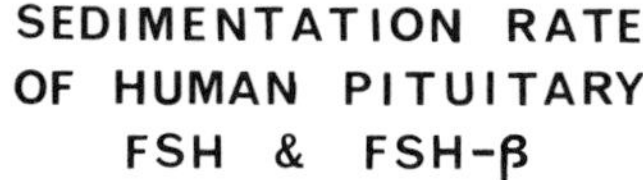

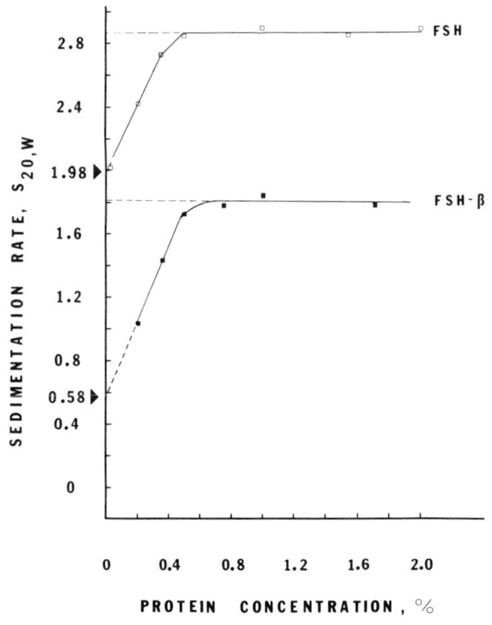

FIG 10. Concentration dependence of the sedimentation rates of FSH and FSH- β .

Extrapolation to zero protein concentration revealed two $S_{20,w}$ values of 0.6 and 1.8, a condition which is virtually diagnostic of interacting systems involving association-dissociation equilibria with very rapid forward and backward reactions. The sedimentation rates, however, do not fit into a simple monomer-dimer model. This behaviour suggests a random aggregation of the β-subunit similar to that suggested for the α-subunit of ovine FSH (22).

A 0.2 % solution of FSH-β in 0.1 M phosphate buffer of pH 7.0 containing 8 M urea was centrifuged in a 30 mm double sector cell at 48,000 rpm for 4 hr, in an AN-E rotor. Photographs of the sedimentation boundary were taken at 8 min intervals, however, the protein boundary did not move from the meniscus for 4 hr. These findings indicate that in the presence of urea, the β-subunit exists in the unaggregated form.

Table 3. Amino acid and carbohydrate analyses of pituitary FSH and its subunits

Amino acids	Human			Equine[1]			Ovine[2]		
	FSH[a]	α[b]	β[b]	FSH	α[a]	β[a]	FSH	α	β
	g/100 g protein								
Asp	6.6	8.7	8.7	7.8	6.9	10.3	5.4	4.1	6.1
Thr	7.6	6.3	7.0	9.1	8.3	10.6	5.7	5.4	6.0
Ser	6.1	5.1	4.2	5.5	3.6	5.9	3.2	3.0	3.4
Glu	11.2	11.4	11.2	9.4	10.5	8.8	6.8	6.4	6.2
Pro	5.8	7.4	10.3	7.0	6.2	5.3	3.3	4.0	2.8
Gly	2.3	3.4	2.2	3.5	2.8	4.2	1.6	1.3	1.6
Ala	3.3	4.8	4.6	4.4	3.2	4.5	2.7	3.2	2.3
Cys	5.9	5.1	12.0	8.8	8.1	8.2	5.1	5.5	5.7
Val	8.0	5.9	5.8	5.3	5.0	6.0	3.4	3.2	3.6
Met	6.3	6.4	1.3	1.3	1.3	1.0	1.4	3.1	0
Ileu	3.1	3.6	4.1	4.8	5.3	4.6	2.6	1.6	3.5
Leu	6.2	4.8	5.1	5.5	4.9	5.3	3.0	1.7	3.1
Tyr	6.7	1.7	4.3	6.4	6.4	8.8	5.0	4.9	5.7
Phe	4.3	5.4	4.0	5.5	7.3	3.3	3.2	3.6	2.4
His	3.1	3.2	1.6	3.2	3.8	3.4	2.4	2.7	2.1
Lys	6.4	5.6	6.5	8.3	9.5	7.1	6.0	7.3	3.7
Arg	5.4	4.0	3.0	5.5	5.8	3.7	3.6	2.9	4.0
Try	0.9	n.d	n.d						
Carbohydrates									
Fucose	1.2	0.4	1.5	1.0	0.5	1.4	0.8	0.4	1.4
Manose	6.1 (Manose + Galactose)	2.2	6.0	5.7	4.5	5.3	5.4	6.3	4.5
Galactose		1.1	2.3	3.0	2.4	3.0	2.8	1.9	3.5
N-Ac-Gluc-NH4	5.3 (N-Ac-Gluc-NH4 + N-Ac-Galac-NH4)	6.4	4.1	5.3	5.6	6.4	6.2	6.5	6.9
N-Ac-Galac-NH4		tr	tr	2.4	1.3	1.4	1.1	1.1	0.9
Sialic acid	5.0	1.7	3.3	6.8	5.6	7.4	5.9	4.0	8.0

1. Landefeld & McShan; personal communication. Values corrected to the first decimal place.
2. Grimek & McShan; personal communication. Values corrected to the first decimal place.
a. Average of 24, 48 and 72 hr hydrolysates.
b. 24 hr hydrolysates.
n.d = not determined.

D. Amino acid, carbohydrate and N- and C-terminal analyses

In Tables 3 and 4 the amino acid and carbohydrate analyses of FSH-β from human, equine and ovine pituitaries (Landefeld, T, and McShan, W. H; Grimek, H, and McShan, W. H - personal communication) are compared. It is interesting to note that similar to FSH-β, Asp and Glu are the predominating

Table 4. Amino acid and carbohydrate analyses of FSH-β

	Human	Equine* (g/1oo g protein)	Ovine**
Amino acids			
Asp	8.7	10.3	6.1
Thr	7.0	10.6	6.0
Ser	4.2	5.9	3.4
Glu	11.2	8.8	6.2
Pro	10.3	5.3	2.8
Gly	2.2	4.2	1.6
Ala	4.6	4.5	2.3
Cys	12.0	8.2	5.7
Val	5.8	6.0	3.6
Met	1.3	1.0	0
Ileu	4.1	4.6	3.5
Leu	5.1	5.3	3.1
Tyr	4.3	8.8	5.7
Phe	4.0	3.3	2.4
His	1.6	3.4	2.1
Lys	6.5	7.1	3.7
Arg	3.0	3.7	4.0
Try	n.d.		
Carbohydrates			
Fucose	1.5	1.4	1.4
Mannose	6.0	5.3	4.5
Galactose	2.3	3.0	3.5
N-Ac-Glucosamine	4.1	6.4	6.9
N-Ac-Galactosamine	tr	1.4	0.9
Sialic acid	3.3	7.4	8.0

*Landefeld & McShan - personal communication. Values corrected to the first decimal place. ** Grimek & McShan - personal communication. Values corrected to first decimal place. n.d = not determined.

amino acids in equine and ovine FSH-β. Similarly, the Lys/Arg ratios of equine and oFSH-β are either ≥ 1, as is observed for the hFSH-β. Minor differences between human, equine and ovine lie in the content of Pro, Cys, Met, Tyr, and Phe. Significant differences exist between the α subunits. Ovine FSH-α does not contain as much glutamic acid as equine or human FSH-α. There are also differences in the content of Met, Tyr, Cys, Pro and Thr. All the subunits contain mannose in much larger amounts than galactose, and higher amounts of N-acetyl-glucosamine than galactosamine. Human FSH and its subunits contain less amount of carbohydrate than those of ovine and equine source.

The reduced and carboxymethylated FSH-β showed micro-heterogeneity at the N-terminal with Val as the predominant N-terminal residue as determined by Dansyl (23) and Edman techniques (24).

The release of amino acids with time from the C-terminus of FSH-β by carboxypeptidases A & B is shown in Fig 11.

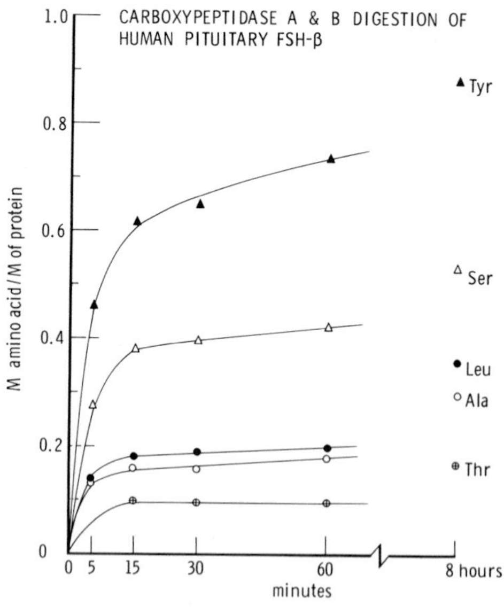

FIG 11. Amino acids released during digestion of FSH-β with carboxypeptidases A & B.

The release of Tyr was followed by Ser, Leu, Ala and Thr. However, during sequence analyses, the C-terminal peptide showed leucine as the C-terminal amino acid residue. In addition to this, C-terminal determination of a previous batch of FSH-β had yielded Leu-Ala-Thr at the C-terminal end. These results indicate the possibility of either microheterogeneity at the C-terminus or that a dipeptide Tyr - Ser is lost during purification procedures.

1. <u>Primary amino acid sequence of FSH-β</u> : The FSH-β has been reduced, carboxyaminomethylated and digested with trypsin.

The amino acid and end group analyses as well as partial sequences of the tryptic peptides have shown considerable homology with the tryptic peptides of ovine and equine FSH-β prepared in the laboratory of Prof. McShan at the University of Wisconsin. However, these tryptic peptides of FSH show significant differences from the tryptic peptides of the β-subunits of hCG, LH or TSH (25-27).

Amino acid sequences of the tryptic and thermolytic peptides of the FSH-α were established by subtractive Edman method. Primary amino acid sequence of human FSH-α is given below:

LINEAR AMINO ACID SEQUENCE OF FSH-α

```
                                                                           10
ALA - PRO - ASX - VAL - GLX - ASX - CYS - PRO - GLX - CYS - THR - LEU - GLX - GLX - ASX -
<-------------------------------- Th-1 ---------------------------->  <--------- Th-2 -------
<---------------------- T-1 ---------------------> <------ T-2 -----> <---- T-3 ------------
                         20                                                              30
PRO - PHE - PHE - SER - GLX - PRO - GLY - ALA - PRO - ILEU - LEU - GLX - CYS - MET - GLY -
---------> <--------------- Th-3 ----------------> <--------- Th-4 ---------> <--- Th-5 ---
           <- - - - - - - - - - - - - Th-4a - - - - - - - - - - - - - - - - ->
--------------------------------------------------------------------------> <--- T-4 ---
                                                        40
CYS - CYS - PHE - SER - ARG - ALA - TYR - PRO - THR - PRO - LEU - ARG - SER - LYS - LYS -
---------> <------------------------- Th-6 --------------------------> <------- Th-7 -------
           <- - - - Th-6a - - -> <- - - - - - - - Th-6b - - - - - - - - ->
---------> <------- T-5 -------> <----------------- T-6 -----------------> <------ T-7 ----->
                        50                                                                 60
THR - MET - LEU - VAL - GLX - LYS - ASX(CHO) - VAL - THR - SER - GLX - SER - THR - CYS - CYS -
---------> <------------ Th-8 --------------> <------------------ Th-9 ---------------------->
<-------------------- T-8 ---------------> <------------------ T-9 ----------------------> <-T-10->
                                                       70
VAL - ALA - LYS - SER - TYR - ASX - ARG - VAL - THR - VAL - MET - GLY - GLY - PHE - LYS -
<------ Th-10 ------> <------ Th-11 -----> <-- Th-12 --> <-------------- Th-13 -----------------
                                                          <- - - - - - Th-13a - - - - - ->
<----- T-11 -----> <-------- T-12 --------> <--------------------- T-13 ------------------->
                         80                                                              90
VAL - GLX - ASX(CHO) - HIS - THR - ALA - CYS - HIS - CYS - SER - THR - CYS - TYR - TYR - HIS -
---------------------------------- Th-13 -------------------------------------> <--- Th-14 ---
<-------------------------- T-14 ---------------------> <--- T-15 ---> <------ T-16 ----> <------ T-17 ------
LYS - SER
---------->
-----> <-T-18->
```

COMPLETE AMINO ACID SEQUENCE OF HUMAN FSH-α AS DERIVED FROM THE SEQUENCES OF THE TRYPTIC AND THERMOLYTIC PEPTIDES BY SUBTRACTIVE EDMAN METHOD

ACKNOWLEDGEMENTS

This study was supported by grants HD-06543 and CA-13908 and contract NICHD-72-2763 from National Institutes of Health, Bethesda, Maryland; grant M72-189 from the Population Council, Rockefeller University, New York; and grant 670-0455 A from The Ford Foundation, New York.

REFERENCES

1. Roos, P. (1968). Acta Endocrinol. (Copenhagen). Suppl. 131, 1
2. Papkoff, H., Mahlmann, L. J. and Li, C. H. (1967). Biochemistry 6, 3976.
3. Peckham, W. D. and Parlow, A. F. (1969). Endocrinology 84, 953.
4. Saxena, B. B. and Rathnam, P. (1967). J. Biol. Chem. 242, 3769.
5. Rathnam, P. and Saxena, B. B. (1972) In "Gonadotropins", B. B. Saxena, C. G. Beling and H. M. Gandy (Eds). pp 167. Wiley-Interscience, New York.
6. Davis, B. J. (1964). Ann. N. Y. Acad. Sci. 121, 404.
7. Steelman, S. L. and Pohley, F. M. (1953). Endocrinology 53, 604.
8. Saxena, B. B. and Rathnam, P. (1968). In "Gonadotropins 1968", E. Rosemberg (Ed). pp 3, Geron-X Inc. California.
9. Rathnam, P. and Saxena, B. B. (1970). J. Biol. Chem. 245, 3725.
10. Parlow, A. F. (1961). In "Human Pituitary Gonadotropins", A. Albert (Ed). pp. 300. Charles C. Thomas, Illinois.
11. Greenspan, F. S., Li, C. H., Simpson, M. E. and Evans, H. M. (1949). Endocrinology 45, 455.
12. Sayers, M. A., Sayers, G. and Woodbury, L. A. (1948). Endocrinology 42, 379.
13. McKenzie, J. M. (1958). Endocrinology 63, 372.
14. Lyons, W. R. and Page, E. (1935). Proc. Soc. Exp. Biol. Med. 32, 1049.

15. Rathnam, P. and Saxena, B.B. (1971). In "Gonadotropins and ovarian development", W.R. Butt, A.C. Crooke and M. Ryle (Eds). pp 107, E & S Livingstone, Edinburgh.
16. Swaminathan, N. and Bahl, O.P. (1970). Biochem. Biophys. Res. Comm. 40, 422.
17. Morgan, F.J. and Canfield, R.E. (1971). Endocrinology 88, 1045.
18. Nureddin, A., Hartree, A.S. and Johnson, R. (1971). In "Gonadotropins", B.B. Saxena, C.G. Beling and H.M. Gandy, (Eds), pp 167. Wiley-Interscience, New York.
19. Saxena, B.B. and Rathnam, P. (1971). J. Biol. Chem. 246, 3549.
20. Reichert, L.E., Jr., Rasco, M.A., Ward, D.N., Niswender, G.D. and Midgley, A.R. (1969). J. Biol. Chem. 244, 5110.
21. Pierce, J.G., Bahl, O.P., Cornell, J.S. and Swaminathan, N. (1971). J. Biol. Chem. 246, 2321.
22. Papkoff, H. and Ekbald, M. (1970). Biochem. Biophys. Res. Comm. 40, 614.
23. Gray, WR and Hartley, B.S. (1963). Biochem. J. 89, 59.
24. Edman, P. (1950). Acta Chem. Scand. 4, 283.
25. Bahl, O.P. (1973). J. Biol. Chem. 248, 6810.
26. Shome, B. and Parlow, A.F. (1973). J. Clin. Endocr. Metab. 36, 618.
27. Parlow, A.F. and Shome, B. (1973). Abst. No. 23, The Endocrine Society 55th Meeting, p. A-60.

CHEMICAL ASPECTS OF HIGHLY PURIFIED HUMAN PITUITARY FOLLICLE STIMULATING HORMONE

J. F. Kennedy

INTRODUCTION

We have been studying the chemistry of human pituitary follicle stimulating hormone since 1967; this has required the preparation of a material of high purity. We describe in the present paper, some of our recent work on the purification of human FSH, analysis of its components, structural identification of its carbohydrate moieties, fragmentation into its subunits and other related aspects of the problem.

PURIFICATION OF HUMAN FSH

Microheterogeneity, being a well-recognized phenomenon among glycoprotein hormones, purification in terms of absolute singular chemical identity may not be possible. Hence absolute purity of a preparation may have to be defined in terms of the chemical structure which is congruent with its maximal biological activity.

The procedure for purification of hFSH has been described in our earlier publications (1-3). Briefly, hFSH was prepared from CM1, a material extracted from acetone-dried human pituitary powder (1). A solution of CM1 in 0.001 M disodium hydrogen phosphate was treated twice with calcium phosphate, and the supernatant containing hFSH activity was adsorbed onto DEAE-cellulose (2). Ethanolic precipitation of the material eluted from the column yielded CP-1. Fractionation of CP-1 on Bio-gel P-150 in 0.01 M sodium phosphate buffer pH 7.0 yielded a heterogeneous protein peak from which the appropriate hFSH-active fraction CP-150 was obtained; this was the preparation which we used routinely. More recently the CP-1 has been subjected to column fractionation on DEAE-cellulose (3) prior to chromatography on Bio-gel P-150. Using 0.15 M ammonium acetate as the eluent, a heterogeneous peak containing all the hFSH activity was obtained; a larger amount of inactive protein was retained by the column at this molarity and could be eluted with 0.2 M ammonium acetate. Pooling of the appropriate fractions yielded CPD, and gel filtration of this on Bio-gel P-150 in 0.01 M sodium phosphate buffer, pH 7.0 showed it to contain a low molecular weight proteinaceous impurity, in addition to the high molecular weight material (CPD-150). Reversal in the order of use of the DEAE-cellulose and Bio-gel columns did not affect the potency of the final product. CPD-150 appeared to be the material of maximum potency, although it has been found to contain a small amount of LH activity. More recently, the latter two fractionation steps, have been modified (4); elution of the DEAE-cellulose column with a stepwise gradient of 0.075, 0.125 and 0.25 M ammonium acetate yielded peaks — I, hLH but no hFSH; II, 70 % of the hFSH activity together with a trace of hLH activity (CPD) and III, 30 % of the hFSH together with inactive protein. Further fractionation of peak II on Sephadex G-100 in 0.01 M sodium phosphate buffer, pH 7.5 containing 0.2 M ammonium acetate yielded two peaks, the one eluted first containing the hFSH activity (CPDS). Although both CPDS and CPD-150 exhibit equivalent FSH activity, the former is to be preferred because of its lower LH activity. Table 1 summarizes the hFSH activities of the fractions at the various stages of purification.

Table 1. Activities of hFSH preparations at various stages of purification.

Preparation	*In vivo* biological activity IU/mg.
Pituitary powder	2
CM-1	140
CP-1	700
CP-150	1,500
CPD	10,000
CPD-150	11,000
CPDS	12,000

Unlike the experience of some investigators that maximal activity is exhibited by solutions kept frozen, but not lyophilized, CPD-150 has proved to be remarkably stable (4) to lyophilization (activity retention: biological 84 %, immunological 94 %), dialysis and lyophilization (88 %, 76 %) and to concentration by rotary evoporation under vacuum (102 %, 98 %). Whereas the stability of CPDS to such conditions has yet to be tested, its properties may be considered analogous to those of CPD-150.

A comparison of the physico-chemical behaviour of CP-150 and CPDS on gel-filtration and on sedimentation analysis showed that these two proteins are largely homogeneous with respect to molecular size, despite the fact that the former is less active than the latter.

COMPONENT ANALYSIS OF HUMAN FSH

Whereas the qualitative composition analysis of glycoproteins presents little problem, as is well-known, quantitative analysis is fraught with difficulty. In particular, the amino acid analysis rather than the carbohydrate analysis has proved to be much more problematic. A number of technical advances have been made for analysis of these, though each of these has got its own drawbacks.

Component analyses of CPDS and the less active CP-150 are shown in Table 2, and it can be seen that they are strikingly similar. Earlier studies have demonstrated that all the neuraminic acid units are N-acetylated and that none are N-glycolylated (5), and also that all the 2-amino-2-deoxyhexose units are N-acetylated (6). Further, with the exception of glycine, the amino acid analyses are virtually identical. The carbohydrate analyses show similar L-fucose, mannose and 2-amino-2-deoxygalactose values. They do, however, vary particularly in their D-galactose and N-acetylneuraminic acid (NANA) contents, the more active material containing the larger amount of these units. It is well-known both from our own studies on hFSH (6) and from general studies on circulating glycoproteins that the NANA units occupy the terminal non-reducing positions of the carbohydrate moieties and that the D-galactose units occupy penultimate positions. Furthermore, it is well established that the NANA units are essential for manifestation of biological activity _in vivo_ (5, 7). Thus on the basis of these analyses, it is conceivable that the

Table 2. Comparison of compositional analyses of hFSH preparations

Component	No. of residues/mole hFSH M. Wt. 35,000	
	CPDS	CP-150
Aspartic acid	15	19
Threonine	17	18
Serine	14	12
Glutamic acid	25	25
Proline	12	14
Glycine	11	17
Alanine	11	12
Half-cystine	15	14
Valine	13	15
Methionine	3	3
Isoleucine	7	7
Leucine	11	13
Tyrosine	12	8
Phenylalanine	8	8
Histidine	7	6
Lysine	12	13
Arginine	8	8
D-Galactose	13	9
Mannose	19	20
L-Fucose	2	2
2-Acetamido-2-deoxygalactose	2	1
2-Acetamido-2-deoxyglucose	15	19
N-Acetylneuraminic acid (by acid)	11	6
N-Acetylneuraminic acid (by enzyme)	11	-

highly active hFSH contains on an average, a fuller complement of N-acetylneuraminosyl-D-galactosyl-units than does the less active hFSH. The latter, however, does not contain excessive extraneous glycoprotein or protein and the material removed between the CP-150 and CPDS stages is chemically similar in composition to pure hFSH. It is also noteworthy that the material with higher activity does contain 2-amino-2-deoxy-galactose. Since this carbohydrate occurred to such a small extent compared to 2-amino-2-deoxyglucose in the less pure CP-150, it was possible that its presence represented impurity at this stage of purification. The fact that CPDS contains the galacto-isomer strengthens the case for this carbohydrate being an integral unit of hFSH. Due to shortage of purified material for analysis, configurations for all carbohydrate units have been assumed to be D, just like amino acids are assumed to be in L-form in their natural existence in proteins; the exception to this appears to be fucose, which exists in L-form.

STRUCTURAL IDENTIFICATION OF THE CARBOHYDRATE MOIETIES OF HUMAN FSH

Structurally, the carbohydrate portion of the macromolecule is more elusive than the protein portion on account of its greater complexity and the much greater number of variables (8). In addition to sequence, the hydroxyl group involved in linkage and the stereochemistry of carbon-1 of each unit have to be determined.

Periodate oxidation analysis is a well-known method of carbohydrate structural identification. Experimentally, the technique, as applied to hFSH (9), involves oxidation with aqueous sodium metaperiodate, destruction of excess periodate with ethylene glycol, reduction of oxidised hFSH with sodium borohydride, destruction of excess borohydride by acidification to pH 4.0, gel filtration to isolate the modified hFSH, acidic hydrolysis to liberate the polyols etc, and identification of the latter by various ion-exchange and gas-phase chromatographic techniques. The compounds identified (9) from modified CPDS are shown in Table 3, and the carbohydrate linkage data which may be deduced from this information is shown in Table 4. Any criticism that the results have been significantly distorted by incomplete oxidation or over-oxidation is refuted. Over-oxidation would give rise to a large number of acidic species - such were not found in the final analysis. Incomplete oxidation would

Table 3. Periodate oxidation analysis of hFSH (CPDS)

Component	Moles/mole hFSH, M. Wt. 35,000	
	Before oxidation	After oxidation
D-Galactose	13.4	4.7
Mannose	19.4	6.5
L-Fucose	2.0	0.0
2-Acetamido-2-deoxygalactose	1.6	n.d
2-Acetamido-2-deoxyglucose	14.5	0.3
N-Acetylneuraminic acid	10.6	1.2
Propane-1,2-diol	-	1.5
Ethane-1,2-diol	-	12.0
Glycerol (including glyceraldehyde)	-	10.6
Erythritol	-	0.0
Threitol	-	0.0
Glyceraldehyde	-	3.9

Table 4. Comparison of periodate oxidation analysis data for hFSH preparations

Carbohydrate residue	Linkage type*	% of total residues	
		CP-150	CPDS
D-Galactose	1- & 3-linked or bp	41	35
	1- & 2- or 1- & 6-linked or tnr	59	65
Mannose	1- & 3-linked or bp	20	33
	1- & 2- 1- & 6- linked or tnr	80	67
L-Fucose	1- & 2-linked or tnr	100	100
2-Acetamido-2-deoxyhexose	1- & 6-linked or tnr	87	98

*bp, branch point; tnr, terminal non-reducing

give rise to excessive amounts of intact carbohydrate for each type of unit, whereas in the final analysis L-Fucose and 2-amino-2-deoxyglucose were both virtually completely oxidised. It is possible, however, that the D-galactosyl units were incompletely oxidised on account of their close proximity to the acidic N-acetylneuraminic acid units. Comparison of the carbohydrate linkage data (9, 10) for high and low activity preparations (Table 4) reveals a remarkable identity, again suggesting that chemically the two hFSH preparations are not vastly different from one another.

Methylation analysis has been applied extensively to the structural identification of polysaccharides and oligosaccharides. However, it has not been applied generally to glycoproteins, since a number of problems arise, not the least of which is the likely loss of small molecular weight fragments via alkaline elimination at the glycopeptide linkage during methylation. However, we have avoided such problems, and experimentally (6) our technique consists of methylation with methyl iodide and methylsulphinyl carbanion, gel filtration to isolate all fragments irrespective of molecular size, infra-red analysis, acidic hydrolysis to liberate the individual carbohydrate units, conversion of the partially methylated monosaccharides to volatile derivatives by reduction and acetylation, and identification by gas-phase chromatography and mass spectrometry. The various carbohydrates identified in the final analysis together with the structural data thereby achieved, are shown in Table 5.

Table 5. Methylation analysis data for hFSH.

Methylation Product Identified	Carbohydrate Structure in HFSH
1,5-Di-*O*-acetyl-2,3,4-tri-*O*-methyl-L-fucitol	1-linked L-fucopyranose
1,2,5-Tri-*O*-acetyl-3,4,6-tri-*O*-methyl-D-galactitol	1- and 2-linked D-galactopyranose
1,5-Di-*O*-acetyl-2,3,4,6-tetra-*O*-methyl-D-mannitol	1-linked D-mannopyranose
1,5,6-Tri-*O*-acetyl-2,3,4-tri-*O*-methyl-D-mannitol	1- and 6-linked D-mannopyranose
1,3,4,5-Tetra-*O*-acetyl-2,6-di-*O*-methyl-D-mannitol	1-, 3- and 4-linked D-mannopyranose
1,5,6-Tri-*O*-acetyl-3,4-di-*O*-methyl-2-(*N*-methyl)acetamido-2-deoxy-D-glucitol	1- and 6-linked 2-acetamido-2-deoxy-D-glucose
1,5,6-Tri-*O*-acetyl-3,4-di-*O*-methyl-2-acetamido-2-deoxy-D-glucitol	1- and 6-linked 2-acetamido-2-deoxy-D-glucose

Any criticism that this data is distorted on account of incomplete methylation is refuted on the basis that such a situation would give rise to a whole spectrum of methyl derivatives for each carbohydrate unit, and would also indicate that many unit types were involved in branch points. Methylation analysis data confirms that obtained from periodate oxidation analysis and also allays any ambiguity which cannot be resolved by the latter alone.

In an attempt to identify the anomeric configuration of the carbohydrate linkages we have employed a series of glycosidases (5), but many of these were inactive against intact hFSH, even when applied in different orders. However, use of neuraminidase liberated all the neuraminic acid units indicating that all these units occupy terminal positions of the carbohydrate moieties. The neuraminic acid-free, but not the intact hFSH, was susceptible to galactose oxidase and to L-fucosidase indicating either that the D-galactose and L-fucose units occupy in the carbohydrate sequences, positions adjacent to and protected by the neuraminic acid units, or that the actions of these enzymes on the intact hormone are inhibited by the acidic nature of the NANA units. In conjunction with the periodate oxidation and methylation data, it may be concluded that the D-galactose residues are adjacent to the NANA residues and that the L-fucose residues occupy solely terminal non-reducing positions. A noteworthy result of the enzymic studies was our original demonstration that whereas the NANA-free hormone (5) is inactive _in vivo_ (9) it is active in follicular stimulation _in vitro_, where the target organ, the ovary is exposed to it directly (10) and also retains immunological activity (7).

FRAGMENTATION OF HUMAN PITUITARY FOLLICLE STIMULATING HORMONE

Both the phenomena of subunit formation (12) and the relationships of activities of glycoprotein hormones to their structures have been reviewed recently (13). Reports available on the biological activity of these subunits, indicate that they are completely devoid of activity _in vivo_ (14).

However, we have preferred a different approach to fragmentation in that we have sought to produce fragments which retain biological activity thereby narrowing down the possible location of and simplification of the structural identification of the active site(s) of hFSH. Some success has been achieved using mild acidic hydrolysis of CP-150; it was found that hydrochloric acid, pH 0, at 20°for 1 hr gave rise to two types of fragments which were separable by gel filtration on Sephadex G-25 using water as eluent (15). One of the fractions had a high molecular weight, whereas the other was totally included in the gel and therefore of molecular weight lower than that of the α - and β -subunits. The mild nature of these conditions is remarkable, particularly as the NANA units (the units generally) considered to be the most acid labile in glycoproteins) are not released by them. Time/release studies have shown that maximal release of this carbohydrate can only be achieved using pH 1.0 (HCl) at 80° for 30 min. Of further importance was the finding that both the high and low molecular weight fragments possessed, to various degrees biological acaivity, both *in vivo* and *in vitro* and also immunological activity. This situation has now been found (10) to hold good for the highly active hFSH preparation CPDS, and again permits an analogy of the chemical and additionally to a certain extent the biological, behaviours of the two preparations. Complete component analyses of both fragment types arising from CPDS showed that they both contained a full spectrum of the carbohydrate and amino acid units occurring in the original hFSH, but that the compositions of the two fractions were different.

Our second fragmentation technique has involved the use of a detergent - sodium dodecyl sulphate (SDS) (16). Fractionation of hFSH, after treatment with 0.5 % SDS, on Bio-gel P-150 using 0.1 % SDS as eluent gave two fragments of dissimilar molecular weights both of which were lower than that of the intact untreated hFSH. The larger fragment was biologically active *in vivo* and therefore presumably *in vitro*, whilst the smaller although inactive *in vivo* was active in follicular stimulation when presented to the ovary *in vitro*. Both fragments exhibited immunological activity. Thus biologically active fragments amenable to further investigation have been produced, and evidence for their ability to recombine to reform the original hFSH was also obtained.

CONCLUSIONS

From all the studies on the carbohydrate moieties of FSH, it may be concluded that the various carbohydrate units contribute to the structures described in Table 6. Since the subunits of other glycoproteins hormone have each been shown

Table 6. Summary of structural data for carbohydrate moieties of hFSH.

α-L-fucopyranosyl-(1→; D-mannopyranosyl-(1→;
→6)-D-mannopyranosyl-(1→; →→3,4)-D-mannopyranosyl-(1→;
→2)-D-galactopyranosyl-(1→;
→6)-(2-acetamido-2-deoxy-D-galactopyranosyl)-(1→
→6)-(2-acetamido-2-deoxy-D-glucopyranosyl)-(1→
5-amino-3,5-dideoxy-D-*glycero*-α-D-*galacto*-nonulosyl-(2→

---

to contain a subunit, it is very likely that each of the subunits of hFSH contain carbohydrates, i.e., that intact hFSH contain at least two separate carbohydrate moieties. Clearly the next stage in our work is to examine these moieties separately. Other structure/activity relationships of hFSH have been described elsewhere (5, 7, 17).

REFERENCES

1. Hartree, A. S. (1966). Biochem. J. 100, 754.
2. Barker, S.A., Gray, C.J., Kennedy, J.F. and Butt, W.R. (1969). J. Endocr. 45, 275.
3. Butt, W.R., Lynch, S.S. and Kennedy, J.F. (1972) In "Structure-activity relationships of protein and polypeptide hormones", M. Margoulies and F.C. Greenwood (Eds).

International Congress Series 241, Excerpta Medica, pp. 355.

4. Butt, W.R. and Lynch, S.S. (unpublished observations).
5. Chaplin, M.F., Gray, C.J. and Kennedy, J.F. (1971). In "Gonadotropins and ovarian development" , W.R. Butt, A.C. Crooke and M. Ryle (Eds), Livingstone, Edinburgh, pp. 77.
6. Kennedy, J.F. and Chaplin, M.F. (1972). Biochem. J. 130, 417.
7. Butt, W.R., Lynch, S.S., Chaplin, M.F., Gray, C.J. and Kennedy, J.F. (1971). In "Gonadotropins and ovarian development," W.R. Butt, A.C. Crooke and M. Ryle (Eds). Livingstone, Edinburgh, pp 171.
8. Kennedy, J.F. (1972). In "Structure-activity relationships of protein and polypeptide hormones, Part 2, M. Margoulies, and F.C. Greenwood (Eds). International Congress Series 241, Excerpta Medica, Amsterdam, pp 360.
9. Kennedy, J.F. and Butt, W.R. (1969). Biochem. J. 115, 225.
10. Kennedy, J.F., Chaplin, M.F. and Stacey, M. J. Endocr (submitted for publication).
11. Ryle, M., Chaplin, M.F., Gray, C.J. and Kennedy, J.F. (1971). "Gonadotropins and ovarian development", W.R. Butt, A.C. Crooke and M. Ryle (Eds). Livingstone, Edinburgh, pp 98.
12. Butt, W.R. and Kennedy, J.F. (1972). In "Structure-activity relationships of protein and polypeptide hormones", Part 1, M. Margoulies and F.C. Greenwood (Eds), International Congress Series 241, Excerpta Medica, Amsterdam, pp. 115.
13. Kennedy, J.F. (1973). Endocrinologia Experimentalis, 7, 5.
14. Kennedy, J.F. (1973). Chem. Soc. Reviews. (in press).
15. Kennedy, J.F. and Chaplin, M.F. (1973). J. Endocr. 57, 501.
16. Kennedy, J.F., Butt, W.R., Robinson, W. and Ryle, M. (1972). In "Structure-activity relationships of protein and polypeptide hormones," Part 2, M. Margoulies and F.C. Greenwood (Eds). International Congress Series 241, Excerpta Medica, Amsterdam, pp. 348.

17. Kennedy, J. F., Ramanvongse, S., Butt, W. R., Robinson, W., Ryle, M and Shirley, A. (1972). In "Structure-activity relationships of protein and polypeptide hormones", Part 2, M. Margoulies and F. C. Greenwood (Eds). International Congress Series 241, Excerpta Medica, Amsterdam, 1972, pp. 351.

CHARACTERIZATION OF AN OVINE PITUITARY GLYCOPROTEIN WITH DUAL GONADOTROPIC ACTIVITY

G. Sreemathi and S. Duraiswami

INTRODUCTION

In the poineering days of research on gonadotropins, there was some discussion as to whether the mammalian pituitary secretes one or two gonadotropins (1-3). Experimental evidence obtained thereafter suggested that pituitary FSH and LH are distinct hormones (4-7). While impressive evidence in support of such a concept continued to accumulate from a variety of biological, chemical and immunological studies (6-9), doubts were being voiced as to whether the pituitary actually produces a variety of molecular species of glycoproteins with different kinds of gonadotropic activity (10, 11). Hellema (12) surveying the field has referred to the behaviour of gonadotropins as "chaemeleonic".

The present report summarizes the results of studies carried out in our laboratory on an ovine pituitary glycoprotein which support the concept that monodisperse functional complexes of FSH and LH may be secreted by the pituitary.

ISOLATION OF AN OVINE PITUITARY GLYCOPROTEIN WITH DUAL GONADOTROPIC ACTIVITY

It was demonstrated earlier that gel chromatography on Sephadex G-100 is a convenient means of analyzing pituitary extracts (13). Following gel filtration of lyophilized Koenig-King extracts of ovine pituitaries, gonadotropic activity was recovered in the major protein peak P 1-2 (K_d= 0.25) and in another fraction P 1-1 (K_d = 0.07) that preceded P 1-2 either as a 'shoulder' or as a distinct peak (14). Disc electrophoresis at pH 8.6 showed that while the original extract as well as P 1-1 are polydisperse, P 1-2 is homogeneous (15). The conclusion that P 1-2 is indeed monodisperse was arrived at, on the basis of several physico-chemical criteria (16). Further, an immunochemical study also established the homogeneity of this protein (15).

The experimentally determined physical parameters for P 1-2 are presented in Table 1. The molecular weight at infinite dilution is 63,000. Interestingly enough, the carbohydrate composition is also at variance with the values reported for other ovine pituitary gonadotropin preparations (Table 2). The data summarized in Tables 3, 4 and 5, when taken in conjunction with our earlier report (14) indicate that, notwithstanding its monodisperse nature, P 1-2 has both FSH (0.4 x NIH-FSH-S3) and LH (1.5 x NIH-LH-S14) activities; as an 'ovulating hormone', it is twice as potent as the ovine standard.

Table 1. Physico-chemical parameters of P1-2

$S_{20,W}$	D^o ($x10^7$ cm)	V	Stokes radius (A^o) A	Stokes radius (A^o) B	M^+	M^{++} a	M^{++} b
4.13	6.414	0.7504	34	30 ± 1	63,000	67,777	71,104

A: from sedimentation data. B: estimated from K_d value on G-100. M^+: molecular weight at infinite dilution. M^{++} : molecular weight of a 0.8 % (w/v) solution (a) at the meniscus; and (b) at the bottom of the cell.

Table 2. A comparison of the carbohydrate composition* of P1-2 and RP1-2** with other ovine pituitary gonadotropin preparations§.

Component	P1-2	RP1-2	Ovine LH	Ovine FSH
Neutral hexoses	2.20	2.30	6.10, 6.50, 5.00	5.70, 12.50
Hexosamine	0.50	0.48	6.70, 7.80, 7.80	4.50, 9.00
Fucose	0.20	0.23	--	--
Sialic acid	0.30	0.35	-- 0.40, 0.50	2.80, 5.00

*Expressed as percentage of total dry weight of sample. ** RP1-2 : material reconstituted from the two fractions obtained from P1-2 by ammonium sulfate fractionation. § Values for ovine FSH and LH taken from Geschwind (7).

Table 3. Assay of LH potency of P1-2 by the ovarian ascorbic acid depletion method.

Assay Number	Relative potency in terms of NIH-LH-S-14	95 % confidence limits	Lambda	Design
1	1.338 *	1.032 - 1.685	0.220	2 x 3
2	1.289 **	0.950 - 1.689	0.142	2 x 2
3	1.971 *	1.476 - 2.493	0.169	2 x 2
4	1.597 *	1.178 - 2.116	0.271	3 x 2
5	1.744 **	1.322 - 2.136	0.264	2 x 2
6	1.666 *	1.316 - 1.110	0.197	2 x 2
7	1.000 **	0.782 - 1.319	0.194	2 x 2
8	1.103 ***	0.801 - 1.514	0.149	2 x 2
9	1.618 §	1.352 - 1.894	0.170	2 x 2

Mean relative potency = 1.482 (in terms of NIH-LH-S14. U/mg dry weight).
*The sample for assay was obtained by pooling individual fractions corresponding to P1-2 following gel filtration of the crude extract. **The sample for assay was obtained by pooling fractions of P1-2 following reachromatography on G-100.
*** P1-2 sample assayed was lyophilized following rechromatography. § Sample assayed was lyophilized and dissolved in phosphate buffer (pH 7.4) and stored in deep freeze for two months.

Table 4. Ovulation inducing ability of P1-2 and its derivatives.

Sample	Dose (μg)	Average No. ova shed/rat (± S.E.)	% rat ovulated
NIH-LH-S-14	1.0	0.0 (6)	0
	2.0	0.2 ± 0.0 (8)	25
	4.0	21.2 ± 6.6 (10)	80
P1-2	1.0	2.2 ± 1.1 (6)	50
	2.0	26.6 ± 15.3 (10)	80
	4.0	63.6 ± 18.5 (10)	90
ASF-FSH*	2.0	3.7 ± 1.2 (8)	75
	4.0	25.6 ± 8.8 (10)	100
ASF-LH*	2.0	15.8 ± 2.2 (10)	90
	4.0	14.0 ± 3.1 (10)	60
Reconstituted P1-2	2.0	30.2 ± 10.8 (10)	80
	4.0	62.8 ± 20.2 (10)	80
PMSG	15 IU	No response	--

24 day old female rats (Holtzman strain) were injected sc with 15 IU of PMSG at 0730 hr. They were given 7.5 mg phenobarbital each sc on day 26 at 1300 hr. NIH-LH or test sample was injected at 1500 hr on the same day (i.e. day 26) by ip route. Autopsy was done on day 27, and the tubal ova counted.
*ASF-FSH and ASF-LH represent the fractions obtained on ammonium sulfate precipitation - see text for details.

Table 5. FSH activity of P 1-2 and its derivatives in the hCG augmentation assay

Sample	Dose (μg)	Response (ovarian weight in mg $\pm$ SE)
P 1-2	140	80.2 $\pm$ 4.8 (10)
	420	148.4 $\pm$ 6.2 (8)
ASF-FSH	140	78.1 $\pm$ 5.3 (8)
	420	148.4 $\pm$ 3.8 (9)
ASF-LH	140	43.2 $\pm$ 4.7 (10)
	420	47.8 $\pm$ 6.8 (10)
Reconstituted P 1-2	140	78.5 $\pm$ 5.8 (10)
	420	149.5 $\pm$ 4.9 (10)
HCG-injected control	-	41.2 $\pm$ 2.8 (15)

Numbers in paranthesis refer to the number of animals in each group.

SIGNIFICANCE OF THE OBSERVATIONS ON P 1-2

There have been very few reports in the literature on the possibility of the existence of a monodisperse pituitary glycoprotein such as P 1-2, which may still possess both FSH and LH activities. Duraiswami et al. (17) observed that a purified preparation of oFSH also had 'intrinsic' LH activity. A similar conclusion was drawn by Papkoff (18) with respect to one of his FSH preparations. Bettendorf et al. (19) could identify on isoelectric-focusing of a human pituitary extract, three distinct protein components of which one, with a pI of 5.0, showed both FSH and LH activities. In apparent confirmation of the above observation, Reichert (20) has reported that hFSH prepared by iso-electric focusing in a pH gradient of 3-6 had significant LH activity. Since hLH was found not to be iso-electric at pH values lower than 6, the possibility of this preparation being contaminated with LH appears to be ruled out. In the light of our observations on P 1-2, additional information on the physico-chemical characteristic of this material should prove of great interest.

Licht and Papkoff (20) have recently examined the extent to which the gonadotropic activity of ovine LH in the lizard is a reflection of the intrinsic activity of this molecule as distinct from residual contamination by FSH. These authors found that repeated precipitation of LH by ammonium sulfate, designed to remove traces of FSH or FSH-β -subunits, did not affect the activity of the LH preparation in the lizard, Anolis - carolinensis. Treatment of the ovine LH with an FSH antiserum shown to be highly effective in blocking FSH activity, did not in any way alter the gonadotropic activity in the lizard. It was therefore concluded that the ovine LH molecule has intrinsic gonadotropic activity in the lizard, even though its potency is considerably less than that of FSH.

In a recent study on human hypophyseal gonadotropin-secreting cells using immuno-histological techniques, Phifer et al. found that the same cells of the anterior pituitary reacted to both FSH and LH antisera, indicating that FSH and LH are produced in the same adenohypophyseal cell. This appears to be true in the case of the rat pituitary also (22,23).

The idea that the pituitary may actually put out a complex of FSH and LH does not appear to be far-fetched. In a thought-provoking review published in 1968, Nalbandov (11) has pointed out that the independent physiological existence of FSH and LH has never been clearly established and adduced cogent arguements in support of the idea that the pituitary does not secrete LH and FSH separately, but secreted a FSH-LH complex.

In recent years, several reports on the existence of multi-enzyme complexes, in prokaryotes as well as eukaryotes, have appeared in the biochemical literature (24). An example is the fatty acid synthetase complex which, though comprised of a group of seven functional enzymes, can yet be isolated in a homogeneous form. In view of the fact that P 1-2 was isolated from an extract from which other investigators, using more elaborate procedures, have isolated FSH and LH respectively (25-27), it would appear that what we have isolated is a functional complex of these two hormones as present in the pituitary.

FURTHER STUDIES ON THE NATURE OF P 1-2

If the glycoprotein isolated by us is indeed an FSH-LH complex, it should be possible to dissociate it and recover the two gonadotropins as independent, homogeneous entities. However, attempts to dissociate and separate the 'sub-units' by the counter-current distribution procedure of Papkoff and Samy (28) were unsuccessful. But, it was found possible to dissociate P 1-2, similar to ovine LH (29) on exposure to low pH. Thus, as illustrated in Fig 1, incubation of P 1-2 in 0.05 M glycine buffer, pH 2.3 followed by gel filtration on G-100, yielded two major peaks, G-II (K_d = 0.54) and G-III (K_d = 1.06). The material in these peaks could be recovered in stable form following neutralization to pH 7.5. Analysis by disc electrophoresis showed that while G-II consists of a major and a minor component, G-III is made up of several components (16). On the basis of bioassays, G-III was found to be devoid of any gonadotropic activity, whereas both FSH and LH activities were associated with the G-II fraction. It is of interest that while G-II was comparable to P 1-2 with respect to LH potency, it was no more than a third as active as the parent molecule when assayed for FSH activity (16). If the original P 1-2 were merely an adventitious mixture of FSH and LH together with other inert proteins, then removal of the inert proteins in the G-III fraction should be looked upon as a purification step. In such a case the potency of G-II with respect to both FSH and LH should have increased as compared to P 1-2. The assay data, however, do not support this possibility. Attempts to reconstitute P 1-2 by reassociation of G-II and G-III at an alkaline pH were only partially successful (Figure 1).

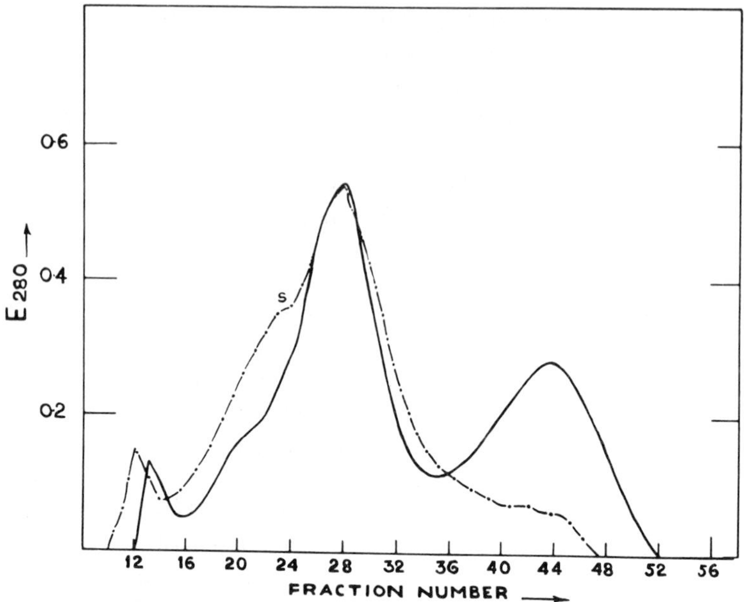

FIG 1. Elution pattern of P 1-2 treated with 0.05 M glycine buffer pH 2.2. Column equilibrated with the same buffer. ____.____.____. recovery of reconstituted P 1-2. G-II and G-III were incubated in and chromatographed with 0.05 M phosphate buffer, pH 7.7. The same results were obtained when 0.05 M glycine buffer, pH 8.6 was substituted for the phosphate buffer. The shoulder marked S(K_d = 0.25) represents reassociated material.

The criterion for reassociation was the recovery of a component with a partition co-efficient of 0.25 from samples subjected to gel chromatography on Sephadex G-100.

A characteristic property of FSH that sets it apart from all other pituitary hormones is its solubility in 50 % saturated ammonium sulfate (4). Advantage was taken of this observation in designing another approach to the problem of dissociating P 1-2. An aqueous solution of P 1-2 was brought to 50 %

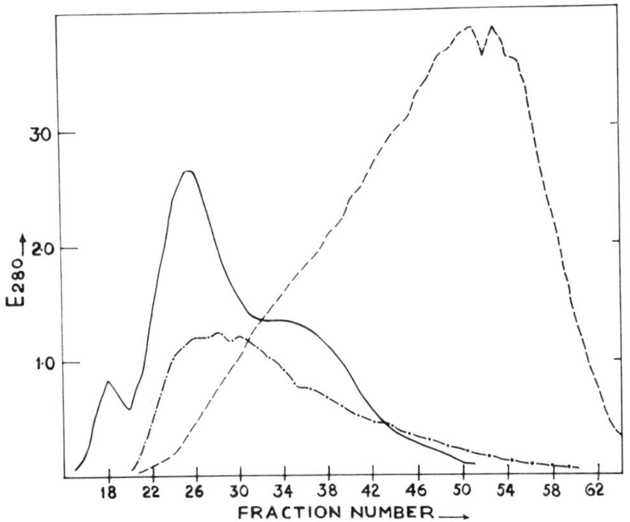

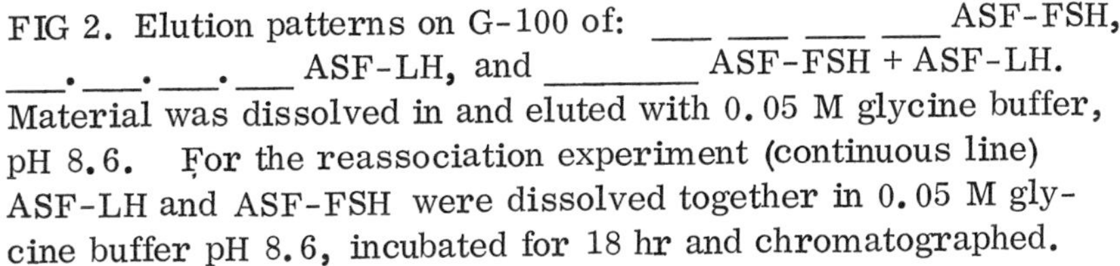
FIG 2. Elution patterns on G-100 of: ___ ___ ___ ___ ASF-FSH, ___.___.___.___ ASF-LH, and ________ ASF-FSH + ASF-LH. Material was dissolved in and eluted with 0.05 M glycine buffer, pH 8.6. For the reassociation experiment (continuous line) ASF-LH and ASF-FSH were dissolved together in 0.05 M glycine buffer pH 8.6, incubated for 18 hr and chromatographed.

saturation with ammonium sulfate and the resultant precipitate (designated ASF-LH) was recovered by centrifugation. The supernatant was brought to 90 % saturation to yield another precipitate (ASF-FSH). The two fractions were dissolved in 0.05 M glycine buffer, pH 8.6 and dialyzed against the same buffer to remove the salt. Samples were then subjected to gel chromatography on G-100 (Fig 2) and to disc gel electrophoresis at pH 8.6 (Fig 3). From the electrophorograms, it is apparent that both ASF-LH and ASF-FSH are heterogeneous. Gel filtration does not reveal this heterogeneity. However, it is of interest that ASF-FSH is retarded on the column to a significantly greater extent than ASF-LH (Fig 2). Also presented in the

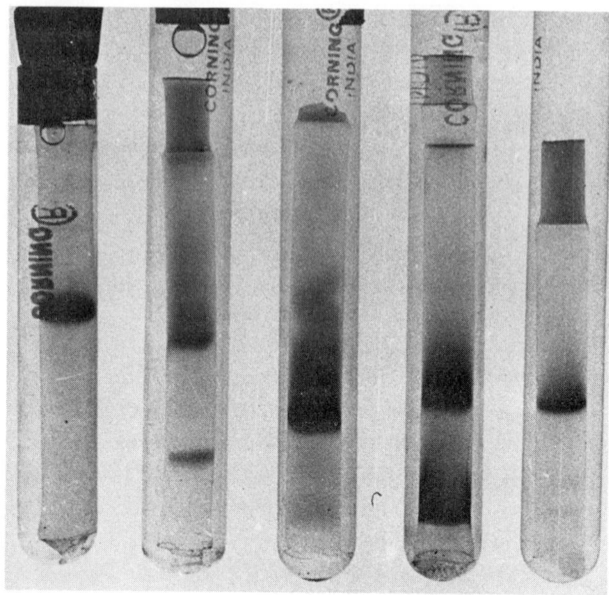

FIG 3. Disc electrophoretic patterns of (left to right) P 1-2, ASF-LH, ASF-FSH, ASF-LH + ASF-FSH (incubated material, before gel filtration) and RP 1-2, respectively run in the usual manner at pH 8.6. Migration towards the anode (top to bottom). Length of the gels 5.5 cm.

same figure is the typical results of attempts to reconstitute the original material (P 1-2) by dialyzing ASF-LH and ASF-FSH together in glycine buffer, pH 8.6. Judging by the fact that virtually all of the sample loaded on the column is recovered in the major protein peak ($K_d = 0.25$), it is clear that a significant recombination of the two fractions to give P 1-2-like material has occured. This is confirmed by the results of disc gel electrophoresis (Fig 3). That the reconstituted material (RP 1-2) is indistinguishable from P 1-2 is also demonstrated by the data on carbohydrate composition (Table 2).

The biological properties of the two ammonium sulfate fractions as well as of RP 1-2 have been compared with P 1-2 in Tables 4 and 5. It is remarkable that, with respect to biological activity, the reconstituted material is identical to P 1-2. As is to be anticipated, ASF-FSH has the follicle stimulating activity. However, its potency is no different from that of P 1-2 - a rather surprising result since removal of 'inert' protein (with respect to FSH activity) by way of ASF-LH fraction which constitutes a purification step, should have resulted in increased potency. What is of even greater interest is that ASF-LH exhibits no biological activity. LH activity, as judged by the ovulation test is, surprisingly enough, found in ASF-FSH. The potency, however, is only half that of the parent molecule. That these results are not due to loss of biological activity during handling would be evident from the observation that on recombination of ASF-FSH and ASF-LH to yield RP 1-2 full biological potency is restored.

CONCLUSION

Taken together, the evidence obtained so far is strongly suggestive of a rather complex structure for the monodisperse P 1-2. That it is not similar to any of the pituitary or urinary gonadotropins reported in the literature is evident. It is pertinent to point out that the isolation of P 1-2 involved minimal processing of the crude extract. Judging by the pattern of biological responses obtained with P 1-2 and its derivatives, it appears justifiable to raise the question whether our preparation represents a specific molecular species of pituitary 'ovulating' hormone. The limited number of components obtained by ammonium sulfate fractionation warrants the hope that studies currently in progress will furnish an early and decisive answer to the above question.

ACKNOWLEDGEMENTS

The work reported here was aided by grants from the Indian Council of Medical Research, New Delhi. It is a pleasure to acknowledge our indebtedness to Dr. M.R.N. Prasad for making available equipment and facilities financed by grants from the Ford Foundation and the Ministry of Health & Family Planning, Government of India, Dr. Mahalaxmi Atreyi (Department of Chemistry) for the sedimentation data. Thanks are also due to Mr. E.A. Daniels for photography.

REFERENCES

1. Aschheim, S. and Zondek, B. (1927). Klin. Wschr. 6, 1322.
2. Fevold, H.L., Hisaw, F.L. and Leonard, S.L. (1931). Am. J. Physiol. 97, 291.
3. Engle, E.T. (1932). In "Sex and internal secretion", pp 794. Williams and Wilkins Co., Baltimore.
4. Li, C.H. and Evans, H.M. (1948). In "The Hormones", G. Pincus and K.V. Thimann (Eds). Vol. I, pp 631, Academic Press, New York.
5. Steelman, S.L. and Segaloff, A. (1959). Recent Prog. Horm. Res. 15, 115.
6. Geschwind, I.I. (1964). In "Gonadotropins - their chemical and biological properties and secretory control", H.H. Cole, (Ed). pp. 1. W.H. Freeman & Co.,
7. Geschwind, I.I. (1969). Gen. Comp. Endo. Suppl. 2, pp. 180.
8. Albert, A. (Ed) (1961) "Human Pituitary Gonadotropins", pp 355, C.C. Thomas, Springfield.
9. Saxena, B.B., Beling, C.G. and Gandy, H.M. (Eds). (1972). "Gonadotropins", pp 107, Wiley-Interscience, New York.
10. Meyer, R.K. (1964). In "Gonadotropins", H.H. Cole (Ed). pp. 37, W.H. Freeman & Co., San Francisco.
11. Nalbandov, A.V. (1968). In "La Specificite Zoologique des hormones hypophysaires et de leurs activities", 177, 335. Coll. Internat. C.N.R.S.

12. Hellema, M.J.C. (1971). J. Endocrinol. 49, 393.
13. Bullemma, M.L. and Duraiswami, S. (1969). Indian. J. Exptl. Biol. 7, 75.
14. Sreemathi, G., Duraiswami, S. and Uberoi, N.K. (1971). Ind. J. Exptl. Biol. 7, 75.
15. Sreemathi, G. and Duraiswami, S. (1972). Experientia 28, 1359.
16. Duraiswami, S. and Sreemathi, G. (1974). Proc. Ind. Natl. Sci. Acad. (in press).
17. Duraiswami, S., McShan, W.H. and Meyer, R.K. (1964). Biochim. Biophys. Acta. 86, 156.
18. Papkoff, H. (1965). Acta Endocrinol. 48, 439.
19. Bettendorf, G., Breckwoldt, M., Czygan, P.J., Fock, A. and Kumasaka, T. (1968). In "Gonadotropins", E. Rosemberg, (Ed). pp. 13, Geron-X, Los Altos, California.
20. Reichert, L.E., Jr., (1971). Endocrinology 88, 1029.
21. Licht, P. and Papkoff, H. (1973). Gen. Comp. Endocrinol. 20, 172.
22. Phifer, R.F., Midgley, A.R., Jr., and Spicer, S.S. (1972). In "Gonadotropins", B.B. Saxena, C.G. Beling and H.M. Gandy (Eds). pp. 9, Wiley-Interscience, New York.
23. Phifer, R.F., Midgley, A.R. and Spicer, S.S.. (1973). J. Clin. Endo. Metab. 36, 125.
24. Reed, L.J. and Cox, D.J. (1970). In "The Enzymes", P.D. Boyer (Ed). Edn. III, Vol I, pp 213, Academic Press, New York.
25. Ward, D.N., Adams-Mayne, and Wade, J. (1961). Acta Endocrinol. 36, 73.
26. Ward, D.N., McGregor, R.F. and Griffin, A.C. (1959). Biochim. Biophys. Acta. 32, 305.
27. Hashimoto, C., McShan, W.H. and Meyer, R.K. (1966). Biochemistry 5, 3419.
28. Papkoff, H. and Samy, T.S.A. (1967). Biochim. Biophys. Acta. 147, 175.
29. Li, C.H. and Starman, B. (1964). Nature 202, 291.

PURIFICATION AND CHARACTERIZATION OF URINARY HCG

H. van Hell

INTRODUCTION

Evidence for the existence of a micro-heterogeneity in hCG was presented by van Hell et al. (1,2), Hamashige et al. (3-5), Yogo (6), Bell et al. (7) and Ashitaka et al.(8). Attempts to separate the various components of this system from each other were made by Moritz (9), Brossmer et al. (10) and ourselves (11). Moritz (9) found isoionic points for HCG from pH 2.2 to pH 7.3 by isoelectric focusing. Using a similar technique Brossmer et al. (10) isolated several hCG preparations with isoionic points ranging from pH 4.00 to pH 5.22. The most potent preparation obtained had an isoionic point of pH 4.2, a biological potency of 7600 IU/mg and a N-acetyl neuraminic acid (NANA) content of 8.3 %.

The procedure for the preparation of the components of this microheterogeneous system of hCG will be presented and the properties of these components discussed. As it was suggested that most, if not all, glycoproteins carrying NANA are subject to microheterogeneity (12), the present study may also have value as a blueprint for the investigation of other glycoproteins. (This work is part of a thesis by H. van Hell, Groningen University, June 16, 1972, Holland).

MATERIALS AND METHODS

A. Starting material

HCG with a potency of about 1500 IU/mg ("crude hCG")was obtained by subjecting urine from healthy pregnant women (collected from the 2nd week after the first missed period up to the 14th week inclusive) to a selective adsorption and desorption process with a technical absorbent followed by precipitation with ethanol (four volumes).

B. Purification procedure

The present purification procedure consists of five steps as shown in the flow sheet in Figure 1. Fractionation with ethanol and chromatography on CM-Sephadex were performed as previously described (2). The final separation was accomplished by combining gel filtration in a salt solution with successive isoelectric focusing and gel filtration. The first gel filtration step was

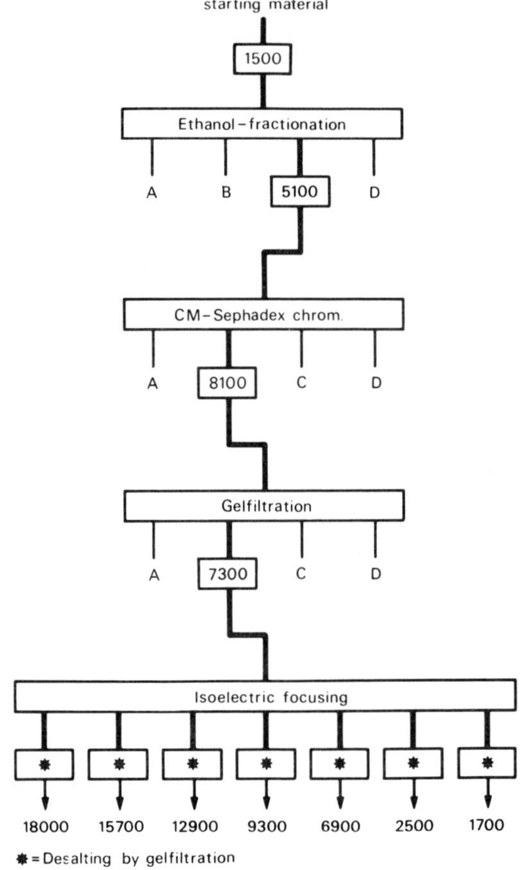

FIG 1. Flow-sheet of the purification of hCG. The heavy lines represent the purification route of the main preparations. The numbers recorded represent the biological potencies of the preparations.

performed at 4° with Sephadex G-100, equilibrated and eluted with 0.05 M ammonium-acetate buffer of pH 4.5 using a column of 5.7 x 4 cm and a load of 0.8 mg protein/ml gel. The elution rate was 4.4 ml/cm^2/hr. Isoelectric focusing was essentially performed as described in the LKB instruction manual 1-8100-EO1. Pooled fractions were dialyzed for 48 hr, lyophilized and finally subjected to gel filtration on Sephadex G-100 in distilled water and again lyophilized.

C. Analysis

1. Assays : The biological potency was estimated using the seminal vesicle test described previously (2). The immunoassay used was the double-antibody solid phase (DASP) radioimmunoassay for hCG and LH as developed by den Hollander and Schuurs (13) and den Hollander et al (14).

2. Physicochemical analyses : Amino acid analysis and the determination of the NANA-content were performed as described by Goverde et al. (15). Two dimensional immunodiffusion (Ouchterlony method) and starch-gel immunoelectrophoresis were carried out as described by Schuurs et al (16).

RESULTS & DISCUSSION

A. Purification

Results obtained on fractionation using ethanol and CM-Sephadex chromatography were consistent with those described previously (2). Gel filtration in 0.05 M ammonium-acetate apparently removed only small amounts of impurities, as the biological potency of the preparation obtained was not significantly increased over that of the starting material (Figure 1). In Figure 2 the elution pattern after isoelectric focusing is presented. The preparations obtained after dialysis and lyophilization were subjected to gel filtration on Sephadex G-100 in distilled water in order to remove the last traces of ampholine. The elution profiles shown in Figure 3 indicate that most of these preparations were still heterogeneous, most probably with respect to the various hCG components. Therefore, from each preparation obtained by isoelectric focusing, two or three preparations could be recovered

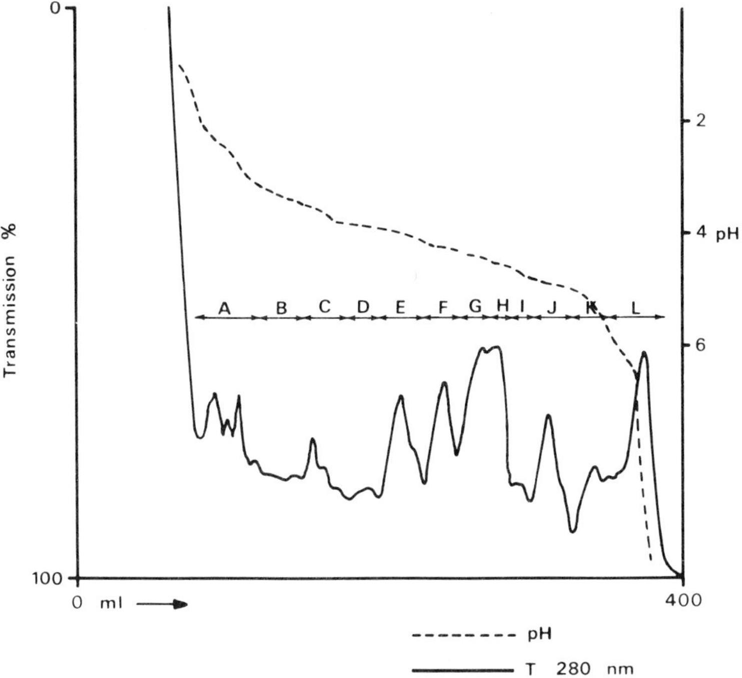

FIG 2. Isoelectric focusing of hCG preparation. 600 mg hCG (biological potency : 8100 (6900-9400) IU/mg) was focused in 440 ml solution containing 2 g Ampholyte (pH range 3-5). LKB 8102 column at $0^{o} \pm 1^{o}$ was used. Pooling of the fractions is indicated as a line between the arrow heads.

after final gel filtration. The properties of these final preparations are described below and are given in Tables 1 and 2.

The biological activity that could be recovered in the final preparation was 83 %. The biological potencies of the preparations recorded in Table 1 which range from 1700 to 18000 IU/mg could apparently be correlated with their NANA-contents. All the preparations were found to be immunochemically identical in an immunodiffusion experiment using an antiserum to highly purified hCG. However, using a mixture of antisera to crude hCG, the preparations PR17B, PR18B, PR19B, PR20B and PR22B showed in an immunodiffusion experiment at 8-16 mg preparation per ml only trace amounts of impurities. No impurities could be detected in the preparations PR14B, PR21B and PR24B using 1, 2 and 4 mg preparation/ml. The outcome of the statistical analysis of the results of the two radioimmunoassays used (Table 2) was unsatisfactory, as the relative potencies of the preparations to one another in one assay were significantly different from those of the other assay. However, the preparations PR18B - PR22B were found to be the most potent. This increased potency was rather unexpected, since all the preparations were found to contain only hCG. It should be noted that preparations such as PR14B and

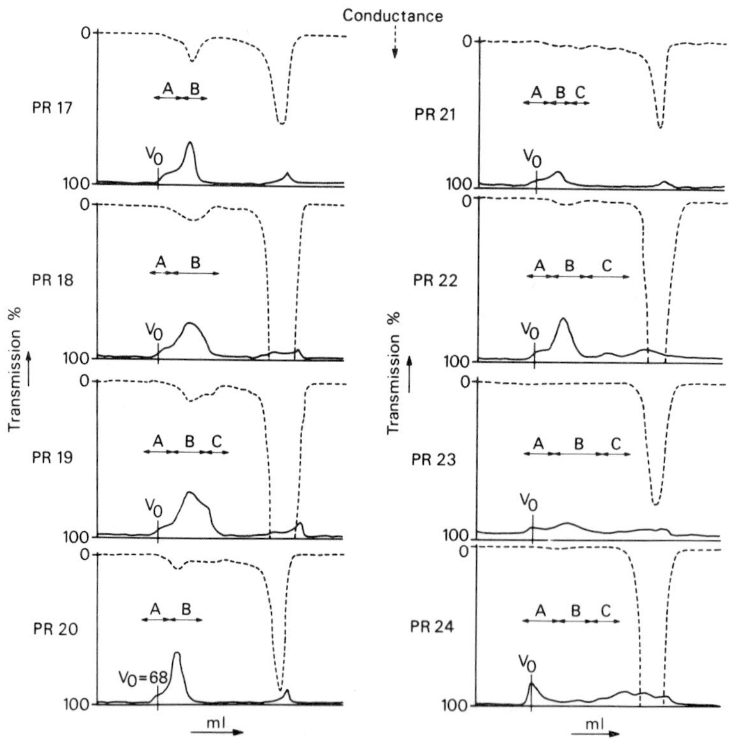

FIG 3. Gel filtration on Sephadex G-100 of some hCG preparations obtained after isoelectric focusing. The column (65 x 2 cm) was equilibrated and eluted with distilled water. The elution rate was 3.0 ml/cm^2/hr.

Table 1. Biological potencies and NANA-content of hCG preparations obtained by isoelectric focusing.
Preparations PR14B through PR24C were obtained after gel filtration of preparations C through L (see Fig 2). NANA-contents recorded are the results of duplicate analyses. The relative S.D. of the average value was 3.6 %. Two average values are significantly different if the quotient of the largest and the smallest value is larger than 1.084.

Preparation	NANA	Biol. pot., IU/mg	Yield %	
	%	95% conf. lim.	weight	biol.act.
PR 14 A		15000	0.3	0.7
B	10.7	15100 (11900-19000)	0.7	1.5
C		11000 (6000 -16000)	0.7	1.1
PR 16 A	10.5	18000 (14000-24000)	0.5	1.1
B		17000 (13000-23000)	0.9	2.0
PR 17 A		11400 (9300 -13900)	1.0	1.5
B	10.3	15700 (12600-19400)	6.6	14
PR 18 A		12900 (9800 -16700)	0.4	0.8
B	10.5	14100 (11500-17100)	10	19
PR 19 A		9700 (7100 -14300)	0.4	0.5
B	9.2	9300 (7400 -11900)	12	15
C		7000 (5600 - 8600)	2.0	1.9
PR 20 A	9.1	8900 (6800 -11500)	3.0	3.7
B		8000 (6500 - 9900)	7.2	7.9
PR 21 A		6600 (4700 - 9100)	0.3	0.2
B	8.6	6900 (5100 - 9500)	1.6	1.6
C		3300 (1900 - 4500)	0.3	0.2
PR 22 A		6800 (4900 - 9500)	0.3	0.3
B	7.8	7100 (5200 -10200)	8.0	7.7
PR 23 A		550 (330 - 790)	0.2	0.02
B		2500 (1900 - 3600)	3.2	1.1
PR 24 A		3800 (2700 - 5800)	0.3	0.1
B	2.9	1700 (1300 - 2300)	1.0	0.2
C		1700 (1200 - 2300)	1.3	0.3
		Total	62	83

Table 2. Immunopotencies and NANA-content of hCG preparations obtained by isoelectric focusing. The immunopotencies of the preparations were estimated using a RIA for hCG. The labelled material used was made from preparation PR20B on January 12, 1972. The two sets of results were obtained on February 28, 1972, and March 14, 1972, using the same solutions of the preparations. These solutions were prepared on February 28. The i/b ratios were calculated using the data of the immunoassays performed on February 28, 1972. Consult Table 1 for data on the NANA-contents.
* Deviation of parallelism of regression lines. RIA = radioimmunoassay.

Preparation	NANA %	Pot. by RIA, IU/mg, 95% conf. lim. febr. 28, 1972	march 14, 1972	i/b
PR 14 B	10.7	6800 (6000-7600)	5900	0.45
PR 16 B		7300 (6500-8300)	4800 (4350-5300)	0.43
PR 17 B	10.3	7700 (6800-8600)	5070 (4580-5610)	0.49
PR 18 B	10.5	7500 (6700-8400)	9000 (8100-9900)	0.53
PR 19 B	9.2	8700 (7700-9700)	7100 (6400-7800)	0.94
PR 20 B		*)	*)	
PR 21 B	8.6	8700 (7700-9800)		1.3
PR 22 B	7.8	8100 (7200-9100)	8800 (7900-9700)	1.1
PR 23 B		6000 (5400-6800)	6000 (5500-6700)	2.4
PR 24 B	2.9	3350 (2980-3770)	4270 (3870-4720)	2.0

PR24B amount to only about 1% of the starting material. Impurities present in these preparations may have escaped detection by the antisera as these were raised against crude hCG preparations which may have contained particular inpurities in very low concentrations. Therefore, the immunodiffusion experiments are not completely conclusive.

Table 3. Relationship between the isoionic points and the Ra value of hCG preparations obtained by isoelectric focusing. Preparations PR14B through PR24B were obtained after gel filtration of the preparations C through L. The bands present in the starch-gel electrophorogram were characterized by their Ra-values (2) which are recorded in the fifth column. The amount of napthalene black stainable material in each band is expressed as a % of the total amount of stainable material in the whole gel pattern. This % is shown in rectangles. The position of the rectangle corresponds to the Ra-value.

Relationship between the isoionic points and the Ra values of HCG components

I.I.P.	Relevant final preparation	% of total density (Ra 0.3 – 0.4 – 0.5 – 0.6 – 0.7 – 0.8)	Ra values
3.5-3.8*)	PR 14 B	100	0.74
3.8	PR 16 A	38; 62	0.69; 0.74
4.0	PR 17 B	20; 80	0.70; 0.64
4.3	PR 18 B	100	0.64
4.4	PR 19 B	21; 79	0.53; 0.60
4.5	PR 20 A	80; 20	0.53; 0.60
4.7	PR 21 B	100	0.54
4.8	PR 22 B	100	0.47
5.2	PR 23 B		0.48; 0.38; 0.28; 0.20
5.9-10.8**)	PR 24 B	100	0.38

B. Characterization

As highly purified preparations could be obtained by isoelectric focusing (Fig 1), the isoionic point can be used for the characterization of the various hCG preparations. Since the preparation used for isoelectric focusing did not contain impurities that could be detected by immunodiffusion this material was considered to contain mainly hCG. The peaks observed in the elution pattern at 280 nm after isoelectric focusing therefore essentially represent

Table 4. Comparison of the amino acid composition of hCG preparations (expressed as residues per 100 amino acids).

Amino-acid	Preparations		
	PR18B	PR22B	Canfield (1)
Aspartic acid	7.8	7.6	8.0
Threonine	7.6	7.8	7.4
Serine	8.8	8.8	8.9
Glutamic acid	8.2	8.2	7.9
Proline	12.7	12.8	12.2
Glycine	6.2	6.2	5.6
Alanine	5.8	5.9	5.7
Cystine	4.2	4.0	3.9
Valine	7.6	7.9	7.4
Methionine	2.0	1.9	1.4
Isoleucine	3.2	3.1	2.5
Leucine	7.2	7.2	6.6
Tyrosine	3.1	2.6	3.0
Phenylalanine	2.8	2.7	2.8
Lysine	4.4	4.6	4.4
Histidine	2.0	1.9	1.9
Arginine	6.4	6.5	6.6
Total	100.0	99.7	96.6

zones of focused hCG material (Fig 2). However, at least eight zones with isoionic points from pH 3.8 to 5.9 could be distinguished (Table 3). It appeared that most of the materials isolated from the symmetrical peaks in the elution pattern showed only one band after starch-gel electrophoresis (Preparations PR18B and PR24B in Table 3). A relationship between the isoionic points and the mobility of the bands can be observed in starch-gel electrophoresis (Table 3); the mobilities increase with increasing acidity of the hCG material. It may be concluded that nine hCG components are discernible by starch-gel electrophoresis - each band is considered to represent a component - with isoionic points ranging from pH 3.8 to pH 5.9. Two of the preparations isolated by the procedure described in Fig 1 (PR18B , Table 3) with isoionic points differing by half a pH unit were found to have virtually identical amino acid compositions (Table 4). Compared with the average amino acid composition as calculated for hCG by Canfield et al. (17) from the results of a number of investigators, a difference was noted only in the content of methionine and possibly isoleucine. These results, together with the finding that the various hCG components are immunochemically identical suggest that these components have an identical protein chain. As the NANA residues are the only charged molecules in the carbohydrate chains of hCG, the differences in the isoionic points of the various components (Table 3) must be mainly due to differences in the contents of NANA. This, however, is not in agreement with the properties of the four most potent preparations obtained by the procedure given in Fig 1. The NANA contents of these preparations (PR14B, PR16A, PR17B, PR18B, Table 1) and their biological potencies were not significantly different from each other (relative S.D. for the NANA content : 3.6 %), but they were focused at different pH values (Table 3). No explanation can be offered at this time for the discrepancy.

SOME PROPERTIES OF HCG COMPONENTS

The chemical evidence obtained so far, indicates that the various hCG components differ only in their NANA content; however, the other parts of the carbohydrate chains were not investigated. Most NANA residues can be expected to be situated at the outside of the molecule as it is a charged hydrophilic residue at the terminal of the carbohydrate chains. It can therefore be expected to affect the properties of the hCG components.

A. Influence of NANA on the biological potency

The relationship between the NANA content and the biological potency of hCG as estimated in a test measuring a chronic growth response (such as the ventral prostate weight assay and the seminal vesicle weight assay) has been firmly established by several investigators (15, 18, 19) and the results of the present studies.

Van Hell et al. (19) showed that the removal of about 60 % of the NANA residues from hCG, by degradation with bacterial neuraminidase reduced the biological potency from 11,110 IU/mg of the native material to 1.3 IU/mg. After 60 % desialylation, approximately 3.6 % NANA still remained bound to the molecule. The present results show that an apparently pure hCG preparation with a NANA content of 2.9 % (Table 1) still had a biological potency of 1700 IU/mg. Comparison of these observations suggests that the different NANA residues do not have the same effect on the biological activity of hCG. It would be most interesting in this respect to study the location of the NANA residues on the carbohydrate chains in preparations such as those listed in Table 1.

B. Influence of NANA on the immunochemical potency

Statistical analysis of the results given in Table 2 showed that the immunopotencies of the preparations listed are not similar. It is unlikely that impurities are present in such high amounts as to cause differences in immunopotency. Furthermore, evidence was presented that the various hCG components have identical protein moieties. The differences in immunopotencies can therefore only be caused by differences in the carbohydrate moieties of the components. Nothing is known about the differences in the contents of carbohydrate other than NANA. They may affect the outer structure of the molecule and consequently the affinity of the antibodies for these molecules. Differences in affinity may be reflected in differing immunochemical potencies. Using haptenic complement fixation inhibition, Mori (18) found that the carbohydrate moiety of hCG is not essential for its immunochemical activity. However, this author probably might have used multicomponent hCG, so that differences in structure could not be detected. In the radioimmunoassay, Vaitukaitis and Ross (20) found an altered immunoreactivity of urinary FSH after desialylation. These authors suggested that the altered immunoreactivity could reflect an altered tertiary structure of the molecule. The present results suggest that the NANA residues in the hCG molecule do contribute to the immunoreactivity of hCG. No data are yet available to conclude the way in which,or to what extent the NANA residues affect immunoreactivity. In this context a remark may be added about the limited reproducibility of the radioimmunoassay when preparations such as those recorded in Table 2 are assayed. Upon standing in solution, the labelled preparation and the preparations to be tested may lose NANA and this loss may affect the assay.

ACKNOWLEDGEMENTS

I gratefully acknowledge fruitful discussion with Dr. A. H. W. M. Schuurs on the immunochemical work and thank Mr. F. C. den Hollander for his work on the radioimmunoassays.

I thank Mr. J. Kouwenberg, who performed the bio-assays, and Mr. A. Delver for the statistical treatment of the results and helpful discussions. I am also indebted to Mr. B. C. Goverde and Mr. F. J. N. Veenkamp for the NANA-determinations and the amino acid analysis. I want to thank Mr. J. I. van Lieshout for his skilled and devoted technical assistance.

REFERENCES

1. Van Hell, H., Goverde, B. C., Schuurs, A. H. W. M., Jager, E. De., Matthijsen, R. and Homan, J. D. H. (1966). Nature (London). 212, 261.
2. Van Hell, H., Matthijsen, R. and Homan, J. D. H. (1968). Acta Endocrinol. (Copenhagen) 59, 89.
3. Hamashige, S., Astor, M. A., Arquilla, E. R. and van Thiel, D. H. (1967). J. Clin. Endo. 27, 1690.
4. Hamashige, S. and Astor, M. A. (1969). Fert. Steril. 20, 1029.
5. Hamashige, S., Alexander, J. D., Abravanel, E. V. and Astor, M. A. (1971). Fert. Steril. 22, 26.
6. Yogo, I. (1969). Endocrinol. Jap. 16, 215.
7. Bell, J. J., Canfield, R. E. and Sciarra, J. J. (1969). Endocrinology 84, 298.
8. Ashitaka, Y., Tokura, Y., Tane, M., Mochizuki, M. and Tojo, S. (1970). Endocrinology 87, 233.
9. Moritz, P. M. (1969). In "Protides of Biological Fluids" Vol. 16, pp 701, H. Peeters (Ed). Pergamon Press.
10. Brossmer, R., Merz, W. E. and Hilgenfeldt, U. (1971). FEBS Letters 18, 112.
11. Van Hell, H. and Schuurs, A. H. W. M. (1970). In "Gonadotrophins and Ovarian Development", W. R. Butt, A. C. Crooke and Margaret Ryle (Eds). pp 70, E & S Livingstone, Edinburgh and London.
12. Gottschalk, A. (1969). Nature (London). 222, 452.
13. Hollander, F. C. den and Schuurs, A. H. W. M. (1971). In "Radioimmunoassay Methods", K. E. Kirkham and W. M. Hunter (Eds) pp 419, Livingstone, E & S, Edinburgh.

14. Hollander, F. C. den, Schuurs, A. H. W. M. and Van Hell, H. (1972). J. Immunol. Methods. 1, 247.
15. Goverde, B. C., Veenkamp, F. J. N. and Homan, J. D. H. (1968) Acta Endocrinol. (Copenhagen) 59, 105.
16. Schuurs, A. H. W. M., de Jager, E. and Homan, J. D. H. (1968) Acta Endocrinol. (Copenhagen) 59, 120.
17. Canfield, R. E., Morgan, F. J., Kammerman, S., Bell, J. J. and Agosto, G. M. (1971). Rec. Prog. Horm. Res. 27, 121.
18. Mori, K. F. (1970). Endocrinology 86, 97.
19. Van Hall, E. V., Vaitukaitis, J. L., Ross, G. T., Hickman, J. W. and Ashwell, G. (1971) Endocrinology 88, 456.
20. Vaitukaitis, J. L. and Ross, G. T. (1971). J. Clin. Endocrinol. 33, 308.

CHEMISTRY OF HUMAN CHORIONIC GONADOTROPIN

F. J. Morgan, S. Birken and R. E. Canfield

INTRODUCTION

Although human chorionic gonadotropin was one of the first glycoprotein hormones to be clearly identified and used in a clinical setting, until recently it was not the object of as intense medical research as the pituitary glycoprotein hormones. HCG is readily available and relatively stable under conditions of experimental manipulation, and it has had widespread use as an investigative agent in reproductive biology. This contribution is intended as a brief review of the chemistry of hCG, with emphasis on areas of current interest.

PURIFICATION AND PROPERTIES OF URINARY HCG

HCG is a glycoprotein containing approximately 30 % carbohydrate. This was evident from early studies (1), and was clearly established by Got and Bourillon (2) who devised purification procedures for urinary hCG and reported amino acid and carbohydrate compositions which compare very favourably with currently accepted values. Several methods have been described for the purification of hCG (3-6). The method currently employed in the authors' laboratory has been reviewed in detail elsewhere (6).

HCG preparations from several laboratories have very similar amino acid compositions (5). The purified hCG migrates as a single broad acidic band on polyacrylamide-gel electrophoresis. Iso-electric focusing shows that hCG preparations possess bands of different isoelectric points, and that removal of sialic acid residues converts this pattern to a single band (7). This evidence, together with the structural determinations indicates that purified hCG contains essentially a unique protein species and that the heterogeneity observed, usually by electrophoretic technique, is largely due to differences in the sialic acid content. Other forms of carbohydrate microheterogeneity may exist, but have not been demonstrated experimentally. A summary of the properties of purified hCG is given in Table 1.

Table 1. Properties of hCG and its subunits *

Property	hCG	hCG$_{\alpha}$	hCG$_{\beta}$
Biological activity** IU/mg	10,000-15,000	nil	nil
Carbohydrate (by weight)	~ 30 %	~ 25 %	~ 30 %
Sialic acid (by weight)	~ 10 %	~ 4 %	~ 10 %
Amino acids	237	92	145
Molecular weight			
Polypeptide	25,690	10,185	15,505
Total	~ 39,000	~ 15,000	~ 25,000
$E^{1\%}_{280\,nm}$ ¶	3.6	4.3	2.1
ε ($M^{-1}cm^{-1}$) ¶	1.41×10^4	0.64×10^4	0.56×10^4

* Approximate values are given when estimates in the literature make exact figures uncertain. ** Ventral prostate weight assay/2nd International Std hCG. ¶ Morgan et al. (14).

SUBUNIT STRUCTURE OF HCG

A. Separation of subunits

HCG resembles luteinizing hormone in many biological and structural features. HCG similar to LH (8) is comprised of two non-identical, non-covalently-bound glycoprotein subunits. Canfield et al. (9) first showed that S-carboxymethylated hCG could be separated into two approximately equal fractions by polyacrylamide gel electrophoresis. These two fractions had strikingly different amino acid compositions, which together accounted for the composition of the intact hCG, and were interpreted as being non-identical subunits analagous to those of LH. Subsequently, methods were devised for the preparative separation of the α and β subunits from native hCG by anion exchange chromatography in urea-containing buffers (10, 11). The method now employed in the authors' laboratory has been described in detail elsewhere (12). In the case of hCG, the β subunit has a significantly larger molecular weight than the

α subunit (5, 11, 12). The final purification of the subunits by gel filtration on Sephadex G-100 takes advantage of this phenomenon to free the subunit preparation from any undissociated hCG or the complementary subunit. The major properties of hCG-α and hCG-β subunits are given in Table 1.

B. Biological activity of subunit preparations

Preparations of either hCG subunit have low activities in conventional assay systems (5, 11). An analysis of the fractions from our large-scale subunit preparations leads to the conclusion that this residual activity can be explained entirely on the basis of contamination with native hormone (13). HCG-β subunit (approximately 200-400 IU/mg) from the ion exchange chromatography step is finally purified by chromatography on Sephadex G-100. When serial fractions from this step are tested for biological activity by the ventral prostate weight bioassay, the total activity applied to the column emerges as a symmetrical peak in the elution position of hCG, ahead of the protein peak of the hCG-β subunit and there is no indication of any biological activity in this peak. The biological activity of some batches of the hCG-β subunit prepared by this method (e.g. CR 115) has been as low as 5 IU/mg, or approximately 0.05 % of the initial activity. Furthermore, antiserum which reacts with the intact hCG or hCG-α, but not with hCG-β, has been shown to neutralize the biological activity in hCG-β subunit preparations (14). These findings, which implicate contamination of the β-subunit with native hCG have been further supported by the absence of binding of the highly purified hCG subunits to membrane receptors in vitro (15). These hCG subunits prepared by ion exchange chromatography and gel filtration have been examined by SDS-gel electrophoresis and have been shown to be free of the complementary subunit within the limits of this system (13).

AMINO ACID SEQUENCE OF HCG

A. The hCG- α subunit

Our proposal for the amino acid sequence of the hCG α subunit (16, 17) is shown in Fig 1. It was determined from a combination of tryptic, chymotryptic and cyanogen bromide peptides. The linear amino acid sequence of the major component is in complete agreement with the proposal of Bahl et al. (18), although amide assignments were not given in their case.

```
                                        10                                          20
Ala-Pro-Asp-Val-Gln-Asp-Cys-Pro-Glu-Cys-Thr-Leu-Gln-Glu-Asp-Pro-Phe-Phe-Ser-Gln-

                                        30                                          40
Pro-Gly-Ala-Pro-Leu-Ile-Glx-Cys-Met-Gly-Cys-Cys-Phe-Ser-Arg-Ala-Tyr-Pro-Thr-Pro-

                                        50      *                                   60
Leu-Arg-Ser-Lys-Lys-Thr-Met-Leu-Val-Gln-Lys-Asn-Val-Thr-Ser-Glu-Ser-Thr-Cys-Cys-

                                        70                                  *       80
Val-Ala-Lys-Ser-Tyr-Asn-Arg-Val-Thr-Val-Met-Gly-Gly-Phe-Lys-Val-Glu-Asn-His-Thr-

                                        90
Ala-Cys-His-Cys-Ser-Thr-Cys-Tyr-Tyr-His-Lys-Ser
```

Fig. 1 Amino acid sequence of hCG- α subunit (18). The sequence proposal of Bahl et al. (19) is identical, except that amide assignments are not given, and the NH_2 terminal heterogeneity is not noted. hLH-α lacks the three NH_2 terminal residues, but is otherwise identical (21). Site of carbohydrate attachment is marked with an asterisk.

The amide assignment of glutamic acid at position 27 is still uncertain. We have found heterogeneity at the amino terminus of the α-chains in our preparations (17, 19). Approximately 30 % of the chains lack three NH_2-terminal residues, Ala-Pro-Asp, and another 10 % lack two residues, Ala-Pro. We have found no COOH-terminal heterogeneity, nor have we isolated any peptide whose composition suggested multiple forms of hCG. Bahl et al. (18) also have not reported any heterogeneity. It is of interest that a recent report (20) suggests that the amino acid sequence of hLH- α is the same as that of hCG- α , except that it lacks entirely the NH_2-terminal tripeptide

Ala-Pro-Asp. This is in striking agreement with the finding of Pierce and colleagues that the α subunit of all the glycoprotein hormones would be similar, if not identical (21).

B. The hCG- β subunit

The sequence of hCG- β consisting of 145 amino acids, as determined in our laboratory (17,22) is shown in Fig 2. We found no heterogeneity either at the NH_2-terminus or the COOH-terminus, nor is there any evidence of multiple forms of hCG-β. Although our proposal is similar to that of Bahl et al. (18) there are several important differences. Our sequence contains a region 89-95 (our numbering) which is not present in the alternative proposal. This region contains two half-cystine residues and is homologous with the similar region in LH- β. The hCG- β sequence then contains twelve half-cystine residues in agreement with the compositional data (11) and equal to the number in the β-subunits of the other glycoprotein hormones (21). From position 26, our sequence Cys-Ile-Thr-Val-Asn-Thr-Thr- differs from that of Bahl et al. (18) who have reported the sequence - Cys-Ile-Asn-Val-Thr-Thr-. We find valine at position 55 instead of leucine, an additional arginine at 95, and an additional serine at 121. There is a serine at 138 in place of a proline. The terminal Ser-Leu-Pro-OH sequence in the proposal of Bahl et al. (18) is not found in our material. These changes result in a total of 145 residues instead of 139. Asparagine 13 and asparagine 30 have carbohydrate attachments and conform to the well-recognised Asn-X-Thr attachment site. Our sequence around residue 30 renders the site of carbohydrate attachment homologous with that of bovine thyrotropin-β (21).

Ninety-four of the 115 residues of hLH- β (i.e., 82 %) are identical with those of hCG- β ; it is not necessary to postulate any gaps to make this alignment (Fig. 2). HCG- β, however, possesses an additional 30 residues at the COOH-terminal end of the molecule which are found neither in hLH- β subunits nor in the β subunits of any of the other glycoprotein hormones. It has an unusual composition with a high proportion of proline and serine residues and contains only one bond, between residues 133 and 134, potentially susceptible to trypsin. This bond

```
                        10       *                     20
CG  Ser-Lys-Glu-Pro-Leu-Arg-Pro-Arg-Cys-Arg-Pro-Ile-Asn-Ala-Thr-Leu-Ala-Val-Glu-Lys-Glu-Gly-Cys-Pro-Val-
                                         *
LH  Ser-Arg-Glx-Pro-Leu-Arg-Pro-Trp-Cys-Glx-Pro-Ile-Asx-Ala-Thr-Leu-Ala-Val-Glx-Lys-Glx-Gly-Cys-Pro-Val-

                *                    40                               50
CG  Cys-Ile-Thr-Val-Asn-Thr-Thr-Ile-Cys-Ala-Gly-Tyr-Cys-Pro-Thr-Met-Thr-Arg-Val-Leu-Gln-Gly-Val-Leu-Pro-
                *
LH  Cys-Ile-Thr-Val-Asx-Thr-Thr-Ile-Cys-Ala-Gly-Tyr-Cys-Pro-Thr-Met-Arg-Met-Leu-Leu-Glx-Ala-Val-Leu-Pro-

                                       60                                70
CG  Ala-Leu-Pro-Gln-Val-Val-Cys-Asn-Tyr-Arg-Asp-Val-Arg-Phe-Glu-Ser-Ile-Arg-Leu-Pro-Gly-Cys-Pro-Arg-Gly-

LH  Pro-Val-Pro-Glx-Pro-Val-Cys-Thr-Tyr-Arg-Asx-Val-Arg-Phe-Glx-Ser-Ile-Arg-Leu-Pro-Gly-Cys-Pro-Arg-Gly-

                  80                                 90                                 100
CG  Val-Asn-Pro-Val-Val-Ser-Tyr-Ala-Val-Ala-Leu-Ser-Cys-Gln-Cys-Ala-Leu-Cys-Arg-Arg-Ser-Thr-Thr-Asp-Cys-

LH  Val-Asx-Pro-Val-Val-Ser-Phe-Pro-Val-Ala-Leu-Ser-Cys-Arg-Cys-Gly-Pro-Cys-Arg-Arg-Ser-Thr-Ser-Asx-Cys-

                                     110                                 120  *
CG  Gly-Gly-Pro-Lys-Asp-His-Pro-Leu-Thr-Cys-Asp-Asp-Pro-Arg-Phe-Gln-Asp-Ser-Ser-Ser-Ser-Lys-Ala-Pro-Pro-

LH  Gly-Gly-Pro-Lys-Asx-His-Pro-Leu-Thr-Cys-Glx-Asx-Ser-Lys-Gly

       *         130     *                       *     140
CG  Pro-Ser-Leu-Pro-Ser-Pro-Ser-Arg-Leu-Pro-Gly-Pro-Ser-Asp-Thr-Pro-Ile-Leu-Pro-Gln
```

Fig. 2 Amino acid sequence of hCG-β subunit. The sequence given is that of the authors (18, 23); differences between this proposal and that of Bahl et al. (19) are discussed in the text. Attachment of carbyhydrate chain is marked with an asterisk. Human LH-β is shown for comparison. The hLH-β amino acid sequence is that of Closset et al. (28); the hLH-β amino acid sequence of Shome and Parlow (29) differs from this in some residues.

was not reported cleaved by trypsin in the proposal of Bahl et al. (18), and although we find that it is susceptible to tryptic cleavage, the rate of cleavage appears to be quite slow. It is possible that this 30 residue fragment of the molecule may represent a region resistant to proteolytic digestion in vivo, serving to protect the molecule from degradation either in the circulation or at the membrane receptor.

Although it was formerly difficult to distinguish immunologically between intact hCG and hLH, specific radioimmunoassays which discriminate between hCG and hLH have been developed on the basis of antisera to the respective β subunits (23). This implies that there are significant differences between some of the antigenic determinants on hCG-β and LH-β. The 30 residue fragment at the COOH-terminal of hCG-β is the most obvious structural difference between the two hormones.

CARBOHYDRATE COMPONENTS OF HCG

A. Carbohydrate composition of hCG and its subunits

Carbohydrate compositions of our preparations of hCG and its subunits (Table 2) correspond reasonably closely with those reported by Bahl and co-workers (10,24). Only the usual

Table 2. Carbohydrate composition of hCG *

Carbohydrate	hCGα	hCGβ
Mannose	6.6	3.0
Galactose	3.2	6.3
Fucose	ND**	trace
Glucosamine	8.5	7.0
Galactosamine	ND**	2.5
Sialic acid	3.5	7.3

* g/100 g (dry weight); data from batch CR117.

** ND = not detected.

sugars existing in serum glycoproteins were found. HCG has a high content of sialic acid and variations in this content from sample to sample of hCG are responsible for most, if not all, of the electrophoretic heterogeneity seen in preparations of hCG and its subunits.

Morell et al. (25) have shown in hCG and other glycoproteins that galactose residues, exposed when the terminal sialic acid molecules are removed from the glycoprotein, are recognized by specific receptors in hepatocytes which rapidly remove desialyated glycoproteins from circulation. This finding provides an explanation for the loss of in vivo biological activity when sialic acid is removed, for the retention of activity by asialo hCG in in vitro systems, and for dissociation between biological and immunological activity, the latter being unaffected by removal of sialic acid.

Bahl (26) has isolated several glycopeptides from hCG and demonstrated that they have two similar types of large branched carbohydrate chains of the type recognised in serum glycoproteins. These carbohydrate chains are attached to the hCG-polypeptide chains at asparagine residues. In a later communication Bahl (24) assigned these structures (designated Structure Structure I and Structure II) to the α and β subunits respectively; the hCG-α subunit contained two identical carbohydrate moieties of Structure I type, while hCG-β had two of Structure II type. Bahl (26) also showed that approximately 3 serine residues in hCG were destroyed by treatment with alkali and postulated the existence of three small carbohydrate side chains, of the type NANA-galactose-N-acetyl-galactosamine attached to serine residues by O-glycosidic linkages.

B. Sites of carbohydrate attachment

The hCG α subunit possesses two points of carbohydrate attachment, at asparagine 52 and asparagine 78. The amino acid sequences at these points both conform to the well established Asn-X-Thr pattern of carbohydrate attachment. It has been claimed that the two carbohydrate side chains in the α subunit have identical structures (24).

HCG- β subunit contains two asparaginyl-linked carbohydrate side chains at positions 13 and 30. Bahl (24) has proposed that these carbohydrate side chains have identical structures, somewhat different from those of the α -subunit. Carbohydrate side chains have been found by Closset et al. (27) in similar positions in the hLH- β subunit, although Shome and Parlow (28) were not able to detect the presence of carbohydrate at residue 13. Bovine and porcine LH- β have carbohydrate residues only at asparagine 13 (29,30); bovine thyrotropin- β possesses carbohydrate residues in the position homologous to residue 30, but there is no carbohydrate at residue 13 (21).

We have detected the presence of four carbohydrate side chains attached to serine residues in the COOH-terminal portion of hCG- β . The proposal of Bahl et al. (18) includes similar though not identical features with three serine-linked carbohydrate chains. In our proposal carbohydrate is attached at serine residues 121, 127, 132 and 138. There are insufficient reports in the literature, of sequences around the attachments of carbohydrate at serine residues to define an amino acid sequence pattern related to the specificity of the glycosyl transferase involved in the formation of O-seryl glycosidic linkages. Bahl et al (18) noted the proximity of proline residues to the site of serine carbohydrate attachment in their proposal of hCG- β sequence. The occurrence in our proposal, of the sequence pattern Pro-X-Pro before the serine residues 127, 132 and 138 is suggestive of a sequence, that may reflect the specificity for a glycosyl transferase. However, it cannot be the only type of recognition pattern as a sequence Ser-Ser-Ser precedes the carbohydrate attachment at serine 127.

RECOMBINATION OF SUBUNITS

HCG- α and β subunits recombine, when incubated in solution, to form native hCG as demonstrated by elution position on gel filtration and by the regain of biological activity (5, 11). This property is exploited in forming hybrid glycoprotein hormones (31) and in the formation of specific-subunit-labeled hCG (19,32). A similar association process is perhaps part of the assembly of glycoprotein hormones following the synthesis of the α and β subunits. Since the use of conventional bioassay to make a detailed study of the rates of association and dissociation is generally impracticable, a quantitative approach to this study has been made using the fluorescent dye 1,8-anilinonaphthalene-sulfonic acid (ANS) (33,34). The quantum yield of fluoresceince of ANS is markedly increased in non-polar solvents or when it binds to hydrophobic regions in proteins. ANS binds to hCG with an increase in fluorescence; however, there is no increase in fluorescence yield in the presence of either subunit alone. This provides a method for measuring the concentration of hCG in the presence of the subunits and of estimating the rate of association or dissociation under varying experimental conditions. Preliminary experiments, employing the technique of Hummel and Dreyer (35), indicate that each mole of hCG binds one mole of ANS (Morgan et al. - unpublished results).

STRUCTURE-ACTIVITY RELATIONSHIPS

The analysis of those sites on the hormone, crucial for the interaction of hCG with its receptor and the expression of biological activity is in a rudimentary state. Neither subunit alone possesses any activity in conventional assay systems (11, 13) nor do they bind <u>in vitro</u> to cells (36) or to membranes (15). A major part of the biological activity is restored on recombination of the subunits (11,13). The β subunit, as in all glycoprotein hormones, seems necessary for the specific activity which, however, is expressed only when the β subunit is combined with an α subunit. Alpha subunits from other hormones can substitute for hCG-α and generate hCG activity (31) but their relative efficiency in this regard is not accurately known.

HCG maintains a significant degree of biological activity when iodinated by the chloramine-T method (37). When such preparations are examined by SDS-gel electrophoresis which effectively separates the subunits, the radioactivity is found localized in the hCG- α subunit (32,38). Similar findings have been reported for LH (39,40). Such preparations are thus, less than adequate for following the fate of the intact molecule or the β subunit. HCG labeled specifically on either or both subunits can be prepared by labelling individual subunits of hCG with different isotopes, followed by appropriate recombinations. HCG, labeled on both the subunits with ^{125}I, and hCG labeled on the α subunit with ^{125}I and the β subunit with ^{131}I, has been prepared and shown to be biologically active (32). *In vivo* studies with these preparations have shown no evidence of dissociation of the α from the β subunit at the ovarian end for periods of upto 4 hr after injection.

Such experiments demonstrate the feasibility of producing modified preparations of hCG, which have not lost their biological activity, and can be used for the detailed study of the mode of action of gonadotropins. Three-dimensional structural information, derived either from crystals or measurements made in solution, may enable one to make even more sophisticated approaches to modification of significant residues.

Addendum

After this paper was written and presented, we became aware of a revised proposal for the hCG- β subunit structure (41) in which some of the discrepancies noted in Section on 'The amino acid sequence of hCG- β ', are resolved. However, the two proposals still do not agree in all details, especially with regard to the COOH-terminal region.

ACKNOWLEDGEMENTS

Supported by NIH research grant AMO 9579, NIH Contract 70-2251 NICHD, and a grant from the Population Council, New York.

REFERENCES

1. Gurin, S., Bachman, C. and Wilson, D.W. (1940). J. Biol. Chem. 133, 467.
2. Got, R. and Bourillon, R. (1960). Biochim. Biophys. Acta. 42, 505.

3. Van Hell, H., Matthijsen, R.M. and Homan, J.D.H. (1968). Acta. Endocrinol. 59, 89.
4. Bahl, O.P. (1969). J. Biol. Chem. 244, 567.
5. Canfield, R.E., Morgan, F.J., Kammerman, S., Bell, J.J. and Agosto, G.M. (1971). Rec. Prog. Horm. Res. 27, 121.
6. Canfield, R.E. and Morgan, F.J. (1973). In "Methods in Investigative and Diagnostic Endocrinology", S.A. Berson and R.S. Yalow (Eds). Vol. 2B, pp 727, North-Holland Publishing Co., Amsterdam.
7. Graesslin, D., Weise, H.C. and Braendle, W. (1973). FEBS Letter 31, 214.
8. Papkoff, H. and Samy, T.S.A. (1967). Biochem. Biophys. Acta. 147, 175.
9. Canfield, R.E., Bell, J.J. and Agosto, G.M. (1970). In "Gonadotropins and Ovarian Development". W.R. Butt, A.C. Crooke and M. Ryle (Eds). pp. 161, E.S. Livingstone, Edinburgh.
10. Swaminathan, N. and Bahl, O.P. (1970). Biochem. Biophys. Res. Comm. 40, 422.
11. Morgan, F.J., and Canfield, R.E. (1971). Endocrinology 88, 1045.
12. Morgan, F.J., Canfield, R.E., Vaitukaitis, J.L. and Ross, G.T. (1973). In "Methods in Investigative and Diagnostic Endocrinology". S.A. Berson and R.S. Yalow (Eds). Vol 2B, pp 733, North-Holland Publishing Co., Amsterdam.
13. Morgan, F.J., Canfield, R.E., Vaitukaitis, J.L. and Ross, G.T. (1974). Endocrinology (in press).
14. Rayford, P.L., Vaitukaitis, J.L., Ross, G.T., Morgan, F.J. and Canfield, R.E. (1972). Endocrinology 91, 144.
15. Catt, K.J., Dufau, M.L., and Tsuruhara, R. (1973). J. Clin. Endo. Metab. 36, 73.
16. Morgan, F.J. and Canfield, R.E. (1972). Proc. 4th Internl. Congr. Endocrinol, Washington, D.C., Abstracts, pp 177.
17. Morgan, F.J., Birken, S. and Canfield, R.E. (1973). Mol. Cell. Biochem. (in press).
18. Bahl, O.P., Carlsen, R.B., Bellisario, R. and Swaminathan, N. (1972). Biochem. Biophys. Res. Comm. 48, 416.

19. Canfield, R.E., Morgan, F.J., Kammerman, S. and Ross, G.T. (1972). In "Structure-activity relationships of protein and polypeptide hormones". M. Margoulies and F.C. Greenwood (Eds). Part 2, pp 341, Excerpta Medica, Amsterdam.
20. Sairam, M.R., Papkoff, H. and Li, C.H. (1972). Biochem. Biophys. Res. Comm. 48, 530.
21. Pierce, J.G., Liso, T.H., Howard, S.M., Shome, B. and Cornell, J.S. (1971). Rec. Prog. Horm. Res. 27, 165.
22. Morgan, F.J., Birken, S. and Canfield, R.E. (1973). FEBS Letter 31, 101.
23. Vaitukaitis, J.L., Ross, G.T. and Reichert, L.E., Jr., (1973). Endocrinology 92, 411.
24. Bahl, O.P. (1971). In "Structure-activity relationships of protein and polypeptide hormones". M. Margoulies and F.C. Greenwood, (Eds). Part 1, pp 99, Excerpta Medica, Amsterdam.
25. Morell, A.G., Gregoriadis, G., Scheinberg, I.H., Hickman, J. and Ashwell, G. (1971). J. Biol. Chem. 246, 1461.
26. Bahl, O.P. (1969). J. Biol. Chem. 244, 575.
27. Closset, J., Hennen, G. and Lequin, R.M. (1973). FEBS Letter 29, 97.
28. Shome, B. and Parlow, A.F. (1973). J. Clin. Endo. Metab. 36, 618.
29. Maghuin-Rogister, G. and Dockier, A. (1971). FEBS Letter 19, 209.
30. Maghuin-Rogister, G. and Hennen, G. (1972). FEBS Letter 23, 225.
31. Pierce, J.G., Bahl, O.P., Cornell, J.S. and Swaminathan, N. (1971). J. Biol. Chem. 246, 2321.
32. Morgan, F.J., Kaye, G.I. and Canfield, R.E. (1974). Israel, J. Med. Sci. (in press).
33. Aloj, S.M., Ingham, K.C. and Edelhoch, H. (1973). Arch. Biochem. Biophys. 155, 478.
34. Aloj, S.M., Edelhoch, H., Ingham, K.C., Morgan, F.J., Canfield, R.E., and Ross, G.T. (1973). Arch. Biochem. Biophys. (in press).
35. Hummell, J.P. and Dreyer, W.J. (1962). Biochem. Biophys. Acta. 63, 530.

36. Channing, C. P. and Kammerman, S. (1973). Endocrinology 92, 531.
37. Midgley, A.R., Jr., (1966), Endocrinology 79, 10.
38. Morgan, F.J., Kammerman, S. and Canfield, R. F. (1972) In "Gonadotropins", B.B. Saxena, C.G. Beling and H.M. Gandy, (Eds). pp. 211, Wiley-Interscience, New York.
39. Yang, K. P. and Ward, D.N. (1972). Endocrinology 91, 317.
40. Gospodarowicz, D. (1973). J. Biol. Chem. 248, 5042.
41. Carlsen, R.B., Bahl, O.P. and Swaminathan, N. (1973). J. Biol. Chem. 248, 6810.

PURIFICATION AND CHARACTERIZATION OF HUMAN CHORIONIC GONADOTROPIN IN HYDATIDIFORM MOLE

P.K. Chan, C.Y. Lee and L. Ma

INTRODUCTION

Hydatidiform mole is a placental disorder where there is pathological accumulation of interstitial fluid within the chorionic villi, so that the latter take on the form of isolated cysts, resembling very much in appearance a huge cluster of grapes (the Chinese have aptly named this condition grape pregnancy).

Hydatidiform mole is potentially malignant and is relatively common in the Far East, especially in Hong Kong where the incidence is 1 : 242 deliveries as compared with 1: 2,000 in European countries (1). Such patients have abnormally high levels of hCG in their blood and urine. It was suspected that endocrine disturbances probably play an important role in effecting certain metabolic changes associated with hydatidiform mole. Thus, differences have been reported on the profiles and levels of acid and alkaline phosphatases and lactic dehydrogenase isoenzymes (2) as well as lipoprotein content in the sera of women with molar and normal pregnancies (3).

Urinary hCG has been extensively studied (4-6) and its sequence has been recently reported (7); Chorionic gonadotropin from different sources are reported to differ in their physical and chemical properties (7). In order to understand the significance of these differences, we have attempted to purify hCG from the molar tissue. The following is a report on its fractionation and characterization.

MATERIALS AND METHODS

Hydatidiform moles obtained on hysterectomy were removed to the laboratory within two hours of operation. The tissues thoroughly cleaned with 0.9 % saline and rinsed with distilled water were homogenized, lyophilized and stored until further use at 4°.

A. Fractionation procedure

The fractionation of hCG involved four steps, i.e., salt precipitation, column chromatography on Sephadex G-200, DEAE Sephadex A-50 and Sephadex G-100. All steps were performed at 4 $\pm$ 1° unless otherwise specified. The fractions obtained at each step were assayed for immunoreactivity and their protein contents were determined by the Folin-Ciocalteu method with bovine serum albumin as standard.

Five gm of freeze-dried molar tissue were suspended in 500 ml of 0.15 M ammonium sulphate solution, adjusted to pH 4.0 with HCl and stirred overnight. It was centrifuged at 10,000 g for 20 min, the cell debris discarded, and the supernatant adjusted to pH 3.0 with freshly prepared 0.5 M H_3PO_4. After centrifugation again at 10,000 g for 20 min, the precipitate was discarded and to the supernatant 30 gm of ammonium sulphate per 100 ml was added and stirred for 2 hr before re-centrifugation at 10,000 g for 30 min. The precipitate was dissolved in 0.2 M K_2HPO_4 solution, dialysed against running cold water for one day and lyophylized.

Crude product ($\sim$500 mg) was dissolved in the equilibration buffer and filtered through a Sephadex G-200 column. Of the active fraction (G-200-2) obtained, 100 mg was dissolved in 5 ml of buffer, and applied to a DEAE Sephadex A-50 column; the active fractions were pooled, dialysed against 0.01 M NH_4HCO_3 for one day, lyophylized and further purified on Sephadex G-100.

B. Immunoassays

The commercial immuno-hCG kit (UCG titration kit from Wampole Labs, Stamford, Conn, USA) with a stated sensitivity of 0.8 IU/ml was used to determine the potency of the eluted fractions. The diluent used for serial dilution was composed of 0.9 % NaCl, 0.1 % bovine serum albumin in 0.01 M Na_2HPO_4 buffer at pH 8.

C. Polyacrylamide-gel electrophoresis

Disc electrophoresis was performed following the method of Davis (8), using 7 % and 7.5 % (w/v) gels at pH 8.9 and 5.0 respectively. 100 µg of protein in 0.1 ml of 10 % sucrose solution was applied to a column (0.5 x 7 cm). Electrophoresis was carried out at room temperature (22 ± 2°) at a constant current of 3 mA per tube for 2-3 hr until the tracing dye had reached the end of the column.

D. Isoelectric focusing

The isoelectric point of the purified hCG sample was determined by isoelectric focusing on an LKB 8100 column with a capacity of 110 ml. The column, containing 2 mg of the final product together with 1 % ampholine of pH values ranging from 3-10, was stabilized by a sucrose density gradient. After isoelectric focusing for 3 days, the content in the column was eluted at a flow-rate of 50 ml/hr. 3 ml fractions were collected and their optical density at 280 nm was read. The pH value of each fraction was determined.

E. Molecular size determination

A Sephadex G-200 (40-120 μ) column (2.3 x 30 cm) equilibrated with 0.05 M NH_4HCO_3 was used at room temperature. 3-5 mg of each of the active products and the protein markers were dissolved in 2 ml of 0.05 M NH_4HCO_3 buffer and applied to the column. The gel filtration was carried out at room temperature (22 ± 2°).

The molecular weight of the subunits of molar hCG was determined by sodium dodecyl sulphate (SDS) gel-electrophoresis (9). The sample (1 mg/ml) was incubated in an incubation mixture (4 M urea, 1 % SDS and 1 % (v/v) 2-mercaptoethanol in 0.01 M NaH_2PO_4 at pH 7) for 1 hr at 37°. About 50 μg of protein was subjected to electrophoresis under a potential of 8 mA/tube for 5 hr, the proteins were stained with Coomassie brilliant blue; Chymotrypsinogen A was used as the marker.

RESULTS AND DISCUSSION

HCG activity was found between the second and the third major protein peaks of the Sephadex G-200 column (Figure 1). On DEAE-Sephadex chromatography most of the protein was eluted between 0.1 M and 0.2 M NaCl; but the active fraction was eluted off the column earlier (Figure 2). This step effected a ten-fold purification of hCG, a finding in good agreement with that of

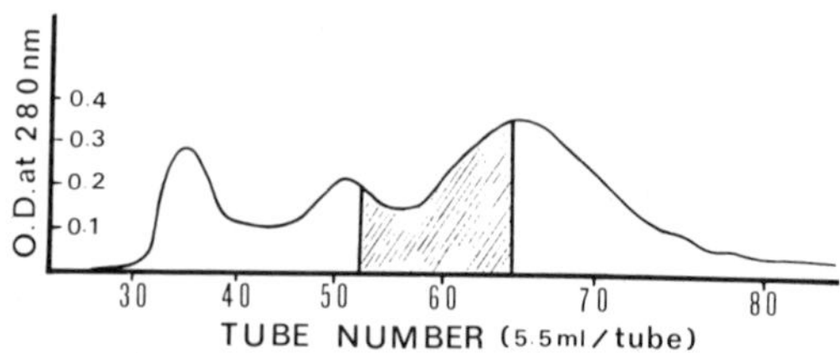

FIG 1. Chromatography of crude hCG on Sephadex G-200. The column (2 x 150 cm) was developed with 0.05 M NH_4HCO_3, the active fraction is indicated by the shaded area. The flow-rate was 10 ml/hr. The 5.5 ml fractions (G-200-2) were pooled, dialysed, and lyophilized.

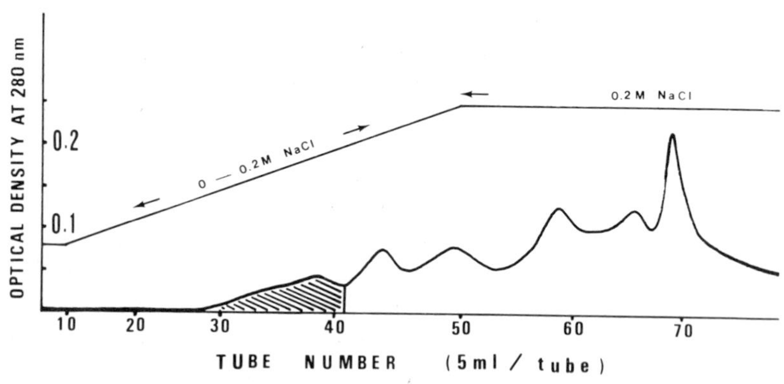

FIG 2. Chromatography of partially purified molar hCG (G-200-2) on DEAE Sephadex A-50.
The column (2 x 30 cm) was eluted initially with 50 ml of 0.04 M tris-phosphate buffer of pH 8.6 followed by NaCl gradient (0-0.2 M) elution, in the same buffer as indicated. Flow-rate was 30-40ml per hr. The active (5 ml fractions) fractions (shaded area) were pooled, dialysed, and lyophilized.

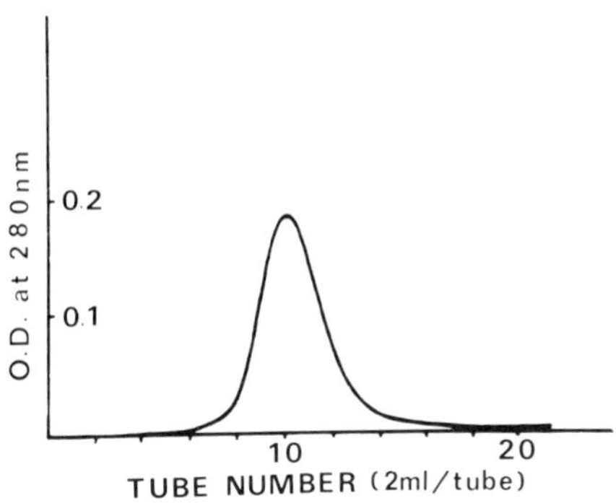

FIG 3. Re-chromatography of purified hCG on Sephadex G-100. 5 mg of the protein was applied. The column (1.4 x 28 cm) was developed with 0.05 M NH_4HCO_3. Flow-rate : 14 ml/hour.

Reisfeld and Hertz (10) and Pala et al. (11). Minor contaminants which were not fractionated by DEAE-Sephadex A-50 were removed by chromatography on Sephadex G-100 (Figure 3).

The yield of the final product is 0.27 % on a dry weight basis and 19.7 % by immunoactivity. The specific activity, as determined by haemagglutination method, after the four major steps is as follows : salt precipitation, 1000 IU/mg; Sephadex G-200 chromatography, 1600 IU/mg; DEAE Sephadex A-50, 15700 IU/mg; and Sephadex G-100, 21000 IU/mg.

The disc electrophoretic pattern of the final product on polyacrylamide gel is shown in Fig 4. Only one band was observed at alkaline pH, but an additional minor band appeared at pH 5. Heterogeneity is a common feature in hCG preparations and some workers (4, 12) have suspected that hCG exists in many forms rather than as a single entity. However, our result does not appear to confirm this thesis.

The pI of urinary hCG as determined by free boundary electrophoresis was found to be 3.0 (10) while that of molar hCG and urinary hCG isolated from patients with trophoblastic disorders was higher (13, 14). By isoelectric focusing,the pI of molar hCG was found to range from 3.5 to 5, with an absorption maximum at pH 4.2. Pala et al. (11) obtained essentially similar results by isoelectric focusing in polyacrylamide gel. The fact that the pI of molar hCG is higher than that of normal hCG suggested that the sialic acid content would be different in these two molecules.

By gel exclusion chromatography, the apparent molecular weight of molar hCG was found to be 63,000, the same as reported by Pala et al. (11); but this is higher than that reported for normal urinary hCG - 37,000 - 59,000 (6, 15). The final hCG product dissociated into two subunits when subjected to SDS-gel electrophoresis in 4 M urea. The apparent molecular weights of these subunits were found to be 26,000 and 31,000.

The final product was treated with dansyl chloride, hydrolysed, and analysed by thin layer chromatography on polyamide sheets

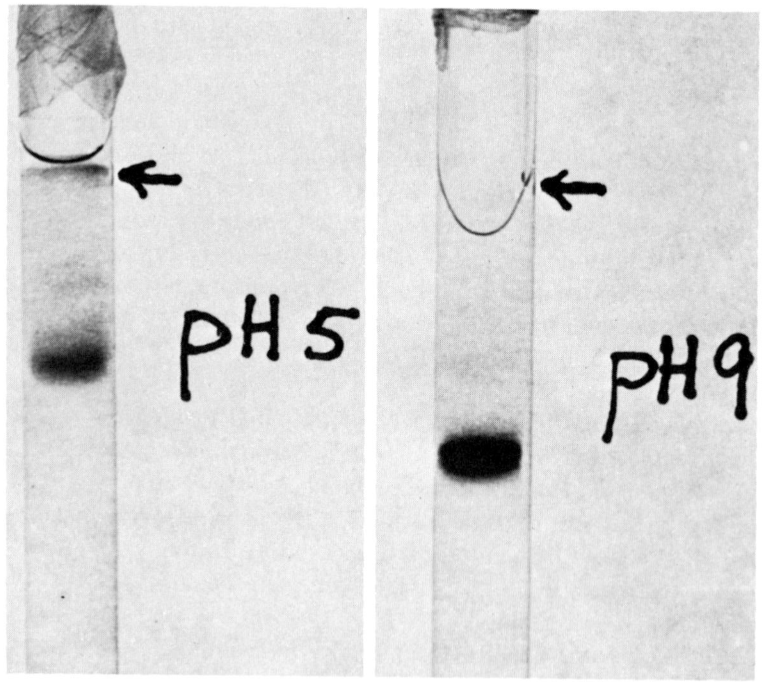

FIG 4. Polyacrylamide-gel electrophoresis of purified molar hCG. About 100 µg/tube of hormone was used. The stacking solutions and gels used are described in the text.

(Cheng Chin Trading Co. Taipei, Taiwan) and by high voltage paper electrophoresis (16). Preliminary results revealed that there are two N-terminal amino acids, serine and alanine.

In view of the above findings, it seems that the molecular size of molar hCG is higher than that of normal urinary hCG. However, these two forms of hCG have identical N-terminal amino acids albeit different charges. It is suggested that while they possess similar protein structures, they differ in their carbohydrate moieties.

To resolve the discrepancy relating to heterogeneity of hCG, it seems appropriate to carry out comparative studies on hCG from the urine and chorionic tissues of pregnant women and molar patients, especially with respect to their amino acid composition and carbohydrate contents. We believe that such comparative studies on a molecular basis will also be useful for the better understanding of this placental disorder and the role of hCG in late pregnancy. The purification of hCG from normal placenta by immunological precipitation is now in progress.

ACKNOWLEDGEMENT

We are grateful to Professor C.H. Li for his advice and to Drs. C.C. Yu, S.U. Lok, Donald S.H. Ko and Wai Chee Li for their help in various ways. The technical assistance of Mrs. A.S.K. Lee is also acknowledged. This work is supported by research grants from this University and the World Health Foundation (Hong Kong).

REFERENCES

1. Chun, D., Braga, C., Chow, C. and Lok, L.S.U. (1964). J. Obstet. Gynec. Brit. Comm. 71, 180.
2. Ma, L. and Lok, L.S.U. (1969). Clin. Chim. Acta. 25, 263.
3. Choi, M. and Ma, L. (1968). Far East. Med. J. 4, 235.
4. van Hell, H., Matthijsen, R. and Homan, J.D.H. (1968). Acta Endocrinologica 59, 89.
5. Ashitaka, Y., Tokura, Y., Tane, M., Mochizuki, M. and Tojo, S. (1970). Endocrinology 87, 233.
6. Bahl, O.P. (1969). J. Biol. Chem. 244, 567.
7. Bahl, O.P., Carlsen, R.B., Bellisario, R. and Swaminathan, N. (1972). Biochem. Biophys. Res. Commun. 48, 416.

8. Davis, B.J. (1964). Annals N.Y. Acad. Sci. 121, 404.
9. Dunker, A.K. and Reuckert, R.R. (1969). J. Biol. Chem. 244, 5074.
10. Reisfeld, R.A. and Hertz, R. (1960). Biochim. Biophys. Acta. 43, 540.
11. Pala, A., Meirinhi, M. and Benagiano, G. (1973). J. Endocr. 56, 441.
12. Canfield, R.E., Morgan, F.J., Kammerman, S., Bell, J.J. and Agosto, G.M. (1971). In Rec. Prog. Horm. Res. 27, 121.
13. Hammond, J.M., Bridson, W.E., Kohler, P.O. and Chrambach, A. (1971). Endocrinology 89, 801.
14. Kaplan, G.N., Maffezzoli, R.D. and Chrambach, A. (1972). J. Clin. Endo. 43, 370.
15. Mori, K.F. (1970). Endocrinology 86, 97.
16. Woods, K.R. and Wang, K.T. (1967). Biochim. Biophys. Acta. 133, 369.

IDENTIFICATION AND CHEMICAL CHARACTERIZATION OF THE PITUITARY GONADOTROPINS IN REPTILES AND AMPHIBIANS

Paul Licht and Harold Papkoff

INTRODUCTION

Information on the chemistry of gonadotropins of the non-mammalian vertebrates comes from indirect studies based on the use of purified mammalian hormones. Such studies have led to speculation that reptiles and amphibians might possess only a single gonadotropin molecule (perhaps an FSH/LH complex) rather than two separate molecules as exist in mammals. While these approaches may give insight into the physiology of the gonadal tissue, they obviously cannot provide definitive answers regarding the chemistry or physiology of the animals'own hypophysial hormones.

Chemical fractionation of the pituitaries of chicken (1,2) and turkey (3,4) has demonstrated that these avian species have a separate FSH- and LH-like gonadotropin. In contrast, studies on fish led to the conclusion that the teleost might possess only a single gonadotropin (5,6). These data suggest that the divergence of a single gonadotropin into a separate FSH and LH might have occurred early in the evolution of tetrapods, at least within the Reptilia; this hypothesis, however, is in conflict with conclusions of physiological studies (7,8). Direct chemical information on the gonadotropins of reptiles and amphibia, the two major "intermediate" groups in tetrapod phylogeny, is obviously critical to our understanding of the relationships among the pituitary glycoprotein hormones.

To gain an insight into the evolution of the vertebrates gonadotropins and the physiology of reproduction in lower vertebrates, we have undertaken purification of the gonadotropins from reptiles and amphibians.

EXPERIMENTAL

The American bullfrog (Rana catesbeiana) and the snapping turtle (Chelydra serpentina) were chosen as representatives of amphibia and reptilia. These choices were based primarily on the availability of the two species from commercial sources (frog-leg and turtle-soup industries).

A. Bioassay :

The comparative approach posed several major problems. First, it was essential to develop techniques for handling small amounts of tissue for both fractionation and bioassay. However, the most fundamental problem was that of biological identification and quantification of the non-mammalian gonadotropins. Previous experience and our own results demonstrated that the standard mammalian bioassays for FSH and LH [e. g., Steelman-Pohley and ovarian ascorbic acid depletion (OAAD) tests in rats] were of no use for comparative studies as these were insensititive to non-mammalian hormones (9, 10). Hence, our efforts were focused on developing sensitive and discriminative bioassays in non-mammalian species for the frog and reptilian gonadotropins. These led to the adoption of four different types of bioassays that appeared to vary in their specificity for gonadotropins - two of the assays (the Anolis lizard and the frog ovulation) being highly specific for one of the gonadotropin while the other two assays, being equally sensitive to both FSH and LH. These were used to construct a biological profile of materials obtained from fractionation of the pituitary gland and the details of the bioassays are given elsewhere (9, 10). The potential gonadotropic specificity of each assay was elucidated using highly purified ovine FSH and LH (Table 1). The tests in the hypophysectomized lizard (Anolis carolinensis) utilized testis weight to quantify gonadotropic potencies, but routine histological examination also provided information on the qualitative actions of hormones in regard to spermatogenesis and androgenesis (11, 12). Both gonadotropins may show the same "complete" spectrum of actions in this assay but FSH is at least 2000 times more potent (13). Similar results have also

Table 1. Specificities of non-mammalian gonadotropin assays for FSH and LH.

Assay	Minimal effective dosage (μg)*	
	FSH	LH
Lizard (*Anolis*) : testis weight, spermatogenesis, androgenesis	0.01	20
Frog ovulation *in vitro*	> 100	0.5
Frog (*Hyla*) spermiation	0.5	1
Chick testis ^{32}P uptake	1	1

*Based on tests with highly purified ovine hormones : LH = 2 x NIH-LH-S1; FSH = 50 x NIH-FSH-S1.

been obtained with a variety of other reptiles, including snakes and turtles (7, 8). In contrast, the induction of ovulation in excised fragments of frog ovaries is a highly specific test for mammalian LH (14). Three species of anurans (*Hyla*, *Xenopus* and *Rana*) have been used routinely for these *in vitro* tests with similar results; however, the *Rana* ovaries proved inconvenient because of their relative insensitivity to mammalian LH.

Sperm release (spermiation) in several species of frog (*Hyla* was used for most studies) and ^{32}P uptake in the tests of day-old cockerels provide rapid quantitative measures of total gonadotropin (15, 16). Tests with highly purified mammalian hormones indicated that the two gonadotropins were approximately equipotent in both cases (Table 1), but subsequent studies with frog and turtle hormones suggest that the spermiation test is relatively more sensitive to non-mammalian FSH's than is the chick assay (see below). The chick assay was also modified to measure TSH simultaneously be examining ^{32}P incorporation into the thyroids (17).

From the biological profile obtained above, it could be expected that if only a single gonadotropin existed, then a single fraction should show activity in all four tests in addition to showing a similar proportion of increase in potency through the fractionation steps. Alternatively, if two or more separate

Table 2. Purification of gonadotropin from pituitaries of the snapping turtle.

	Biological potency *			
	FSH	FSH + LH		LH
	Anolis	Frog spermiation	Chick ^{32}P uptake	Ovulation**
I. Alkaline extract	1	1	1	1
II. Amberlite IRC-50 from 0.6 SAS				
IRC-A (glycoprotein from unadsorbed fraction)	[20]	20	6	< 0.1
IRC-C (pH 6 eluate)	1.5	5	0.5	[5]
III. DEAE-cellulose of AS glycoprotein				
A (0.03 M eluate)	10	20	31	[0.1]
B (0.08 M eluate)	[100]	100	14	nil
IV. DEAE-cellulose of IRC-C				
A' (0.03 M eluate)	1.3	8	1	[10]
B' (1 M eluate)	[3.3]	3	0	0.7

* Alkaline extracts represent about 72 % of the total dry weight; thus, all potencies can be expressed in terms of pituitary dry weight by using a correction factor of 1.4. Values are maximal for the three batches of glands. Solid boxes indicate the most potent "FSH" fraction and dashed boxes show the most potent "LH" fraction at each stage of purification.
**Values represent averages of tests in three anurans: Xenopus, Hyla and Rana.
Based on data from Licht & Papkoff (9).

gonadotropins exist, then it should be possible to isolate fractions that are differentially potent in the lizard and frog assays, while being comparably active in the spermiation or chick assays. Potencies in each assay were measured by reference to NIH standard preparations of ovine hormones, but for convenience of present discussion, relative potencies of each fraction have been computed in terms of the alkaline extracts from which they were derived (Tables 2 and 3).

B. Purification procedures

Fractionation procedures were modeled after those used for isolation of gonadotropins from mammalian pituitaries;

Table 3. Purification of gonadotropin from pituitaries of the bull frog

	Biological potency *			
	FSH	FSH + LH		LH
	Anolis	Frog spermiation	Chick ^{32}P uptake	ovulation
I. Alkaline extract	1	1	1	1
II. Amberlite IRC-50 from 0.6 SAS				
IRC-A (glycoprotein from unadsorbed fraction)	[18]	4	0.3	0.1
IRC-C (pH 6 eluate)	0.5	1	0.7	[3]
III. DEAE-cellulose of AS glycoprotein				
A (0.03 M eluate)	1.5	0.2	0.7	0.3
B (0.08 M eluate)	20	10	0.5	nil
C (0.2 M eluate)	[50]	10	0.1	nil
IV. DEAE-cellulose of IRC-C				
A' (0.03 M eluate)	--	0.6	--	[10]
B' (0.08 M eluate)	--	0.2	--	nil

Based on data in Licht and Papkoff (10). See footnotes to Table 2 for explanations of data.

modifications included enabled the recovery of as many other pituitary hormones as possible (9, 10) (Fig 1). After an initial alkaline extraction of the homogenized pituitaries, special attention was focussed on ammonium sulphate fractionation, a step which is essentially used for separating mammalian FSH and LH. In all mammals studies, (both placental and marsupial species), LH has a relatively low solubility in ammonium sulfate solutions and is precipitated at 0.5 to 0.6 saturation, while FSH is more soluble and is precipitated at higher concentrations (mostly between 0.6 - 0.8 saturation). However, with both the turtle and frog materials, all gonadotropic activity in the extract was recovered at an ammonium sulfate concentration of 0.6 saturation (0.6 SAS); the higher salt fraction (0.6 - 0.8 SAS) generally contains very little protein and hormonal activity. This behaviour of gonadotropins was subsequently found to be the general rule for all non-mammalian species examined, including birds, reptiles, amphibia and fish (4, 18).

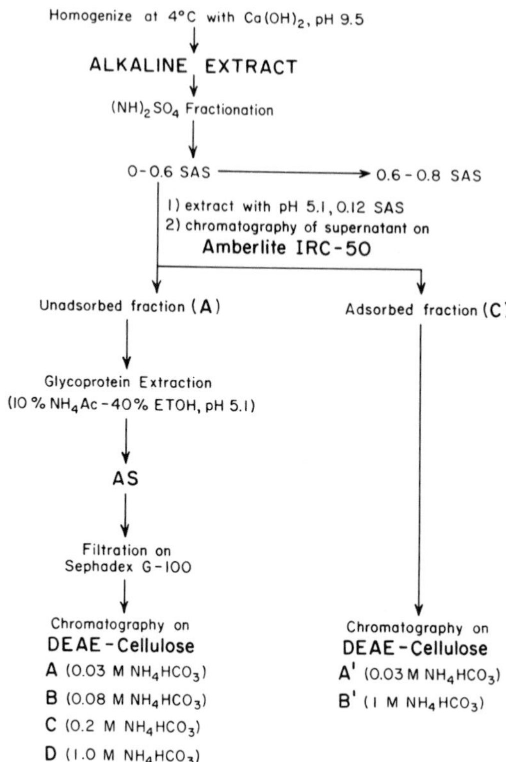

FIG 1. Fractionation scheme for the separation and purification of gonadotropins from pituitaries. Only the major gonadotropin-rich fractions are shown for most steps. From Licht and Papkoff (9).

Further purification of the 0.6 SAS fraction was accomplished primarily by ion-exchange chromatography on Amberlite IRC-50 and DEAE-cellulose. Four distinct fractions were obtained from the IRC-50 column (IRC-A, B, C and D) (Fig 2). In case of both turtle and frog materials, only the unadsorbed fraction (IRC-A) and the pH 6 eluate (IRC-C) contained

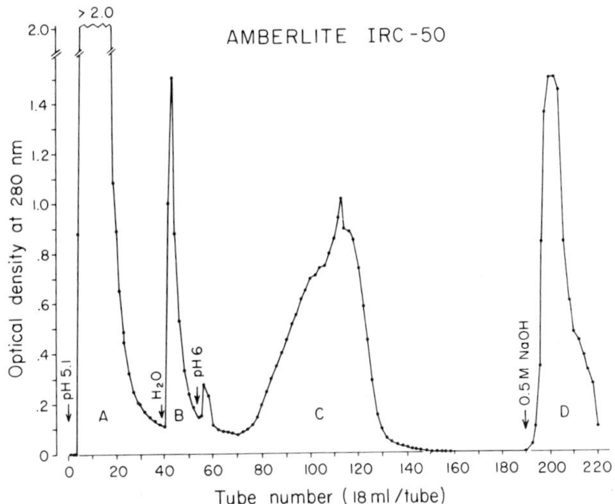

FIG 2. Ion-exchange chromatography of materials from snapping turtle on Amberlite IRC-50. The methods were those described for the preparation of various growth hormones (19,20). 2 g of the 0.6 SAS fraction was loaded and the elution medium was changed at points indicated by arrows to give the four fractions A-D. Only A and C contained appreciable gonadotropic activity.

appreciable activity in any assay; however, these two fractions showed profoundly different biological profiles (Tables 2 and 3), IRC-C fraction showing significant activity in the *in vitro* ovulation test, and IRC-A showing activity in the *Anolis* lizard assay. With the turtle, there was some overlap of this latter activity in the IRC-C fraction. Both IRC fractions were active to different extents in the spermiation and chick assays.

The glycoprotein in the IRC-A fraction was immediately extracted with 10 % ammonium acetate-40 % ethanol at pH 5.1 (21); this effectively extracted all gonadotropic activity and increased its potency by several-fold. Since by our experience growth hormone (GH) yield was found to be reduced by the above

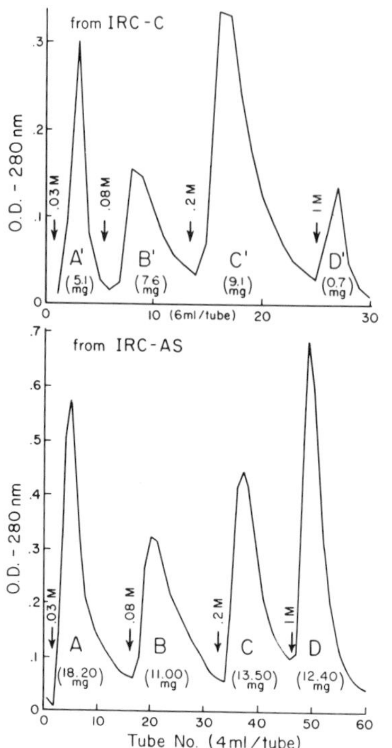

FIG 3. Ion exchange chromatography of bull-frog gonadotropins on DEAE cellulose. Upper : chromatography of the pH 6 eluate from IRC-50 (30 g), and Lower : chromatography of the glycoprotein extract from the unadsorbed IRC-A fraction (55 g). The yield of each fraction is indicated in parentheses.

treatment, this step was avoided for the IRC-C fraction which was known to contain GH.

These results indicate that the turtle and frog possess two qualitatively distinct types of gonadotropins which are largely separated on the Amberlite IRC-50 column. The existence of separate molecular principles was further confirmed by chromatography of the IRC fractions on DEAE-cellulose using stepwise increase in the molarity of the elution buffer (materials were applied in 0.03 M NH_4HCO_3 buffer, pH 6.0) (Fig 3). The four fractions derived from IRC-A and IRC-C glycoprotein fractions were designated DEAE-A, B, C & D and DEAE A'-D' respectively (when using a two-step system, the B', C' and D' fractions were combined and called B'). Bioassay demonstrated that the unadsorbed 0.03 M eluate from DEAE (i.e., DEAE-A or A') was the most potent in ovulation test. Virtually all the gonadotropic activity as measured by the Anolis assay, was contained in the 0.08 M eluate (DEAE-B) in the case of turtle, and in the 0.2 M eluate (DEAE-C) in the case of bull-frog. Thus, almost all residual overlap in activities in the two specific assays that was present in IRC fractions is removed by chromatography on DEAE. At this stage of purification, there is generally less than 1 % cross-contamination between the two types of activity. Although several fractions showed activity in the chick ^{32}P-uptake and the frog spermiation tests, even these indicate a qualitative separation of activities (Table 2 & 3). Total recovery of the two major activities was generally good (~ 50 %).

It is interesting to relate these two distinct pituitary gonadotropins obtained by the above method to the better known FSH and LH of mammals. Thus, on the basis of biological profiles in the four assays, the material derived from IRC-A and DEAE-B, C would resemble FSH, while the IRC-C and DEAE-A' can be compared to mammalian LH. Fig 4 summarizes the distribution of these two activities in turtle and frog pituitaries

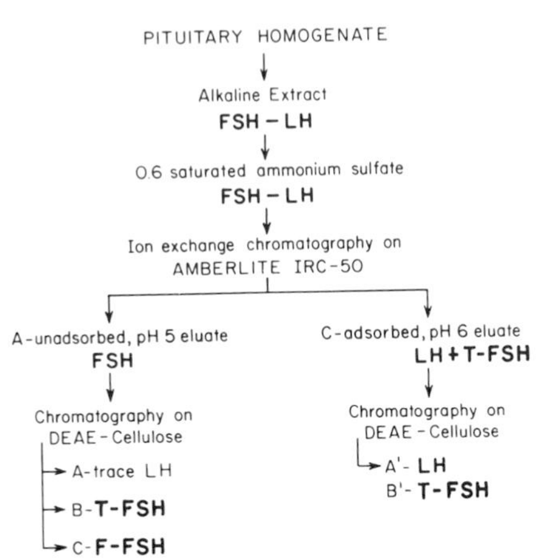

FIG 4. Fractionation of the two types of gonadotropic activity from turtle (T), and bull-frog (B) pituitaries. The major steps of the fractionation scheme are depicted in Fig 1.

in our chemical fractionation scheme and this closely parallels that of the mammalian hormones with comparable activities. Studies with ovine, porcine and marsupial (kangaroo) hormones (4) indicate that virtually all LH is adsorbed on Amberlite IRC-50 (in IRC-C) and unadsorbed on DEAE-cellulose. The FSH is largely unadsorbed on IRC and is then recovered in the 0.2 M eluate from DEAE-cellulose. Thus, a clear homology in biological and chemical behaviour is evident among the reptilian, amphibian and mammalian hormones, and for heuristic purposes we termed the non-mammalian hormones FSH and LH at this stage of our studies. Additional evidence for chemical homologies between the hormones, at least for LH's, is also suggested by further chemical and immunological studies.

C. Further purification and characterization of turtle LH

The LH obtained from the unadsorbed fraction from DEAE-cellulose (i.e., DEAE-A') was further purified by chromatography on sulfoethyl-Sephadex G-50; like mammalian LH, it was adsorbed in 0.03 M NH_4HCO_3 and eluted with 1 M buffer. This eluate was filtered through Sephadex G-100 to obtain the final material. The potency of this material in frog ovulation assay was about 50 times that of initial crude alkaline extract or about five times that of the DEAE-A' fraction from which it was derived (Table 2). However, some TSH activity was still detectable in this LH.

Amino acid analysis of this turtle-LH (T-LH) revealed a marked similarity to ovine LH and a lesser degree of overlap with bovine TSH (Table 4). In general, the turtle hormone shows the high half-cystine value characteristic of mammalian glycoproteins. The difference in proline values of o- and T-LH indicates that this unusually high proline content is characteristic of oLH; turtle LH would more closely resemble human, porcine or rat LH in proline content. Phenylalanine was the major N-terminal group; leucine and glycine in approximately equal but lesser amounts were also found (Table 5); the latter contrasts with the N-terminal analysis for oLH.

The observation that T-LH exhibited a marked decrease in sedimentation coefficient ($S_{20,w}$) when made highly acidic

Table 4. Amino acid composition of turtle LH compared with ovine LH and bovine TSH

Amino acid	Ovine LH *	Turtle LH **	Bovine TSH*
Lysine	12	15	19
Histidine	6	5	6
Arginine	11	9	7
Aspartic	11	17	15
Threonine	16	18	20
Serine	14	14	11
Glutamic	14	16	15
Proline	27	15	14
Glycine	11	14	9
Alanine	15	15	12
1/2 Cystine	22	19	22
Valine	13	13	11
Methionine	7	5	9
Isoleucine	7	9	8
Leucine	14	11	6
Tyrosine	7	13	16
Phenylalanine	8	9	9

*Calculated from structure analysis; Ovine LH - 214 residues;
**Amino acid analysis; 20 hr hydrolysis; uncorrected for hydrolytic destruction; calculated on the basis of 215 residues per mole and rounded to the nearest integer.

(Table 5) as observed for oLH (22), suggests that T-LH may have a subunit nature comparable to the α and β components of mammalian LH. Furthermore, the resemblance in $S_{20,w}$ values between turtle and ovine hormones at both pH's used suggests a similarity in the molecular weights of the subunits in the LH of the two species.

Table 5. Sedimentation properties and N-terminal groups of turtle LH

	Turtle	Sheep
Sedimentation coefficient ($S_{20,w}$)		
pH 7.5	2.76	2.55
pH 1.3	1.78	1.76
N-terminal groups (Dansyl)	Phenylalanine	Phenylalanine (α)
	Leucine Glycine	Serine (β)
	Threonine, Alanine, Aspartic, Serine } traces	

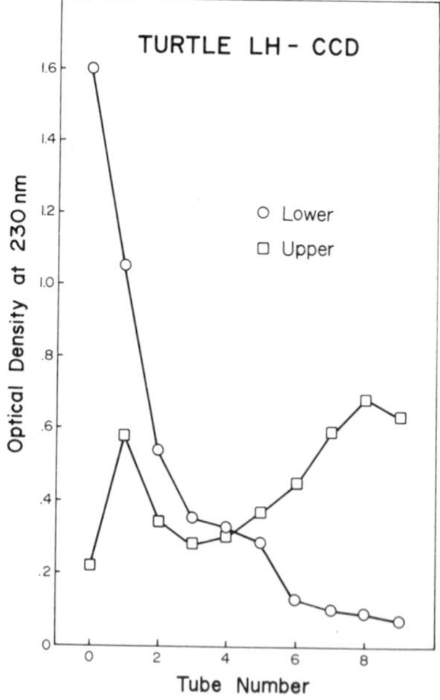

FIG 5. Counter-current distribution pattern for LH from the snapping turtle in a solvent system consisting of 40 % $(NH_4)_2SO_4$: 0.2 % dichloroacetic acid : n-propanol : ethanol (60:60:27:33).

Application of counter-current distribution technique used for the dissociation and isolation of ovine LH subunits (23) to the turtle LH (Fig 5) again yielded results similar to those obtained with the ovine molecule, the α -subunit appearing in the lower phase and the β -subunit in the upper, organic phase.

A preliminary biological test gave additional evidence for the presence of homology in the subunit composition between turtle and ovine LH. Ovine LH-β was mixed with T-LH in acidic medium under conditions that would lead to dissociation of the latter if it were composed of subunits. Both of the materials, alone, were relatively inactive in the Parlow OAAD test for LH; but following neutralization and incubation, the solution showed a significant enhancement of bioactivity. The potency of the mixture was at least four times greater than that of either component alone. We interpret these results as an evidence for the T-LH possessing a subunit that is closely similar to oLH-α , which on combination with the oLH-β leads to subsequent reconstitution of activity.

D. Immunological relatedness of LH from different species

Additional evidence for chemical homologies among the LH molecules of reptiles, birds and mammals was derived from immunological studies done in collaboration with Drs. Brian Follett and Bruce Goldman. The antisera used in these studies were prepared in rabbits against (i) oLH (prepared by Niswender); (ii) bLH-β subunit (prepared by Goldman); (iii) chicken-LH (2); and (iv) a mixture of the two snapping turtle gonadotropins. Biological tests done in our laboratory confirmed that immunologic cross-reaction exists between heterologous hormones. The antiserum to snapping turtle gonadotropin was able to inactivate LH from other species of turtles and alligators, but not the mammalian LH. The avian LH antisera and mammalian LH-β antisera also blocked the activity of turtle and alligator LH. When the T-LH was tested by radioimmunoassay with the chicken and the two mammalian LH antisera, reasonably high cross-reactions with parallel slopes were observed (24). In both cases, however, the antisera also cross-reacted with some fractions from the turtle that lacked LH activity, indicating that their specificity is not confined only to the biologically active T-LH.

E. Phylogenetic survey of reptilian gonadotropins

The results of the above study thus, suggest that the separation of the FSH- and LH-like molecules probably occurred early in the evolution of tetrapods, certainly by the time Reptilia came into existence. However, further comparative investigations into representatives of other families of turtles, and especially the other two orders of reptiles - Crocodilia and Squamata - indicate that considerable restraint must be exercised in generalizing from the results of a few species. Pronounced diversity is apparent in the chemistry of the gonadotropins among extant reptiles.

When pituitaries from diverse sources before and after neuraminidase-treatment were tested for their activity in the Anolis assay (presumably) reflecting FSH activities) it was found that sialic acid was important for the biological activity of gonadotropins from some mammals, birds, reptiles (lizards and snakes), amphibia and fish (12). Noteworthy exceptions were the chelonian reptiles and a few amphibia (newts). Tests with representatives from three families of turtle suggested that the FSH in these reptiles was insensitive to neuraminidase (either sialic acid was lacking or not important for biological activity). However, subsequent studies in our laboratory have shown that this generalization was premature since most families of turtles, including the most primitive members of both chelonian suborders are dependent on sialic acid; i.e., desialylation causes marked reduction in the gonadotropic potency of the pituitary. The three families that were initially studied belong to a single modern family assemblage (Superfamily Testudinoidea). Thus, the loss of sialic acid dependence has apparently occurred rather recently in the evolution of the turtle FSH and independently among some amphibia.

A more important divergence in the chemistry of gonadotropins is evident in the nature of the LH activity (14). Using the frog ovulation test, it is possible to demonstrate that all groups of living turtles possess LH activity; pituitary concentrations are relatively uniform. Studies with two crocodilians (Caiman and Alligator) also indicate a comparably high level of this LH in this reptilian order. In marked contrast, we have been unable to detect any activity in the pituitaries of snakes or lizards, using dosages up to 1500 times those required to detect activity in chelonians and crocodilians. Consistent with these findings are immunological measurements with antisera to chicken and mammalian LH which indicate only trace amounts of reactive material in lizard and snake glands (24, Licht, P., Follett, B. K., Goldman, B. and Papkoff, H - unpublished data) Since these antisera are not specific for T-LH (see above) it is not clear whether even these low levels of reaction are due to an LH in snakes. Thus, there appears to have been a major divergence between Squamata and other reptiles with regard to LH structure or concentration. The possibility exists that squamate reptiles lack the gonadotropin that is homologous to the LHs of the other tetrapods; this conclusion would be consistent with earlier physiological studies indicating that FSH acts as a complete gonadotropin in snakes and lizards.

In addition to the apparent lack of LH activity, the gonadotropic activity in the snakes shows a different chromatographic behaviour from both FSH and LH of other vertebrates. Studies in progress on alligators, indicate that the FSH- and LH-like activities in them behave on fractionation similar to that of the turtle and mammalian hormones (Farmer, Licht and Papkoff - unpublished data). However, in the case of the rattlesnake (Crotalus atrox), all of the gonadotropic activity (which can only be measured by Anolis assay) is adsorbed on IRC-50 Amberlite (eluted with pH 6.0 buffer), also subsequently on DEAE-cellulose. Thus, it behaves like LH on Amberlite IRC-50 and like FSH on DEAE-cellulose (Farmer, Licht and Papkoff - unpublished data).

A broad comparative approach is clearly required before the nature of non-mammalian gonadotropins and the evolution of gonadotropin chemistry and physiology can be elucidated. In this regard, it is important to consider the long evolutionary history of many of the lower vertebrate orders and attention must be given to possible major divergence within each order. Any generalization based on a few species would be premature.

ACKNOWLEDGEMENTS

Work described herein was supported in part by grant GB-35241X from the National Science Foundation. Harold Papkoff is a career development awardee of the NIH and Paul Licht is a Miller Professor. Dr. Susan Farmer assisted in several aspects of the chemical fractionation studies.

REFERENCES

1. Stockell Hartree A. and Cunningham, F.J. (1969). J. Endocrinol. 43, 609.
2. Follett, B.K., Scanes, C.G. and Cunningham, F.J. (1972). J. Endocrinol. 52, 359.
3. Wentworth, B.C. (1971). Biol. Reprod. 5, 107.
4. Farmer, S.W. and Papkoff, H. (1973). Endocrine Soc. Mts. Abstract 334, Chicago, Ill.
5. Burzawa-Gerard, E. and Fontaine, Y.A. (1972). Gen. Comp. Endocrinol. Suppl. 3, 715.
6. Donaldson, E.M., Yamazaki, F., Dye, H.M. and Philleo, W.W. (1973). Gen. Comp. Endocrinol. 18, 469.
7. Licht, P. (1972). Gen. Comp. Endocrinol. 19, 273.
8. Licht, P. (1972). Gen. Comp. Endocrinol. 19, 282.
9. Licht, P. and Papkoff, H. (1974). Gen. Comp. Endocrinol. (in press).
10. Licht, P. and Papkoff, H. (1974). Endocrinology (in press).
11. Licht, P. and Pearson, A.K. (1969). Gen. Comp. Endocrinol. 13, 367.
12. Licht, P. and Papkoff, H. (1972). Gen. Comp. Endocrinol. 19, 102.
13. Licht, P. and Papkoff, H. (1973). Gen. Comp. Endocrinol. 20, 172.
14. Licht, P. (1974). Gen. Comp. Endocrinol. (in press).
15. Licht, P. (1973). Gen. Comp. Endocrinol. 20, 522.
16. Licht, P. (1973). Gen. Comp. Endocrinol. 20, 592.
17. Breneman, W.R. (1973). Gen. Comp. Endocrinol. 20, 41.
18. Papkoff, H. and Licht, P. (1972). Proc. Soc. Exptl. Biol. Med. 139, 372.

19. Papkoff, H. and Li, C.H. (1958). J. Biol. Chem. 231, 367.
20. Papkoff, H., Li, C.H. and Liu, W.K. (1962). Arch. Biochem. Biophys. 120, 434.
21. Stockell Hartree, A. (1966). Biochem. J. 100, 754.
22. Li, C.H. and Starman, B. (1964). Nature 202, 291.
23. Papkoff, H. and Samy, T.S.A. (1967). Biochem. Biophys. Acta. 147, 175.
24. Scanes, C.G., Follett, B.K. and Goos. H.J.Th. (1972). Gen. Comp. Endocrinol. 19, 596.

SOME ASPECTS OF CHEMISTRY AND BIOLOGY OF PISCINE GONADOTROPINS

B.I. Sundararaj and T.S.A. Samy

INTRODUCTION

While remarkable progress has been made in unravelling the chemical structure of mammalian gonadotropins, there is paucity of data on the chemical nature of gonadotropins in submammalian vertebrates; however, limited progress has been made on the chemistry of piscine pituitary gonadotropins. Extraction and purification of gonadotropins have been attempted with varying degrees of success in teleost fishes such as the Pacific salmon (1-5), dffferent species of carp (6-12), the mudfish (13), the Whitefish, Coregonus lavaretus and the roach, Gardonus sp. (14). Gonadotropins from pituitaries of an elasmobranch fish, Scyliorhinus canicula (15) and from the African lungfish, Protopterus annectens (16) have been partially purified.

The purification of gonadotropins from fishes has posed many problems, the primary one being the assay of their activity. Since they are inactive in the mammalian systems, lower vertebrates have to be used for their bioassay. The methods used by various investigators for assaying piscine gonadotropins are as follows: spermiation assay in frog (17) and goldfish (19); gonadal hydration test in the goldfish (7); uptake of ^{32}P in the testes of the eel (18); ovulation assay in carps (9, 10) and catfish (21); adenyl cyclase activity in the goldfish ovary (20) and augmentation of ^{32}P uptake in day-old chick testes (5);

CATFISH GONADOTROPIN

Ammonium sulphate at 50 % saturation is known to precipitate mammalian LH, while full saturation is required for precipitating FSH (22-25). We have used this procedure to isolate the pituitary gonadotropins of the catfish, Heteropneustes follilis. Pituitaries collected from decapitated catfish of either sex during the pre-spawning (May-June) and the spawning periods (July-August) were stored in ice-cold acetone at -10°, and later acetone-dried powder was prepared from these. It was then homogenized with

0.9 % saline in a glass homogenizer and stirred for 2 hr at 4°. Various fractions obtained by precipitation at different saturations of $(NH_4)_2 SO_4$ were either dissolved or suspended in water, dialyzed against the same and lyophilized. The fractions were bioassayed using intact female gravid catfish as described previously (21,26). The flow-sheet of the purification method used is depicted in Fig 1. The saline extract was adjusted to 30 % saturation of ammonium sulphate and the biological activity was detected only in the precipitate. The residue was extracted with 0.1M sodium phosphate-saline (0.9 % NaCl) buffer, pH 7.5 and the extract was adjusted to 50 % saturation of ammonium sulphate; the resulting precipitate (fraction D) was considerably more active than the starting material (A). Further increase in ammonium sulphate saturation did not yield any active fractions. Fraction D was subjected to chromatography on Sephadex G-200 and eluted with 0.01 M ammonium acetate, pH 9.0. Three fractions were obtained: fractions I and III were inactive, and fraction II had low biological activity.

Table 1 and Figure 2 show the yields and biological activities of the various fractions obtained. Fraction D, the yield of which was 14.2 % was highly active even at a dose of 10 µg (4.26 µg protein); fraction A, on the other hand, had very little activity even at 100 µg (34 µg protein) level. Approximately, fraction-D is at least five times more potent than the starting material.

Of the three fractions obtained by chromatography of fraction D on Sephadex G-200, only the second fraction had low biological activity in the ovulation assay and the yield was around 54 %. This loss of biological activity of the gonadotropin following chromatography on Sephadex G-200 is puzzling. Similar loss of activity has been reported by other investigators also, following chromatography on Sephadex G-25 (5).

The above data show that the catfish pituitary gonadotropin resembles mammalian LH more closely than FSH in its solubility property in ammonium sulphate solution as well as in its ability to induce ovulation in the catfish. This is in contrast to turtle gonadotropin which behaves like mammalian LH in its solubility properties but resembles mammalian FSH in its biological activity. (27).

We have used only this ovulation bioassay to test the biological activity of the various catfish pituitary fractions. It is, however, necessary to test the biological activity of all the fractions in other

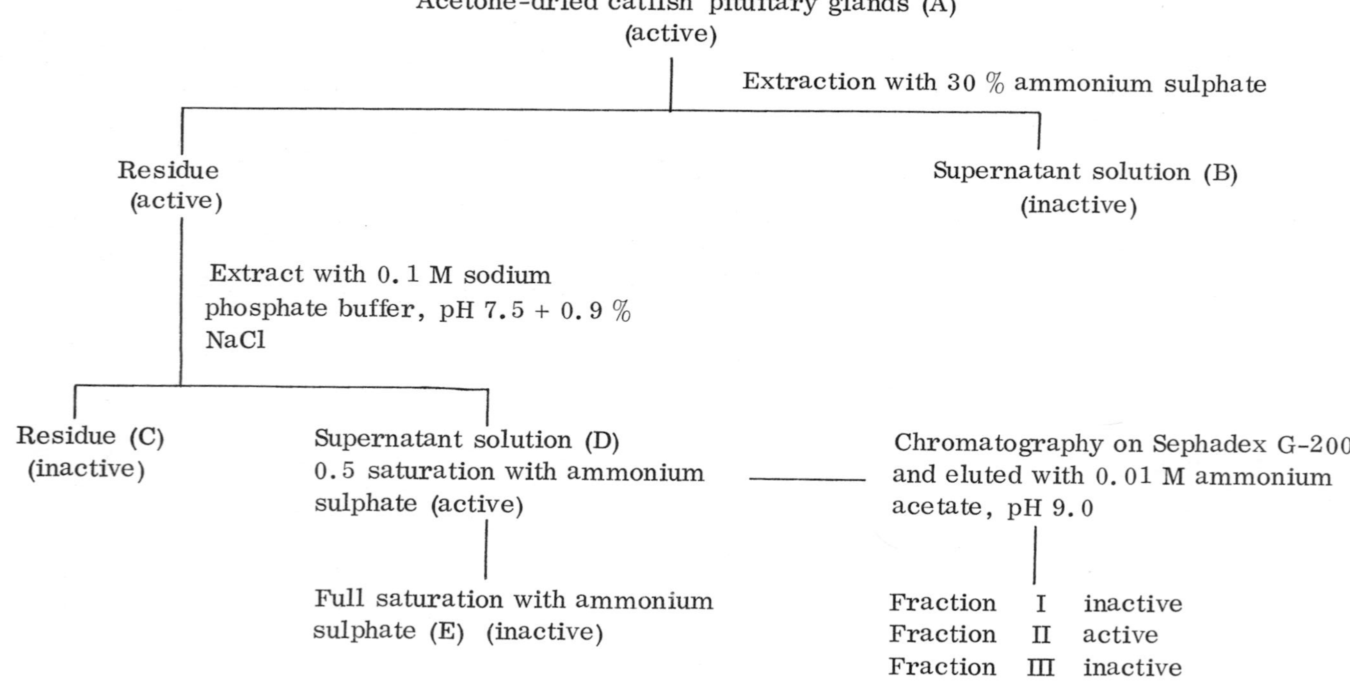

FIG 1. Procedure for isolation of an active gonadotropic material from the pituitary glands of the catfish, <u>Heteropneustes fossilis.</u>

Table 1. Yields and biological activities of gonadotropin fractions of catfish, *Heteropneustes fossilis.*

	Fraction	Yield (mg)	Protein (mg)	Biological activity
A	Starting material (acetone-dried fish pituitaries)	300.0	102.0	+
B	30 % ammonium sulphate extract	3.7	0.9	-
C	0.1 M sodium phosphate containing 0.9 % NaCl, pH 7.5 extract of 30 % ammonium sulphate	74.0	44.5	-
D	Ammonium sulphate 0.5 saturation	34.0	14.5*	+
E	Full ammonium sulphate 1.0 saturation	2.8	1.2	-

* Highly active fraction; yield is about 14.2 % of the starting material.

bioassay systems notably, the stimulation of spermatogenesis in the lizard (28), before drawing any conclusion regarding the presence or absence of FSH avtivity in the fractions.

According to Licht and Papkoff (28), salmon gonadotropin (SG-G100) is largely inactivated by desialylation when tested in lizard testis bioassay, thus resembling mammalian FSH. Nevertheless, our studies on the catfish gonadotropin show that it resembles mammalian LH rather than FSH. Thus, interspecific variations within Pisces may exist as in Amphibia and Reptila (28). The effect of neuraminidase treatment on the biological activity of catfish gonadotropin would throw light on its chemical nature.

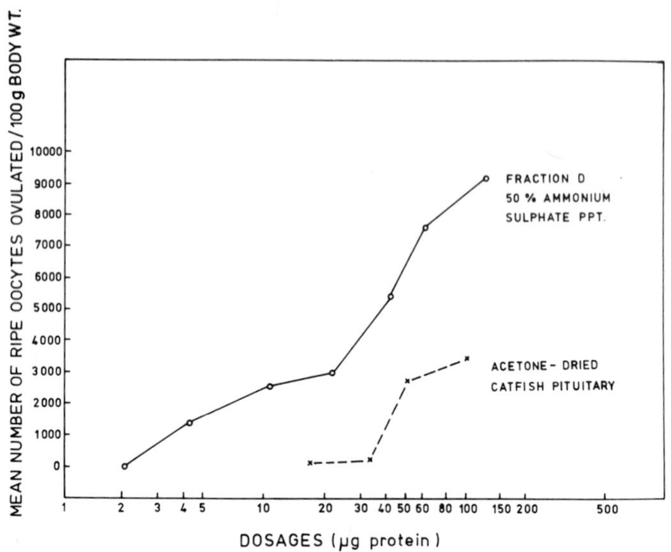

FIG 2. Log-dose-response curves for number of ripe eggs ovulated by the intact gravid catfish after a single injection of fraction D (50 % ammonium sulphate precipitate) and acetone-dried catfish pituitary powder.

BIOLOGICAL ACTIONS OF PISCINE GONADOTROPINS

The biological activities of carp-gonadotropin (c-GTH)and salmon gonadotropin (s-GTH) & (SG-G100) and (SG-DEAE-3) have been extensively investigated not only in the teleost fish but also in other lower vertebrates such as amphibians, reptiles and even birds.

A. In teleost fishes

Goldfish, *Carassius auratus*, has been used as a recipient for both c-GTH and s-GTH. In the hypophysectomized goldfish, c-GTH at a dose level of 1 µg/g body weight not only restores spermatogenesis and spermiation in the male (29) but also restores vitellogenesis in the female (12). s-GTH (SG-G100) similarly is effective in inducing spermatogenesis (9 injections of 10 μg/g body weight) and spermiation (3 μg/g body weight) in the hypophysectomized male goldfish as well as in inducing vitellogenesis (9 injections of 50 μg/g body weight) and ovulation (30 μg/g body weight) in the hypophysectomized female goldfish (19,30). Goldfish being a carp, it obviously needs a higher dosage of s-GTH than c-GTH to bring about an equivalent response. Fontaine et al. (31) have interestingly shown that c-GTH is 36 times more potent than s-GTH in stimulating adenyl cyclase activity in homogenates of ovaries from the goldfish. This suggests the existence of partial biological specificity of teleost gonadotropin.

In the catfish, *Heteropneustes fossilis*, both s-GTH and carp pituitary Sephadex G-100 fractions have been tested for biological activity. s-GTH (SG-G100) induces spermatogenesis in the hypophysectomized catfish even at a daily dose level of 33 ng/g body weight for 30 days. Further, the seminal vesicles which are androgen-sensitive also become secretory. A single dose of s-GTH (30 ng/g body weight) induces spermiation (32). In the female hypophysectomized catfish, s-GTH induces vitellogenesis (2-5 μg/g body weight/day for 23 days), maintains the gravid ovaries (15 - 75 ng/g body weight/day for 20 days) and also induces ovulation (1 - 1.5 μg/g body weight) (26). Thus s-GTH acts as a complete gonadotropin in the catfish. Puntius carp pituitary Sephadex G-100 fraction II induces vitellogenesis in the female hypophysectomized catfish (1.8 - 7 μg/g body weight/day for 23 days), maintains gravid ovaries (2 - 10 ng/g body weight/day for 20 days) and also induces ovulation (1.5 - 2 μg/g body weight). All the reproductive processes in the hypophysectomized female catfish can be initiated and/or maintained by the puntius carp pituitary Sephadex G-100 fraction II. The first and third fractions have no gonadotropic activity at the dose levels tested (33). Between s-GTH and puntius carp pituitary fraction II, the latter even though chromatographed only once, is more effective than the former. Since phylogenetically, catfish and carps belong to the same order (Cypriniformes) it is not surprising that they respond to carp pituitary fraction better than salmon gonadotropin.

SG-G100 also induces vitellogenesis and sexual behaviour in the female guppy, Poecilia reticulata (34). Funk and Donaldson (35) have reported that in the juvenile male pink salmon, *Oncorhynchus gorbuscha*, complete sexual maturation is attained by September of the year of hatching with thrice-weekly treatments of

1 and 10 µg of SG-G100 per 100 g body weight. As mentioned earlier, partially-purified catfish gonadotropin has so far been tested only on ovulation, its effects on spermatogenesis and vitellogenesis have yet to be examined.

B. In other vertebrates

There is paucity of data on the action of piscine gonadotropins in higher vertebrates. c-GTH is active in inducing spermiation in the frog (17) and a rapid swelling of the testes tissue in larval toad, *Alytes obstetricans* (18). Extracts of pituitary glands from a few teleost fishes stimulate spermiation and ovulation in frogs (36).

Licht and Donaldson (37) reported that salmon gonadotropin (SG-100) in doses of 100 or 200 µg/day maintained the normally enlarged testes, spermatogenic activity and enlarged accessory sexual structures in surgically hypophysectomized lizard, *Anolis carolinensis*. Administration of 100 µg of SG-G100 on alternate days for 15 or 29 days promoted testicular growth and spermatogenesis in lizards with regressed gonads. SG-DEAE-3 was five times more potent than SG-G100. Fish gonadotropin is not effective beyond reptilia and the latter may have receptors capable of recognizing both piscine and mammalian gonadotropins. SG-G100, however, has been reported to have an effect on the uptake of radioactive phosphorous into the testes of day-old chicks (5).

Piscine gonadotropic preparations, with the exception of lungfish GTH, are inactive in mammals (12). Saline extracts of the pituitary of the African lungfish, *Protopterus annectens*, has been shown to give a positive response only in the Steelman-Pohley assay (16).

C. Heterotropic activity of piscine gonadotropin

Another little understood biological activity of piscine gonadotropin is its heterotropic action on the adrenal cortical tissue. In the hypophysectomized gravid catfish, *H. fossilis*, maturation and ovulation are not only induced by ovine LH, hCG, and SG-G100 but also by corticosteroids notably 11-deoxy-corticosterone (DOC) and cortisol (compound F) (38). Further, DOC, compound F and 11-deoxycortisol are very potent ovulating agents of catfish oocytes *in vitro*, whereas LH and SG-G100 have only a marginal effect (39, 40 and Goswami and Sundararaj - unpublished results). That gonadotropin, be it LH or SG-G100, stimulates the adrenal is shown by the fact that co-culture of catfish oocytes and adrenal cortical tissue in the presence of LH or SG-G100 produces a maturation response significantly greater than that obtained in the absence of either adrenal cortical tissue or LH or SG-G100 (Goswami, Sundararaj & Donaldson - unpublished results; Sundararaj and Goswami - unpublished results). These results suggest that piscine gonadotropin has not only a gonadotropic effect but also an 'adrenocorticotropic effect'. SG-G100 also activates the catfish thyroid (Sundararaj - unpublished results). This is comparable to the stimulation of teleost thyroid by mammalian gonadotropins (41). These heterotropic actions noticed in the catfish could be due to contamination with other pituitary hormones. But this seems unlikely inasmuch as the heterotropic actions of SG-G100 are shared by ovine LH. Thus, receptors which are able to recognize piscine gonadotropin or ovine LH must be present not only in the gonad but also in the adrenal cortical tissue. The specificity of receptors to gonadotropin in the adrenal cortical tissue may vary with changes in the sexual cycle and the titers of gonadal hormones.

CONCLUSION

In teleost fishes, the evidence accumulated hitherto by investigations in a few species supports, at least tentatively, that all testicular and ovarian functions are regulated by a single gonadotropin (5, 6, 8, 18, 19, 26, 29, 30, 32, 33). But interspecific variations in the chemical nature of the gonadotropic hormones may be more prevalent than hitherto suspected. Nevertheless, generalizations may have to wait until investigations covering more teleost species have been completed.

ACKNOWLEDGEMENT

Supported in part by grants M69.91 from the Population Council, Rockefeller University, New York, U.S.A, and GF-34379 from the National Science Foundation, Washington, D.C., U.S.A., to B.I. Sundaraj, and grants from the Ministry of Health & Family Planning, Govt. of India, and the Ford Foundation to N.R. Moudgal.

REFERENCES

1. Otsuka, S. (1956). Endocr. Jap. 3, 272.
2. Robertson, O.H. and Rinfret, A.P. (1957). Endocrinology 60, 559.
3. Schmidt, P.J., Mitchell, B.S., Smith, M. and Tsuyuki, H. (1965). Gen. Comp. Endocrinol. 5, 197.
4. Gronlund, W. (1969). M.Sc., Thesis, Univ. of Washington, Seattle.
5. Donaldson, E.M., Yamazaki, F., Dye, H.M. and Philleo, W.W. (1972). Gen. Comp. Endocrinol. 18, 469.
6. Fontaine, Y.A. and Gérard, E. (1963). C. R. Acad. Sci. 256, 5634.
7. Clemens, H.P. and Grant, F.B. (1964). Zoologica 49, 193.
8. Burzawa-Gérard, E. and Fontaine, Y.A. (1966). Ann. Endocrinol. 27, 305.
9. Sinha, V.R.P. (1969). J. Chromat. 44, 624.
10. Sinha, V.R.P. (1971). J. Fish. Biol. 3, 263.
11. Burzawa-Gérard, E. (1971). Biochimie 53, 545.
12. Burzawa-Gérard, E. and Fontaine, Y.A. (1972). Gen. Comp. Endocrinol. Suppl. 3, 715.
13. Hattingh, J. and Du Toit, P.J. (1973). J. Fish. Biol. 5, 41.
14. Breton, B. (1968). Ph.D. Thesis, Universite de Lyon.
15. Scanes, C.G., Dobson, S., Follett, B.K. and Dodd, J.M. (1972). J. Endocrinol. 54, 343.
16. Burzawa-Gérard, E. (1969). Colloq. Int. Cent. Nat. Rech. Sci. 177, 351.
17. Fontaine, M. and Chauvel, M. (1961). C.R. Acad. Sci. 257, 822.
18. Burzawa-Gérard, E. and Fontaine, Y.A. (1965). Gen. Comp. Endocrinol. 5, 87.
19. Yamazaki, F. and Donaldson, E.M. (1968). Gen. Comp. Endocrinol. 10, 383.
20. Fontaine, Y.A., Burzawa-Gérard, E. and Delerue-Lebelle,N. (1970). C.R. Acad Sci. 271, 780.
21. Sundararaj, B.I. and Anand, T.C. (1972). Gen. Comp. Endocrinol. Suppl. 3, 688.
22. Li, C.H. (1949). Vitamins and Hormones 7, 223.
23. Papkoff, H. (1969). In "Reproduction in Domestic Animals" H.H. Cole and P.T. Cupps (Eds). p 67, Academic Press, New York.

24. Papkoff, H., Gospodarowicz, D., Candiotti, A. and Li, C.H. (1965). Arch. Biochem. Biophys. 111, 431.
25. Papkoff, H., Gospodarowicz, D. and Li, C.H. (1967). Arch. Biochem. Biophys. 120, 434.
26. Sundararaj, B.I., Anand, T.C., and Donaldson, E.M. (1972) Gen. Comp. Endocrinol. 18, 102.
27. Papkoff, H. and Licht, P. (1972). Proc. Soc. Exp. Biol. Med. 139, 372.
28. Licht, P. and Papkoff, H. (1972). Gen. Comp. Endocrinol. 19, 102.
29. Billard, R., Burzawa-Gérard, E. and Breton, B. (1970). C.R. Acad. Sci. 271, 1896.
30. Yamazaki, F. and Donaldson, E.M. (1968). Gen. Comp. Endocrinol. 11, 292.
31. Fontaine, Y.A., Salmon, C., Fontaine-Bertrand, E., Burzawa-Gérard, E. and Donaldson, E.M. (1972). Can. J. Zool. 50, 1673.
32. Sundararaj, B.I., Nayyar, S.K., Anand, T.C., and Donaldson, E.M. (1971). Gen. Comp. Endocrinol. 17, 73.
33. Sundararaj, B.I., Anand, T.C. and Sinha, V.R.P. (1972). J. Endocrinol. 54, 87.
34. Liley, N.R. and Donaldson, E.M. (1969). Can. J. Zool. 47, 569.
35. Funk, J.D. and Donaldson, E.M. (1972). Can. J. Zool. 50, 1413.
36. Pickford, G.E. and Atz, J.W. (1957). "The Physiology of the Pituitary Gland of Fishes", New York Zoological Society, New York.
37. Licht, P. and Donaldson, E.M. (1969). Biol. Reprod. 1, 307.
38. Sundararaj, B.I. and Goswami, S.V. (1966). J. Exp. Zool. 161, 287.
39. Goswami, S.V. and Sundararaj, B.I. (1971). J. Exp. Zool. 178, 467.
40. Sundararaj, B.I., Goswami, S.V. and Donaldson, E.M. (1972). J. Fish. Res. Bd. Canada 29, 435.
41. Fontaine, Y.A. (1969). Gen. Comp. Endocrinol. Suppl. 2, 417.

STUDIES ON HYPOTHALAMIC GONADOTROPIN-RELEASING FACTORS

Raghavan M.G. Nair and John A. Colwell

INTRODUCTION

Neurohumoral substances from the hypothalamus enter and travel through the hypophyseal portal circulation, reach the anterior pituitary gland, and control its vital secretory processes (1-4). It is now well established that secretion of the gonadotropins, LH and FSH, is controlled by neurohumoral substances designated LH/FSH-releasing factor(s) or hormone(s) (5-8). Attempts to isolate these hypothalamic hormones reached fruition when Schally et al. (9) reported obtaining homogeneous LRF from 165,000 porcine hypothalami. This material stimulated the release of LH and FSH *in vivo* and *in vitro* in doses of a few nanograms and was found to be a polypeptide with an amino acid composition (determined by acid hydrolysis) His 1, Arg 1, Ser 1, Glu 1, Pro 1, Gly 2, Leu 1, Tyr 1. Amoss et al. (10) reported the same amino acid composition for the ovine hormone. However, determination of the constituent amino acids after HCl hydrolysis in the presence of thioglycolic acid (11), indicated a tryptophan moiety also in the peptide hormone (12). Subsequently the complete amino acid sequence of the porcine LRF, Glu-His-Trp-Ser-Tyr-Gly-Leu-Arg-Pro-Gly-NH_2, has been determined by the use of the combined Edman-dansyl procedure coupled with the selective tritiation method for C-terminal analysis, and mass spectral fragmentation after derivatization (12). Their decapeptide was then synthesized (13), and the pure synthetic and native hormone preparations were found to be similar in chromatographic and electrophoretic mobilities and other physical and chemical properties. Both preparations released LH and FSH, *in vivo* and *in vitro* at nanogram levels similar to porcine LRF. The primary structure of oLRF was determined to be the same as that of porcine (14). This structure was determined by analysis of two aliquots of 200 nano moles LRF each, using hydrolysis of the peptide with chymotrypsin or pyrrolidone carboxylyl peptidase followed by Edman-^{14}C-dansylation and mass spectrometry. The structure was confirmed by a total synthesis of LRF by solid-phase methodology and the synthetic product was found identical with the native LRF (15). Many workers (16-20) have reported the syntheses of LRF by both classical and solid-phase methods and these preparations were found to be biologically active.

This presentation provides a description of the isolation and structural degradation of the second batch of LRF and the structure-activity relationships of its various synthetic analogues.

ISOLATION

LRF was isolated from powdered, defatted hypothalami (porcine or bovine), utilizing a modified sequence of operations as given below: 2N acetic acid extraction followed by Sephadex (G-25, fine) filtration, phenol extraction, countercurrent distribution I (CCD I), CM-cellulose chromatography, CCD II, and CCD III.

Batches of 20,000 hypothalami were extracted with 2N acetic acid 5 times at 8°, using about 3 liters of the extracting liquid each time (21). The extracts were centrifuged and lyophilized, and the yield from 240,000 hypothalami (5.3 kg after defatting) was 2 kg. The residue after extraction was inactive in doses up to 500 μg.

The crude lyophilizate was suspended in 1 N acetic acid, centrifuged at 30,000 xg, and a 100 gm equivalent of the extract was subjected to gel filtration on a large column of Sephadex G-25 (fine - 15.5 x 180 cm). The elution pattern was followed by estimating protein by Lowry method (22) or by recording O.D. at 278 nm, and also by assaying for LRF-activity. A pool of large number of fractions showing LRF activity yielded 731 gm of material (Table 1); it was active _in vivo_ in rats, at a dose of 150 μg.

Phenol extraction and chromatographic purification on CM-cellulose were carried out as previously described (21). The crude material obtained after Sephadex filtration, was extracted with 4 liters of redistilled phenol and the active fractions were re-extracted into the aqueous phase by addition of redistilled

Table 1. Purification of LRF by gel filtration

Fraction No.	PEAKS I a	I b	II a	II b	III a	III b	IV a	IV b	V a	V b
500-700 O.D., 1.7	--	--								
750-850 O.D., 0.3			--	--						
850-950 O.D., 0.45					--	10 %				
950-1150 O.D., 1.3							120 IU	60 %		
1350-1750 O.D., 2.0									55 IU	8 %

a = Pressor activity (units); b = LRF activity (%). Gel filtration on a column (15.5 x 180 cm) of Sephadex G-25 (fine), solvent 1 M acetic acid, fraction size 25 ml. Assays were carried out with 50 μg doses/rat, for LRF-activity. Pressor assays were performed by the method of Dekanski (31).

diethylether. The yield at this stage was 179 gm and it showed LRF-activity in doses of 10 μg/rat; the residue was inactive even at doses up to 100 μg.

A. Counter-current distribution (CCD)

An automatic glass apparatus (Spectrum Medical Industries, Los Angeles, CA) consisting of 400 cells, with a 3 ml capacity in the lower phase and up to 5 ml in the upper phase, was used for the final stages of purification. At the early stages, purification was carried out in a macro-unit of 100 cells, with 50 ml capacity in each phase. Modifications were introduced in the automatic robot of the macro-unit, for complete separation and draining of the viscous upper phase (23).

1. Distribution I : The LRF-activity concentrated by the phenol extraction was further purified by CCD in the macro-

unit with 100 cells using the system 0.1 % acetic acid : 1-butanol : pyridine - 11:5:3 (23). Applying the single withdrawal method, and arranging 250 transfers, the LRF-activity was obtained in fractions 130-230. Eventhough a large quantity of the material (179 gm) was applied and distributed equally in the first ten tubes, the mean K-value for the LRF-activity was found to be 2.0, which was identical to the K-value found for LRF, in analytical runs, in the same solvent system. Lysine-vasopressin was found in fractions 60-99 (mean K = 0.76). The yield after this purification was 2.7 gm and significant LRF-activity was shown in doses of 0.2 μg/rat; other fractions were inactive in doses up to 20 μg.

The next step of purification was carried out by ion exchange chromatography on CM-cellulose column (2.8 x 80 cm), as described previously (21). The LRF-activity was located in fractions 190-229 and this on lyophilization yielded 138 mg of material which was active at doses of 5 ng. Fractions 10-35, 50-70 and 95-155 gave peaks at 278 nm, but were inactive in doses 4-15 times larger than those utilized for LRF.

2. Distribution II : The material obtained from above was further purified by CCD in the 400-cell analytical unit using the same solvent system as in distribution I. After 400-transfers, small aliquots of the first 250 cells were analyzed by the Folin-Lowry method. Since no peptide material was revealed in the first 250 cells at this stage, the distribution was continued for an additional 400 transfers, by recycling. The main LRF-activity occured in fractions 600-654 with a mean K value of 2.06 for the partition coefficient, in good agreement with the previous experiments. The yield after lyophilization of the LRF-active fractions was 55.4 mg and it was active *in vivo* at doses of 2 ng.

3. Distribution III : Since the partition coefficient in the previous CCD was 2.06, a different solvent system (1-butanol: acetic acid:water - 4:1:5) in which the K-value for LRF is 0.22 was selected for the next run. Using the 400-cell apparatus, a total of 900 transfers were given and instead of recycling, fresh upper phase solvent was continually introduced by the automatic

filling device, collecting the emerging fractions in the fraction collector. Folin-Lowry analyses of 100 µl aliquots of the upper phase of fractions 400-900 revealed no peptide material, but fractions 215-269 (K = 0.22), 110-150 (K = 0.10), 155-180 (K = 0.13) and 0-40 (K = 0.006) indicated separate peaks. The peptide peak with a K-value of 0.22, was pooled together and lyophylized, to yield 11.5 mg of material which was active in vitro in doses as small as 0.5 ng. This material was found to be homogeneous by thin-layer chromatography (TLC) on cellulose under different solvent systems and also by thin-layer electrophoresis (TLE). The overall recovery of LRF-activity from the 2 N acetic acid extract, after six purification steps was 64 % and the purification factor, through these six steps after the extraction, was about 200,000. The over-all purification of the LRF-activity was about 500,000 times.

ASSAYS

LRF-activity was determined in vivo by stimulation of the release of LH in ovariectomized rats previously treated with estrogen and progesterone (24). The rats (3-5 per group) were anesthetized with 150 mg of urethane per 100 g of body weight given ip. One hour later the samples were injected into the jugular vein in a volume of 0.5 ml of acidified saline (with 0.01 M acetic acid). Twenty minutes after the injection, blood was collected from the abdominal aorta and the serum was assayed for LH (in triplicates) by the double-antibody radioimmunoassay (25); LH concentration was expressed in terms of NIH-LH-S14. The increase of serum LH over the saline control was used as the index of LRF-activity (26).

FSH-RF activity was measured by a specific assay based on stimulation of FSH release in vitro by pituitaries of male rats (27), the FSH released being measured by the method of Steelman and Pohley (28). NIH-FSH-S8 was used as the reference standard and 5-8 rats per group were used. The significance of differences between groups was calculated by the new Duncan's multiple range test (29). In some experiments the FSH released was also measured by radioimmunoassay for FSH (30). The location of the LRF-activity on the chromatograms or CCD curves is based on assays carried out on a large number of fractions with the use of one single dose level of the liquid aliquot. Pressor assays were performed as described by Dekanski (31).

ELUCIDATION OF THE STRUCTURE OF LRF

A. General methodology

Amino acid analyses were performed in an automatic Beckman-Spinco model 120-C analyzer, provided with micro-cuvettes and 1-MV range card. The samples were hydrolyzed in 6 N HCl for 22 hr in evacuated sealed tubes in the presence of 5 % (v/v) thioglycolic acid (11) or using pure p-toluene sulfonic acid, instead of 6 N HCl and also a scavenger-like tryptamine (32). The digestion with chymotrypsin (Armour, Lot XIN-10705) was carried out in 0. 1 M ammonium acetate buffer pH 8.3 at 37° for 22 hr (E:S-ratio = 1:20). After neutralization with glacial acetic acid, the hydrolysate was freeze-dried and the chymotryptic fragments separated by preparative TLC on pre-washed cellulose (33), using the solvent system 1-butanol:acetic acid :water - 4:1:5. The amino acid sequences of the major chymotryptic peptides were determined by Edman-dansyl degradation on a micro-scale (33,34). When arginine was expected during dansylation, 5-10 nmoles of the peptide were dansylated to permit identification by TLC on silica gel. After dansylation the peptides were hydrolyzed at 100° in 6N HCl, in sealed evacuated tubes for 16 hr. When DNS-Pro (DNS=diemthylaminonaphthalenesulfonyl) was expected, the time of hydrolysis was brought down to 3 hr. For DNS-Trp, conditions suggested by Matsubara and Sasaki (7) were utilized. To determine if any free carboxyl group was present in LRF, the hormone was treated with (^{14}C) diazomethane and the resultant radioactivity was measured (35,36). Derivatization reactions, like acetylation and permethylation before and after methanolysis, were carried out according to the methods described previously (34, 37-40). The methods lead to acetylation of -NH_2 groups (-$NH_2 \rightarrow$ -$NHCOCH_3$), methylation of amide nitrogen [$-CONH_2 \rightarrow -CON(CH_3)_2$, $-CONH- \rightarrow -CON-(CH_3)-$] and hydroxyl and carboxylic acid functions ($-OH \rightarrow -OCH_3$, $-COOH \rightarrow -COOCH_3$). Modification of the arginine moiety was effected by mild hydrazinolysis (41-43). Nanomole quantities (50-150 μg) of the arginine-containing peptide was treated with 20 % aqueous hydrazine in a partially evacuated sealed tube at 80-90° for 1 hr, and the excess reagent removed in vacuum. After checking the purity by TLC, the resultant peptide was subjected to lyophilization and further derivatization reactions. (^{14}C) acetic anhydride and (^{14}C) methyl iodide were used for acetylation and permethylation, respectively, and the completion of derivatization was checked by measurement of the resultant radioactivity in a Tricarb liquid scintillation spectrometer.

High and low resolution mass spectra were recorded in an AE1 MS 902 mas spectrometer (MS) equipped with PDP-8 computer and MSDS 11 MS data system. Low resolution spectra were also recorded on a Hitachi-Perkin Elmer RMU-4 instrument. The direct inlet probe was used for the peptides and their derivatives. Probe samples were prepared by placing 5-10 μg portions of a concentrated solution of the corresponding peptide or its derivative in aqueous methanol at the quartz tip of the direct insertion probe and removal of the solvent under slight vacuum in a desiccator, taking care to avoid splattering of the solution during evacuation. Spectra were recorded at ion source temperatures 225-300°, 70 ev ionizing energy and resolving power 15,000-20,000 for high resolution and 1500-3000 for low resolution studies. An initial background scan was performed for each set of experiments; the probe was then introduced into the ion source of the MS by using the standard vacuum-lock system. The temperature of the ion source was gradually increased from 200 to 300° and at each 15° interval the probe tip was moved into the ion source, the spectrum monitored on the oscilloscope, and the relevant spectra recorded.

B. Results and comments

The amino acid composition of the pure LRF preparation after hydrolysis under controlled conditions as described above,

Table 2. Amino acids composition of LRF

Amino acid	Micromoles per 20 μg *	Amino acid ratios **	Integral residues
Tryptophan	0.00878	0.99	1
Histidine	0.00915	1.03	1
Arginine	0.00801	0.91	1
Serine	0.00798	0.90	1
Glutamic acid	0.00815	0.92	1
Proline	0.00905	1.03	1
Glycine	0.01796	2.02	2
Leucine	0.00840	1.0	1
Tyrosine	0.00685	0.77	1
Total			10

* Hydrolyzed by the method of Matsubara and Sasaki (11). Total amino acid content = 68 % dry weight. ** Leucine = 1.0

indicated the presence of 2 moles of glycine and one mole each of histidine, arginine, tryptophan, serine, glutamic acid, proline, leucine and tyrosine (Table 2). Edman-dansyl degradation showed that the amino-terminal group is blocked, in agreement with previous results (12). Intense peaks at 111

Table 3. Mass spectral fragmentation pattern of free LRF

Mass units m/e	Relative intensity	Probable assignment
111, 112	49.6	(pyro)Glu
97	52.4	Pro
83	54.6	Pyrrolidone ring
82	39.6	Phenoxy ring
117	8.7	Indole ring
154	16.1	Pro-Gly
253, 210	12.5	Arg-Pro and its decomposition
269, 226	11.6	Leu-Arg and its decomposition
220	15.3	Tyr-Gly
273, 255	12.2	Trp-Ser, Trp-dehydro-Ser
248	22.4	(pyro)Glu-His
326, 283	7.5	Gly-Leu-Arg and decomposition
305	11.3	(pyro)Glu-His-Gly or (pyro)Glu-His-Trp less 129 m/e
280, 281	6.4	unexplained
368	4.8	unexplained
567	5.0	unexplained

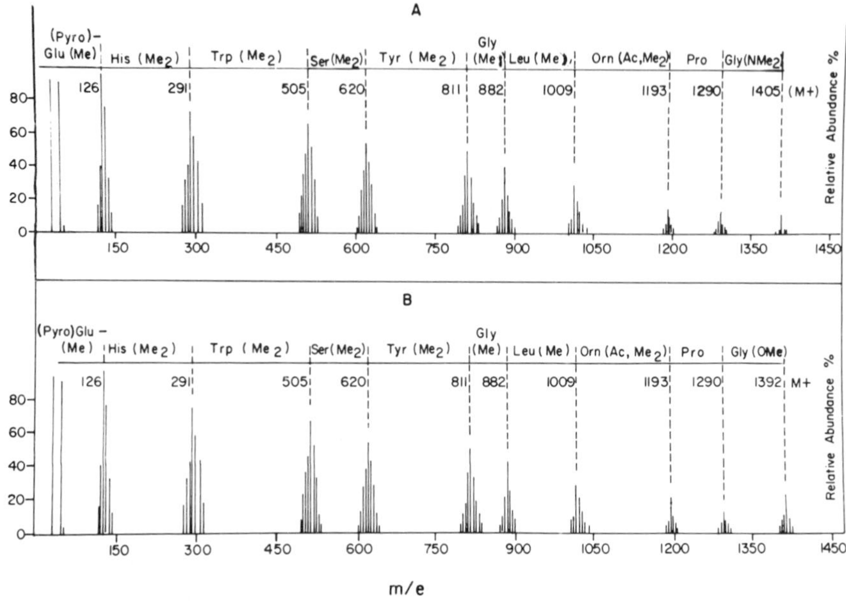

FIG 1. Sequence spectra of LRF after derivatization and mass spectrometry.

mass-units due to (pyro) glutamyl moiety (Table 3), during mass spectral fragmentation of free LRF and at 126 m/e due to N-methyl-(pyro)-Glu in the mass spectra of permethylated LRF (Fig 1), reinforced our conclusions that the N-terminus of the hormone is occupied by a (pyro) glutamyl moiety.

Esterification of LRF with (^{14}C) diazomethane failed to show any resultant radioactivity, indicating the absence of any free carboxyl group in the molecule. This showed that the C-terminus of LRF is also blocked. Mass spectral fragmentation of the hormone after permethylation yielded a prominent peak of 115 mass units (Fig 1) due to trimethylglycylamide. A similar fragmentation of LRF after methanolysis and permethylation yielded the peak of monomethylglycyl methylester (102 mass units). One of the major chymotryptic fragments,

Table 4A Cleavage of LRF with chymotrypsin

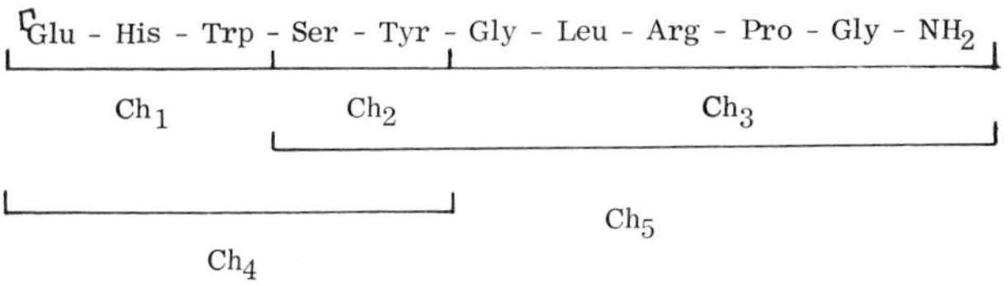

pGlu - His - Trp - Ser - Tyr - Gly - Leu - Arg - Pro - Gly - NH_2

Ch_1 Ch_2 Ch_3

Ch_5

Ch_4

Table 4B. Edman-Dansyl degradation of the chymotryptic fragments

Fragments	N-terminal amino acid	Sequence from step II onwards					
	I	II	III	IV	V	VI	VII
Ch_1	---	---	---	---	---	---	---
Ch_2	Ser	Tyr	---	---	---	---	---
Ch_3	Gly	Leu	Arg	Pro	Gly	---	---
Ch_4	---	---	---	---	---	---	---
Ch_5	Ser	Tyr	Gly	Leu	Arg	Pro	Gly

Ch_3 (Table 4), after similar derivatization reactions yielded the same peak of 102 mass units due to N-methylglycylester. This suggested that glycylamide forms the C-terminus of LRF, which on methanolysis was converted to a methylester and on subsequent permethylation yielded the N-methyl glycylmethylester. Permethylation without methanolysis on the other hand, gave rise to the trimethylglycylamide.

Mass spectral fragmentation of underivatized LRF showed a disorderly fragmentation pattern with peaks of several diketopiperazines, few tripeptide moities and their decomposition. The most important ones were (pyro) Glu-His 248 m/e, Leu-Arg 269 m/e, Arg-Pro 253 and 210 m/e, Pro-Gly 154 m/e and Gly/Leu-Arg 326 m/e (Table 3).

Chymotryptic digestion of LRF and subsequent separation of the hydrolytic fragments by TLC on cellulose, revealed three major and two minor spots when sprayed with chlorinetolidine reagent (33). The peptide spots in the main channel corresponding to those in the marker were recovered with 0.2 N acetic acid and lyophilized. The three major fragments Ch_1,

Ch_2, and Ch_3 (Table 4) after acetylation and permethylation yielded orderly mass spectral fragmentation patterns, showing the respective amino acid sequences Glu-His-Trp, Ser-Tyr and Gly-Leu-Arg-Pro-Gly. Fragment Ch_1 indicated peaks due to N-methyl (pyro) Glu, N:N-dimethyl His and Dimethyl-Trp-methylester (126, 165 and 245 m/e respectively). The parent molecular ion (M^+ = 536 m/e) corresponding to the pentamethyl monomethylester was obtained, even though the intensity was, as expected, very low. The (pyro) glutamyl N-terminus and the subsequent His-Trp sequence were confirmed by this study. Edman-dansyl sequential degradation of this fragment (Ch_1) did not show any result, presumably because the N-terminal moiety is blocked. After incubation with pyrrolidone carboxylyl peptidase, Ch_1 was subjected to Edman-dansyl procedure and the ◻Glu-His-Trp sequence was obtained. The other major peptidases Ch_2 and Ch_3 after Edman-dansyl degradation yielded the respective amino acid sequences, Ser-Tyr and Gly-Leu-Arg-Pro-Gly-NH_2.

Mass spectra of LRF after modification of arginine and N- and O-permethylation gave a sequential fragmentation pattern (Fig 1) yielding also the parent molecular ions (1405 m/e after permethylation and 1392 m/e after methanolysis and permethylation) of very low intensity. The fragmentation pattern exhibited the sequence: methyl(pyro) Glu, dimethyl His, dimethyl Trp, dimethyl Ser, dimethyl Tyr, methyl Gly, methyl Leu, monoacetyl dimethyl Orn, unsubstituted Pro and trimethyl glycylamide (Fig 1A). The peaks due to N-methyl (pyro) glutamyl moiety and its decomposition were identical to both derivatization products of LRF, indicating that the N-terminal pyrrolidone ring was not opened during methanolysis as expected (34), but was N-methylated during permethylation. The other sequence ions also were common for both derivatives (Fig 1A and B) except those at the C-terminal portion. Hence, the spectra are non-identical as are the two molecular ions. This is explained by the difference in the N-methylation of the C-terminal glycylamide before, and the carboxy methylation after, methanolysis (34,37). However, these two derivatives (Fig 1A and B) showed the same sequence: ◻Glu-His-Trp-Ser-Tyr-Gly-Leu-Arg-Pro-Gly-NH_2. The amino acid sequence of the chymotryptic fragments of LRF, as determined either by derivatization and mass spectrometry or by Edman-dansyl sequential degradation, also corresponded with the total sequence obtained for the intact hormone. These studies, in agreement with the structural work on the first batch of LRF (12), proved the amino acid sequence <Glu-His-Trp-Ser-Tyr-Gly-Leu-Arg-Pro-Gly-NH_2, for both batches of the hormone.

CONFIRMATION OF THE STRUCTURE OF LRF BY SYNTHESES

The decapeptide corresponding to the sequence <Glu-His-Trp-Ser-Tyr-Gly-Leu-Arg-Pro-Gly-NH_2 was synthesized by Merrifield's solid-phase method (44,45) with slight modifications. Starting with the C-terminal glycine which is esterified in its N-tertiarybutyloxycarbonyl form, to a polystyrene-cross-linked resin, the synthesis was continued step by step, by coupling the appropriate protected amino acids one by one (13). Side-chain functional groups of the amino acids involved in the synthesis were also protected. Thus during the synthesis, arginine was used as T-Boc-nitro-arginine; lysine, carbobenzoxy-lysine; histidine, tosyl-histidine; glutamic as the gamma-benzylester; serine and tyrosine, O-benzyl protection. Coupling was achieved with dicyclohexylcarbodiimide. Stepwise synthesis was carried out in the methylene chloride and/or dimethylformamide medium. Deprotection of the N-T-Boc group was effected by treating with 4 N HCl-dioxan containing 4 % mercaptoethanol for protection of the secondary amino group in tryptophan. For the cleavage of the peptide from the resin, ammonolysis in absolute methanol was carried out. The resultant protected peptide was purified and then fully deprotected using liquid anhydrous HF at 0°, after addition of anisole as a scavenger in the reaction medium, for saving the seryl and tyrosyl -OH groups. The crude synthetic peptide was purified by Sephadex filtration and then by counter-current distribution. The electrophoretic and chromatographic mobilities and the biological activities of the pure synthetic and native LRF-preparations were compared and were found similar. These investigations confirmed the primary structure of LRF to be <Glu-His-Trp-Ser-Tyr-Gly-Leu-Arg-Pro-Gly-NH_2 (Fig 2).

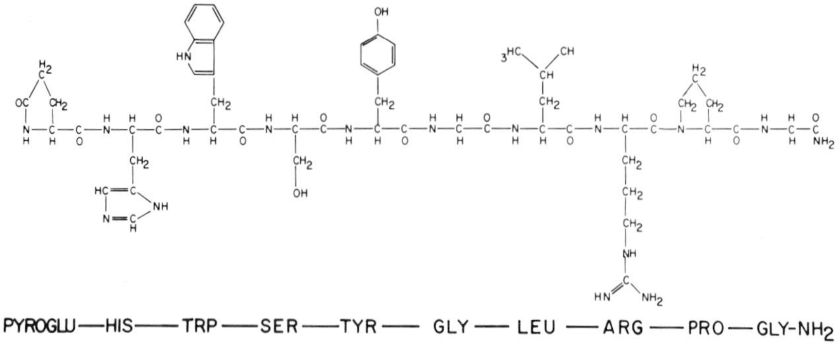

PYROGLU—HIS—TRP—SER—TYR—GLY—LEU—ARG—PRO—GLY-NH$_2$

FIG 2. Structural formula of LRF.

Table 5. Synthetic LRF and its analogues

Peptide	LH/FSH release	Reference No.
<Glu-His-Trp-Ser-Tyr-Gly-Leu-Arg-Pro-Gly-NH$_2$	Active (100%)	13, 15, 18, 68
___H-His-Trp-Ser-Tyr-Gly-Leu-Arg-Pro-Gly-NH$_2$	Inactive	67
<Glu-___-Trp-Ser-Tyr-Gly-Leu-Arg-Pro-Gly-NH$_2$	Inhibits in vitro	66, 62
<Glu-His-Trp-Ser-Tyr-Gly-Leu-Arg-Pro-Gly-OH	Inactive (1%)	17
<Glu-His-Trp-Ser-Tyr-Gly-Leu-Arg-Pro-NH$_2$	Active (11%)	65
<Glu-His-Trp-Ser-Tyr-Gly-Leu-Arg-Pro-NHCH$_2$CH$_3$	Active (150%)	61
<Glu-His-Trp-Ser-Tyr-Gly-Leu-Arg-___-Gly-NH$_2$	Very little activity (3%)	67
<Glu-His-Trp-Ser-Tyr-Gly-Leu-Arg-Pro-Gly-NH(CH$_3$)	Active (80%)	61
<Glu-His-Trp-Ser-Tyr-Gly-Leu-Pro-Arg-Gly-NH$_2$	Inactive	67
<Glu-His-Trp-Ser-Tyr-D-Ala-Leu-Arg-Pro-Gly-NH$_2$	Active (300%)	62
<Glu-His-Trp-Ser-Tyr-Ala-Leu-Arg-Pro-Gly-NH$_2$	Little activity (3%)	62
<Glu-His-Trp-Ser-Tyr-Gly-___-Arg-Pro-Gly-NH$_2$	Active (42%)	19
<Glu-His-Trp-Ser-Tyr-Gly-___-___-Pro-Gly-NH$_2$	Inactive	19
<Glu-His-Trp-Ser-Phe-Gly-Leu-Arg-Pro-Gly-NH$_2$	Active (60%)	68
<Glu-His-Trp-Ser-Tyr-Gly-Leu-Lys-Pro-Gly-NH$_2$	Active (22%)	19
<Glu-His-Trp-Ser-Tyr-D-Val-Leu-Arg-Pro-Gly-NH$_2$	Active (30%)	63
<Glu-Gly-Trp-Ser-Tyr-Gly-Leu-Arg-Pro-Gly-NH$_2$	Inhibits in vitro	66
<Glu-Trp-Trp-Ser-Tyr-Gly-Leu-Arg-Pro-Gly-NH$_2$	Active (40%)	63
<Glu-Asp-Trp-Ser-Tyr-Gly-Leu-Arg-Pro-Gly-NH$_2$	Inhibits in vitro	63
<Glu-___-Trp-Ser-Tyr-Gly-Leu-Arg-Pro-NHCH$_2$CH$_3$	Inhibits in vitro	68
<Glu-___-Trp-Ser-Tyr-D-Ala-Leu-Arg-Pro-Gly-NH$_2$	Greatly inhibits	63
<Glu-His-Trp-Ser-Tyr-D-Leu-Leu-Arg-Pro-Gly-NH$_2$	Active (60%)	63
<Glu-His-Trp-Ser-Tyr-D-Pro-Leu-Arg-Pro-Gly-NH$_2$	Active (10%)	63
<Glu-His-Trp-Ser-Tyr-NH$_2$	Very little activity	*
<Glu-His-Trp-NH$_2$	Inactive	*
___-___-H-Ser-Tyr-Gly-Leu-Arg-Pro-Gly-NH$_2$	Inactive	*
<Glu-___-Trp-Ser-Tyr-D-Ala-Leu-Arg-Pro-NHCH$_2$CH$_3$	Greatly inhibits	*

* Nair, unpublished.

STRUCTURE-ACTIVITY RELATIONSHIPS

The confirmation of the primary structure of LRF and the establishment of its biological activity offered innumerable opportunities for the study of structure-activity relationships in the molecule. Several workers in this field are interested in finding analogs of LRF, which instead of stimulating would inhibit the release of LH and FSH. Syntheses of powerful antagonists of LRF would thus form the basis of new contraceptive method. Table 5 summarizes the various agonistic and a few antagonistic analogs that have been synthesized and these exhibit ample variations in the constituent amino acids of LRF and corresponding variations in biological activity, thus giving an insight into the structure-activity relationships of the LRF molecule. Thus it is evident that any replacement for Glu results in almost complete loss of the LRF-activity. However, it might be possible to replace the pyrrolidone ring with linear molecules containing a $-CH_2-CO-NH-\overset{|}{C}H-CO \rightleftharpoons -CH_2-C(OH)=N-CH-CO-$ system, which permit each proton transfer and enhancement of the transport processes. The imidazole ring in position 3 of LRF seems to be crucial for the biological activity, as evidenced by virtually complete loss of LRF-activity, when changes in these positions occur. However, the tripeptide <Glu-His-Trp-NH_2 by itself is devoid of LRF-activity ($<$ 1 part in 100,000 of the parent molecule). On replacement of the hydroxyl groups of serine and/or tyrosine by a variety of groups, the activity is decreased with increase in size of the substituent group. Tyrosine at position 5 can be substituted by phenylalanine with 60 % retention of activity. Substitution of glycine and leucine can be made with only moderate to small loss of LRF-activity. Glycine, when replaced with alanine having the D-configuration, enhances the LRF-activity to a very great extent. But L-alanine, instead of glycine, does not make the molecule appreciably active. Arginine^8 can be replaced by lysine, a similar basic amino acid, with retention of much activity. However the Arg-Pro sequence is essential for the biological activity: Pro^8-Arg^9-LRF is inactive. The C-terminal amide function also is very essential for the LRF-activity; the LRF-free acid is inactive. Replacement of the glycylamide moiety with straight chain amides like methylamide or ethylamide retains the activity. Elimination of histidine from the second position renders the molecule inactive and also anti-LRF-active. The inhibition of LRF-activity is very predominent wh when histidine at position 2 of the decapeptide is absent and other moieties like D-alanine at position 6 and/or NH-CH_2CH_3 at 10 are present.

These investigations indicate that the initial Glu-His-Trp sequence in the molecule is essential for the functional part of LRF. Tyrosine, arginine and probably serine which can be replaced by similar amino acids with much retention of the activity, are responsible for the proper binding of LRF to the receptor sites of the gonadotroph cell membranes. The rest of the amino acids are involved in transport mechanisms. It is now well-established that pituitary is the major target organ for the hypothalamic hormones (46,47). The functional part of the molecule after binding to the appropriate cell membrane activates the adenyl cyclase-cyclic AMP system (48,49) which in turn triggers the mechanism of LH synthesis and release.

There is now good evidence that LRF regulates the release of both LH and FSH from the anterior pituitary of several species of animals including man (50,51). Preliminary clinical evaluations using synthetic LRF in volunteers, indicated (Figs 3, 4 & 5) that both gonadotropins are released from the pituitary into the peripheral circulation. However, in all cases, more LH was released (Fig 3,4 & 5) by a given amount of LRF, than was FSH (52,53). LRF, with its intrinsic FSH-releasing activity, has been successfully used for the induction of ovulation in women with secondary amenorrhea (54). Preliminary studies with LRF on men with oligospermia and azoospermia, resulted in increased spermatogenesis (55,56), even though the improvement was of small magnitude. Thus there is convincing evidence for the LH and FSH-releasing activity of this decapeptide which is now being extensively used for various clinical studies (57-59). Such investigations suggest that LRF alone may regulate both LH and FSH-release, a concept that is also supported by the fact that plasma LH and FSH levels vary in parallel during the menstrual cycle (60), including the hormonal surge which occurs just prior to ovulation. However, it

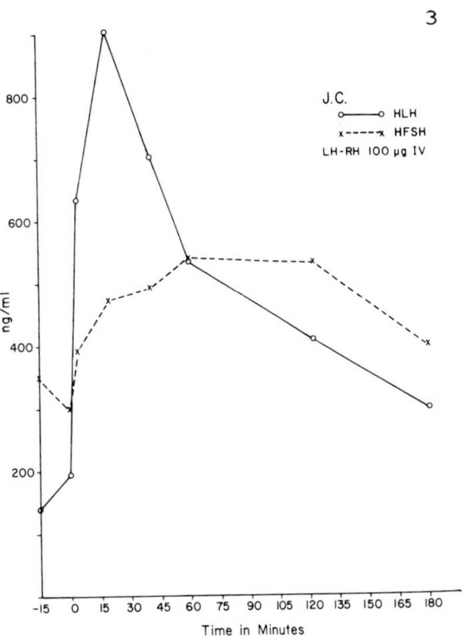

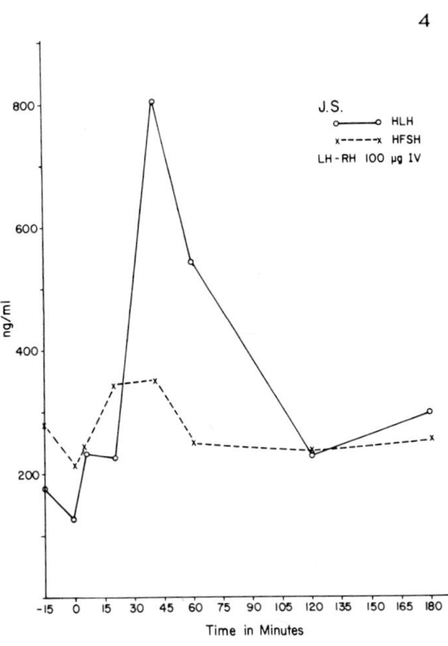

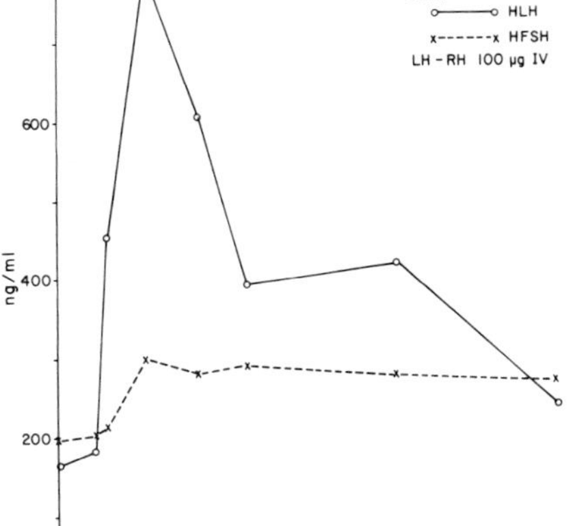

FIG 3,4 & 5. Plasma LH and FSH levels in humans (male volunteers), after administration of pure synthetic LRF intravenous. LH and FSH levels were determined by radioimmunoassay, using RIA kits for human LH and FSH supplied by NIH.

may be somewhat premature, at this stage, to propose that LRF is the sole hypothalamic controller of the secretion of LH and FSH. Further studies on the purification, isolation and characterization are necessary.

ACKNOWLEDGEMENTS

The authors are grateful to the National Pituitary Agency, National Institutes of Health and especially to Drs. A. E. Wilhelmi and A. F. Parlow for generous gifts of the Human and Rat radioimmunoassay kits for LH and FSH. The skillful technical assistance of Mrs. Anne Greene is acknowledged, as is the typing of the manuscript by Miss Denise Downs.

This study was supported by funds from Veterans Administration and Medical University of South Carolina Grant GR-54.

REFERENCES

1. Harris, G. W. (1955). In "Neural control of the pituitary gland", Arnold, E. (Ed).
2. Schally, A. V., Arimura, A., Bowers, C. Y., Kastin, A. J., Sawano, S. and Redding, T. W. (1968). Rec. Prog. Horm. Res. 24, 497.
3. Harris, G. W. (1971). Proc. Soc. Endocrinol 54, ii-xxi.
4. Guillemin, R. (1967). Ann. Rev. Physiol. 29, 313.
5. Harris, G. W. and Naftolin, F. (1970). Br. Med. Bul. 26, 3.
6. Blackwell, R. E. and Guillemin, R. (1973). Ann. Rev. Physiol. 35, 357.
7. McCann, S. M., Dhariwal, A. P. S. and Porter, J. C. (1968) Ann. Rev. Physiol. 30, 589.
8. Schally, A. V., Arimura, A., Kastin, A. J., Matsuo, H., Baba, Y., Redding, T. W., Nair, R. M. G., Debeljuk, L., and White, W. F. (1971). Science 173, 1036.
9. Schally, A. V., Arimura, A., Baba, Y., Nair, R. M. G., Matsuo, H., Redding, T. W., Debeljuk, L. and White, W. F. (1971). Biochem. Biophys. Res. Comm. 43, 393.
10. Amoss, M., Burgus, R., Ward, D. N., Fellows, R. E., Guillemin, R. (1971). Biochem. Biophys. Res. Comm. 44, 205.

11. Matsubara, H. and Sasaki, R. M. (1969). Biochem. Biophys. Res. Comm. 35, 175.
12. Matsuo, H., Baba, Y., Nair, R. M. G., Arimura, A. and Schally, A. V. (1971). Biochem. Biophys. Res. Comm. 43, 1334.
13. Matsuo, H., Arimura, A., Nair, R. M. G. and Schally, A. V. (1971). Biochem. Biophys. Res. Comm. 45, 822.
14. Burgus, R., Butcher, M., Amoss, M. (1972). Proc. Nat. Acad. Sci (USA). 69, 278.
15. Monahan, M., Rivier, J., Burgus, R., Amoss, M., Blackwell, R., Vale, W., Guillemin, R. (1971). C.R. Acad. Sci. Ser. D, 273, 508.
16. Geiger, R., Konig, W., Wissman, H., Giesen, K. and Enzmann, F. (1971). Biochem. Biophys. Res. Comm. 45, 767.
17. Sievertsson, H., Chang, J. K., Bogentoft, C., Currie, B. L, Folkers, K., and Bowers, C. Y. (1971). Biochem. Biophys. Res. Comm. 44, 1566.
18. Sievertsson, H., Chang, J. K., Klaudy, A., Bogentoft, C., Currie, B. L., Folkers, K. and Bowers, C. (1972). J. Med. Chem. 15, 222.
19. Chang, J. K., Sievertsson, H., Currie, B. L., Bogentoft, C, Folkers, K., and Bowers, C. Y. (1972). J. Med. Chem. 15, 623.
20. Rivaille, P., Robinson, A., Kamen, M. and Milhaud, G. (1971). Helv. Chim. Acta. 54, 2772.
21. Schally, A. V., Redding, T. W., Bowers, C. Y. and Barrett, J. F. (1969). J. Biol. Chem. 244, 4077.
22. Lowry, O. H., Rosebrough, N. J., Farr, A. L. and Randall, R. J. (1951). J. Biol. Chem. 193, 265.
23. Schally, A. V., Nair, R. M. G. and Carter, W. H. (1971). Analytical Chemistry 43, 1527.
24. Ramirez, V. D. and McCann, S. M. (1963). Endocrinology 73, 193.
25. Niswender, G. D., Midgley, A. R., Jr., Monroe, S. E., Reichert, L. E., Jr. (1968). Proc. Soc. Exp. Biol. Med. 128, 807.
26. Schally, A. V., Nair, R. M. G., Redding, T. W. and Arimura, A. (1971). J. Biol. Chem. 246, 7230.

27. Schally, A. V., Mittler, J. C. and White, W. F. (1970). Endocrinology 86, 903.
28. Steelman, S. L. and Pohley, F. M. (1953). Endocrinology 53, 604.
29. Steel, R. G. D. and Torrie, J. H. (1960). In "Principles and procedures of statistics", R. G. D. Steel and J. H. Torrie (Eds). McGraw-Hill Book Co.
30. Daane, T. A. and Parlow, A. F. (1971) Endocrinology 88, 653.
31. Dekanski, J. (1952). J. Pharmacol. Chemother. 7, 567.
32. Liu, T. Y. and Chang, Y. H. (1971). J. Biol. Chem. 246, 2842.
33. Nair, R. M. G., Kastin, A. J. and Schally, A. V. (1971). Biochem. Biophys. Res. Comm. 43, 1376.
34. Nair, R. M. G., Barrett, J. F., Bowers, C. Y. and Schally, A. V. (1970). Biochemistry 9, 1103.
35. Nair, R. M. G., Redding, T. W. and Schally, A. V. (1971). Biochemistry 10, 3621.
36. Nair, R. M. G., Redding, T. W. and Schally, A. V. (1971). Fed. Proc. 30, 1563.
37. Nair, R. M. G., Kastin, A. J. and Schally, A. V. (1972). Biochem. Biophys. Res. Comm. 47, 1420.
38. Thomas, D. W., Das, B. C., Gero, S. D. and Lederer, E. (1968). Biochem. Biophys. Res. Comm. 32, 199.
39. Agarwal, K. L., Kenner, G. W. and Sheppard, R. C. (1969). J. Am. Chem. Soc. 91, 3096.
40. Morris, H. R., Williams, D. H. and Ambler, R. P. (1971). Biochem. J. 125, 189.
41. Thomas, D. W., Das, B. C., Gero, S. D. and Lederer, E. (1968). Biochem. Biophys. Res. Comm. 32, 519.
42. Nair, R. M. G. and Schally, A. V. (1972). Int. J. Peptide Protein Res. 4, 421.
43. Shymyakin, M. M., Ovchinnikov, Y., Vinogradova, E. I., Feigina, M. Y., Kiryushkin, A. A., Aldanova, N. A., Alakhov, Y. B., Lipkin, V. M. and Rosinov, B. V. (1967). Experientia 23, 428.
44. Merrifield, R. B. (1963). J. Amer. Chem. Soc. 85, 2149.
45. Merrifield, R. B. (1964). Biochemistry 3, 1385.

46. Nair, R.M.G., Redding, T.W., Kastin, A.J. and Schally, A.V. (1973). Biochem. Pharmacol. 22, 1915.
47. Redding, T.W. and Schally, A.V. (1973) Life Sciences 12, 23.
48. Kaneko, T., Saito, S., Oka, H., Oda, T. and Tanaihara, N. (1973). Metabolism 22, 77.
49. Zor, U., Kaneko, T. and Schneider, H.P. (1969). Proc. Natl. Acad. Sci (USA) 63, 918.
50. Schally, A.V., Arimura, A., Kastin, A.J., Debeljuk, L., Matsuo, H., Baba, Y., Nair, R.M.G., Redding, T.W. (1972). In "Currents in reproductive biology", J.T. Velardo (Ed). Oxford University Press.
51. Kastin, A.J., Gual, C. and Schally, A.V. (1972). Rec. Prog. Horm. Res. 28, 201.
52. Kastin, A.J., Schally, A.V., Gual, C., Midgley, A.R., Bowers, C.Y. and Diaz-Infante, A. (1969). J. Clin. Endocrinol. Metab. 29, 1046.
53. Kastin, A.J., Schally, A.V., Gual, G., Midgley, A.R., Bowers, C.Y. and Gomez-Perez, F. (1970). Am. J. Obst. Gynec. 108, 177.
54. Zarate, A., Canales, E., Schally, A.V., Ayala-Valdes, L. Kastin, A.J. (1972). Fertility and Sterility 23, 672.
55. Schneider, H.P.G. and Dahlen, H.G. (1972). Life Sciences 11, 623.
56. Bergada, C., Mancini, R.E., Rivarola, M.A., Vilar, O., Calamera, J.C., Bianculli, C., Schally, A.V. and Kastin, A.J. (1972). Prog. Sociedad Argentina de Endocrinologia y Metabolismo, Dec. 22-24.
57. Marshall, J.C., Harsoulis, P., Anderson, D.C., Mc Neilly, A.S., Besser, G.M. and Hall, R. (1972). Brit. Med. J. 4, 643.
58. Hashimoto, T., Miyai, K., Izumi, K. and Kumahara, Y. (1972). New Eng. J. Med. 287, 1059.
59. Roth, J.C., Kelch, R.P., Kaplan, S.L. and Grumbach, M.M. (1972). J. Clin. Endo. Metab. 35, 926.
60. Cargille, C.M., Ross, G.T., Rayford, P.L. (1968). In "Gonadotropins", E. Rosemberg, (Ed). pp 355, Geron-X.
61. Fujino, M., Kobayashi, S., Obayashi, M., Shinagawa, S., Fukuda, T., Kitada, C., Nakayama, R. and Yamazaki, I.

(1972). Biochem. Biophys. Res. Comm. 49, 863.

62. Monahan, M., Rivier, J., Vale, W., Guillemin, R. and Burgus, R. (1972). Biochem. Biophys. Res. Comm. 47, 551.
63. Monahan, M., Vale, W., Rivier, C., Grant, G. and Guillemin, R. (1973). 55th Annual Meeting of Endocrine Society, Abstract #194.
64. Nair, R.M.G., Kastin, A.J. and Schally, A.V. (1972). 20th Annual Conf. on Mass spectrometry and allied topics, June 4-9, pp. 78.
65. Rivier, J., Monahan, M., Vale, W., Grant, G., Amoss, M., Blackwell, R., Guillemin, R. and Burgus, R. (1972). Chimia 26, 300.
66. Vale, W., Grant, G., Rivier, J., Monahan, M., Amoss, M., Blackwell, R., Burgus, R. and Guillemin, R. (1972). Science 176, 933.
67. Yanaihara, N., Yanaihara, C., Hashimoto, T. and Sakagami, M. (1972). 92nd Annual Meeting of the Pharmaceutical Society of Japan at Osaka, Abstracts, pp. III-95.
68. Coy, D.H., Coy, E.J. and Schally, A.V. (1973). J. Med. Chem. 16, 827 and 83.

RECENT ADVANCES IN THE PHYSIOLOGY AND CHEMISTRY OF GONADOTROPIN-RELEASING FACTORS

S.M. McCann, P.G. Harms, C. Libertun, S.R. Ojeda, R. Orias, R.L. Moss, C.P. Fawcett and L. Krulich.

INTRODUCTION

In this communication we would like to review research from our laboratory directed toward an understanding of the complex control system which regulates the secretion of gonadotropins and prolactin, with particular emphasis on the role played by the hypothalamic releasing and inhibiting hormones. Early work on these hormones, for example, a study of their effects on target organs using bioassay, laid the framework of our current understanding of the hypothalamic control of gonadotropin and prolactin release. A quantitative understanding of these relationships had to await the development of sensitive methods of measurement of the hormones, such as radioimmunoassay. The observations described here are based on the measurement of plasma concentration of the hormones by radioimmunoassay.

HYPOTHALAMIC REGIONS CONTROLLING GONADOTROPIN AND PROLACTIN RELEASE

A. Effects of electrical or electrochemical stimulation of the hypothalamus and preoptic region on gonadotropin release

It has been known since mid-30's that ovulation can be induced by hypothalamic stimulation. With radioimmunoassay of plasma concentrations of gonadotropins, it has been possible to quantitate the release of both LH and FSH. In proestrus rats, in which the spontaneous release of LH had been blocked by Nembutal, electrochemical stimulation of a band of tissue extending from the medial preoptic region through the anterior hypothalamus to the median eminence, led to an increase in plasma LH, indicative of LH release. On the other hand, FSH release resulted from stimulation of a more caudally-located region extending from the anterior hypothalamic area to the median eminence. Stimulation of the preoptic region was followed by increase in LH only, FSH release being unmodified; in two animals, stimulation in the anterior hypothalamic area resulted in increases in plasma FSH, with the absence of any change in LH (1). Thus, it would appear that the LH-controlling region extends more rostrally in the preoptic area, than the overlapping FSH-controlling region.

B. Effects of hypothalamic lesions on the release of gonadotropins and prolactin

1. Median eminence lesions : Early work indicated that a drastic curtailment of gonadotropin release followed the placement of lesions in the median eminence and these lesions were also accompanied by signs of increased prolactin release. Measurements by radioimmunoassay have borne out these early conclusions and demonstrated a dramatic decrease in the release of both FSH and LH in castrate animals; however, the decrease in plasma LH of approximately 95 % was greater than the decrease in FSH of 75 %. This could either mean that the pituitary has some autonomous capability to release FSH or that the lesions may not have been complete, even though no intact tissue was seen in the median eminence region. In dramatic contrast to the effects on gonadotropins were the effects on prolactin, the plasma titer of which, instead of being decreased, was markedly elevated. Thus, in agreement with earlier work, it appears that the hypothalamus exerts a net stimulatory effect on the release of FSH and LH on the one hand, and a dramatic inhibitory effect on the release of prolactin, on the other (2).

Surprisingly, immediately following median eminence lesions, there was a discharge of all three hormones as indicated by rapid elevation in plasma titers. We believe that this is the result of the release of stored releasing hormones from the injured tissue (2).

2. Suprachiasmatic lesions : Lesions in the suprachiasmatic region have been known, for over 20 years, to block ovulation and to induce a state of constant vaginal cornification. Examination of the ovaries has demonstrated that they are filled with large follicles. These rats appear poised on the brink of ovulation but unable to release an ovulatory quota of gonadotropins. It has been postulated that these lesions destroy that part of the brain involved in the stimulatory feedback of gonadal steroids which normally brings on the ovulatory discharge of gonadotropins (3). Recent

studies by radioimmunoassay further support this thesis. In animals with intact brains and which are under the influence of estrogen, progesterone can induce a release of LH and FSH. The suprachiasmatic lesions prevented the release of LH in response to progesterone treatment, whereas the release of FSH still occurred (4). These results are in accord with the stimulation experiments cited above and suggest that the hypothalamic centers controlling FSH release are located slightly more caudally than those controlling LH release.

HYPOTHALAMIC GONADOTROPIN-RELEASING FACTORS

With the realization that a corticotropin releasing factor governed the release of ACTH, it became of interest to search for similar factors regulating the discharge of other pituitary hormones. In 1960, we reported that hypothalamic extracts could induce LH release as evidenced by a depletion of ovarian ascorbic acid (5). This conclusion was reached independently by Harris' group on the basis of the ability of microinjections of hypothalamic extracts to trigger ovulation in both rats and rabbits (6). Shortly thereafter, we reported the FSH-releasing activity of hypothalamic extracts (7). Both the LH- and FSH-releasing factors (LRF and FRF) in hypothalamic extracts were purified by several groups and were reported to be separable, at least partially, one from the other (8-10).

A very important advance was made when Matsuo et al. (11) determined the structure of an LH-releasing peptide isolated from porcine hypothalami; they were able to synthesize this decapeptide. Subsequently, Burgus et al. (12) reported that ovine LRF had a similar structure. Single injections of the synthetic decapeptide LRF or purified LRF promote LH release almost exclusively in normal rats, castrate rats, or castrate rats primed with estrogen and/or progesterone (13, 14). Infusions of the decapeptide enhanced not only LH but FSH release, as reported by Arimura et al. (15), and we have confirmed this finding (16). Similarly, when incubated with pituitaries in vitro, the decapeptide promotes a significant release of both FSH and LH (Sundberg and Fawcett, unpublished data). Apparently, when the gonadotrophs are given long exposure to the decapeptide, FSH as well as LH release is promoted; however, it should be pointed out that the relative increase in FSH release is always less than that of LH.

In earlier work utilizing bioassay, as indicated above, the presence of a separate FRF was demonstrated by us (8, 9) and by several other investigators (10, 17). Utilizing radioimmunoassay, several groups have had difficulty in separating a discrete FRF from LRF in hypothalamic extracts. We have similarly had difficulties in separating the two activities, but have encountered suggestive evidence for a separation following chromotography of hypothalamic extracts (18). Johansson et al. (19) have recently reported a partial separation of the two activities. In addition, the LH to FSH-releasing ratio of hypothalamic extracts appears to be altered at certain stages of the estrous cycle and after estrogen treatment of ovariectomized females (14, 18). Furthermore, on the basis of the lesion and stimulation studies, as well as on the basis of many other studies on the dissociation of LH and FSH release, which occur either naturally or can be experimentally induced, we believe that a distinct FRF will ultimately be isolated.

A. Effect of steroids on the pituitary responsiveness to LRF

Recent studies have shown that single i v injections of physiological doses of estradiol can acutely inhibit the response of the pituitary to the decapeptide in vivo (20). Furthermore, ovariectomy is followed by enhanced sensitivity to purified LRF (13) which suggests that steroids of ovarian origin are continuously suppressing the hypophyseal response to the hypothalamic hormone. In chronically ovariectomized animals, the sensitivity to LRF is enhanced by treatment with large doses of estradiol benzoate, 72 hr prior to the measurements. In these experiments, the sensitization to LRF was observed both in vivo and in vitro (14). In fact, it can be shown in ovariectomized animals that estrogen has a biphasic effect on the pituitary in altering the response to either purified or synthetic LRF. If a single i v injection of estradiol or estradiol benzoate is given, this is followed by an acute inhibition of LH release which is accompanied by a decreased response to LRF in terms of both FSH and LH release. The responsiveness to the hypothalamic hormone then returns to normal, and at approximately 8 to 10 hr after the single injection of estrogen, it becomes supernormal (16, 21). In this situation, the changes in sensitivity were the result of administration of relatively low doses of estrogen (100 ng), which are presumably within the physiological range.

The changes in sensitivity to the releasing factor at the pituitary level appear to play a role during the normal estrous cycle since an enhanced sensitivity to purified LRF has been observed in rats and in man prior to the preovulatory discharge of gonadotropins (13,22,23).

B. Localization of the gonadotropin-releasing factors in the hypothalamus

Gonadotropin-releasing activity can be extracted from a region extending from the medial preoptic area caudally through the anterior hypothalamic area to the median eminence-arcuate region, where the bulk of the activity is concentrated. This has been revealed by making frozen sections of the tissue along three planes at right angles to each other, i.e., frontal, horizontal and sagittal and assaying extracts of these sections for their effect on gonadotropin release from pituitaries incubated in vitro (24,25). Since lesions in the suprachiasmatic area caused a decline in the content of LRF stored in the median eminence, we have postulated that some LRF-secreting neurons have cell bodies in the suprachiasmatic region and long axons extending down to the median eminence region where the secretory products are emptied into the hypophysial portal vessels. Since some LRF remained in the median eminence region after these lesions, we also postulated that other LRF neruons have short axons extending to the median eminence and cell bodies located near it, perhaps in the arcuate nuclei (26). The largest amount of activity was stored in the median eminence region. There was also LRF activity in the hypophysial stalk, but none in the neural lobe proper (24). Thus, the median eminence serves a function analogous to that of the neural lobe, the latter serving as a reservoir for neurohypophyseal hormones. In these studies, small amounts of FSH- as well as LH-releasing activity were found as far forward as the preoptic region (25), whereas in the lesion and stimulation experiments, the FSH-controlling center appeared to be located slightly more caudally than the LH center. We believe that the detection of FSH-releasing activity in this rostral site may be related to the potentiation of the FSH-releasing response by the in vitro system as indicated above.

In recent work, Barry et al. (27) have used fluorescent antibodies to synthetic LRF to localize the site of origin of the decapeptide in the preoptic and hypothalamic region. It is of extreme interest that they found the decapeptide to be localized in exactly the same regions in which we have detected LRF by bioassay; that is, in a region extending from the preoptic region rostrally to the median eminence-arcuate region caudally. Furthermore, they have been able to demonstrate that the decapeptide is localized in the pericarya of neurons in these loci and concentrated in axon terminals in the vicinity of the portal vessels. Thus, there is excellent agreement between bioassay results and results by the immunofluorescence technique suggesting that the decapeptide is localized in the regions previously shown to contain LRF.

POSSIBLE SYNAPTIC TRANSMITTERS INVOLVED IN CONTROLLING RELEASE OF GONADOTROPIN-RELEASING FACTORS AND PROLACTIN-INHIBITING FACTOR

A. Role of catecholamines

Extensive investigations have now been performed in an attempt to determine the possible synaptic transmitters which may mediate the influence of the rest of the CNS on the neurosecretory cells which secrete the releasing factors. As a result of studies both *in vitro* and *in vivo*, it appears that dopamine, and to a lesser extent, norepinephrine, can stimulate the release of gonadotropin-releasing factors and prolactin-inhibiting factor (28, 29). Dopamine, when incubated with pituitaries, at low doses inhibited prolactin release without affecting the release of FSH and LH. The release of the latter was, however, affected at high doses, which destroyed the hormones. Similar effect of dopamine on prolactin release has been shown by others as well (30, 31). When anterior pituitaries were incubated in a coincubation system with ventral hypothalamic fragments, dopamine was capable of stimulating a release of FRF and LRF as well as the prolactin-inhibiting factor (PIF) (28,29). In the *in vivo* experiments, the catecholamines were injected into third ventricular cannulae and it was possible to show that dopamine could stimulate the release of LRF, FRF and PIF (28,32). The stimulatory effect on LRF release could be blocked by estrogen which suggests that this may be one site for the negative feedback of the steroid (33).

Another approach was to inject drugs which could either block adrenergic receptors or alter biosynthesis of catecholamines. This approach lent further support for a role of dopamine as a synaptic transmitter to release PIF (34).

On the other hand, in the case of the gonadotropins, the evidence is not conclusive, although most of it points to norepinephrine as the probable transmitter involved. Thus, drugs which block norepinephrine synthesis impair the post-castration rise of gonadotropins, interfere with the stimulation of gonadotropin release brought about by either estrogen or progesterone and block the preovulatory surge of gonadotropins (34-36). The noradrenergic synapse may lie in the suprachiasmatic region since inhibitors of norepinephrine synthesis blocked LH release from preoptic but not median eminence stimulation (37). However, the dopamine receptor blocker, pimozide, has an effect in inhibiting FSH and LH release which would be consistent with the participation of a dopaminergic synapse (Ojeda, S.R., Krulich, L., & McCann, S.M - unpublished data).

B. Other putative transmitters

There is a possibility that cholinergic synapses may also be involved in controlling gonadotropin and prolactin release, since atropine given either subcutaneously or into the third ventricle can block gonadotropin and prolactin release. For example, the drug blocks the preovulatory discharge of FSH, LH and prolactin in the rat. The post-castration rise of gonadotropin is also blocked (38), but the situation is complicated by the failure of cholinergic drugs to produce an immediate elevation in gonadotropins. These drugs do produce delayed increments in plasma LH (39).

Serotonin has been shown to inhibit gonadotropin and to stimulate prolactin release in several studies (28, 32). In our laboratory no effects have been observed with the inhibitor of serotonin synthesis, parachlorophenylalanine, casting doubt on the physiological significance of serotonin in the control of these hormones; however, in a recent abstract, Kordon et al. (40) have reported that parachlorophenylalanine can block the suckling-induced rise in prolactin which suggests that it may be involved in mediating suckling-induced prolactin increases.

The pineal hormone melatonin has effects similar to serotonin; that is, it stimulates prolactin and inhibits gonadotropin release. We have recently observed that pinealectomy blocks the early morning discharge (0400-0500 hr) of prolactin which occurs in male rats and in general leads to lower levels of the hormone than those found in normal animals, which suggests a role for the pineal in the control of prolactin release (41). The effects of pinealectomy on gonadotropin release, by contrast, have been quite small (42).

THE POSSIBLE ROLE OF PROSTAGLANDINS IN MEDIATING GONADOTROPIN AND PROLACTIN RELEASE

Inhibitors of prostaglandin (PG) synthesis can block ovulation, but there has been controversy as to the locus of action (43, 44). In recent studies from our laboratory, it has been possible to show that injection of PGs, either into the third ventricle, or in larger doses peripherally, can alter gonadotropin and prolactin release in castrate female rats (45). PGE_1 elevated prolactin release, perhaps by stimulating the discharge of prolactin-releasing factor, or, alternatively, by inhibiting the release of prolactin-inhibiting factor. On the other hand, PGE_2 caused the discharge of LH apparently by stimulating the release of LRF. $PGF_{1\alpha}$ and $F_{2\alpha}$ were without effect. If the animals were primed with estrogen, PGE_1 had a significant LH-releasing action which was less than that of E_2.

Injection of PGE_1 and E_2 into the pituitary itself produced much smaller but significant increases in prolactin and LH respectively. These results suggest that prostaglandins may participate in the control of gonadotropin and prolactin release by actions on both the hypothalamus and pituitary. Studies are under way to determine the mechanism of the releasing action of these agents, and to determine if they play an essential role in the release of the pituitary hormones.

POSSIBLE ROLE OF CYCLIC NUCLEOTIDES IN CONTROL OF PIF AND LRF RELEASE

In other studies, third ventricular injections of cyclic AMP or dibutyryl cyclic AMP have been shown to result in a lowering of plasma prolactin levels, whereas similar injections into the pituitary were without effect (46). It appears that cyclic AMP may be involved as a second messenger to control the release of PIF, perhaps mediating the response to dopaminergic input. In contrast, to the effects of cyclic nucleotides on prolactin, their effects on LH release have been shown to be small. LH release was produced only by third ventricular injections of relatively large doses which also produced behavioral effects.

RELATIONSHIP OF THE LH CONTROLLING CENTER TO MATING BEHAVIOR

In normal animals, the preovulatory surge of gonadotropins is followed several hours later by the onset of mating behaviour. It occurred to us that the discharge of LRF into the portal vessels might be accompanied by a local discharge of the hormone from its storage sites in the preoptic area. The LRF might then have an influence on the mating center which lies in juxtaposition to the presumed cell-bodies of the neurons secreting LRF in the preoptic area. To test this hypothesis, we injected LRF s c in a dose of 500 ng into ovariectomized, estrogen-primed rats. The s c route was chosen because of the ease of administration and lack of disturbance to the animal. The dose was one previously shown to produce a considerable discharge of LH (47). The animals were primed with a dose of estrone which did not by itself produce mating behaviour. Within 2 hr of administration of LRF, nearly all of the animals came into behavioral receptivity and exhibited lordosis. The effect appeared to be specific for LRF since ovulating doses of LH, large doses of FSH or a large dose of thyrotropin-releasing factor were ineffective in inducing mating behavior (48). If these effects carry over to the human, they will obviously have profound significance.

REFERENCES

1. Kalra, S. P., Ajika, K., Krulich, L., Fawcett, C. P., Quijada, M., and McCann, S. M. (1971). Endocrinology 88, 1150.
2. Bishop, W., Fawcett, C. P., Krulich, L., and McCann, S. M. (1972). Endocrinology 91, 643.
3. Barraclough, C., (1966). Rec. Prog. Hormone Res. 22, 503.
4. Bishop, W., Kalra, P. S., Fawcett, C. P., Krulich, L., and McCann, S. M. (1972). Endocrinology 91, 1401.
5. McCann, S. M., Taleisnik, S., and Friedman, N. M. (1960). Proc. Soc. Exp. Biol. Med. 104, 432.
6. Harris, G. W. (1961). In "Control of Ovulation", C. A. Villee, (Ed), p. 56, Pergamon Press, New York.
7. Igarashi, M., Nallar, R., and McCann, S. M. (1964). Endocrinology 75, 901.

8. Dhariwal, A. P. S., Nallar, R., Batt, M., and McCann, S. M. (1965). Endocrinology 76, 290.
9. Dhariwal, A. P. S., Watanabe, S., Antunes-Rodriques, J., and McCann, S. M. (1967). Neuroendocrinology 2, 294.
10. Schally, A. V., Saito, T., Arimura, A., Muller, E. E., Bowers, C. Y., and White, W. F. (1966). Endocrinology 79, 1087.
11. Matsuo, H., Baba, Y., Nair, R. M. G., Arimura, A., and Schally, A. V. (1971). Biochem. Biophys. Res. Comm. 43, 1334
12. Burgus, R., Butcher, M., Ling, N., Monahan, M., Rivier, J., Fellows, R., Amoss, M., Blackwell, R., Vale, W., and Guilleman, R. (1971). Curr. Rev. Acad. Sci. 273, 1611.
13. Cooper, K. J., Fawcett, C. P., and McCann, S. M. (1973). J. Endocrinol. 57, 187.
14. Libertun, C., Cooper, K. J., Fawcett, C. P., and McCann, S. M. (1974). Endocrinology (in press).
15. Arimura, A., Debeljuk, L., and Schally, A. V. (1972). Endocrinology 91, 529.
16. Orias, R., Libertun, C., and McCann, S. M. (1974). Endocrinology (in press).
17. Jutisz, M. (1970). In "The Human Testis", p. 207, Plenum Press, New York.
18. Fawcett, C. P. (1973). Discussion of paper #24, Proc. of the Conference on Hypothalamic Hypophysiotropic Hormones, Acapulco, Serono Research Foundation, C. Gual & E. Rosemberg (Eds). p. 111, Excerpta Medica, Amsterdam.
19. Johansson, K. N. G., Currie, B. L., Folkers, K., and Bowers, C. Y. (1973). Biochem. Biophys. Res. Comm. 50, 8.
20. Negro-Vilar, A., Orias, R., and McCann, S. M. (1973). Endocrinology 92, 1680.
21. Cooper, K. J., Fawcett, C. P., and McCann, S. M. (1974). Proc. Soc. Exp. Biol. Med. (in press).
22. Martin, J. E., Tyrey, L., Everett, J. W., and Fellows, R. E. (1973). Fed. Proc. 32, 163.
23. Yen, S. S. C., Van den Berg, G., Rebar, R., and Ehara, Y. (1972). J. Clin. Endo. Metab. 35, 931.
24. Crighton, D. B., Schneider, H. P. G., and McCann, S. M. (1970). Endocrinology 87, 323.
25. Quijada, M., Krulich, L., Fawcett, C. P., Sundberg, D. K., and McCann, S. M. (1971). Fed. Proc. 30, 97 (abs).

26. Schneider, H.P.G., Crighton, D.B., and McCann, S.M. (1969) Neuroendocrinology 5, 271.
27. Barry, J., Dubois, M.P., Poulain, P., and Leonardelli, J. (1973). Curr. Rev. Acad. Sci. Paris 276, 3191.
28. McCann, S.M., Kalra, S.P., Kalra, P.S., Bishop, W., Donoso, A.O., Schneider, H.P.G., Fawcett, C.P., and Krulich, L. (1972). In "Brain-Endocrine Interaction · Median Eminence: Structure & Function, K.M. Knigge, D.E. Scott & A. Weindle (Eds). p. 224, Karger, Basel.
29. Quijada, M., Illner, P., Krulich, L., and McCann, S.M. (1974). Neuroendocrinology (in press).
30. Birge, C.A., Jacobs, L.S., Hammeo, C.T., and Daughaday, W.H. (1970). Endocrinology 86, 120.
31. MacLeod, R.M. (1969). Endocrinology 85, 916.
32. Porter, J.C., Kamberi, I.A., and Ondo, J.G. (1972). In "Brain-Endocrine Interaction. Median Eminence: Structure & Function" K.M. Knigge, D.E. Scott, and A. Weindl (Eds). p. 245, Karger, Basel.
33. Schneider, H.P.G., and McCann, S.M. (1970). Endocrinology 87, 249.
34. Donoso, A.O., Bishop, W., Fawcett, C.P., Krulich, L., and McCann, S.M. (1971). Endocrinology 89, 774.
35. Kalra, P.S., Kalra, S.P., Krulich, L., Fawcett, C.P., and McCann, S.M. (1972). Endocrinology 90, 1168.
36. Ojeda, S.R., and McCann, S.M. (1973). Neuroendocrinology 12, 295.
37. Kalra, S.P., and McCann, S.M. (1973). Endocrinology, 93, 356.
38. Libertun, C., and McCann, S.M. (1973). Endocrinology, 92, 1714.
39. Libertun, C. (1973). Proc. of the 55th Meeting of the Endocrine Society.
40. Kordon, C.A., Blake, C.A., and Sawyer, C.H. (1972). Proc. IV Int. Cong. of Endocrinology. #51 (abs).
41. Rønnekleiv, O., Krulich, L., and McCann, S.M. (1973). Endocrinology 92, 1339.
42. Rønnekleiv, O., McCann, S.M. (1973). The Physiologist 16, 3.
43. Behrman, H.R., Orczyk, G.P., and Greep, R.O. (1972). Prostaglandins 1, 245.
44. Tsafriri, A., Lindner, H.R., Zor, U., and Lamprecht, S.A. (1972). Prostaglandins 2, 1.

45. Harms, P. G., Ojeda, S. R., and McCann, S. M. (1973). Science 181, 760.
46. Ojeda, S. R., Harms, P. G., and McCann, S. M. (1974). Endocrinology (in press).
47. Zeballos, G., and McCann, S. M. (1974). Proc. Soc. Exp. Biol. Med. (in press).
48. Moss, R. L., and McCann, S. M. (1973). Science 181, 177.

GONADOTROPINS : A CORRELATION OF THEIR BIOLOGICAL AND IMMUNOLOGICAL ACTIVITIES

Shanta S. Rao, B. Dattatreya Murthy and Anil R. Sheth

The two important properties with which gonadotropins - for that matter any protein hormone - are endowed with are: a characteristic biological property and a specific immunological reactivity.

Immunodiffusion in an agar matrix - with or without recourse to electrophoresis has been used to study antigenic constituents of gonadotropins. The earlier work on the immunology of gonadotropins has been reviewed by Rao (1,2). During the last couple of years better antigenic resolution of several protein hormones has been achieved by employing electrophoresis in starch (3) and polyacrylamide (4) gels followed by immunodiffusion in agar.

Immunological techniques have been utilized for the detection and estimation of microquantities of gonadotropins. Complement fixation test has been used for the estimation of both ICSH (5) and hCG (6). Also, passive haemagglutination (7, 8) and haemagglutination inhibition (9) techniques have been used to detect and estimate hCG. The latter forms the basis for the extensively used hCG detection test during early pregnancy and also in pathological conditions like chorio-carcinoma and molar pregnancy. In addition, radioimmunoassays have been extensively used to quantify gonadotropins.

A number of bioassays (10) employing a variety of parameters such as increase in weights of gonads and accessory reproductive organs, and measuring the biochemical changes in the target organ have been used for estimating the potency of gonadotropins. The precision, sensitivity, reproducibility and specificity of the bioassays varies according to the strain of animals used, mode of administration of hormone, the procedure adopted to measure the end-organ response etc. For instance, Purandare et al. (11) from our laboratory have observed that Swiss mice were suitable for the ovarian ascorbic acid depletion assay for LH, as compared to six other strains of mice available locally.

An exciting development in the field of *in vitro* bioassays, has been the use of receptor assay to measure the intrinsic biological activity of natural and modified tropic hormones at the target cell level (12). These assays in addition to being economical, precise, and more sensitive than bioassays, eliminate variations caused by such factors as species differences (13), variation in sialic acid content and differential metabolism of the hormones seen in in vivo systems.

The loss of biological activity has been shown not necessarily to destroy the immunological reactivity of the gonadotropin (14, 15). If the biological active site on the molecule of the gonadotropin is near its antigenic determinant group, then the antiserum can be expected to inhibit the biological activity (16). These studies thus suggest that these two properties are evidently contributed by different sites on the gonadotropin molecule (14).

An attempt has been made in our laboratory to dissociate the sites responsible for biological and immunological activities of hCG and the same is reported here.

EXPERIMENTAL

A. Biological and immunological properties of hCG

We used for the studies, hCG isolated in our laboratory according to the method of Albert (17). A semi-purified preparation was purposefully used as we were interested in finding out whether the impurities in a crude preparation would contribute to the antigenic properties of hCG.

The crude hCG was fractionated by zone electrophoresis on Pevicon by the procedure of Bocci (18) but with a slight modification. We used as the vehicle barbital buffer, pH 8.6 and of an ionic strength 0.0784 and containing 0.0017 M of the disodium salt of EDTA. HCG dissolved in the buffer and dialyzed against the same buffer was subjected to preparative zone electrophoresis at 4°. At the end of the run the block was cut into 48 segments each of 0.5 cm width. The polyacrylamide disc-gel electrophoretic patterns of some of the hCG fractions obtained from the electrophorogram are illustrated in Figure 1. Fraction 5 showed two slow moving bands while fraction 10 gave a dark and diffused band. On the other hand, the three prominent bands given by fraction 18 migrated more rapidly than those observed in fractions 5 and 10. Fractions 22, 26 and 33 did not show major differences in their electrophoretic patterns, but they appeared to be considerably different from earlier fractions.

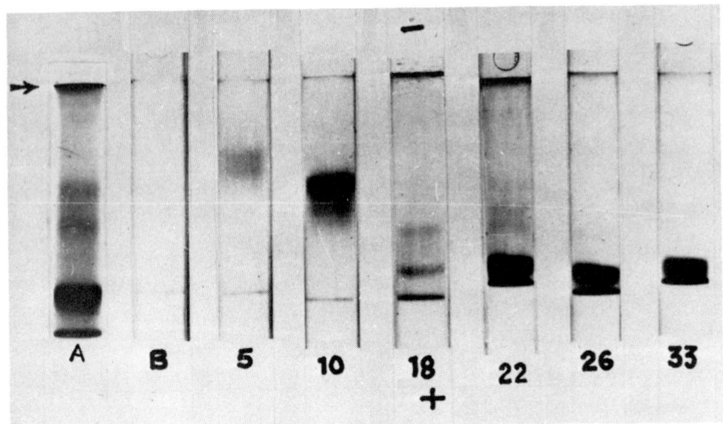

FIG 1. Disc electrophoresis on polyacrylamide gel.
A. Electrophoretic pattern of crude hCG; B. Control gel (normal saline was applied). Numbers 5 to 33 refer to electrophoretic patterns of hCG fractions obtained from Pevicon electrophorogram. → Junction of the spacer and separation gels. Gel columns were stained with amido black.

1. Biological activity : The biological activity of the hCG fractions was assessed at two dose levels i.e., 8 µg and 16 µg, by the method described by Diczfalusy (19). The relative responsiveness of hCG fractions revealed two peaks of biological activity in fractions 8-13 and 15-18 (Fig 2A). Fractions after 18, when injected at higher dose levels (upto 120 µg) were inactive.

2. Immunological activity : In both passive haemagglutination inhibition and haemagglutination tests an antiserum of high degree of specificity to hCG was used. The former technique, revealed that the maximum immunological activity was present in hCG fractions 17-21 (Fig 2A). Four equal aliquots (0.5 ml) of the antiserum to hCG were absorbed with fractions 9, 17, 21 (1 mg per ml) and normal saline. The precipitates obtained, were separated by centrifugation at 3000 rpm at 4° for 20 min. Absolute amount of antibody protein precipitated by fractions 9, 17 and 21 were 435, 790, 845 µg respectively.

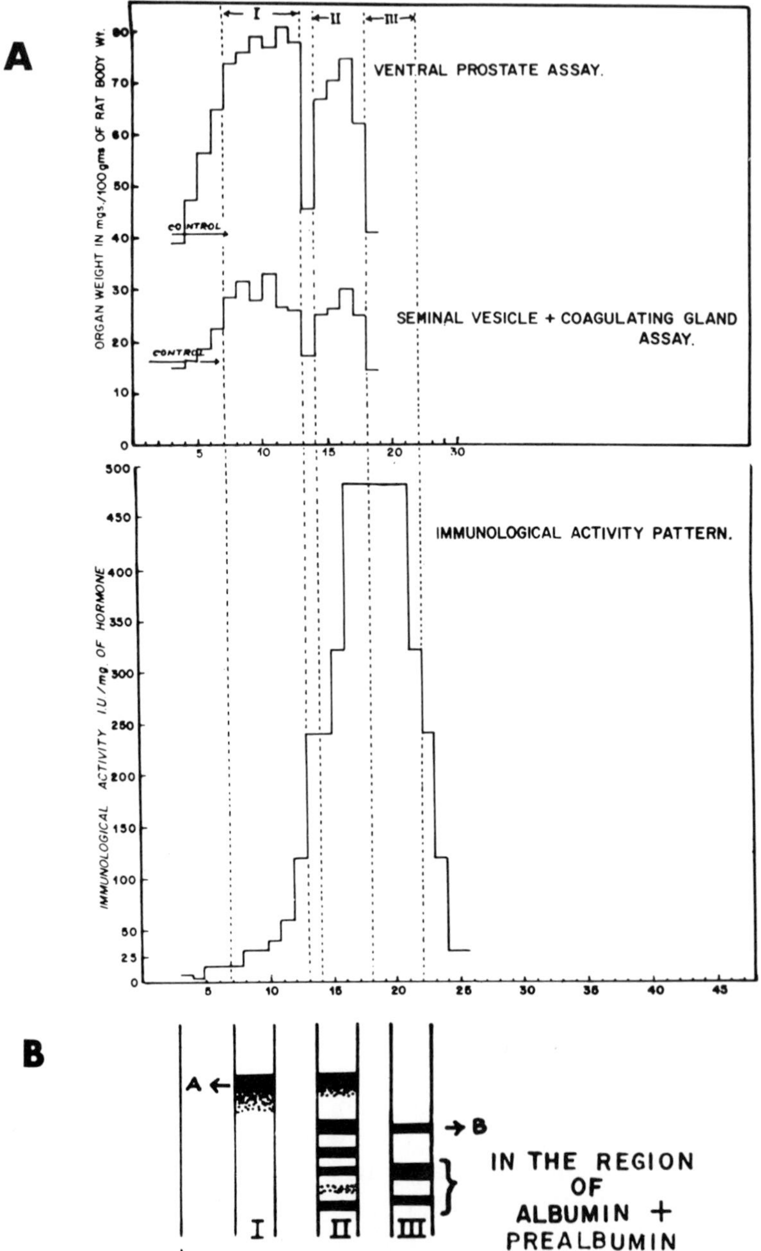

FIG 2 (A) Patterns of biological and immunological activity of individual hCG fractions obtained from Pevicon electrophorogram. (B) Disc electrophoresis pattern of Fraction I, II & III obtained from Pevicon electrophorogram.

The antibody titre in the supernatants was determined by the haemagglutination technique. Following absorption of antiserum aliquots with fractions 17 and 21, no antibody could be detected in the supernatant. On the other hand, that absorbed with fraction 9 continued to show the presence of high antibody titre (Fig 3).

The individual fractions from the Pevicon electrophorogram were pooled into three major fractions (fractions I, II & III) (Fig 2B) according to their activity pattern, and these were further subjected to polyacrylamide disc gel electrophoresis, using tris-glycine buffer, pH 8.3. The results are presented in Fig 2B.

The electrophoretic patterns of FR-I and III were found to be very different, while FR-II was found to share the properties of both FR I and III. The active components A and B eluted from FR-I and II respectively were assessed for their activity by radioimmunoassay. Using anti-hCG serum and labeled NIH-hCG,

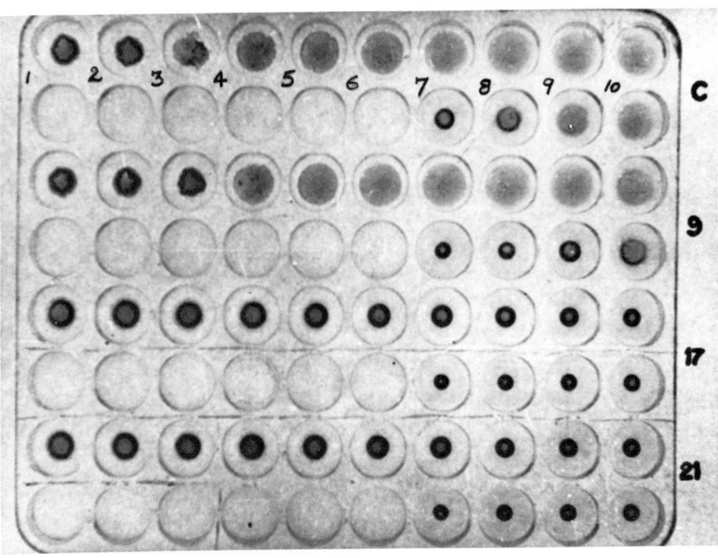

FIG 3. Haemagglutination patterns using antisera absorbed with normal saline (C) and fractions 9, 17 and 21. Titers: C = 1:4096; 9 = 1:1024; 17 = -Ve; 21 = -Ve.

component B was found to exhibit a very high immunological reactivity as compared to component A, the ratio of activity being 17.86 (B/A = 339.4/19). Even in an assay system using anti-hCG β serum, the component B was found to be more active than component A, the ratio being 3.61 (B/A = 90.0/24.9). Thus it was possible to separate by using the above methods, the component B possessing negligible biological activity, but higher immunological reactivity and specificity, from component A with high biological, but low immunological activity.

It is reasonable to expect that component A on further purification would yeild a hCG, which is more active biologically when compared to hCG preparations made by several other investigators. It is important to note that the purified preparations displayed a higher index of discrimination (Biopotency/immunopotency) (20-22). During purification of hCG, attention is generally focused on the biological activity of the hormone purified, thus neglecting the component having higher immunological activity but low biological activity (for e.g. component B). The results of our work indicate that it would be essential to carry out the purification, keeping in view which type of activity is desirable in the hCG to be obtained. The two components of hCG obtained in our study, should on further purification be useful in studying the structure-activity relationship of hCG.

Several attempts have been made to study the physico- chemical characteristics and immuno- and biological properties of hCG purified by different procedures. Variable results were obtained by many investigators (23-26) and this has led to the conclusion that hCG may consist of multiple components. Our earlier work also indicated that hCG has LH- and FSH-like principles, each with a characteristic immunological activity (27). Ashitaka et al. (28) also have obtained similar results and have further reported that their preparation was not immunologically and biologically homogeneous. Recently, Metthies et al. (29) by gel filtration on Sephadex G-100 showed that the biologically active hCG present in urine may not be identical with the molecule possessing immunological activity. They further showed that the physico-chemical procedures involved in the purification of hCG might introduce artifacts in biological and immunological characteristics of hCG.

Our recent findings as well as those of others reported here strongly suggest that methods used for the extraction and purification of gonadotropins would influence their biological and immunological activity. It is conceivable that the biological and immunological activity can be separated to a large extent or selectively inactivated by specific procedures.

ACKNOWLEDGEMENTS

We are grateful to Dr. D.R. Bangham, National Institute for Medical Research, London for the gift of 2nd IRP-hCG; to the World Health Organization for the supply of Pevicon, and to the National Institute of Health, Bethesda for providing reagents for radioimmunoassay.

REFERENCES

1. Rao, S.S. (1964). Fifth All India Conference on Family Planning, Patna, January 1964.
2. Rao, S.S. (1968). Proc. W.H.O. Symp. on Immunology of Reproduction, Geneva.
3. Schuurs, A.H.W.M., Jager, E.de., Homan, J.D.H. (1968). Acta Endocrinologica 59, 120.
4. Kosugiyama, M., Mori, J. and Nagasawa, H. (1970). Endocrinologica Japonica 17, 251.
5. Trenkle, A., Moudgal, N.R., Sadri, K.K., and Li, C.H. (1961). Nature (Lond) 192, 260.
6. Brody, S. and Carlstrom, G. (1960). Lancet 2, 99.
7. Rao, S.S. (1959). Proc. West Point Conference on Mechanisms concerned with Conception. New York.
8. Rao, S.S. and Shahani, S.K. (1961). In S.K. Shahani's M.Sc., thesis, Univ. of Bombay.
9. Wide, L. and Gemzell, C.A. (1960). Acta Endocrinol (kbh) 35, 261.
10. Loraine, J.A. and Bell, E.T. (1966). In "Hormone Assays and their clinical application" 2nd edition, Williams and Wilkins Co., Baltimore.
11. Purandare, T.V., Sadri, K.K. and Rao, S.S. (1969). Ind. J. of Exptl. Biol. 7, 10.
12. Dufau, M.L., Catt, K.J. and Tsuruhara, T. (1972). Endocrinol. 90, 1032.
13. Parlow, A.F. (1968). In "Gonadotropins", p. 59, Geron-x, Inc., Los Altos, California.

14. Rao, S.S., Shahani, S.K., Munshi, S.R. and Rangnekar, K.N. (1967). Presented in the Vth International symposium on Comparative Endocrinology, Delhi, November 1967. Gen. & Comp. Endo. Suppl. 2, 171, (1969), Prasad, M.R.N. (Ed). Academic Press, New York.
15. Munshi, S.R. and Rao, S.S. (1967). Ind. J. Exptl. Biol. 5, 135.
16. Rao, S.S., Munshi, S.R. and Purandare, T.V. (1972). Ind. J. Med. Res. 60, 1220.
17. Albert, A. (1955). Proc. Staff Met, Mayo Clin. 30, 552.
18. Bocci, V. (1962). J. Chromatography 8, 218.
19. Diczfalusy, E. (1954). Acta Endocrinologica (kbh) 17, 58.
20. Robyn, C. (1969). Acta Endocrinologica (kbh) suppl. 142, 130.
21. Bahl, O.P. (1969). J. Biol. Chem. 244, 575.
22. Schuurs, A.H.W.M. (1969). Acta Endocrinologica (kbh). suppl. 142, 130.
23. Brody, S. (1969). In "Foetus and Placenta", Klopper and Diczfalusy, E. (Eds). Blackwell, Oxford, and Edinburgh.
24. Hellema, M.J.C. (1971). J. Endocrinol. 49, 393.
25. Van Hell, E., Matthijsen, R. and Homen, J.D.H. (1968). Acta Endocrinologica 59, 89.
26. Hamashige, S., Alexander, J.D., Abravanel, E.V. and Astor, M.A. (1971). Fert. Steril. 22, 26.
27. Shahani, S.K. and Rao, S.S. (1964). Acta Endocrinologica (kbh) 46, 317.
28. Ashitaka, Y., Tokura, Y., Tane, M., Mochizuki, M. and Tojo, S. (1970). Endocrinology 87, 233.
29. Matthies, D.L., Petrusz, P. and Diczfalusy, E. (1971). Acta Endocrinologica 67, 445.

IMMUNOSORBENTS OF GONADOTROPINS AND THEIR ANTIBODIES

K. Muralidhar, T.S.A. Samy and N.R. Moudgal

INTRODUCTION

Water insoluble derivatives of functional macromolecules and ligands of biological interest like steroids, sugars etc have been prepared and studied by many investigators (1). Such immobilized biomolecules have been used in affinity chromatography (2), solid state macromolecular synthesis (3), fermentation technology, isolation and purification of biologically active molecules and complex biological structures like drug receptors, immunocompetent cells, polysomes synthesizing a specific protein etc. (4,5). These have also been used as models of functional membranes (6). Immunosorbents have found additional applications in radioimmunoassays (7) and in a variety of immunological studies (2). Some of the major methods of preparing immobilized biomolecules involve physical adsorption or covalent linkage to inert supports, intermolecular cross-linking or entrapping in polymeric matrices (1, 8) etc.

Many interesting and fruitful results have been obtained by the use of the above principles and methods in the isolation and purification of hormones (9-13) and hormone antibodies (14, 15) localization of hormone receptors, and purification of hormone receptors (16, 17).

We describe here the preparation and uses of some immunosorbents of LH, FSH and of their antisera. A preliminary account of this study has been reported earlier (13).

METHODOLOGY

A. Preparation of antibody polymer immunosorbent

The polymerization of serum was carried out with ethylchloroformate, essentially according to Avrameas and Ternynck (18); more than 99 % of the protein could be recovered in the polymeric form. The washed polymer could be stored at 4°, merthiolate being added at 1 : 10000 dilution.

B. Preparation of erythrocyte immunosorbent

Sheep erythrocytes were prepared and used according to conventional methods described for protein coating (19). This usually involves formalinization, treatment with tannic acid followed by protein adsorption. The use of LH coated erythrocytes for purification of FSH antiserum (a/s) has been described earlier by us (20).

C. Solid phase radioimmunoassay procedure

LH a/s polymer at suitable dilution was incubated with standards or rat serum samples at 37° for 1 hr followed by addition of ^{125}I-LH-β, prepared by the method of Greenwood et al. (21). Incubation was continued for an additional 10-12 hr. After counting for total radioactivity, a pinch of silicic acid (column chromatography grade, Mallinckrodt Chemical Works, New York) and 0.5 ml of 0.05 M phosphate -EDTA buffer, pH 7.5 were added. The tubes after centrifugation and removal of supernatant were counted for bound radioactivity in a Packard autogamma spectrometer.

D. Extraction of pituitary hormones

Pituitaries either fresh or stored at -20° of rats and monkeys were homogenized in 0.01 M phosphate buffered saline, pH 7.5, centrifuged at 10,000 g for 30 min and the clear supernatant taken as a source of pituitary LH and FSH.

APPLICATIONS OF IMMUNOSORBENTS

A. Purification of anti-LH and FSH sera

It has been our general experience, that antisera to FSH and LH are contaminated with other non-specific antibodies directed against serum and tissue protein contaminants present in the antigens used for immunization. In addition, a/s raised to FSH generally shows the presence of antibodies to LH also. Classical procedures of purification involving addition, in small amounts, of dilute solutions of the contaminating antigen, removes only the precipitating type of antibodies. Further, this results in the a/s having an excess of the contaminating antigen and other impurities. While the use of specific purified contaminants in amounts at equivalence would partially overcome the above difficulties, the use of the contaminants in the form of an immunosorbent would obviate all these difficulties. For example, polymerized normal sheep serum (NSS) has been used to purify a/s to gonadotropins. A sufficiently large excess of NSS polymer was incubated with LH a/s or FSH a/s for a period of 2 to 3 hr at 4°, the removal of NSS antibodies from the a/s being confirmed by the micro double-diffusion test. Additional advantages of the immunosorbent method are, its reusability, the quickness of the absorption process and the removal of both soluble and precipitating type of antibodies. The polymer can be recycled at least 2-3 times by treatment each time with 3 M potassium iodide and washing with buffers. The efficiency of the immunosorbent, however, decreases with each cycle.

LH-coated erythrocytes have been found to be very efficient in our hands in the complete removal of LH antibodies from FSH a/s; this process, however, does not reduce the FSH antibody titre, showing thereby the two antibody species to be entirely different. Moreover, leaching of LH from erythrocytes is also not observed, if careful handling is maintained. The process involves incubation of FSH a/s with coated erythrocytes at 4°overnight, followed by centrifugation. The number of treatments with coated erythrocytes varies from batch to batch depending upon the extent of contamination. Sensitive radio-hormone binding test was used to monitor the completion of removal of the contaminant. As shown in Figure 1, in a homologous radioimmunoassay system for ovine FSH using FSH a/s purified by the above method, LH does not interfere, indicating that even traces of LH antibodies have been removed.

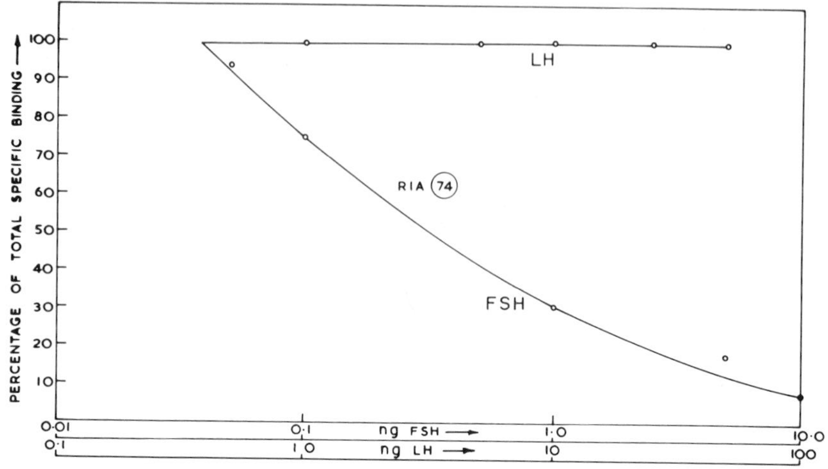

FIG 1. Standard curve for the homologous radioimmunoassay of ovine FSH. Note that LH in the range 0.1 - 100 ng does not interfere.

B. Solid-phase radioimmunoassay of rat serum LH

A number of workers have employed immunosorbents in a variety of forms (7) for the purposes of radioimmunoassay. Polymerized antibodies were first applied for the radioimmunoassay of hCG by Donini (22) and later for steroids by Michail et al. (23). Recently Isozima et al. (24) described a similar procedure using hCG antiserum polymers made with glutaraldehyde. A comparison of assay conditions using polymerized antibodies employed by various workers is given in Table 1. Donini's filtration procedure is tedious and could be expensive when used for routine assay. Cellulose, which was used by the Japanese workers for giving mass to the polymer gave in our hands, high non-specific values. We therefore, used a centrifugation procedure (at 3000 rpm for 15 min at 4°) to separate the polymer pellet; settling of polymer particles was greatly aided by the addition of a pinch of silicic acid. For maintaining

Table 1. A comparison of radioimmunoassay conditions using polymerised antibodies employed by different investigators.

Assay conditions	Donini (20)*	Michail et al (21)	Isozima et al (22)	Present work
Polymerising agent	ECF**	ECF	ECF Glutaraldehyde	ECF
Temperature of assay	4°	Room temperature	37°	37°
Duration of assay	48 hr	2 hr	1 hr	2-12 hr
Shaking	No	No	Yes	No
Incubation volume	0.5 ml	1 ml	0.9 ml	0.3 ml
Nonspecific carrier	Buffer with 0.25% BSA	Buffer	Cellulose or normal rabbit serum	1:100 BSA polymer
Separation	Filtration on oxoid cellulose acetate filters	Centrifugation as such	Centrifugation as such	Centrifugation with a pinch of silicic acid
Hormone measured	hCG	Estrogens	hLH	oLH and rat serum LH.

*the numbers in paranthesis refer to individual references. ** ECF = Ethylchloroformate.

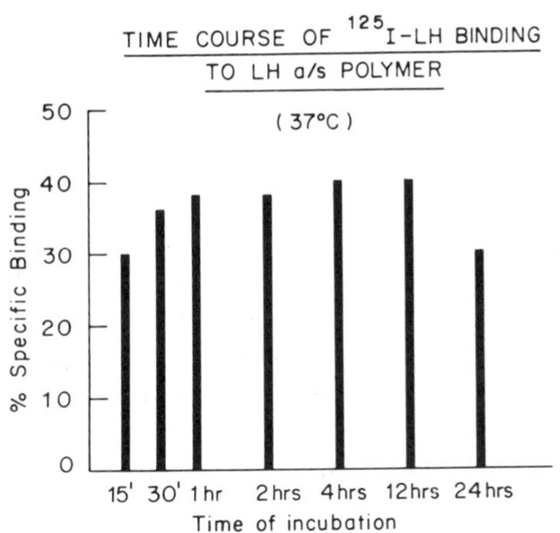

FIG 2. Time course of ^{125}I-LH binding to LH a/s polymer. Aliquots of 1:500 diluted LH a/s polymer were incubated with a known amount of label for varying intervals of time. They were processed as described for bound radioactivity.

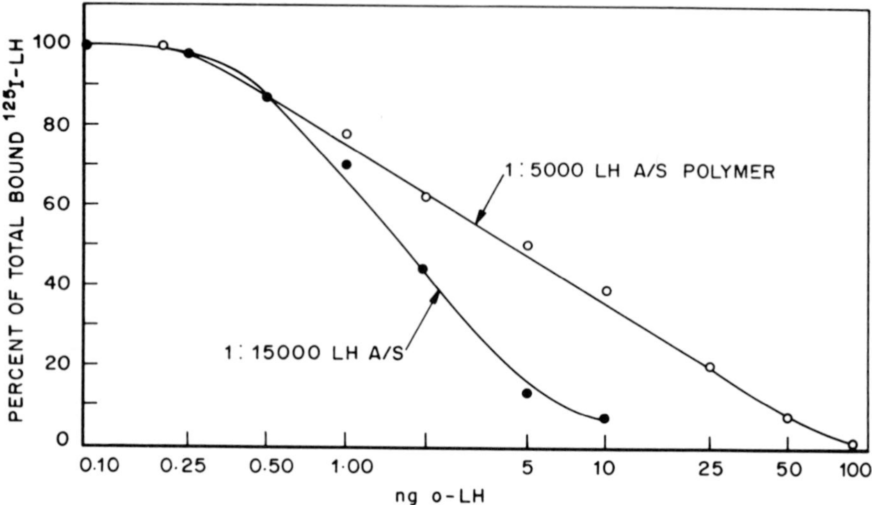

FIG 3. Comparison of standard curves of homologous radioimmunoassay for sheep LH using either a/s polymer or double antibody technique. The incubation time (12 hr) and temperature (37°) with standards and label was same for both the systems.

an uniform density of polymer suspension, the a/s polymer was diluted with a suspension of 0.5 % bovine serum albumin polymer. Earlier studies from our laboratory have shown that radioimmunoassay can be carried out at 37° without appreciable loss in sensitivity (25). At this temperature, the polymer binds maximally within 2-4 hrs (Fig 2). A comparison of the standard curves for the radioimmunoassay of sheep LH using double antibody technique and immunosorbent technique is shown in Fig 3. A compromise between sensitivity of the assay and slope of the standard curve can be achieved by selecting a suitable dilution of the polymer (1:5000 as used in this case). Notwithstanding that this would mean higher consumption of a/s per assay, the fact that the use of second antibody is not necessary would ensure an overall economy.

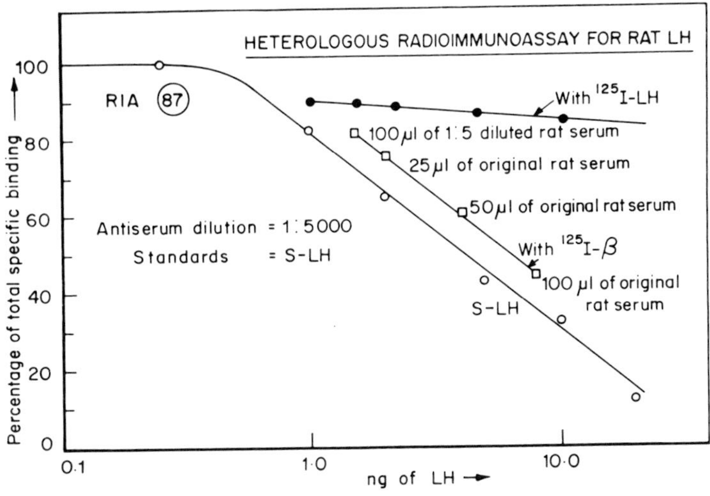

FIG 4. Figure showing the effectiveness of rat serum LH to inhibit the binding of ^{125}I ovine LH-β to ovine LH a/s. Note that rat LH is unable to compete in the same system with labelled whole ovine LH. □———□ inhibition curve with ^{125}I ovine LH-β as labeled hormone. •———• inhibition curve with ^{125}I ovine LH as labeled hormone. o———o standard curve with oLH, with ^{125}I-oLH-β as label.

Using this procedure, we have developed a new heterologous system of radioimmunoassy for rat serum LH. It is known that the β-subunit of oLH confers the species cross-reactivity to oLH (26). A heterologous radioimmunoassay system comprising of oLH a/s and labeled oLH, which was not useful earlier in measuring rat serum LH, could thus be employed for assaying rat LH, by merely changing the labeled hormone to oLH-β (Fig 4). Using this system, serum samples withdrawn at periodic intervals from lactating rats whose litter size had been reduced from an initial 8 to 2 pups on day 4 of lactation were analyzed for LH concentration (Table 2). A steep rise in LH levels could be observed following reduction in suckling stimulus. While the response of prolactin levels to stress, like

Table 2. Serum levels of luteinizing hormone in lactating rats following reduction of pups *

Time after reduction of pups	LH** (ng/ml)
2 hr before	3.3
2 hr	4.0
4 hr	4.2
8 hr	19.25

*Number of pups reduced from 8 to 2 on day 4 of lactation.
** Standard used was oLH of high purity. For details see text.

suckling etc is well documented (27), the reciprocal relationship between prolactin and LH during lactational stress is evident from the above results. Thus the modified solid phase radioimmunoassay has proved to be a fast, simple and reliable technique to obtain assessment of hormonal levels of serum samples.

C. Isolation of gonadotropins from sheep, rat and monkey pituitaries

Conventional techniques of protein hormone purification require large amounts of source material and involve a number of steps. On the other hand, immunosorbents of hormone antisera have been effectively used for the isolation of hormones from small amounts of starting material. Thus Akanuma et al. obtained insulin from plasma using anti-insulin antibodies linked to Sepharose (11). Monkey growth hormone and prolactin were separated from each other using immunosorbent of antiserum to human placental lactogen (9). Similar work has been reported on somatomammotropin (12). We have reported earlier, results of preliminary attempts to isolate pituitary LH and FSH using immunosorbents of the respective antisera (13).

The procedure used essentially follows the principles of affinity chromatography.

1. Preliminary experiments with standard samples: Well characterized rabbit a/s to oLH was polymerized and its capacity to bind standard oLH was assessed by incubating a known amount of a/s polymer with LH in 0.1 M phosphate buffered saline (PBS), pH 7.5, for 1 hr at 4° with constant stirring; the suspension was centrifuged and the pellet washed repeatedly with 0.1 M PBS till the washings were free of any protein. The antibody polymer-hormone complex was then suspended in KI solution prepared in 0.1 M tris, pH 8.5 and kept stirred for 1-2 hr at 4°. It was then centrifuged at 10,000 g for 30 min, the supernatant filtered through a Millipore (0.45 μ) and the clear filtrate dialysed against water. The dialysed solution was directly tested for biological and immunological activity by ovarian ascorbic acid depletion (OAAD) test of Parlow (28) and quantitative precipitin test respectively. Protein measurements were made by the method of Lowry et al (29). As shown in Table 3, 80 percent of the absorbed material could be dissociated with 5.5 KI, of which more than 70 percent could be accounted for, in terms of immunological activity; it was also found to be biologically active.

Table 3. Assessment of the recovery of bound LH from its antibody polymer

Amount of LH (μg)		Dissociating agent used	LH recovered (μg)	% yield by quantitative precipitin test
Loaded	Bound			
2000 *	210	5.5 M KI in 0.1 M tris, pH 8.5 ***	160	76
300 **	190	4 M guanidine-HCl ***	145	76
350 **	200	5.5 M KI in 0.1 M ¶ tris pH 8.5	160	80

0.5 ml of LH a/s polymer was used in each experiment. * NIH-LH-S8 was used; ** LH used was obtained through the courtesy of Profs. C. H. Li and H. Papkoff; *** Carried out at 22°; ¶ Carried out at 3-4°.

Table 4. Average ovarian ascorbic acid depleting activity in various samples : a representative data.

Group	Average OAAD activity (%)
Saline control	0.0
NIH-LH-S12 , 1 μg	5.0
NIH-LH-S12 , 2 μg	14.0
NIH-LH-S12 , 4 μg	40.0
Rat pituitary extract (crude) (350 μg protein)	50.0
Rat LH - isolated	
36 μg protein	13.0
72 μg protein	29.0
144 μg protein	50.0
Monkey pituitary extract (crude) (110 μg protein)	30.0
Monkey LH - isolated	
42 μg protein	8.0
56 μg protein	35.0
84 μg protein	45.0

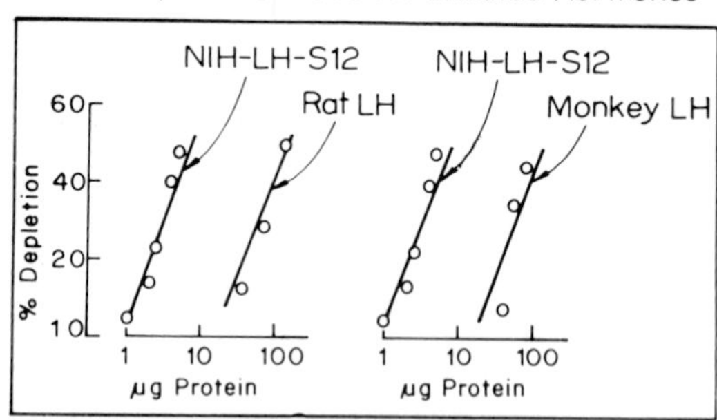

FIG 5. OAAD assay results for isolated rat LH and monkey LH in the form of log dose-response curve.

2. Experiments with pituitary extract: On the basis of the above preliminary data, the immunosorbent was used for isolation of LH and FSH from small amounts of starting material like 50 to 100 rat pituitaries or 4 to 5 monkey or sheep pituitaries. Extracts of pituitaries from sheep or rat were treated with oLH a/s polymer while that of monkey pituitaries, with hCG a/s polymer. Further processing was exactly like the one described for standard LH.

The OAAD activities of LH standards, pituitary extracts and isolated material is presented in Table 4 and Fig 5. While we could account for, in terms of immunological activity 70-80 % of the isolated protein, the isolated materials were less active biologically in terms of NIH-LH-S12; however, the rat LH isolated was equal in potency to NIAMD-rat LH RP-1. Hence modifications were introduced in our procedure to improve biological activities. Thus, reducing the KI concentration resulted in a three-fold increase in the biological activity of the LH without affecting the yield (Table 5).

Table 5. Effect of KI concentration on the yield and biological activity of isolated LH.

In each case 0.5 ml of LH a/s was incubated with 200 μg of highly purified LH. Both unpolymerized and polymerized antisera bind LH to the same extent (0.5 ml binds ~ 140-160 μg LH in each case.

KI	Protein dissociated (μg)	Relative biological activity index *
5.5 M	150	1
4.0 M	115	1.5
3.0 M	146	2.3
3.0 M + 0.01 M $Na_2S_2O_3$	104	2.8

* Expressed as ratio of biological activity of a sample/biological activity of sample using 5.5 M KI.

Table 6. Isolation of LH from rat pituitaries

Number of pituitaries	Polymer equivalent	Yield* (μg) NIH-LH-S12 equivalent
50	1 ml	38
1000	5 ml	700
30	1 ml	25
80	2 ml	64

*Based on bioassay data. 100 pituitaries approximately yielded 150 μg protein.

As is evident from Table 6, hundred rat pituitaries on an average yielded 150 μg of protein of which 80 percent could be accounted for as LH in terms of immunological activity. Disc electrophoretic pattern of the isolated LH as given in Fig 6 indicates the presence of one major band and two minor bands. That the method by itself is very effective in purification is indicated by the reduction in the number of bands with isolated FSH, compared to the number of bands exhibited by the starting material (NIH-FSH).

During the progress of this work, Gospodarowicz reported on the single step purification of LH from sheep pituitary (10), using antibodies linked to Sepharose, and 6 M guanidine hydrochloride as the dissociating agent; this brought about the dissociation of the isolated material into its subunits. However, dialysis against buffers at neutral or alkaline pH resulted in recovery of 50 % of activity.

The method of isolating hormones by use of immunosorbents thus appears promising as indicated by the variety of species for which it has been applied. By this method, small amounts of pure hormones required for radioimmunoassay standards could be easily obtained. Presently the conditions for dissociation of the bound hormone are being modified in order to obtain hormone samples which could be used as standards in bioassay also. Use of more specific bioassays for these

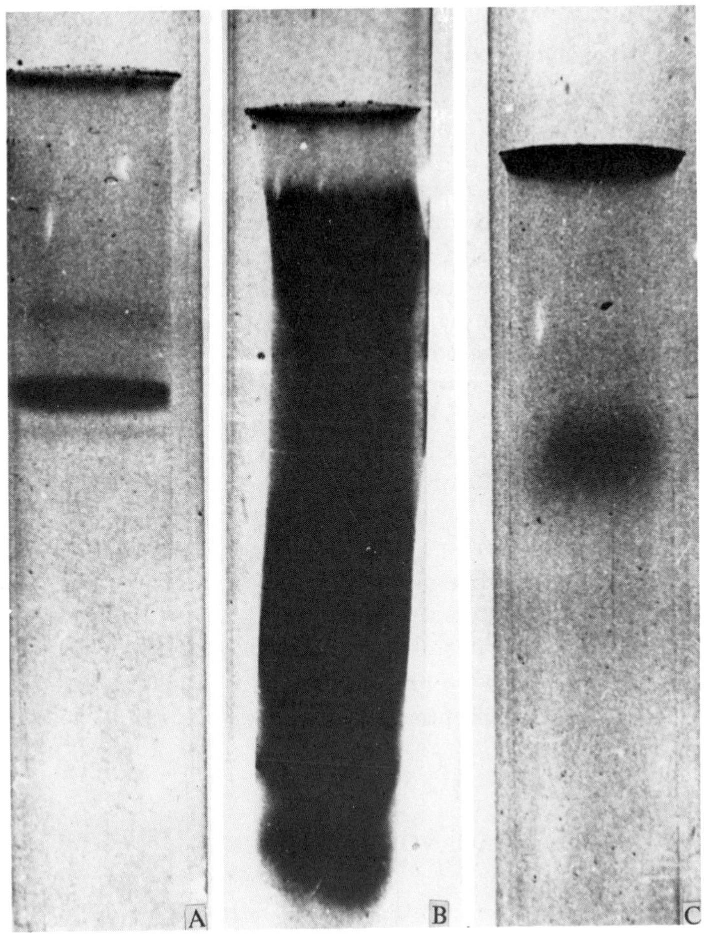

FIG 6. Disc electrophoretic pattern of (A) isolated rat LH, (B) NIH-FSH-S1, (C) sheep FSH purified from NIH-FSH-S1. Electrophoresis was run at acid pH essentially according to Reisfeld et al (32) using 10 % acrylamide gel. Staining was with 0.5 % amido black. Approximately equal amounts were loaded (~ 100 μg).

hormones would obviously yield a better quantitative information on the quality of the product.

GENERAL COMMENTS

As is evident from the foregoing, immunosorbents could be used in many types of studies like purification of antisera, solid phase radioimmunoassays and hormone isolation. Further, use of appropriate immunosorbents of antisera in studies on biosynthesis of protein hormones using *in vitro* systems should make it easier for monitoring the newly formed hormone. Immunoprecipitation has been used earlier by Samli and Geschwind (30) for following pituitary hormone biosynthesis and by Delovich et al. (31) for similar studies on L-chains of immunoglobulins.

Another possible usage is in the purification of antigens by use of the principle of negative absorption. Using antiserum to the proteins present along with the required antigen as immunosorbent, it should be possible to obtain purified antigen. Thus, we have obtained PMSG-enriched serum by treating pregnant mare serum with an immunosorbent made of normal horse serum.

ACKNOWLEDGEMENTS

Supported by generous grants from the Ministry of Health and Family Planning, Government of India, Indian Council of Medical Research, New Delhi, and The Ford Foundation, New York.

REFERENCES

1. Weetal, H.H. In "The Chemistry of Biosurfaces", M.L. Hair (Ed). Vol. II, pp 597, Marcel Dekker, Inc, New York.
2. Cuatrecasas, P. (1971). Ann. Rev. Biochem. 40, 259.
3. Marshall, G.R. and Merrifield, R.B. In "Biochemical aspects of solid state chemistry" G.R. Stark (Ed). pp 111.

Academic Press Inc., New York.
4. Winegard, L. B. (Ed). In "Enzyme Engineering" (1972). Interscience Publishers.
5. Cuatrecasas, P. (1971). In "Methods in Enzymology", W. B. Jakoby (Ed). Vol. 22, pp 345.
6. Goldman, R., Goldstein, L. S. and Katchalski, E. (1971) In "Biochemical aspects of solid state chemistry", G. R. Stark (Ed). pp. 1, Academic Press, New York.
7. Diczfalusy, E. (Ed). (1969). In "Methods in reproductive Endocrinology", Karolinska Symposium on Immunoassay of Gonadotropins.
8. Silman, I. H. and Katchalski, E. (1966). Ann. Rev. Biochem. 35, 873.
9. Guyda, H. J. and Friesen, H. G. (1971). Biochem. Biophys. Res. Comm. 42, 1068.
10. Gospodarowicz, D. (1972). J. Biol. Chem. 247, 6491.
11. Akanuma, Y., Kuzuya, T., Hayashi, M., Ide, T. and Kuzuya, N. (1970). Biochem. Biophys. Res. Comm. 38, 947.
12. Weintraub, B. D. (1970). Biochem. Biophys. Res. Comm. 39, 83.
13. Muralidhar, K., Anantha Samy, T. S. and Moudgal, N. R. (1972). Proc. IV Intl. Cong. Endocrinol. Washington, D. C. Abstract No. 244.
14. Sato, N. and Cargille, C. M. (1972) Endocrinology 90, 302.
15. Cuatrecasas, P. (1969). Biochem. Biophys. Res. Comm. 35, 531.
16. Cuatrecasas, P. (1972). Proc. Natl. Acad. Sci. (USA). 69, 1277.
17. Dufau, M. L. and Catt, K. J. (1973). Nature New Biology, 242, 246.
18. Avrameas, S. and Ternynck, T. (1967). J. Biol. Chem. 242, 1651.
19. Kabat, E. A. and Mayer, M. M. (1964). In "Experimental Immunochemistry", C. C. Thomas Springfield, USA.
20. Jagannadha Rao, A., Moudgal, N. R., Madhwa Raj, H. G., Lipner, H. G. and Greep, R. O. (1974) J. Reprod. Fert. (in press).

21. Greenwood, F.C., Hunter, W.M. and Glover, J.S. (1963). Biochem. J. 89, 114.
22. Donini, P. (1969). In Karolonska Symposium on "Immunoassay of Gonadotropins", E. Diczfalusy (Ed). pp. 257.
23. Michail, G., Chung, H.W., Ferin, M., Vande Wiele, R.L. (1970). In "Immunological Methods in steroid determination". F.G. Peron and B.V. Caldwell (Eds). Appleton Century Crofts, pp 113.
24. Isozima, S., Naka, O., Koyama, K. and Adachi, H. (1970) J. Clin. Endo. Metab. 31, 693.
25. Moudgal, N.R., Moyle, W.R. and Greep, R.O. (1971). J. Biol. Chem. 246, 4983.
26. Moudgal, N.R., Jagannadha Rao, A., Maneckjee, R., Muralidhar, K., Venkatramaiah, M. and Sheela Rani, C.S. (1974). Rec. Prog. Horm. Res. Vol. 30. 47.
27. Meites, J. and Clemens, J.A. (1972). Vitamins & Hormones 30, 166.
28. Parlow, A.F. (1961). in "Human Pituitary Gonadotropins" A. Albert, (Ed). C.C. Thomas Springfield, USA, pp 300.
29. Lowry, O.H., Rosebrough, N.J., Farr, A. and Randall, R.J., (1951). J. Biol. Chem. 193, 265.
30. Samli, M.H., Lai, M.F. and Geschwind, I.I. (1971). Endocrinology 88, 540.
31. Delovitch, T.L., Boyd, S.L., Tsay, H.M., Holme, G. and Sehon, A.H. (1973). Biochem. Biophys. Acta 299, 621.
32. Reisfeld, R.A., Lewis, U.J., and Williams, D.D. (1962). Nature 195, 281.

THE USE OF GRANULOSA CELL CULTURES AND SHORT-TERM INCUBATIONS IN THE ASSAY FOR GONADOTROPINS

Cornelia P. Channing

INTRODUCTION

It has been shown that granulosa cells harvested from medium sized follicles of the mare (1), pig (2,3), monkey (4-6), human (7) and rabbit (8) can respond to low doses of gonadotropins. LH, FSH and chorionic gonadotropin (CG) can stimulate progestin secretion as well as morphological luteinization; the latter involves an increase in cell size, cytoplasmic-nuclear ratio, cytoplasmic lipid droplets and granules. Since these cells form a normal target tissue for gonadotropins and they are also extremely sensitive in culture to gonadotropins, they make a physiologically relevant test system.

Granulosa cells harvested from large preovulatory follicles from pig (2), mare (1) and monkey (4)luteinize spontaneously in culture. However, in the monkey granulosa cells harvested only during or immediately after the LH surge (but not before) luteinize (9). This spontaneous luteinization does not last for more than 6 days in culture; however, it can be maintained even upto 20 days if small amounts of LH, FSH or dibutyryl cyclic AMP (dbcAMP) are added to the cultures (5). This enables the granulosa cell cultures to be used as an assay system not only for gonadotropins responsible for initiating luteinization, but also for those responsible for maintaining the cells in a luteinized state, once the process has been initiated. Granulosa cells harvested from monkey follicles have also been shown to respond to suggested mediators of gonadotropin action such as cyclic AMP (5, 10) and prostaglandins (PGs) of the E series (11). Thus, the long-term cultures consisting of viable cells bridge the gap between the _in vivo_ and the short-term _in vitro_ experiments.

LH and FSH stimulate cyclic AMP production in culture within 5 min (12) and this parallels the degree of luteinization (13). Porcine granulosa cells can bind iodinated hCG and the ability of various tropic hormones to displace this labelled hCG is proportional to their gonadotropic activity (14).

The use of the above parameters in assaying serum LH and CG has been described here. Further, in this presentation our studies on the influences of the gonadotropins of different species, and their subunits, PGs and cyclic AMP on luteinization of monkey granulosa cells in culture have been summarized.

LUTEINIZATION OF RHESUS MONKEY GRANULOSA CELLS

A. Effect of hCG, asialo hCG and hCG subunits

Potencies of tropic hormones and their derivatives have been estimated in granulosa cell cultures, using progestin secretion and morphological luteinization as parameters and hCG rather than LH as standards (6). Rhesus monkeys were given a series of sc injections of PMSG in 10 % gelatin to induce multiple medium-sized follicles (5, 6, 15). Granulosa cells obtained from such ovaries yielded enough cells for about 60 Leighten tube cultures using about 10 x 10^6 cells/culture on a coverslip measuring 10.5 x 35 mm. The cells were grown in a tissue culture medium containing 15 % male and non-midcycle female monkey serum (about 1:1 v/v) the balance being made up of medium 199 containing Earles Salts and 25 mM Hepes buffer (5, 6). Each agent or tropic hormone to be tested in this system was added to duplicate cultures, the cultures being grown at 37.5° and the medium changed on alternate days. The hormone solutions were added at each medium change. The degree of morphological luteinization (4) was assessed by examining the percent covering of the cells on the coverslip on alternate days.

While a dose of 0.1 ng/ml of hCG (14,000-16,000 IU/mg) brought about a barely detectable morphological luteinization, 1 ng/ml of hCG brought about a clear-cut stimulation, the maximal stimulation being seen within 6-8 days at a dose of 100 ng/ml. Luteinization could be maintained only if hCG was present throughout the culture period, since it was lost 4-6 days after its removal (5). It was demonstrated in 7 experiments, that desialization of hCG to an extent of 95 % did not affect its ability to bring about luteinization. Highly purified α and β subunits (CR114 obtained from Dr. R. Canfield) of hCG had no detectable morphological effects at a dose of 1 μg/ml demonstrating that the subunits had less than 1 % of the activity of native hCG.

Table 1. Potency estimates of hCG, asialo hCG, LH and α and β subunits of hCG and LH in monkey granulosa cell cultures.

Hormone preparation	Potency estimate in terms of hCG or oLH	
	Number of determinations	Average potency*
hCG	8	1.0
Asialo hCG (95 % desialylated)	7	1.2 (0.7-2.0)
α-hCG subunit	4	< 0.01
β-hCG subunit (CR-114)	2	< 0.001
o-LH (NIH-oLH-S17)	12	1.0
oLH (HP)	4	2.02
α-oLH subunit (HP)	6	< 0.04
β-oLH subunit (HP)	6	< 0.02
α-oLH subunit (DNW)	2	< 0.015
β-oLH subunit (DNW)	2	< 0.014

* Potency of hCG derivatives are expressed using native hCG as a standard whose potency is defined as 1.0. Potencies of subunits of LH are expressed using native oLH (either NIH-LH having potency of 1.0 or oLH obtained from H. Papkoff having a potency of 2.02) as standards (6, 10).

The potency of hCG and its derivatives could be more quantitatively assessed by an estimation of their ability to stimulate progestin secretion in granulosa cell cultures. The average secretion rate which reached a maximum with hCG (6) between 6 and 8 days or the total secretion rate over a 12-day period has been employed as a potency estimate of tropic activity; the latter assessment is advantageous since it obliterates variation in day-to-day secretion rates. The potency of native hCG has been defined as 1.0 and that of other derivatives compared with it. Effect of hCG on progestin secretion paralleled its effect on morphological luteinization (Table 1). Asialo hCG had a potency equal to or slightly greater than hCG, whereas the purified subunits had less than 1 % of the activity of the native hormone. Asialo hCG, but not the subunits of hCG have been shown to bind to granulosa cells (14). Dufau et al. (16) have made similar observations on activities of hCG and its subunits using the rat testis. Thus sialic acid appears not to be required for expression of activity of hCG at the target cell.

B. Effects of ovine LH and its subunits

Using granulosa cells obtained from PMSG-treated monkeys, we have demonstrated that oLH is able to stimulate morphological luteinization and progestin secretion, while the subunits of LH are inactive (10) (Table 1).

C. Comparison of activities of mammalian, reptilian and piscine gonadotropins

An advantage of using the monkey granulosa cell cultures is that, it is possible to test in this system the gonadotropic activities of various species. Using this system we have shown that rhesus monkey (Rh) LH, FSH and CG, human LH, FSH and CG, ovine and bovine LH and FSH, and surprisingly turtle (T) gonadotropin are active in stimulating luteinization and progestin secretion (Tables 2 and 3). Turtle gonadotropin was active, but piscine (salmon) gonadotropin was inactive at a dose of 100 μg/ml (17). Chicken gonadotropin (Table 2) showed intermediate activity. The chick LH of Follett had some activity in the primate granulosa cell system equivalent to that obtained in the OAAD; however, it was only a small fraction (0. 15 x NIH-oLH-S1) compared to the activity of this LH in the chicken ^{32}P uptake assay, which was 1.35 U/mg (Tables 2 and 3). Standard bioassays for the various hormones were used: the Parlow ascorbic acid depletion assay (OAAD) for LH (18), the hCG-augmentation assay for FSH (19), the mouse uterine weight assay to measure total gonadotropin activity (20), the lizard testicular assay for turtle gonadotropin (21), the ^{32}P-uptake into the 1-day old chick testis to measure bird gonadotropin (22), and the McKenzie assay (23) for TSH activity.

Attempts to determine potencies per se of the various gonadotropins in relation to one another are difficult because of lack of knowledge on the appropriate choice of a standard. It is clear from Table 2 that both LH and FSH of primate and non-primate

Table 2. Effects of human, monkey, ovine and turtle gonadotropins on the progestin secretion rate in replicate cultures of granulosa cells harvested from PMSG-treated monkeys.

No.	Gonadotropin added (U or μg/ml)	Progestin secretion rate over a 12-day period (ng/culture)		
		Value 1	Value 2	Average
M135	Control	246	375	309
	0.2 mU (0.03 μg) RhLH	12,948	12,604	12,791
	2.0 mU (0.05 μg) RhTSH	6,309	4,139	5,224
	0.2 IU (0.1 μg) RhCG	13,569	8,858	11,198
	2.0 mU (0.04 μg) RhFSH	6,309	4,139	5,224
	0.38 mU (0.1 μg) hLH	32,713	23,875	23,392
		18,811	18,170	
	1.4 IU (0.1 μg) hCG	14,403	13,094	13,748
	20 U (0.1 μg) hFSH	6,729	7,740	7,234
	2.0 mU (1 μg) oLH	2,909	4,532	3,720
	1 μg t-GTH	936	844	890
	10 μg t-GTH	6,846	7,175	7,010
M159	Control	612	359	485
	0.38 mU (0.1 μg) hLH	>9,375	>9,375	>9,375
	0.038 mU (0.01μg) hLH	6,998	6,242	6,620
	0.1 mU (0.1 μg) oLH	2,305	779	1,542
	1.0 mU (1.0 μg) oLH	3,907	9,375	6,641
	1.0 mU (1.0 μg) bLH	8,839	4,652	6,745
M153	Control	13	42	27
	0.38 mU (0.1 μg) hLH	1,888	1,632	1,760
	0.1 mU (0.1 μg) oLH	181	299	240
	1.0 mU (1.0 μg) oLH	2,796	1,966	2,367
	0.025 mU (0.01 μg) oLH	779	318	548
	0.25 mU (0.1 μg) oLH	1,066	1,666	1,386
	1.0 mU (1.0 μg) oFSH	877	1,289	1,083
	1 μg Bird LH	50	37	43
	5 μg Bird LH	265	291	278

Gonadotropins were added to the cultures at each change of medium on alternate days. Progestin content of the media at each medium change was determined and totalled over a 12-day period to give the values shown in the table. Data on turtle gonadotropin (t-GTH) are taken from Channing et al (17) and others are unpublished. Units are expressed in terms of the appropriate NIH-oLH or NIH-oFSH standards except in the case of hCG which is expressed in terms of the 2nd IRP-hCG(obtained from Dr. D. Bangham, W.H.O.)

origin are potent in this system. Furthermore hLH and RhLH appear to be more active compared to oLH whether expressed on a weight basis or on the basis of NIH-oLH-S1 units. Differences in potencies of the primate or oLH cannot be explained entirely by differences in purity of the gonadotropins and they may be due to some inherent differences in the molecules themselves.

Highly purified human and monkey FSH, which was virtually devoid of contaminating LH showed stimulatory activity. The NIH-oFSH which had contaminating LH (1 %) showed an activity greater than that predicted for FSH alone (Tables 2 and 3). Highly purified oFSH obtained from Papkoff (50 x NIH-oFSH-S1) was also

Table 3. Source and bioassay potencies of various gonadotropins employed for these studies.

Donor *		Hormone	Potency
W. D. Peckham	(24)	RhLH (WDP X p 101 A)	6.7U/mg
	(25)	RhFSH (WDP XI 2 B)	115 IU /mg
	(26)	RhCG (WDP XI, p23 #29)	5000 IU/mg
	(25)	RhTSH (WDP X, p 103, #31)	39 U/mg
	(27)	hFSH (WDP X, p 15 #28 32)	200 U/mg
A. S. Hartree	(28)	hLH (DEAE-I, 19-1-65)	3.8 U /mg
H. Papkoff	(29)	oLH (HP-G3-206)	2.02 U/mg
	(30)	oFSH (HP)	50 U/mg
	(31)	Turtle GTH (T-GTH)	0.8-1.0 U/mg**
R. Canfield	(32)	hCG	13,000-16,000 IU /mg
W. H. McShan		oLH	2.5 U/mg
J. D. Pierce	(33)	bLH	1 U/mg
B. K. Follett	(34)	Chicken LH	0.153 U/mg (OAAD) 1.35 U/mg §

* Numbers in parantheses refer to the original references of the donors detailing the method of preparation and assay. **Potency was estimated in the lizard assay. § Potency was estimated by the ^{32}P uptake assay in chicks.

active in this system (17). The activity of the monkey TSH in this system was accounted for by its high LH contamination (Dr. W. D. Peckham, personal communication).

D. Effect of cyclic AMP and prostaglandins

Earlier studies have clearly demonstrated that dbcAMP and cyclic AMP could stimulate luteinization and progestin secretion in monkey granulosa cell cultures (35). Addition of imidazole, a stimulant of phosphodiesterase activity, inhibits spontaneous luteinization of monkey granulosa cell cultures and stimulation of luteinization by LH (5). On the other hand, addition of small amounts of aminophylline, a phosphodiesterase inhibitor, potentiates the luteinizing action of small doses of LH (9). These results give credence to the suggestion that cyclic AMP is the mediator of luteinization.

Prostaglandins of the E series could stimulate granulosa cell luteinization in terms of morphology and progestin secretion (11), while PGFs were weak in causing luteinization. Since addition of PGs along with LH inhibited the action of the latter (11) it is probable that they are not the sole mediators of LH action, particularly in porcine granulosa cell suspensions their effects together with LH were more than additive in stimulating cyclic-AMP production (12). Inhibitors of prostaglandin action such as 7-oxa-13 prostynoic acid, which by themselves have no effect on granulosa cell luteinization, inhibited the action of PGE_2 and hCG on luteinization (36). When the inhibitor was mixed with the PG or LH agonist there was severe cellular necrosis thus complicating interpretation of such data.

LUTEINIZATION OF PORCINE GRANULOSA CELLS IN CULTURE

A. Effects of LH, FSH and hCG

Granulosa cells harvested from large preovulatory porcine follicles luteinize spontaneously in culture and in some instances can respond to exogenous LH, FSH (2,35) hCG and choriocarcinoma gonadotropin (3,37). Cultures of granulosa cells obtained from medium sized follicles consistently responded to LH or FSH with a stimulation of morphological luteinization and progestin secretion (2). As in the monkey granulosa cell cultures, it is necessary to add the hormones at each change of medium (37). Rabbit granulosa cell cultures may also be used as an assay system for LH (8).

B. Effects of various nucleotides

As was the case in the monkey, dbcAMP or cyclic AMP granulosa cell luteinization in terms of morphology and progestin secretion (9,38). Cyclic AMP when compared to other cyclic nucleotides, tri- and monophosphates was found to have a greater potency in stimulating luteinization and progestin secretion (9).

Similar observations have been made by Jungmann and Halpren with dbcAMP. (personal communication).

EFFECT OF GONADOTROPINS AND OTHER AGENTS ON CYCLIC AMP LEVELS IN PORCINE GRANULOSA CELL SUSPENSIONS

Both LH and FSH can increase cyclic AMP levels in granulosa cells obtained from medium sized follicles (12). Stimulation was specific to gonadotropins since TSH had low activity and ACTH and prolactin were totally inactive. Cells from large follicles (6-12) are best suited for use as they are more sensitive to LH and respond with the greatest magnitude (13); they contain more LH-hCG receptors compared to cells obtained from smaller follicles (39).

This system can also be used to assay inhibitors of gonadotropic action such as a possible follicular fluid inhibitor (40). The follicular fluid is incubated for 48 hr with the cells followed by washing and a post incubation with oLH (1 μg/ml). The inhibitory influence of the fluid on the LH stimulation of cyclic AMP is then measured. Follicular fluid from small follicles appear to have a greater inhibitory influence compared to that from large follicles. Investigation into the nature of the inhibitor is being carried out.

STUDIES ON BINDING OF RADIO-IODINATED HCG TO PORCINE GRANULOSA CELLS

A. Characteristics of gonadotropin binding

Preincubation of cells from large and medium follicles with small amounts of unlabelled hCG, LH or asialo hCG, produced about 95 % inhibition of binding of labelled hCG after 10-30 min of incubation (14, 39); FSH, ACTH and TSH as well as subunits of hCG (14) and LH (Table 4) were unable to inhibit this binding of ^{125}I-hCG indicating the binding to be specific and sensitive.

Sialic acid is not required for binding since asialo hCG was as active as native hCG in inhibiting binding of the iodinated hormone (14). It was a better inhibitor of binding of radioiodinated hCG than the native hCG itself and this perhaps might be due to the sugar moiety in the native hCG bringing about steric hindrance for binding. Binding of gonadotropins to granulosa and other cells has been reviewed extensively elsewhere (41). Suffice it here to

Table 4 Competition of unlabeled oLH and its subunits with ^{125}I hCG for binding to porcine granulosa cells

LH or hCG added	Amount (μg/ml)	^{125}I hCG bound % control		
		Expt 1	Expt 2	Average
hCG	0	100		
	0.001	100		
	0.01	54		
	0.05	21		
	0.1	10		
	0.5	15		
	1.0	10		
NIH-oLH-S18	0	100	100	100
	0.05	106	81	93
	0.1	87	71	79
	1.0	31	31	31
HP-oLH	0	100		
	0.05	85		
	0.1	64		
	0.5	42		
	1.0	21		
oLH-α (HP)	0	100	100	100
	0.05	99	-	99
	0.1	102	102	102
	0.5	88	106	97
	1.0	45	78	61
	10.0	-	34	34
oLH-β (HP)	0	100	100	100
	0.05	99	95	97
	0.1	93	100	96
	0.5	90	97	93
	1.0	83	-	83
	10.0	44	36	40

Granulosa cells were harvested from medium sized (3-5mm) porcine follicles and preincubated for 10 min with either hCG, NIH-oLH (NIH-oLH-S18; 1.03 x NIH-oLH-S1), Papkoff oLH (HP oLH; 2.01 x NIH-oLH-S1) or α or β subunits of Papkoff oLH. Subsequently the cells were incubated with 0.1 μg/ml ^{125}I-hCG (6 x 10^6cpm) for 10 min at 37° as detailed previously[14]. Values are expressed as a percent of cpm bound to cells pre-incubated in the absence of added tropic hormones. Each value shown is the average of 3 separate incubations using a given pool of cells.

say that the granulosa cells have receptors to both LH and hCG and are saturable with respect to the dose of the hormone, time of incubation and have either tight binding or a slow turnover of the hormone at the receptor. Cells from large follicles bind more hCG than those from small follicles (39, 42).

Primate and ovine LH but not reptilian or piscine hormones can inhibit binding of iodinated hCG to its receptor (Channing - unpublished). While turtle gonadotropins have been shown to be biologically potent in the monkey granulosa cell culture, it is unable to displace iodinated hCG from its receptor, which perhaps means that it has, like FSH, a receptor different from that of hCG or LH (17).

B. Assay for LH or CG using inhibition of binding of labelled hCG

Preliminary data on the use of porcine granulosa cell system for the assay of LH activity are presented here. Serum samples and pools of sera from monkeys (obtained from Dr. Knobil and his associates) have been assayed for LH by radioimmunoassay using an anti-hCG serum (Organon antiserum 267, against β-subunit of hCG) as outlined by Karsch et al (24) and Monroe et al. (26,43). An RhLH standard with a potency of 1.9 x NIH-LH-S1 was used.

In our system for each assay granulosa cells were obtained from large porcine follicles and about 5 x 10^6 cells were incubated with labeled hCG as described previously (15,39). The cells could be stored at 4°, suspended in medium 199 or Eagles medium containing 15 % pig serum for at least 4 days. Sera (0.1 - 0.4 ml) or standard hCG or LH were incubated with cells in a total volume of 0.9 ml in medium Y (15 % pig serum in Eagle's medium) for 30 min with shaking at 37°. 0.1 or 0.05 µg of ^{125}I - or ^{131}I-hCG in 0.1 ml of medium Y was added and the cells incubated for another 30 min followed by 4 washes with 0.9 % NaCl containing 1 % bovine serum albumin, pH 7.4 and counting in an autogamma counter. 0.001, 0.005, 0.01 and 1 µg/ml hCG as well as 0.005 and 0.01 µg/ml of RhLH were used as standards in these studies. The hCG, RhLH standards (1.9 U/mg) and hLH (3.8 U/mg) produced parallel curves of inhibition; the extent of inhibition by the unknown serum samples was computed using the hCG standard curve. These could be converted to RhLH values for comparative purposes by multiplying the values with 2 (3.8/1.9). LH estimates by our granulosa cell radioligand assay (GC-RLA-CPC) were comparable to the values obtained by Knobil radioimmunoassay (RIA-EK)(Table 5). However, in a number of instances values obtained by the GC-RLA-CPC were slightly lower than those obtained by the RIA-EK. This could be attributed to the fact that the radioligand assay measures only biologically active hormone, while the RIA measures native hormone as well as subunits. It is probable that subunits or aggregates of LH in addition to native LH are at times found in circulation. Comparison of the values of LH in sera during various physiological states as measured by the two assays may further elucidate this point.

Figure 1 shows the displacement produced by 0.2 ml of preovulatory monkey serum, which is quite significant. Thus this assay has great potential as it measures biologically active

Table 5. Monkey serum LH levels measured by granulosa cell radio-ligand assay (RLA) and radioimmunoassay.

No.	Sample	Volume (ml)	RhLH (ng/ml)	
			Granulosa cell RLA	Radioimmunoassay
P 135A	Ovariectomized monkey serum	0.4	14.5	20
	Ovariectomized monkey serum	0.2	17.5	20
	Female 716 (11/11/72)	0.4	60	>50
P 135B	Female 747 (12/25/72)	0.4	6	2.7
	747 (12/27/72)	0.2	18	38
	747 (12/27/72)	0.1	22	38
	747 (12/26/72)	0.4	<5	2.8
	747 (12/24/72)	0.4	<5	2.6
	747 (12/27 A)	0.2	33	42.7
	747 (12/27 A)	0.05	~40	42.7
	747 (12/27 B)	0.1	40	38.9
	716 (11/11/72)	0.4	20	>50
	716 (11/11/72)	0.1	28	>50
	716 (11/8/72)	0.4	<5	2.1
	716 (11/9/72)	0.4	<5	2.2
P 143	Ovariectomized monkey serum	0.4	25	20
	Low LH monkey serum pool	0.4	<10	9
	Hypophysectomized monkey serum pool	0.4	<10	2

The Rh LH (1.9 x NIH-oLH-S1) and hCG (13-15,000 IU/mg) used as standards were generously donated by Drs. E. Knobil and R. Canfield respectively. In inhibition of hCG-binding, hCG had an activity equivalent to hLH (3.8 x NIH-S1). In order to convert serum values, using an hCG standard curve, to LH values the estimates were multiplied by 2. I am grateful to Dr. E. Knobil and his associates for performing LH radioimmunoassays and providing various monkey serum samples.

hormone and can be done rapidly (in 3-6 hr depending upon the ready availability of cells). Furthermore, it has a high degree of specificity as well as sensitivity. The variables such as time of preincubation and amount of labelled hormone to be used have to be changed in a systematic fashion in order to arrive at the greatest sensitivity possible. Our preliminary results (from 3 experiments) show that other serum constituents do not interfere with the assay since the addition of 0.2 ml/ml of hypophysectomized serum does not displace labelled hCG from the cells nor does it inhibit the binding produced by 0.01 μg/ml hCG. The labelled hormone is reasonably stable if the iodination is carried out for less than 30 seconds, a longer time causing destruction of the hormone and

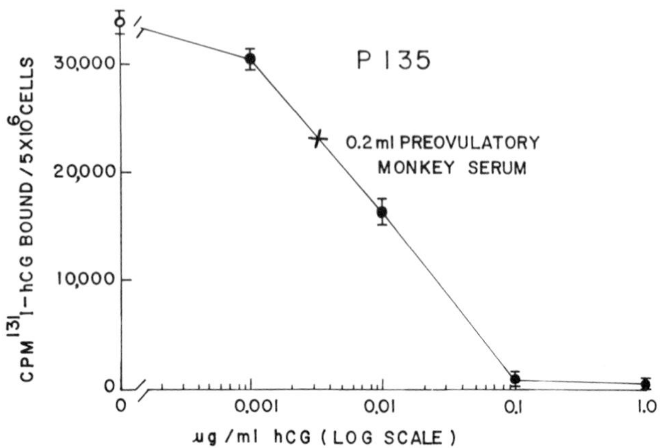

FIG 1. Effect of unlabelled hCG and 0.2 ml preovulatory monkey serum (indicated by an X on the curve) upon binding of ^{131}I-hCG to porcine granulosa cells (cells from large follicles).

a high degree of non-displaceable binding. Finally, in order to get good inhibition of binding it is necessary to add the unlabelled hormone or serum before, rather than after the iodinated hCG (39).

ACKNOWLEDGEMENTS

The collaboration of Drs. Sandra Kammerman, Harold Papkoff, Paul Licht and Edward Donaldson is gratefully acknowledged. The expert technical assistance of Mrs. Viki Tsai, Mrs. Maxine Montgomery and Mr. James Cover is appreciated. Donors of the varióur hormone preparations mentioned in the text are gratefully acknowledged. The co-operation of Dr. Ernst Knobil and his associates in performing monkey serum LH assays is appreciated. Supported by grants HD 03315 from the Institute of Child Health and Human Development, USPHS and by a grant from the Population Council, New York.

REFERENCES

1. Channing, C.P. (1969). J. Endocrinology 43, 415.
2. Channing, C.P. (1970). Endocrinology 87, 156.
3. Van Thiel, D.H., Bridson, W.E. and Kohler, P.O. (1971) Endocrinology 89, 622.
4. Channing, C.P. (1970). Endocrinology 87, 49.
5. Channing, C.P. (1973). Endocrinology (in press).
6. Channing, C.P. and Kammerman, S. (1973). Endocrinology. 93, 1035.
7. Channing, C.P., Butt, W.R. and Crooke, A.C. (1969). Excerpta Medica International Congress Series No. 157, Abs. 306.
8. Shirley, A. and Stephenson, J. (1973). J. Endocrinology 58, 346.
9. Channing, C.P. (1973). In "Regulation of Mammalian Reproduction", S.J. Segal, R. Crozier, P. Corfman and P.A. Condliffe, (Eds). pp. 505.
10. Channing, C.P. (1973). Endocrinology (in press).
11. Channing, C.P. (1972). Prostaglandins 2, 331.
12. Kolena, J. and Channing, C.P. (1972). Endocrinology 90, 1543.
13. Channing, C.P. (1973). In Proceedings of the IV International Congress of Endocrinology, Washington, D.C. June 1972. E.O. Scow. (Ed). (in press).
14. Kammerman, S.K., Canfield, R.E., Kolena, R.E. and Channing, C.P. (1972). Endocrinology 91, 65.
15. Channing, C.P. and Ledwitz-Rigby (1973) In "Methods in Enzymology", J. Hardman and B.W. O'Malley (Eds). Academic Press, New York (in press).
16. Dufau, M.L., Catt, K.J., and Tsuruhara, T. (1970) Biochem. Biophys. Acta 252, 574.
17. Channing, C.P., Licht, P., Papkoff, H. and Donaldson, E.M. (1973). Gen. Comp. Endocrinol. (in press).
18. Parlow, A.F. (1961). In "Human Pituitary Gonadotropins", A. Albert, (Ed). pp 300, Thomas, Springfield, Illinois.
19. Steelman, S.L. and Pohley, R.M. (1953). Endocrinology 53, 604.
20. Brown, P.S. (1955). J. Endocrinology 13, 15.
21. Licht, P. and Pearson, A.K. (1969). Gen. Comp. Endocrinol. 13, 367.
22. Breneman, W.R., Zeller, F.J. and Creck, R.O. (1962). Endocrinology 71, 790.

23. McKenzie, J.M. (1958). Endocrinology 63, 372.
24. Karsch, F.J., Weick, R.F., Butler, W.R., Dierschke, O.J, Krey, L.C., Weiss, G., Hotchkiss, J., Yamaji, T., and Knobil, E. (1973). Endocrinology 92, 1740.
25. Yamaji, T., Peckham, W.D., Atkinson, L.E., Dierschke, D.J. and Knobil, E. Endocrinology 92, 1652.
26. Monroe, S.E., Peckham, E.D., Neill, J.D. and Knobil, E. (1970). Endocrinology 86, 1012.
27. Peckham, W.D. and Parlow, A.F. (1969). Endocrinology 84, 953.
28. Hartree, A.S. (1966). Biochem. J. 100, 754.
29. Papkoff, H., Gospodarowicz, D., Candiotti, A. and Li, C.H. (1965). Arch. Biochem. Biophys. 111, 431.
30. Papkoff, H., Gospodarowicz, D. and Li, C.H. (1967). Arch. Biochem. Biophys. 120, 434.
31. Papkoff, H. and Licht, P. (1972). Proc. Soc. Exp. Biol. Med. 139, 372.
32. Morgan, R.J. and Canfield, R.E. (1971). Endocrinology 88, 1045.
33. Pierce, J.G., Liao, T.H., Howard, S.M. and Shome, B. (1971). Rec. Prog. Horm. Res. 27, 165.
34. Scanes, C.G. and Follett, B.K. (1972). Br. Poult. Sci. 13, 603.
35. Channing, C.P. (1970). Rec. Prog. Horm. Res. 26, 584.
36. Channing, C.P. (1972). Prostaglandins 2, 351.
37. Channing, C.P. and Crisp, T. (1972). Gen. Comp. Endocr. Suppl. No. 3, 3, 617.
38. Channing, C.P. and J.F. Seymour (1970). Endocrinology 87, 165.
39. Channing, C.P. and Kammerman, S. (1973). Endocrinology 92, 531.
40. Ledwitz-Rigby, E. and Channing, C.P. (1973). Biol. Reprod. Abstract.
41. Channing, C.P. and Kammerman, S. (1973). Biol. Reprod. (in press).
42. Schomberg, D.W. and Tyrey, L. (1972). Biol. Reprod. 7, 127. Abstract 79.
43. Monroe, S.R., Neill, J.D., Atkinson, L.E. and Knobil, E. (1970). Endocrinology 87, 453.

GONADOTROPIC CONTROL OF THE DEVELOPMENT OF TESTES AND ACCESSORY ORGANS

M.R.N. Prasad

The dependence of the testis and accessory glands of reproduction on gonadotropins will be discussed with reference to key events in prenatal and postnatal development. The role of gonadotropins in the development, differentiation and function of the fetal testis and accessory organs has been reviewed exhaustively (1-5).

The classical experiments of fetal castration at different stages of development of rabbit by Jost (1) demonstrated the crucial role of the fetal testis in testicular and accessory organ development. He showed that the presence of the fetal testis during days 20-26 was essential for the establishment of the male type of development. The lack of influence of the fetal testis at this stage resulted in feminization. Clear-cut evidence in support of the existence of a pituitary-gonadal axis in the fetus of rabbits was obtained by fetal decapitation experiments (1). In fetuses which were decapitated on day 18 or 19 (before the regression of the Müllerian duct), the genital tract was abnormal in development and this could be prevented by the administration of PMSG to the fetuses on the day of decapitation. Time sequence study of the effect of decapitation of fetuses from days 18 to 24 showed that the presence of the fetal pituitary on days 22-24 was necessary for maintaining the function of the fetal testis. An examination of the pituitary gland of the fetuses during this period showed accumulation of PAS-positive granules from days 19-22 followed by a marked decrease thereafter. Fetal decapitation at the end of the II period of development had no effect on sexual organogenesis. These results indicate that the fetal pituitary produces a gonadotropic substance(s) which stimulate(s) the fetal testis optimally during a limited, but critical period of development and differentiation of the testis and accessory organs.

Anencephalic human fetuses offer a comparable physiological situation for an understanding of the role of gonadotropins during development. Anencephaly results in a marked hypoplasia of the external genitalia (6). In human anencephalic fetuses lacking adenohypophysis, there is a trend towards reduced size of the testis and penis; however, masculinization of the genital tract occurs which may be due to the action of hCG on the fetal testis (2).

Appearance of peak levels of hCG in pregnant women (i.e., 7-9 weeks) coincide with the period of maximal sexual organogenesis in the male fetuses. During this period, the interstitial cells are well developed and genital ducts, urinogenital sinus and external genitalia acquire definite characteristics. The stimulation of Leydig cells of the fetal testis is due to the action of gonadotropins secreted by the fetal pituitary and/or hCG which doubly ensures normal sexual development and differentiation. Even after the decline in the levels of hCG, the interstitial cells of the human fetal testis continue to hypertrophy reaching a maximum at the age of 18 weeks, indicating regulation by the fetal pituitary. Hypospadias occurs if the fetal pituitary is absent in phase III of development (period of stabilization); after the sixth month, interstitial cells normally decrease suggesting a lowering of both fetal pituitary and placental gonadotropins (2). Abramovich and Rowe (7) found high levels of plasma testosterone in early to midterm human male fetuses (12-18 weeks) which parallels the maximal occurence of both Leydig cell hyperplasia and of Δ^5, 3β hydroxysteroid dehydrogenase activity in the fetal testis (8). Similar observations were made by Reyes et al. (9). These studies show that for a period of about two weeks after the formation of the external genitalia,there are high levels of plasma testosterone associated with Leydig cell hyperplasia (7). It is probably that human sexual differentiation parallels that in the guinea pig, in which development of external genitalia occurs during early and mid pregnancy (10). High levels of testosterone occur in the plasma of the umbilical artery of male fetuses of the rhesus monkey and are secreted by the fetal testis (11); the physiological function of testosterone secreted by the fetal testis is to affect the central nervous system regulating reproductive function. It has been demonstrated that testosterone injected to pregnant rhesus monkeys not only masculinizes the reproductive tract (12, 13), but also the areas of the central nervous system which are associated with behaviour (14). It is likely that imprinting of the hypothalamus by testosterone in the human male fetus occurs sometime between 14-18 weeks of gestation when the development of external genitalia has taken place (7); during this period high plasma testosterone levels are found.

Another approach to the study of the role of the pituitary-gonadal axis of the fetus during sexual development is by the use of specific antibodies against luteinizing hormone or testosterone and use of selective inhibitors to block steroidogenesis in the fetal testis. Goldman et al. (15) used rat as the experimental model in which the role of pituitary during masculine development and differentiation is ill-understood; rat fetuses decapitated at the time of sexual development show little inhibition of masculine differentiation, but the embryonic rat testis grafted into adults elicit androgenic activity indicating the role of fetal pituitary in stimulation of the fetal testis (1). Administration of anti-LH/FSH to the pregnant rat during days 13-21 of pregnancy induced hypospadias, nipple development and reduction in ano-genital distance in male rat fetuses. These results demonstrate that the inhibition of masculine development is mediated by the passage of the antibody to LH/FSH through the placental barrier and reducing the level of circulating gonadotropins in the fetus; consequent reduction in steroidogenesis by the fetal testis causes failure of masculinization of the genitalia.

The role of testicular hormones secreted by the fetal testis in masculinization of the genital ducts and development of accessory glands and external genitalia has been clearly demonstrated by Jost (1). These were confirmed by the observations of Neumann et al. (16) who showed that administration of the antiandrogen, cyproterone acetate to pregnant rats from days 13-21 of pregnancy resulted in feminization of male fetuses; the Wolffian ducts were regressed, external genitalia were as in the genetic females and the Müllerian ducts were not resorbed. These studies support the concept of Jost that the fetal testis secretes an androgenic substance which has a crucial role to play during a critical phase of development of sex accessories. Similar results were obtained by the administration of cyanoketone (2α-cyano-4,4, 17α-trimethyl-androst-5-en-17β-ol-3-one), an inhibitor of Δ^5, 3β hydroxysteroid dehydrogenase, and antibodies against testosterone dihydrotestosterone (15).

Steroidogenesis by the fetal testis has been studied extensively in a number of species. Lippsett and Tullner (17) showed that in the rabbit fetal testis testosterone synthesis could be demonstrated prior to the appearance of Leydig cells; the conversion of pregnenolone to testosterone increased with the age of gestation. In the fetal sheep, androgen content of the fetal testis has been demonstrated on the 30th day of gestation, five days before the onset of sexual differentiation (3). Wilson and Siiteri (18) studied the steroidogenic ability of fetal rabbit testis as a function of the age of the embryos using different precursors and demonstrated a parallelism between events during masculinization of the male genital tract and pattern of testosterone synthesis by the fetal testis. They concluded that the enzyme Δ^5, 3β hydroxysteroid dehydrogenase and isomerase crucial in the pathway of testosterone biosynthesis is acquired between days 17-19, while all the enzymes involved in the synthesis of testosterone appear on days 21-23. Testosterone may be the active androgen in mediating differentiation of Wolffian ducts into the epididymis, ductus deferens and seminal vesicles (19).

The fetal testis of rabbit secretes a Müllerian duct-inhibiting substance distinct from testosterone (1); similar studies have also been made in the rat and guinea pig. The chemical nature of Müllerian-inhibiting substance (hormone) is not clearly established; the hormone is non-dialyzable (20) and its secretion is restricted to the fetal or early post-natal period (21). Josso (22) demonstrated by <u>in vitro</u> culture technique that the Müllerian-inhibiting hormone may be produced by the fetal Sertoli cells of the calf-testicular tissue. The Müllerian-inhibiting hormone of the human testis is species-nonspecific in its action (23).

It has been established that mechanisms regulating the release of gonadotropins in the male rat are organized by the secretion of androgens by the neonatal testes (24, 25). It has recently been demonstrated that a pituitary-gonadal feed back system exists soon after birth in the male rat (26). Inhibition of testicular steroidogenesis by administration of antiserum to gonadotropins in the newborn male rat results in failure to mate, when they reach adulthood; since spermatozoa were present in the testes, the failure to mate was attributed to impairment of sexual behaviour (27). These results were further confirmed by the administration of antiserum to gonadotropins on days 1, 3 & 5 postnatally. The fact that masculinization of the behavioral centre did not occur in neonatal male rats treated with antiserum to gonadotropin, suggests that the pituitary gland participates in postnatal sexual differentiation of these centres. Similar conclusions were also drawn by Arai and Serisawa (28) who found that treatment of neonatal male rats with gonadotropic hormones advanced the differentiation of the masculine pattern of release of gonadotropic hormones.

REFERENCES

1. Jost, A. (1953). In Rec. Prog. Horm. Res. <u>8</u>, 379.

2. Jost, A. (1966) In "The Pituitary Gland", G.W. Harris and B.T. Donovan (Eds) Butterworth, London.
3. Jost, A. (1971) In "Hermaphroditism, Genitial abnormalities and related Endocrine disorders." 2nd Rev. Edn., H.W. Jones and W.W. Scott (Eds). p. 16, Baltimore, Williams and Wilkins.
4. Jost, A. (1972). Johns Hopkins Med. J. 13, 38.
5. Jost, A., Vigier, B., Prepin, J., and Perchellet, J. (1973). Rec. Prog. Horm. Res. 29.
6. Bearn, J.G. (1959). Lancet. ii. 464.
7. Abramovich, D.R. and Rowe, P. (1973). J. Endocr. 56, 121.
8. Niemi, M., Ikonen, M., and Herkonene., (1967). In "Endocrinology of the testis", G.E.W. Wolstenholme and O'Connor, (Eds.) London, Churchill.
9. Reyes, F.I., Winter, J.S., and Faiman, C. (1973). J. Clin. Endo. Metab. 37, 71.
10. Brown-Grant, K., and Sherwood, M.R. (1971). J. Endocr., 49, 277.
11. Resko, J.A., Malley, A., Begley, D., and Hess, D.L. (1973). Endocrinology 93, 150.
12. Wells, L.J., and Van Wagenen, G. (1964). Contrib. Embryol. Carnegie Inst. Washington. 35, 93.
13. Phoenix, C.H., Goy, R.W., and Resko, J.A. (1968). In "Perspectives in Reproduction and Sexual behaviour", Diamond, M. (Ed). Indiana Univ. Press. Bloomington, pp 33.
14. Goy, R.W., and Resko, J.A. (1972). Rec. Prog. Horm. Res. 28, 707.
15. Goldman, A.S., Shapiro, B.H. and Root, A.W. (1973). Proc. Soc. Exptl. Biol· Med. 143, 422.
16. Neumann, F., Elger, W., and Steinbeck, H. (1969). J. Reprod Fertil. Suppl. 7, 9.
17. Lippsett, M., and Tullner, W.W. (1965). Endocrinology 77, 273.
18. Wilson, G.W. and Siiteri, P.K. (1973). Endocrinology 92, 1182.
19. Wilson, G.W. (1973). Endocrinology 92, 1192.
20. Josso, N. (1972). J. Clin. Endo. Metab. 34, 265.
21. Josso, N. (1972). Biology of the Neunate. 20, 368.
22. Josso, N. (1973). Endocrinology, 93, 829.
23. Josso, N. (1971). J. Clin. Endo. Metab. 32, 74.
24. Barraclough, C.A. (1967). In "Neuroendocrinology," Martini, L,

and W. F. Ganong. (Eds). 2, 61, Academic Press, New York.
25. Gorski, R. A. (1971). In "Frontiers in Neuroendocrinology" L. Martini, and W. F. Ganong (Eds). p. 237, Oxford. Univ. Press, New York.
26. Gorski, R. A. and Goldman, B. D. (1971). Physiologist. 14, 153.
27. Goldman, B. D., Quadagno, D. M., Shoyne, J., and Gorski, R. A. (1972). Endocrinology 90, 1025.
28. Arai, Y., and Serisawa, P. (1973). Proc. Soc. Exptl. Biol. Med. 143, 656.

GONADOTROPIN REGULATION OF FOLLICULAR DEVELOPMENT IN THE HAMSTER

Gilbert S. Greenwald

An intriguing and still unresolved question in ovarian physiology is what factors determine why one follicle remains quiescent, another matures but ultimately degenerates, and still a third follicle goes on to ovulate. I have been interested in this problem for the past 13 years, using the cyclic hamster as an experimental model (1). Several features of the estrous cycle of the hamster lend themselves to such studies, especially the very predictable 4 day cycle and an easily detectable post-ovulatory marker in the form of a conspicuous vaginal discharge. Further, the ovary responds to single injections of PMS to the extent that superovulation of as many as 70 eggs is possible without recourse to a subsequent injection of hCG (2).

The availability of radioimmunoassays for steroids and gonadotropins now makes it possible to test directly some of the hypotheses that have emerged from this work. The purpose of the present paper is therefore to correlate peripheral hormonal levels with quantitative studies of follicular development in the hamster.

Our colony is maintained on a 14 hr light and 10 hr dark schedule (lights on from 0500 to 1900 CST). Day 1 designates the day of ovulation, with 100% of the animals ovulating by 0200 hr. It is characterized by the afore-mentioned vaginal discharge. Day 4 corresponds to proestrus with behavioral estrus manifested in all females by 1830 hr (3).

By the morning of day 1, the largest healthy follicles have reached the preantral stage and consist of 8-12 layers of granulosa cells. By day 2, these have progressed upto the incipient antrum formation represented by a series of isolated pockets among the granulosa cells. By day 3, a coalesced antral cavity is present. It is noteworthy that this is the first stage at which the histochemical reaction for 3β-OH-dehydrogenase in the theca interna equals that in the interstitium; it is also the earliest stage at which ovulation can be induced by exogenous LH. The number of large follicles maturing under the influence of endogenous gonadotropins - henceforth referred to as "developing follicles" - is approximately 10 per ovary until the morning of day 3. However, between days 3 and 4, the number is halved by follicular atresia resulting in the ultimate ovulation of about 10 eggs (4).

What changes occur in the population of smaller follicles throughout the cycle ? Follicular development at 1500 hr for each day of the cycle has recently been assessed (5). There are no discernible fluctuations in the number of follicles with 2-7 layers of granulosa cells throughout the estrous cycle. The number of preantral follicles with 8-12 layers of granulosa cells present on day 1 gradually move into the larger size categories so that by day 3, a gap exists between antral follicles and those in small preantral stages. The replenishment of developing follicles occuring between 1500 hr of day 4 and that of day 1 is believed to be of considerable importance.

The effect of a single sc injection of 5 or 15 IU PMS given at 0900 hr of day 1 on subsequent follicular development was also determined (5). The former dose results in the ovulation of 14 ova whereas 15 IU PMS leads to superovulation of 44 eggs. On the afternoon of day 1, both doses of PMS lead to the recruitment of twice as many large preantral follicles as in saline injected controls. However, by day 2 the pattern of follicular development in the group treated with 5 IU PMS now resembles that of the normal cyclic hamster, whereas almost twice the normal number of antral follicles are present in the 15 IU PMS group. The conclusion is that high levels of PMS are needed not only to mature more follicles at critical stages of their development,but also to sustain them throughout the cycle.

At what stage, does the preantral follicle becomes dependent on gonadotropins for its further differentiation ? A recent study has been directed towards this question (6). Hamsters were hypophysectomized on day 1 of the cycle and killed at 1 to 28 days thereafter. The largest healthy follicles were found to have 6 to 7 layers of granulosa cells. The conclusion is that the follicle becomes dependent on pituitary hormones considerably before development of the antral cavity and that normally, the developing follicles are the first stage to become hormonally dependent.

In the next experiment we were concerned with what hormonal regimen would restore follicular maturation and ovulation in long-term hypophysectomized hamsters. Accordingly, on day 8 post-hypophysectomy, hamsters were injected subcutaneously for 4 days with various amounts of ovine FSH (NIH-FSH-S7). This was followed on the afternoon of day 4 by a single ip injection of ovine LH (NIH-S-13). The duration of the hormonal treatments therefore simulated the duration of the normal 4 day estrous cycle. The minimal daily requirement to obtain large antral follicles was 100-200 µg FSH. Daily treatment for 4 days with 200 µg FSH, followed by LH, resulted in superovulation of 32 eggs. Thus, elevated and sustained levels of FSH are required for superovulation. If 200 µg of FSH on day 8 post-hypophysectomy was followed by 50 µg of FSH on the next 3 days the animals ovulated 9 eggs - comparable to the number ovulated by intact hamsters. Thus a large pulse of FSH followed by a low maintenance dose of the hormone matures the normal number of follicles. This is consistent with the observed pattern of endogenous gonadotropins during the normal estrous cycle.

The final experiment to be considered involving hypophysectomy, was designed to determine the effects of beginning FSH treatment immediately after hypophysectomy, rather than waiting for one week as in the previous experiments. We felt that an ovary "starved" for gonadotropins for one week might require more FSH to resume follicular development, than one that had just been exposed to gonadotropins. To our surprise, this was not the case. Following hypophysectomy at day 1 when FSH treatment was initiated on day 1 or 2, ovulation did not occur in response to an ovulating dose of LH. However, treatment with 400 µg FSH, commencing on day 1, resulted in superovulation.

The key to this paradox apparently lies in the production of luteal progesterone. The corpora lutea of the estrous cycle function until day 2 (Fig. 1) and progesterone levels are maintained in the absence of the pituitary once the proestrus surge of ovulating hormone(s) has occurred. Thus a transitory phase of luteal "autonomy" exists in the hamster corpus luteum of the cycle. The experiment of administering FSH to long-term hypophysectomized hamsters (day 8-11) was then repeated but concomitantly 1 mg of progesterone was injected daily from days 7-11. Under these circumstances less than half of the animals ovulated (10/24) and follicular development was blocked in the anovulatory group at the 6-7 granulosal stage. From these results it is concluded that progesterone can directly inhibit follicular growth unless high amounts of FSH are available.

Figure 1 shows the pattern of peripheral levels of FSH, LH estradiol and progesterone in the cyclic hamster as determined by radioimmunoassays [gonadotropins (7), estradiol (8), and progesterone (Ridley and Greenwald, unpublished results)]. The most

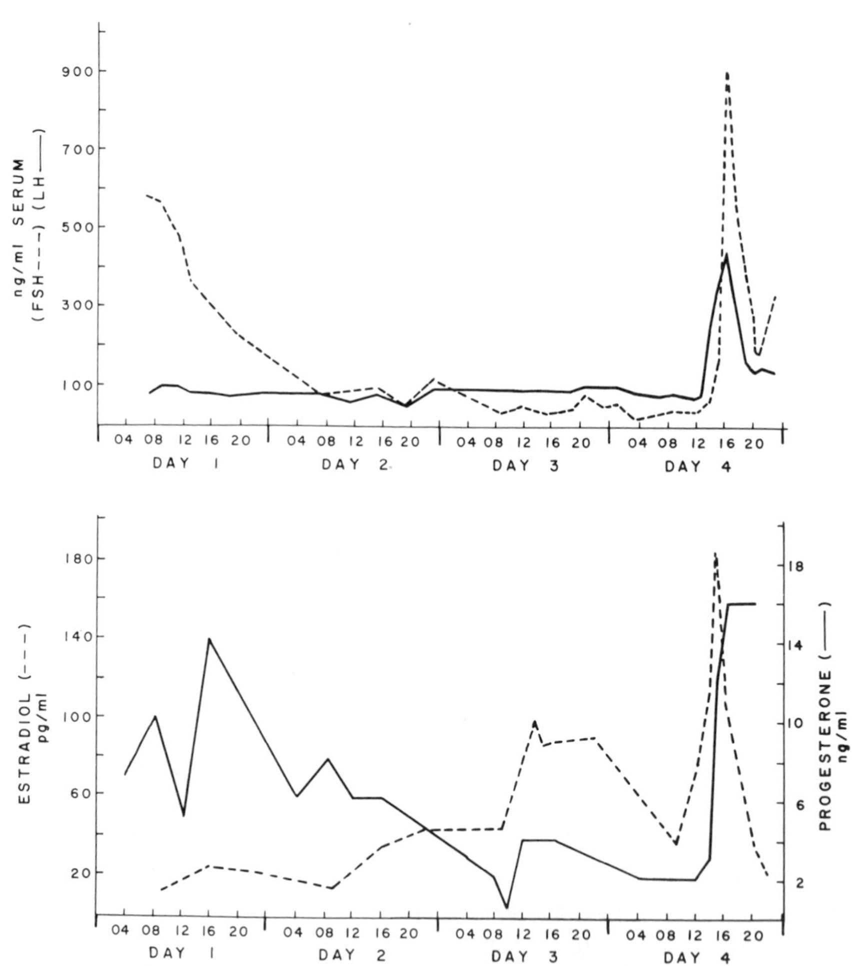

FIG 1. Composite picture of steroid and gonadotropic hormones during the estrous cycle of the hamster. FSH is expressed in terms of NIAMD-rat-FSH-RP-1 and LH as NIAMD-rat-LH-RP-1.

interesting finding is the divergent profiles of FSH and LH. High levels of FSH are found throughout most of day 1 of the cycle. These levels are 2-to 6-fold greater than the levels on day 2 and 5 to 12-fold greater than the mean basal level found on day 3. In contrast, during this same time span, the levels of LH remain relatively low and constant. The high levels of FSH on day 1 are consistent with its presumed role in initiating the growth of the developing follicles. The fall of serum FSH to its lowest values at day 3 may be responsible for the follicular atresia that normally destroys half of the developing follicles between days 3 and 4.

The high peripheral levels of progesterone on days 1 and 2 of the cycle (ca 10 ng/ml) largely represent luteal secretion, in agreement with the findings of Lukaszewska and Greenwald (9). Progesterone drops sharply after 0200 hr of day 3 with the nadir reached at 1000 hr. It is only after the curtailment of this sustained level of progesterone that antral follicles differentiate. There is a dramatic upsurge of progesterone by 1600 hr of day 4, produced both by the preovulatory follicles and the interstitium (3), which is secreted in response to the proestrus surge of LH but not apparently in response to the almost concomitant increase in FSH (Greenwald, unpublished results).

Estradiol levels during the first two days of the cycle do not exceed the values found in plasma of bilaterally ovariectomized hamsters, consistent with the immature status of the developing follicles at this time. Estradiol secretion is initiated on day 3, concomitant with the fall in progesterone and the development of antral follicles. The increase in estradiol on day 3 is not associated with any significant changes in FSH or LH. It is noteworthy that the increase of estradiol on day 3 is in the form of a plateau rather than a sharp peak. Estradiol levels drop by the morning of day 4 and the onset of the LH surge initiates a sharp transitory peak in estradiol between 1400 and 1600 hr.

The final topic to be considered is the effects of unilateral ovariectomy (ULO) on follicular development. In 1920 Arai (10) observed that removal of one ovary each from cyclic rats resulted several weeks later in a compensatory increase in weight of the in situ ovary. My experiments have been directed towards an analysis of follicular development. One ovary from each animal was removed at definite stages of the estrous cycle and the oviduct of the remaining ovary was flushed on day 1 of the next cycle; ovulation was therefore used as the principal endpoint in the above experiment. Typical results of an experiment are shown in Table 1. One ovary was removed between 0800 and 1000 hr on each day of the hamster cycle. It is evident that ULO on the morning of days 1-3 results in a doubling of the number of ovulations from the remaining ovary, accounting for maintenance of the number of ovulations characteristic of the species (4). This compensatory ovulation recurs for at least 10-12 cycles in ULO females and they still maintain their 4 day cycles (11). Compensatory ovulation is blocked by a single sc injection on day 1 or 2 of 10 μg estradiol cyclopentylpropionate but not by 2 mg of progesterone.

Table 1. The effect of unilateral ovariectomy on ovulation from the remaining ovary.

Day of estrous cycle of semispaying	N	No. ova ovulated from remaining ovary at next day 1 ($\bar{X} \pm$ SE)
1	6	12.5 ± 0.43
2	6	11.0 ± 1.31
3	6	11.2 ± 0.40
4	6	5.8 ± 1.24

The important component in the removed ovary is the follicular apparatus. Compensatory follicular development and ovulation takes place in the presence of both ovaries, if one is exteriorized and x-irradiated to prevent the unilateral development of antral follicles (3). The mechanism of compensatory ovulation in the cyclic hamster depends on the prevention of follicular atresia of the developing follicles which normally occurs between days 3 and 4. As previously mentioned, each ovary normally has 10 developing follicles which is reduced to 5 follicles by day 4. This does not occur when one ovary is removed on the morning of days 1-3 (4).

The obvious question is what gonadotropin changes prevent follicular atresia in the ULO hamster ? There have been two leading theories: (1) That there is no change in the level of gonadotropins from the intact animal but in the absence of one ovary the same amount available for two ovaries is now available for

Table 2. Effect of unilateral ovariectomy (ULO) or sham ovariectomy on serum FSH concentrations.

Treatment at 0900 hr of day 3	FSH levels* (ng/ml±SE)					Mean no. ova on day 1
	Day 3 (hr)				Day 4	
	0900	1300	1700	2100	0100	
ULO	85±10	258±24	394±11	383±15	287±30	10.8±2.2
Sham	98±7	105±10	107±12	107±12	132±48	10.4±1.2

*Expressed in terms of NIAMD-Rat FSH-RP-1; (n=5).

utilization by the remaining one (2). The other theory is that ULO lessens the negative feedback action of steroids (in particular, estrogens) and consequently there is increased release of gonadotropins. Other workers have had difficulties in proving either theory, but with the availability of radioimmunoassay and working at carefully circumscribed time intervals, we have preliminary results supporting the idea of increased gonadotropin release. This is the work of one of my associates, Dr. Joseph Bast. Hamsters were sham-ovariectomized or unilaterally ovariectomized at 0900 hr on day 3 of the cycle. Serial blood samples taken via cardiac puncture at 4 hr intervals reveal that there is a significant increase in peripheral levels of FSH in the ULO group (Table 2). We have not yet determined the effects of ULO on LH levels, but prolactin is unchanged. Obviously, considerably more work will be needed to unravel all of the intricacies of compensatory ovulation but we are confident that the current assay procedures and the background gained from our other approaches will enable us to formulate more concrete notions on the factors regulating follicular development in the intact, cycling animal.

ACKNOWLEDGEMENTS

This is a contribution from the Research Professorship in Human Reproduction. The research was supported by grants from the Ford Foundation and NIH (HD00596).

REFERENCES

1. Greenwald, G.S. (1960). Endocrinology 66, 89.
2. Greenwald, G.S. (1962). Endocrinology 71, 378.
3. Norman, R.L. and G.S. Greenwald (1971). Endocrinology 89, 598.
4. Greenwald, G.S. (1961). J. Reprod. Fert. 2, 351.
5. Greenwald, G.S. (1973). Anat. Rec. (in press).
6. Moore, P.J. and G.S. Greenwald. (1973). Am. J. Anat. (in press).
7. Bast, J.D. and G.S. Greenwald. (1973). Biology of Reproduction 9, 74 (abstract).
8. Baranczuk, R. and G.S. Greenwald (1973). Endocrinology 92, 805.
9. Lukaszewska, J.H. and G.S. Greenwald (1970). Endocrinology 85, 1160.
10. Arai, H. (1920). Amer. J. Anat. 28, 59.
11. Chatterjee, A. and G.S. Greenwald (1972). Biology of Reproduction 7, 238.

STUDIES ON FOLLICULAR MATURATION - EFFECT OF FSH-AND LH ANTISERA IN HAMSTERS

A. Jagannadha Rao, C.S. Sheela Rani and N.R. Moudgal

INTRODUCTION

The process of follicular maturation is known to be dependent on both FSH and LH, but their specific roles in this process is not clearly delineated. Hypophysectomy and replacement therapy with individual gonadotropins has been used as a method to study this problem (1-4). Another approach to this study, which is of recent origin has been to use characterized antisera (5-7), to selectively neutralize endogenous gonadotropins. The advantages of using an immunological method over hypophysectomy to deprive an animal of its endogenous gonadotropic support have been discussed in detail earlier (8).

The effects of neutralizing circulating LH on the reproductive cycle of laboratory animals are well-documented (9-13). On the other hand, due to the difficulty experienced in obtaining a specific FSH a/s, which is free of contaminating LH antibodies, definitive studies on the effects of neutralizing FSH specifically are lacking. Thus, for instance, Talaat and Laurence (14) observed that active immunization of rats and rabbits with NIH-oFSH led to follicular degeneration and general cessation of reproductive function; but they could not unequivocally attribute these effects to the lack of FSH alone, as the antigen used by them was definitely known to be contaminated with oLH.

We report here, an account of our preliminary study directed towards an understanding of the involvement of FSH and LH in the process of follicular maturation, using FSH or LH antisera characterized for their specificity.

EXPERIMENTAL

A. Characterization of antisera

Antisera to oFSH (NIH-FSH-S 8 & 9) and LH (NIH-oLH and Papkoff and Li preparations) were raised in monkeys and rabbits respectively. The details of immunization and charactterization procedures have been described elsewhere (15-17). While LH a/s was found to be free of contaminating FSH antibody, FSH a/s was found to contain LH antibody. In addition to using labeled hormone binding and Ouchterlony double diffusion tests, the absence of cross-contaminating antibodies was checked by using appropriate biological end-points. For example, while unabsorbed FSH a/s is able to terminate gestation and affect luteal and interstitial cell function of the pregnant hamsters, the antiserum absorbed with LH is unable to influence the above biological end-points; these parameters have been shown earlier by us to be affected by lack of LH (18).

The FSH a/s used in these studies was a hyperimmune serum obtained from monkeys and was freed of LH antibody contamination using the LH-coated RBC immunosorbent (19); the advantages of using this method over that of absorption with excess LH have been discussed in this volume by Muralidhar et al. The ability of these absorbed antisera to neutralize pituitary FSH and LH of hamsters have been earlier established (16).

B. Studies in pregnant hamsters

Studies by Greenwald (20) have shown that ovaries of hamsters at any stage of pregnancy contain follicles which are ready to ovulate in response to exogenous LH or hCG. We have examined the effect of LH deprivation on the follicular apparatus, as well as the ability of FSH to promote follicular growth in the absence of LH in pregnant hamsters; it was seen that deprival of LH led to the disappearance of both luteal bodies and Graafian follicles, but without affecting the primary follicular population (Figs 1A & B). When exogenous FSH was administered along with LH a/s to pregnant hamsters, it was found to promote follicular growth, but only upto the pre-antral stage (Fig 1C). This shows that even in the total absence of LH, the primary follicles are capable of responding to FSH; however, LH appears to be necessary for the further development of the follicle, i.e., beyond the pre-antral stage. Similarly, using hypophysectomized rats, Lostroh and Johnson (3) were able to

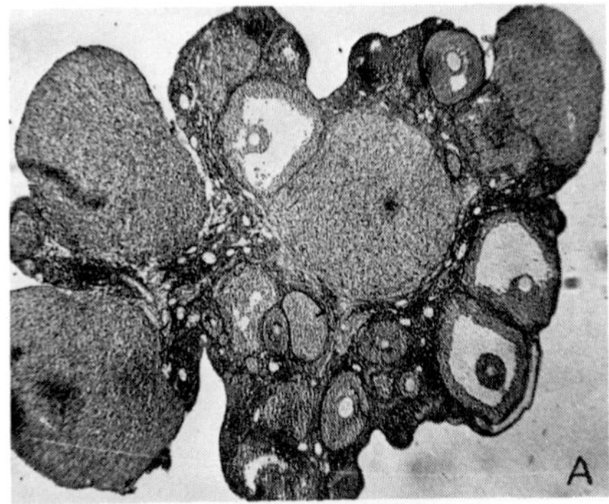

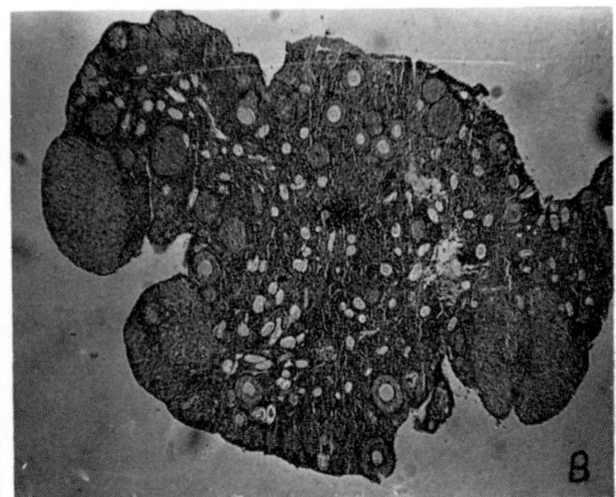

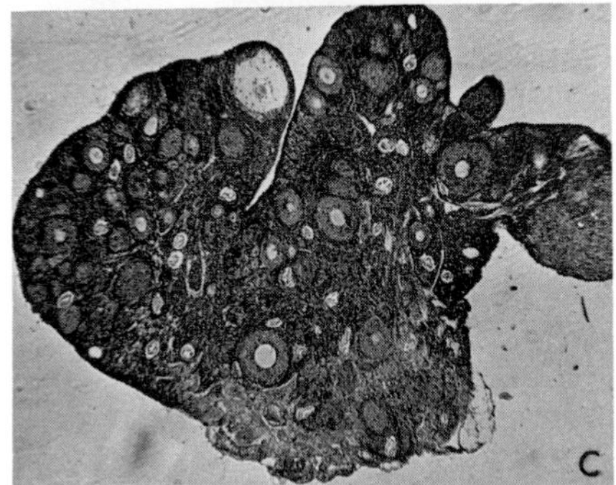

FIG 1. Relative effect of LH and FSH on follicular development as seen in the ovary of pregnant hamster. Treatment was given on day 8 of pregnancy and the animals were autopsied on day 12. The ovaries were excised and processed for histological examination. A: treated with normal rabbit serum; B: treated with LH a/s (0.2 ml); C: treated with LH a/s (0.2 ml) + FSH (NIH-FSH-S 7 - 200 µg) + prolactin (NIH-oPL - 4 mg) (x 8).

demonstrate that a pure FSH preparation (having not more than 1 % LH concentration) was able to promote follicular development, but not beyond the stage of medium-size follicles.

C. Studies in cycling hamsters

In cycling hamsters, on the afternoon of proestrus, LH and FSH are known to appear in the form of a surge (21). Neutralization of the proestrus LH surge using LH a/s has been shown by us to result in blockade of ovulation occuring on the estrus morning, while treatment with FSH a/s at the same time didnot affect the ovulatory process. The significance of this FSH surge and its involvement, if any, in the process of growth and maturation of follicles required for ovulation during the subsequent cycle was therefore examined. Thus, FSH a/s was administered to regularly cycling hamsters on proestrus at 1300 hr and its effects on ovarian cyclicity were studied by following the changes in the vaginal cytology.

It appeared from the normal smear pattern (consisting of two days of diestrus) exhibited by the treated animals during the first cycle, that blockade of FSH did not apparently influence the luteal functionality of that cycle. But from the results presented in Table 1, it appears that neutralization of FSH does lead to an interference with follicular development, which, however, becomes evident only after the first cycle; these animals showed a continuous estrus smear which is atypical (comprising of cornified epithelial cells, leucocytes and a few nucleated cells - in the order of preponderence). Unilaterally ovariectomized animals show an amplification in the process of follicular development and hence these were used as another experimental

Table 1. Effect of LH-and FSH antisera on estrous cycle in hamsters.

Group *	a/s ml	Duration of treatment ** (days)	Vaginal estrus NE/N §	Remarks
I	FSH a/s 0.5 ml	on PE *** only	12/19	Normal smear pattern during first cycle followed by continuous atypical estrus. ¶
II	FSH a/s 0.5 ml	8	8/12	Same as in group I.
III	LH a/s 0.2 ml	12	0/17	Anestrous diestrus.
IV	LH a/s 0.2 ml	8	0/12	Anestrous diestrus.

* Groups I & III comprised of adult cycling animals; group II & IV-unilaterally ovariectomized just before the start of a/s treatment; N = 4. ** Treatment was initiated on proestrus (PE) day in case of hamsters treated with FSH a/s, and on estrus (E) day in case of those given LH a/s. *** Regularly cycling hamsters were included in the experiment and they received the first a/s injection on the day of proestrus. Two more injections of a/s were given on the day of expected proestrus eventhough, the animals ceased to cycle. § NE/N = Number of days on which estrus smear was observed /Total number of days the smear patterns were monitored. ¶ Atypical estrus = Vaginal lavage showed the presence of cornified epithelial cells, leucotyes and nucleated cells in the order of preponderance.

model to study the effects of FSH a/s. Continued administration of FSH a/s to these animals starting from proestrus brought about effects similar to those observed in intact cycling hamsters receiving the a/s only on proestrus. In contrast to the effects of FSH neutralization, LH deprival had significantly different effects, resulting in a continuous anestrus diestrus smear.

Reduction in ovarian and uterine weights following FSH a/s or LH a/s treatments (Table 2) shows that the effects of the latter are much more drastic. Although the uterine weights of the FSH a/s treated animals were significantly reduced compared to that of the controls, they were higher than those of the LH a/s treated animals. These results can be interpreted in terms of differential production of estrogen; compared to the normal levels in controls, FSH a/s treated hamsters could be having minimal levels while the LH a/s treated hamsters could have no estrogen at all. This, however, needs to be confirmed by actual measurements of estrogen levels in these groups of animals. Progesterone in synergism with estrogen is known to influence the uterine condition. Thus, the reduced uterine weights could also be a reflection of the lowered progesterone level which is a consequence of the disruption in luteal functionality; the latter is brought about by the neutralization of either

Table 2. Effect of deprival of endogenous FSH or LH on ovarian and uterine weights in female hamsters.

Treatment	Experimental Model					
	Adult cycling			Unilaterally ovariectomized		
	ovarian weight	uterine weight	% ** redn.	ovarian weight	uterine weight	% redn.
NRS	20.5±4.25	352±67.5	-	34.5±2.7	215±55.2	-
FSH a/s*	13.5±2.2	172± 5.6	51	23.0±3.5	172±65	20
LH a/s	6.6±0.7	63±1.7	80	13.0±1.2	68.7±17	68

*For details of experiment, see Table 1. ** Percent reduction in uterine weight compared to controls. Number of animals in each group is 4. Results are Mean ± S. D. in mg.

LH or FSH. Although FSH deprival has been observed not to affect the normal duration of the diestrus phase in the first cycle, the absence of luteal function during the subsequent cycles is perhaps due to the neutralization of FSH during proestrus, interfering with the process of follicular maturation; this would mean that no ovulable follicle becomes available for LH action and corpus luteum formation.

CONCLUDING REMARKS

The foregoing study makes it evident that gonadotropin antisera characterized for specificity can be used for studying the role of FSH and LH in follicular development. Our results suggest that it may be possible to specify which particular stage(s) of this process is influenced by either of the two gonadotropins or whether there is synergism throughout their action.

The true physiological significance of FSH and LH appearing in a surge form at proestrus has been debated for a long time. The present study suggests, that this FSH has a role in triggering a fresh wave of follicles to develop, some of which reach maturity and ovulate. It may be of interest to note that Welshen (22) has also observed that ovaries of rats at proestrus are more sensitive to FSH action. Further information on estrogen, progesterone and LH levels during the cycle following FSH a/s treatment may enlighten us on the sequence of events.

ACKNOWLEDGEMENTS

Work aided by generous grants from the Indian Council of Medical Research, New Delhi, and the Ford Foundation, New York.

REFERENCES

1. Fevold, A. L., Hisaw, F. C., Hellbaum, A. and Hertz, R. (1933). Am. J. Physiol. 104, 710.
2. Greep, R. O., Van Dyke, H. B. and Chow, B. F. (1942). Endocrinology 30, 635.

3. Lostroh, A. J. & Johnson, R.(1966). Endocrinology 79, 991.
4. Greenwald, G. S. Proceedings of this symposium. pp 206.
5. Li, C. H., Moudgal, N. R., Trenkle, A., Bourdel, G. and Sadri, K. (1962). CIBA Foundation Colloq, on Endocrinol. 14, 20.
6. Bourdel, G. and Li, C. H. (1963). Acta Endocrinologica. 42, 478.
7. Laurence, K. A. and Ichikawa, S. (1968). Endocrinology 82, 1190.
8. Moudgal, N. R. (1973). In "Physiology series, Volume 8, Reproductive Physiology" - MTP International Review of Science, R. O. Greep, (Ed).
9. Moudgal, N. R. and Li, C. H. (1961). Arch. Biochem. and Biophys. 95, 93.
10. Young, W. P., Nasser, R. and Hayashida, T. (1963). Nature (London), 197, 1117.
11. Ely, C. A., Tuercke, R. and Chen, B. L. (1966). Proc. Soc. Exptl. Biol. Med. 122, 601.
12. Schwartz, N. B. and Gold, J. J. (1967). Anat. Rec. 157, 137.
13. Schwartz, N. B. and Ely, C. A. (1970). Endocrinology 86, 1420.
14. Talaat, M. and Laurence, K. A. (1969). Endocrinology 84, 185.
15. Madhwa Raj, H. G. and Moudgal, N. R. (1970). Endocrinology 86, 874.
16. Jagannadha Rao, A. and Moudgal, N. R. (1970). Arch. Biochem. and Biophys. 138, 189.
17. Moudgal, N. R., Jagannadha Rao, A., Maneckjee, R., Muralidhar, K., Venkatramaiah Mukku, and Sheela Rani, C. S. (1974). Rec. Prog. Horm. Res. 30, 47.
18. Jagannadha Rao, A., Madhwa Raj, H. G. and Moudgal, N. R. (1972). J. Reprod. Fert. 29, 239.
19. Jagannadha Rao, A., Moudgal, N. R., Madhwa Raj, H. G. Lipner, H. and Greep, R. O. (1974). J. Reprod. Fert. (in press).
20. Greenwald, G. S. (1967). Amer. J. Anat. 121, 249.
21. Bast, J. D. & Greenwald, G. S. (1973) Biol. of Reprod. 9, 74.
22. Welshen, R. (1973). Acta Endocr. 72, 137.

GONADOTROPINS AND FUNCTIONS OF GRANULOSAL AND THECAL CELLS <u>IN VIVO</u> AND <u>IN VITRO</u>

Sardul S. Guraya

INTRODUCTION

The past few years have witnessed a revival of great interest in determining the functions of granulosal and thecal cells and their relation to gonadotropins, using techniques like histochemistry, biochemistry, autoradiography, electron microscopy etc. The purpose of this paper is to summarize and integrate the results of these studies in order to get an insight into the functions of granulosal and thecal cells during follicular maturation and atresia, ovulation, corpus luteum formation and its regression.

FOLLICULAR GROWTH

A considerable controversy has existed regarding the sites of steroid hormone synthesis in the maturing follicle of mammalian ovary. Theca interna and/or granulosa cells are believed to constitute the site of steroidogenesis in the developing follicle.

A. <u>Theca interna</u>

Secondary or preantral follicles are surrounded by the concentric sheath of undifferentiated stromal elements which do not show any appreciable development of blood vascularity. They contain a few organelles such as small Golgi complex, mitochondria, profiles of granular endoplasmic reticulum and some free ribosomes (1) ; they lack the enzyme activities indicative of steroidogenesis. With the appearance of an antrum in the granulosa, some of the surrounding stromal elements, lying adjacent to the granulosa, begin to hypertrophy or luteinize to form large secretory cells having abundant cytoplasm and vesicular nuclei. These changes are brought about by gonadotropins, especially the luteinizing hormone. These hypertrophied, well vascularized stromal cells, constitute the theca interna around the growing follicle. They generally exhibit greater nuclear and cytoplasmic density. The concentric sheath of undifferentiated stromal elements surrounding the theca interna cells forms the theca externa. The development and differentiation of the theca interna cells greatly vary in different mammalian species (2-8). The hypertrophied theca interna cells in the developing follicles of the rat, rabbit, cat and bat store abundant sudanophilic lipid droplets consisting of phospholipids, triglycerides, cholesterol and its esters. These may constitute the hormone precursors which are mobilized during the preovulatory period (3,6). In contrast to the above, in hamster, guinea pig, marmoset and the human, hypertrophied theca interna cells consist of sparsely distributed lipid droplets having phospholipids, and/or triglycerides, suggesting that these cells might be functioning in the secretion of some steroid hormone rather than in the storage of hormone precursors. In dog, buffalo, cow and rhesus monkey, these cells show relatively less cytoplasmic differentiation and contain some lipid granules consisting mainly of phospholipids. In the growing antral follicles of oppossum, it is hardly differentiated morphologically from the surrounding stromal tissue and no lipids are present; however, during the preovulatory period, its theca interna cells are also hypertrophied to form the thecal gland cells. These comparative studies have suggested that the timing and degree of differentiation of theca interna during the follicular growth as well as the LH content of the gonadotropin complex involved in this process (9) greatly vary.

With the appearance of blood vascularity in the theca interna, its alkaline phosphatase activity is also increased (10-12); the latter is usually correlated to the transport of substances across the cellular membranes, and it greatly varies in different mammalian species. The hypertrophied theca interna cells also possess the ultrastructural features typical of most steroid-secreting cells: tubular smooth endoplasmic reticulum, mitochondria with predominantly tubular cristae, and lipid droplets (1, 13-15). Diffusely distributed lipoproteins demonstrable with histochemical techniques (1, 5-7) apparently are derived from the abundant agranular endoplasmic reticulum of steroid-secreting cells.

The above changes are closely accompanied by the appearance of enzyme activities like Δ^5, 3 β -hydroxysteroid dehydrogenase (HSD) and 17 β -HSD, indicative of the synthesis of steroids (1,6, 7,16,17). Some of the enzymes are believed to be involved in the production of NADPH. Systems for estrogen synthesis have been demonstrated in the theca interna cells but not in the granulosa (18,19); cytological and histochemical data support this finding.

The ability of antral follicles to accumulate estrogen in the follicular fluid parallelling the differentiation of theca interna cells _in vivo_ agrees well with the ability of these cells _in vitro_ to synthesize estrogen from its labeled precursors (18-20).

The preovulatory depletion of cholesterol-containing lipid droplets from the theca interna of rabbit and rat follicle is a result of LH surge increasing synthesis of estrogen during this period; estrogen synthesis has been shown to be stimulated by LH, but not by FSH _in vitro_ (21,22). The secretion of extraordinarily elevated amounts of estrogen in the untreated and PMSG-primed cyclic hamster is related to the preovulatory growth of the follicle (23,24). The theca interna cells besides the estrogens, are also considered to form small amounts of other steroids (1, 19).

B. Granulosa

There has been a considerable controversy about the origin of granulosa cells. But recent ultrastructural studies have indicated their possible origin to be from the undifferentiated stromal cells of the developing mammalian ovary (25,26). Once the granulosa (or follicle cells) are formed around the primordial oocyte, they increase in their numbers by mitosis, possibly in response to some hormones (27), thus forming a multi-layered follicular epithelium. Its development, structure and the number of constituent granulosa cells are greatly variable in the comparable follicles of different mammalian species. The corona radiata around the oocyte and the peripheral granulosal layers lying inner to the basement membrane, however, are differentiated very early during the follicular growth.

The presence of Golgi zone, granular mitochondria, irregular lipid bodies of variable size, and abundant cytoplasmic RNA have been shown in granulosa cells by cytological and histological techniques; lipid bodies containing phospholipids are distributed irregularly among the granulosal cells and their amount varies in different mammals. Glycogen, confined to the cells of the cumulus oophorus, is prominent in mature follicles on the sixteenth day of cycle in guinea pig (11) and in follicle of hibernation in bat (28). The diffusely distributed lipoproteins found in theca interna cells are not seen in the cytoplasm of granulosa cells. Electron microscopy has revealed the presence of a Golgi complex, granular endoplasmic reticulum, several free ribosomes, very little or no agranular endoplasmic reticulum, and mitochondria with simple lamellar cristae (1,29). The granulosal wall of follicles in the guinea pig, but not in any other mammal, has been shown to have nucleoside monophosphatase activity (11, 30-32). Brandau (17) has demonstrated the activity of glyceraldehyde-phosphate dehydrogenase and lactic dehydrogenase in the granulosa of growing follicles, which is considerably increased after FSH treatment but not after hCG. There is low to moderately high activity of the enzyme of the citric acid cycle in the granulosa cells. Several species variations in regard to the presence or absence of acid and alkaline phosphatases in the granulosal layer or follicles have also been reported (10, 11).

Both morphological and histochemical studies show that the granulosa cells are indeed metabolically active in protein rather than steroid synthesis. It may thus be interesting to emphasize that the diffusely distributed lipoproteins, agranular endoplasmic reticulum, and cholesterol-containing lipid granules described for the theca interna cells do not show any appreciable development in the normal granulosa cells. However, some faint sudanophilia and lipid granules similar to those of theca interna may appear in the peripheral granulosal layer of the mature follicles where it may be related to the abortive "luteinization" of these cells (3, 11). Enzyme activities indicative of synthesis of steroid hormones are not seen in the normal granulosa cells *in vivo* (1, 17, 33). However, the granulosa cells in atresia and culture develop such enzyme activity (16, 33-35). According to Lobel and Levy (36) the steroid dehydrogenases were demonstrable in the granulosa of normal follicles in the bovine ovary. The significance of this discrepancy, however, could not be determined. The follicles studied by them might be in very early stage of their atresia, which is difficult to characterize with the techniques available. Brandau (17) also believes that the presence of 3 β -HSD activity in the granulosa of small and medium follicles may perhaps indicate that these cells act as target sites for the action of steroid hormones. They are unlikely to synthesize steroids because they lack the NADPH-producing enzymes typical of the steroid secreting cells.

A basement membrane in the follicle prevents the blood supply from reaching the granulosa cells. This may presumably result in the lack of adequate blood-borne nutrients and oxygen supply to the cells which are essential for luteinization; this in the normal course, becomes available after ovulation as a result of a vascularization of granulosa cells (37, 38). The granulosa cells lysing adjacent to the basement membrane, may develop an incipient luteinization in some mammals because of their proximity with the vascularized theca interna. According to Channing (37, 38), the complete luteinization and subsequent production of progesterone occurs only after ovulation or in culture after prestimulation with LH and FSH. Nicosia (39), and Stoklosowa and Nalbandov (22) have observed a higher rate of progestin secretion by granulosa cells in culture, the former by adding FSH-LH and the latter by adding 10 ng of LH to the culture medium. Brandau et al. (40) are of the opinion that the NADPH-producing enzymes of the granulosa cells of preovulatory follicle are directly induced by LH, while a substrate induction of 3β-HSD occurs after initiation of steroid synthesis.

In vitro studies using the granulosa cells have provided valuable information on the steroid biosynthesis and metabolism (1, 6, 7, 29, 37-39), and these studies indicate the potentiality of the granulosa cells and not necessarily their secretory activity *in vivo.* This is strongly supported by the recent studies of Younglai and Short (19) on the pathways of steroid biosynthesis in the intact Graafian follicle of mares in estrus. They have shown that estradiol-17β in the follicular fluid is derived mainly from the theca interna cells and not from the granulosa cells which have at most an extremely weak aromatizing ability, since in the latter only a small proportion of the labelled androstenedione is converted to estradiol-17β ; *in vitro*, however, their aromatizing ability is pronounced (37, 38, 41, 42). The principal steroid hormones formed by the granulosa cells *in vitro* are progesterone and 17α-hydroxyprogesterone.

OVULATION

It is well-established that ovulation in mammals occurs as a result of endogenous preovulatory LH surge. HCG, PMSG etc., which have LH activity also bring about ovulation when administered. During ovulation, the granulosa, theca interna and surrounding stroma undergo morphological, histochemical and biochemical changes.

A. Granulosa

The granulosa cells of the newly ruptured human follicle do not show any conspicuous cytological and histochemical changes (1,2). However, the process of luteinization has set in and is evident in the form of appearance of fine lipid granules and large lipid bodies similar to those seen in theca interna cells. Blood vascularity also starts developing and it seems to have originated from the thecal layers. The above changes are seen in all species studied such as the human, rabbit, hamster and rat (3, 8). In the rat and rabbit ovary, in addition to the above, there is development of agranular endoplasmic reticulum during the preovulatory period which is presumably derived from diffuse lipoproteins. This has been taken as an indication of the onset of luteinization in steroid secreting cells in the various vertebrate species studied (1,6,43, 44). The comparative studies have shown that the granulosa cells of rodent ovary begin to luteinize earlier than those of human ovary; the significance of these differences, however, are not known.

B. Theca interna

The theca interna cells of newly ruptured follicles of the human, rabbit (1,2), rat, guinea pig and hamster (Guraya, unpublished data) become filled with sudanophilic lipid bodies of variable size, consisting of phospholipids, triglycerides, cholesterol and/or its esters. This storage of cholesterol-containing lipids has been attributed to their inactivity in the release of estrogen, which perhaps is a result of the disruption of theca interna cells during ovulation (1-3). Thus, the drop in estrogen production after the ovulatory surge of gonadotropins in women and immediately after ovulation in rodents (23,24) could be attributed to a sudden change in the metabolism of cholesterol-containing lipids in the theca interna cells; they begin to function in the storage of hormone precursor, rather than in the secretion of hormone (1,2). However, these lipid bodies disappear in the fully differentiated corpus luteum suggesting that they again become active in the production of estrogen. The decline in estrogen synthesis by day 3 of culture of rat ovarian follicles as reported by Stoklosowa and Nalbandov (22) might also be due to the inactivity or degeneration of theca interna cells. They have further suggested that less LH is able to bring about maximal progesterone synthesis, while 10 times the amount of LH is required for maximal estrogen synthesis; the latter was apparently carried out by the luteinized theca interna cells which continued to form a part of their cultured follicles.

C. Stroma

Lying outside the irregularly distributed theca interna cells is the loose surrounding stroma which shows accumulation of blood corpuscles. From the results of the recent studies on the process of ovulation, it has become increasingly clear that the rupture of a follicle is the result of a series of definitive degradative changes in the wall of follicle which are apparently brought about by lysosomal hydrolases, presumably in response to the action of LH (44,45). Further studies are needed to work out the details of origin and nature of these enzymes and of gonadotropic control mechanisms in relation to their activity in bringing about the disintegration of stromal tissue.

LUTEINIZATION

A. Theca lutein cells

The theca interna cells after ovulation are reorganized to form definite groups of cells about the periphery of a developing human corpus luteum and in the base of the folds formed in the wall of the collapsed follicles (1,2). These cells have been designated as the theca lutein or paraluteal cells. The corresponding cells of thecal origin in the corpora lutea of rodents (guinea pig, rat, hamster and rabbit) do not remain distinct, as they are mixed up with the granulosa lutein cells and finally disappear from view as a result of their degeneration (Guraya, unpublished). This may be correlated to the absence of secretion of estrogens by the corpora lutea of rodents both *in vivo* and *in vitro* (20). However, the cell type concerned with the formation of estradiol *in vitro* from rat corpora lutea incubated on day 5 of pregnancy with labeled progesterone (46) is not known.

B. Granulosa lutein cells

Compared to the granulosa cells of the follicle, the granulosa lutein cells are relatively more hypertrophied forming large secretory cells having vesicular nuclei. They also make up the bulk of the human corpus luteum. The most striking features, which develop during the transformation of granulosa cells into granulosa lutein cells are : (a) well-developed cell organelles, especially the pleomorphic mitochondria with a complex system of tubular internal cristae; (b) the development of abundant diffuse lipoproteins (or membranes of smooth reticulum), closely accompanied by the appearance of enzyme activities indicative of the biosynthesis of steroid hormones; (c) under certain physiological situations, appearance of stored lipid droplets in the cytoplasm; and (d) capacity to form progestins (1,20,37,38,44,47,48). The presence of different cell types (theca lutein and granulosa cells) in the human corpus luteum may be related to the multiple steroids obtained with *in vitro* techniques (1).

The functional life span of corpus luteum varies greatly in different mammalian species as well as in various physiological conditions such as nonpregnancy, pseudopregnancy, pregnancy and lactation (6,7,49). A luteotropic hormone(s) whose nature and composition varies in different species is believed to control the functional life of luteal cells (49, 52-56); sheep (50) and swine (51) appear to be exceptions to this. However, in all the species so-far tested, LH has been shown to be luteotropic (20,48,57-63). With the withdrawal of tropic stimulation, the function of luteal cells declines and simultaneously they begin to undergo degenerative changes. This is closely accompanied by the accumulation of sudanophilic lipid droplets of a coarse nature, pigments, and very little phospholipids, and by the drastic alterations in cell organelles especially the membranes of reticulum and mitochondria (1); the agranular endoplasmic reticulum is transformed into inclusion bodies of diverse nature. More or less, similar ultrastructural degenerative alterations have also been reported for the luteal cells of pregnant rat treated with prostaglandin $F_{2\alpha}$ which specifically affects smooth endoplasmic reticulum (64), perhaps by antagonizing the action of luteotropin or by a direct action. The regressing luteal cells also show sharp decrease in activities of the steroid dehydrogenases (1,2). Once the degenerative changes have started, the luteal cells begin to become refractory to gonadotropic stimulation both in vivo and in vitro. Hence, before studying the effects of gonadotropins on steroidogenesis in vitro it is very essential to determine first whether the steroid gland cells to be used have not already developed degenerative changes.

FOLLICULAR ATRESIA

Follicular atresia is a wide-spread phenomenon in the mammalian ovary by which majority of oocytes are lost at various stages of their development (65). Factors causing atresia may be variable, also depending upon the stage of follicular growth. One of the reasons may be the lack of proper gonadotropic support (65, 66) or imperfect balance of various hormones, leading to many degenerative changes (65). Whether these alterations are the cause or response to a subtle beginning of atresia is not clear. The cholesterol-containing lipid droplets, diffuse lipoproteins and some enzyme activities indicative of steroidogenesis develop in the granulosa of atretic secondary and tertiary follicles suggesting that they apparently undergo an incipient luteinization in response to luteinizing and other factors; the degree of their luteinization seem to vary in follicles of different sizes under different physiological situations. Granulosa cells of primordial, primary and small secondary follicles appear to be relatively more resistant to atresia (65). In some mammals they continue to persist after the disappearance of oocyte and form epithelial cords which may develop the histochemical features of steroid-secreting cells (65, 67). These differences in the behaviour of granulosa cells in follicles of variable sizes during atresia in vivo as well as in vitro (68) clearly suggest that they undergo some basic metabolic changes during follicular growth, apparently in response to gonadotropins and other environmental factors (69). Granulosa cells from follicles of variable size in culture, show great differences in their behaviour in relation to luteinization and secretion of progesterone (37,38,70).

A. Significance of follicular atresia :

The granulosa cells and their lipid accumulations in atretic secondary and tertiary follicles degenerate and disappear, leaving behind their hypertrophied thecae which finally form conspicuous patches of interstitial gland cells in the ovarian stroma. These gland cells of thecal origin develop abundant diffuse lipoproteins, cholesterol-containing lipid droplets, intense alkaline phosphatase activity and various enzyme activities indicative of steroidogenesis (1,43,44,65,71) and they also respond to exogenous or endogenous gonadotropins. These ovarian interstitial glands are believed to be capable of synthesizing androgens, estrogens and progesterone depending on the mammalian species.

Interstitial gland cells of thecal origin are of very transient nature in the ovaries of some non-pregnant mammalian species (human, rhesus monkey, cow and buffalo) and they generally revert to the relatively embryonic, compressed stromal tissue; hence no accumulation in their number is seen in such ovaries (43,44). On the other hand, in the ovaries of other mammals showing a considerable development of interstitial gland cells they begin to accumulate rather than revert back immediately to the original stromal tissue.

Since interstitial gland cells derived from theca interna of atretic follicles are present from young to old age and show cycles of abundance and differentiation correlated with the reproductive age and cycle, they seem to be the most important ovarian gland cells. Their secretory products may be of great physiological significance in the initiation of puberty and cyclic ovarian activity in the female.

GENERAL DISCUSSION AND CONCLUSIONS

Correlation of histochemical, biochemical, and electron-microscopic studies has revealed that the theca interna cells during the follicular growth are "luteinized" in response to a luteinizing factor which appears to exhibit species variation (9), and constitute the site for estrogen synthesis. The accumulation of cholesterol-containing lipid droplets in the theca interna cells of some mammalian species such as rat, rabbit, cat and bat suggests that they may be producing relatively less estrogens during follicular growth than those of hamster, marmoset, rhesus monkey, human etc. which do not store such hormone precursors. Species differences regarding the levels of estrogens during follicular maturation have been observed (23,24).

Though the granulosa cells of developing follicles do not appear to secrete steroid hormones *in vivo*, their characteristics show that they function in the synthesis of RNA, proteins, carbohydrates and phospholipids required for the oocyte growth as well as for the formation of zona pellucida and primary follicular fluid (44,45). However, in culture, the granulosa cells are known to luteinize, synthesize progestins (22,37-39), and respond to LH stimulation in vitro. Similarly, they develop incipient luteinization during follicular atresia when the whole structure of the follicle is disorganized or disrupted.

The varied behaviour of granulosa cells from follicles of different sizes during atresia (65) as well as in tissue culture suggests that they undergo structural and metabolic changes apparently in response to changing environmental factors. It has been suggested that the coupling of granulosa cells - an important step in their differentiation in vivo - is not directly dependent on gonadotropins. Merk et al (27) have discussed the roles that gonadotropins, estrogens and nexuses might play in follicular development. Actually, the nature of these alterations in granulosa brought by the above factors during follicular growth are poorly understood and form a promising area for future research (69). It appears that the coordinated effects of estrogen, FSH and LH are required for the normal follicular growth (72); estrogens are apparently provided by the theca interna cells. Berger et al. (73) have also suggested that LH, in addition to FSH, is either directly or indirectly essential for the maturation and function of ovarian follicle. Some additional factors are required for their luteinization besides prestimulation with LH and FSH, which are apparently made available only at ovulation and follicular atresia when blood reaches the granulosa cells, or in culture when sufficient nutrients and oxygen can cause synthesis of ATP and other compounds.

Recently, the follicular oocyte itself has also been implicated in the process of luteinization by Nalbandov and co-workers (22, 74-76). Their in vivo and in vitro studies seem to indicate that the oocyte plays a major role in the differentiation of follicular cells by producing a luteostatic substance which inhibits the luteinization, thus maintaining the integrity of granulosa cells during the follicular growth. They have further suggested that in cases where luteinization occurs in the presence of ovum, such as due to exposure to massive doses of LH, the latter may produce deleterious effect on the ovum and thus the subsequent luteinization of the follicle. However, according to Nicosia (39) the presence of follicular oocytes does not seem to interfere with the morphologic luteinization and progestin biosynthesis of parietal layer and cumulus oophorus granulosa cells. Norman and Greenwald (77) have suggested that the cells forming the cumulus and corona radiata under the normal preovulatory stimuli undergo some change, the nature of which is still not known. Foote and Thibault (78), using in vitro techniques, have shown that nuclear maturation of oocyte depends upon physiological or mechanical isolation of oocyte from granulosa cells, suggesting the influence of the latter over the former (39). The maturation of oocytes has also been attributed to the effect of progestins and gonadotropins, probably LH, by direct or indirect utilization of substrates (39).

The theca interna cells of developing follicles, luteal cells of corpus luteum and interstitial gland cells possess similar cytological and histochemical characteristics which are indicative of steroidogenesis as established by the criteria described earlier. The functional significance of various cell compounds in steroid biosynthesis has already been discussed in detail in earlier reviews (1, 6, 7, 13, 14, 43). The enzyme activity necessary for splitting off the cholesterol side-chain is believed to reside in the mitochondria while most of the other steroid converting enzymes are localized in the membranes of smooth reticulum (or diffuse lipoproteins). The lipid droplets in the steroid gland cells are the stores of potential precursor materials. They greatly vary in their amount in different steroid gland cells as well as under different physiological situations. These precursor materials are converted into steroid hormones when suitable gonadotropic (LH, hCG, PMSG) stimulation becomes available.

The storage of cholesterol-containing lipid droplets is not an autonomous cellular process but is conditioned by gonadotropins (43, 48, 79-82). It is generally believed that prolactin favours cholesterol storage (particularly in the esterified form) in the absence of other hypophyseal factors, and favours utilization in the presence of the LH which antagonizes the ability of prolactin to promote cholesterol storage. The apparent ability of prolactin to act synergistically with other hypophyseal factors, especially LH, in the regulation of synthesis and storage of cholesterol in the esterified form, is of importance in controlling the supply of cholesterol for progesterone synthesis. Zarrow and Clark (81) have stated that the function of prolactin appears to be similar in both the interstitial and luteal compartments. Prolactin causes a significant increase in cholesterol accumulation without stimulating uterine growth. The other hypophyseal hormones are of less importance for expression of the "lipogenic" activity than for the "cholesterogenic" activity of prolactin. The recent studies have shown that the chronic control of esterification and de-esterification of ovarian cholesterol, which is brought about by steroid concentration, appears to be through effects of LH and prolactin on the total activities of cholesterol esterase and cholesterol esters synthetase (83-85). The studies of Flint et al. (86) have indicated that the inhibition of esterification of cholesterol by LH in vitro can be mimicked by cyclic AMP, and this effect of cyclic AMP is prevented by inhibition of the synthesis of steroids from cholesterol. Inhibitors of steriod synthesis block the LH-induced cholesterol ester depletion in vivo, possibly by preventing inhibition of cholesterol ester synthetase.

REFERENCES

1. Guraya, S.S. (1971). Physiol. Rev. 51, 785.
2. Guraya, S.S. (1968). Am. J. Obst. Gynec. 101, 448.
3. Guraya, S.S. (1968). J. Reprod. Fert. 15, 381.
4. Guraya, S.S. (1968). J. Endocr. 39, 237.
5. Guraya, S.S. (1968). Acta. Morph. Neerl. Scan. 7, 51.
6. Guraya, S.S. (1972). Acta. Anat. 82, 284.
7. Guraya, S.S. (1972). Acta. Endocr. (Kbh) 69, 107.
8. Guraya, S.S. (1969). Acta. Vet. Acad. Sci. Hung. 19, 351.
9. Parlow, A.F. (1963). Endocrinology 73, 509.
10. Jacoby, F. (1962). In "The Ovary", S. Zukerman (Ed). Vol. I, pp. 189, Academic Press, New York.
11. Adams, E.C., Hertig, A.T., and Foster, S. (1966). Am. J. Anat. 119, 303.
12. Varma, S.K., and Guraya, S.S. (1968). Experientia. 24, 398.
13. Fawcett, D.W., Long, J.A., and Jones, A.L. (1969). Rec. Prog. Horm. Res. 20, 367.
14. Christensen, A.K., and Gillim, S.W. (1969). In "The Gonads" K.W. McKerns (Ed). pp 415, Appleton-Century-Crofts, New York.
15. Byskov, A.G.S. (1969). Z. Zellforsch. 100, 285.
16. Baillie, A.H., Ferguson, M.M. and Hart, D.M. (1966) In "Developments in Steroid Histochemistry", Academic Press, New York.

17. Brandau, H. (1970). In "Gonadotropins and Ovarian Development", W.R. Butt, A.C. Crooke and M. Ryle (Eds). pp. 307, E & S Livingstone, Edinburgh and London.
18. Short, R.V. (1964). Rec. Prog. Horm. Res. 20, 303.
19. Younglai, E.A., and Short, R.V. (1970). J. Endocr. 47, 321.
20. Savard, K., Marsh, J.M. and Rice, B.F. (1965). Rec. Prog. Horm. Res. 21, 285.
21. Mills, T.M., Davies, P.J.A. and Savard, K. (1971). Endocrinology 88, 857.
22. Stoklosowa, S. and Nalbandov, A.V. (1972). Endocrinology 91, 25.
23. Baranczuk, R. and Greenwald, G.S. (1973). Endocrinology 92, 805.
24. Baranczuk, R. and Greenwald, G.S. (1973). Endocrinology 92, 1547.
25. Stegner, H.E. and Onken, M. (1971). Cytobiologie 3, 240.
26. Guraya, S.S., Stegner, H.E. and Pape, C. (1974). Z. Zellforsch (in press).
27. Merk, F.B., Botticelli, C.R. and Albright, J.T. (1972). Endocrinology 90, 992.
28. Wimsatt, W.A. and Parks, H.F. (1966). In "Comparative Biology of Reproduction", I.W. Rolands (Ed). pp 419, Academic Press, London.
29. Nicosia, S.V. (1972). Fert. Steril. 23, 802.
30. McKay, D.G., Pinkerton, J.H.M., Hertig, A.T. and Danziger, S. (1961). Obst. and Gynec. 18, 13.
31. Novikoff, A.B., Drucker, J., Shin, W. and Goldfisher, S. (1961). J. Histo. and Cytochem. 9, 434.
32. Arvy, L. (1960). Z. Zellforsch. 51, 406.
33. Borzynski, L.J., McDougall, W.J., Gist, R.L., Vogel, M.D. and Norton, D.A. (1971). Com. Biochem. Physiol. 40, 575.
34. Deane, H.W., Lobel, B.L. and Romney, S.L. (1962). Am. J. Obst. Gynec. 83, 281.
35. Rubin, L.B., Deane, H.W. and Hamilton, J.A. (1963). Endocrinology 73, 748.
36. Lobel, B.L. and Levy, E. (1968). Acta Endocr. (Kbh), 59, Suppl. 1.
37. Channing, C.P. (1969). In "The Gonads", K.W. McKerns (Ed). pp 415, Appleton-Century-Crofts, New York.

38. Channing, C.P. (1970). Rec. Prog. Horm. Res. 26, 589.
39. Nicosia, S.V. (1972). Fert. Steril. 23, 791.
40. Brandau, H., Remmlinger, K. and Luh, W. (1967). Acta. Endocr. (Kbh) 56, 433.
41. Ryan, K.J. and Short, R.V. (1965). Endocrinology 76, 108.
42. Ryan, K.J. and Short, R.V. (1966). Endocrinology 78, 214.
43. Guraya, S.S. (1973). Acta. Endocr. (Kbh) 72, suppl. 171. p 1.
44. Guraya, S.S. (1973). Ann. Biol. Anim. Biochem. Biophys. (in press).
45. Guraya, S.S. (1973). Inter. Rev. Cytol. (in press).
46. Zmigrod, A. and Lindner, H.R. (1972). Acta Endocr (Kbh) 69, 127.
47. Rice, B.F., Hammerstein, J. and Savard, K. (1964). J. Clin. Endo. 24, 606.
48. Armstrong, D.T. (1968). Rec. Prog. Horm. Res. 24, 255.
49. Greenwald, G.S. and Rothchild, I. (1968). J. Anim. Sci. 27, 139.
50. Denamur, R., Martinet, J. and Short, R.V. (1966). Acta. Endocr. (Kbh) 52, 72.
51. DuMesnil De Buisson, F., Leglise, P.C., Anderson, L.L., and Rombants, P. (1964). Proc. 5th Intern. Congr. Reprod. Anim. Insem, Artif., Torento, Vol. 3, p. 571.
52. Spies, H.G., Hillard, J. and Sawyer, C.H. (1968). Endocrinology 83, 354.
53. Choudary, J.B. and Greenwald, G.S. (1969). Anat. Rec. 163, 373.
54. Bartosik, D.B. and Romanoff, E.B. (1969). In "The Gonads" K.W. McKerns (Ed). pp 211, Appleton-Century-Crofts, New York.
55. Takayama, M. and Greenwald, G.S. (1973). J. Endocr. 56, 421.
56. Greenwald, G.S. (1973). Endocrinology 92, 235.
57. Hansel, W. and Seifart, K.H. (1967). J. Dairy, Sci. 50, 1948.
58. Nalbandov, A.V. (1970). Biol. Reprod. 2, 7.
59. Raj, H.G.M. and Moudgal, N.R. (1970). Endocrinology 86, 874.
60. Rao, A.J., Raj, H.G.M. and Moudgal, N.R. (1972) J. Reprod. Fertil. 29, 239.
61. Duncan, G.W. and Kirton, K.T. (1971). J. Reprod. Med. 7, 2471.
62. Macdonald, G.J. and Greep, R.O. (1972). Fert. Steril. 23, 466

63. Niswender, G.D., Menon, K.M.J. and Jaffe, R.B. (1972). Fert. Steril. 23, 432.
64. Okamura, H., Yang, S.L., Wright, K.H. and Wallach, E.E. (1972). Fert. Steril. 23, 475.
65. Guraya, S.S. (1973). Proc. Ind. Natl. Sci. Acad (in press).
66. Guraya, S.S. and Greenwald, G.S. (1965). Amer. J. Anat. 116, 257.
67. Guraya, S.S. (1968). Proc. 6th Cong. Intern. Reprod. Anim. Insem. Artif, Paris, Vol. 1, 141.
68. Blandau, R.J. and Odor, D.L. (1972). In "Oogenesis", J.D. Biggers and A.W. Schuetz (Eds). pp 301, University Park Press, Baltimore.
69. Delforge, J.P., Thomas, K., Roux, F., Carneirode Siqueira, J., and Ferin, J. (1972). Fert. Steril. 23, 1.
70. Channing, C.P. and Crisp, T.M. (1972). Gen. Comp. Endo. Suppl. 3, 617.
71. Guraya, S.S. (1974). Acta Anat. (in press).
72. Hisaw, F.L. (1947). Physiol. Rev. 27, 95.
73. Berger, M.J., Taymor, M.L. Karam, K. and Nudemberg, F. (1972). Fert. Steril. 23, 783.
74. El-Fouly, M.A., Cook, B., Nekola, M. and Nalbandov, A.V. (1970). Endocrinology 87, 288.
75. Nekola, M.V. and Nalbandov, A.V. (1971). Biol. Reprod. 4, 154.
76. Nalbandov, A.V. (1972). In "Oogenesis", J.D. Biggers and A.W. Schuetz, (Eds). pp 513, University Park Press, Baltimore.
77. Norman, R.L. and Greenwald, G.S. (1972). Anat. Rec. 173, 95.
78. Foote, W.D. and Thibault, C. (1969). Ann. Biol. Anim. Biochem. Biophys. 9, 329.
79. Armstrong, D.T., Miller, L.S. and Knudsen, K.A. (1969) Endocrinology 85, 393.
80. Armstrong, D.T., Knudsen, K.A. and Miller, L.S. (1970). Endocrinology 86, 634.
81. Zarrow, M.X. and Clark, J.H. (1969). Endocrinology 84, 340.
82. Hilliard, J., Spies, H.G. and Sawyer, C.H. (1969). In "The Gonads", K.H. McKerns (Ed) pp. 55, Appleton-Century-Crofts, New York.

83. Behrman, H.R. and Armstrong, D.T. (1969). Endocrinology 85, 474.
84. Behrman, H.R., Orczyk, G.P., Macdonald, G.J. and Greep, R.O. (1970). Endocrinology 87, 1251.
85. Flint, A.P.F., Grinwich, D.L. and Armstrong, D.T. (1973). Biochem. J. 132, 313.
86. Flint, A.P.F. and Armstrong, D.T. (1973). Biochem. J. 132, 301.

ROLE OF GONADOTROPINS IN OVULATION

Neena B. Schwartz and Charles A. Ely.

INTRODUCTION

The purpose of this essay is to examine evidence relating to the relative roles played by FSH and LH in inducing ovulation in the mature, "ready" follicle. We will not review the extensive literature which deals with the separability of FSH and LH (1-4), but will assume the possibility at least of partial separability of (a) control and secretion rates, as well as (b) measurability in pituitary gland and serum. There are two reasons for making these assumptions: (a) pituitary extracts separated into FSH and LH on the basis of individual bioassays - mainly ovarian ascorbic acid depletion (OAAD) for LH,and hCG-augmentation assays for FSH (5-7) - show differences in chemical composition; (b) simultaneous bioassays and/or immunoassays for pituitary or serum levels of FSH and LH can show vastly differing ratios of the two hormones during various physiological and experimental states (3, 4).

The arguments of this paper will be developed in the following sequence. First, the process of follicle-maturation and preparation for ovulation will be discussed. Second, correlative data linking secretion rates of FSH and LH and ovulation or its blockade will be outlined. Third, data on hormone injections will be described. Next, the data on the use of antigonadotropic sera in studying the problem will be summarized. Then the other events accompanying ovulation, such as steroid secretion, will be summarized in relation to FSH and LH. Finally, we will attempt to draw conclusions regarding the two hormones and their obligatory or redundant roles in inducing ovulation.

CONCEPT OF THE MATURE, RIPE OR "READY" FOLLICLE

Each given follicle in the ovary can remain in the non-proliferating pool indefinitely, or begin to grow by granulosa cell-division, thereby entering the "proliferating" pool (4, 8). At each succeeding stage of follicle size, the follicle may become atretic, and die, or may grow into the next stage, until it becomes mature, and ovulable.

Pituitary hormones are necessary for entrance into the proliferating pool, as evidenced by the reduction in the rate of total loss of follicles within the ovary following hypophysectomy (4). If follicular growth to the point of maturation is to occur in the pre-pubertal or in the hypophysectomized animal, injections of hormones containing both FSH- and LH-like activities must be given (2, 9, 10). Concomitant with this morphological maturation, estrogen secretion occurs (10, 11, 12).

What hormones are responsible for the different stages of follicular maturation occurring during the estrous or menstrual cycles ? For reasons outlined in a paper by Schwartz (4), it is difficult to correlate the normal, hormonal secretion rates with the stages of follicular growth, and it is possible that FSH secretion during a given cycle, particularly in animals with short-cycles such as rodents, is responsible for follicular growth in succeeding cycles (13, 14). However, it is clear that gonadotropins are necessary continuously for the maintenance of follicular morphology and to bring about ovulation during the cycle; hypophysectomy or antiserum to LH or hCG very quickly block follicular maturation, and the follicles show signs of atresia and inability to ovulate (15-18).

It is possible to bring about ovulation of a follicle during the cycle, after it has achieved a given size, but even before it attains that size by normal course, it is possible to bring about ovulation, if higher doses of exogenous LH are administered (19, 20) indicating that the ovulatory threshold is not absolute, and that maturity of a follicle is not an abrupt, short-lived phenomenon. This is also suggested in mammals, such as humans where length of the follicular phase is quite variable (21, 22) or in the rat which normally shows a 4- or 5-day cycle, with a longer period of follicular "maturation" in the latter group (23, 24). However, follicles which have been mature for an overly-long period of time, such as in the persistent-estrus rodent, may not ovulate in response to exogenous LH (25).

CORRELATION OF OVULATION WITH THE SECRETION OF A SURGE OF GONADOTROPIN(S)

In every species in which the measurement has been made, a short-lived, large surge of LH with an abrupt onset has been detected in the blood at a time interval before ovulation, which is species-specific (11, 12, 21, 26-29). Usually, a surge of FSH is also detected at about the same time; however, this is not true in the rabbit (26) and occasionally in the human (21). In the rodent, at any rate, a surge of prolactin also occurs (30).

In a "spontaneously" cycling animal such as the rat, the three surges (LH, FSH and prolactin), and ovulation are all dependent on precedent rising estrogen titers, as demonstrated by the blocking of the surges by ovariectomy or by antiestrogenic compounds administered on the day before the release of the expected surges (30-34). This estrogen secretion, in turn is dependent on secretion of LH, but not FSH, as demonstrated by the effects of hypophysectomy or anti-LH serum on the day of estrogen secretion (15, 16, 30). Interestingly, pentobarbital administered on the same day (vide infra) can also block the LH surge expected the next day and subsequent ovulation, but not the estrogen secretion necessary for uterine and vaginal events (35).

Coitus-induced ovulation apparently occurs because of estrogen induced mating behaviour, with the cervical stimulation inducing LH release (11, 12, 22, 26). In the light of the apparent interchangeability of these two signals as stimuli for ovulation in many species (12, 22), coitus may indirectly substitute for estrogen or vice versa.

On the day of the pre-ovulatory surge in rodents, a series of compounds can prevent both the LH and FSH surge and the subsequent ovulation (12, 24). Barbiturates, such as pentobarbital, have been most widely used (34, 36-39). LH, or FSH, injected exogenously on the afternoon of proestrus can overcome the blockade caused by barbiturate, chlorpromazine or antiestrogen (36, 40, 41).

The correlative data leave no doubt that LH, at any rate, could be the necessary stimulus for ovulation; the role of FSH is somewhat more questionable because of reports that ovulation may occur in the absence of a FSH surge (21, 26).

INDUCTION OF OVULATION IN MATURE FOLLICLES BY GONADOTROPIN INJECTION.

A priori it should be simple to determine the relative roles of FSH and LH in causing ovulation by their administration to animals whose ovaries contain mature follicles and where spontaneous release of the gonadotropin surge(s) is prevented. In practice, however, the situation is more complex.

If absolutely pure FSH and LH were available, as judged by bioassay, physicochemical and immunological criteria, it would just be necessary to inject the materials singly or in combination at a series of doses and check for ovulation. But pure hormones are not available, there is a circularity in defining purity based on bioassays, and there is some ambiguity in definition of the bioassays themselves (1,3,4). The purest FSH hormones available still cause steroidogenesis (42) as well as exhibit OAAD activity (3). The problems with respect to bioassays themselves can be illustrated with two recent articles from the laboratory of Parlow. Even in the acute OAAD test, circulatory life-span of LH's from different species influence assay potencies (43); in the "longer" bioassay of rat uterine weight stimulation, bovine and ovine LH, in contrast to rat LH, reveal different indices of discrimination compared to other bioassays (44). Since ovulation is nothing more than another bioassay of some intermediate duration (between OAAD and chronic ovarian or uterine weight increase), what generalizations are possible using this assay when testing in a given species, the homologous and heterologous hormones having different circulatory life-spans (45).

Having outlined some of the objections and pitfalls, we can briefly state that either LH (or its β subunit) or FSH, is capable of inducing ovulation if injected in sufficiently high doses (9, 10, 20, 40-42, 45-47). In the absence of data on purity of injected materials it is not possible to compare the true ED_{50} of the two hormones; however, some suggestion of synergism exists (40,41).

In an attempt to circumvent the problem of contamination of FSH with LH, as judged by residual activity in the OAAD test, Harrington and co-workers (48) subjected ovine FSH to α-chymotrypsin digestion, thus destroying its ability to cause OAAD (49). The treated FSH, however, retained its ovulating ability, suggesting either that this ability is truly intrinsic to FSH, or that there are two separate sites on contaminating LH causing ovulation and OAAD. Here again, the reader should note that the validity of Harrington's experiment depends on the definition of LH as <u>the</u> hormone which induces OAAD.

USE OF GONADOTROPIN ANTISERA IN THE STUDY OF OVULATION

A. Problems involved in using antiserum

Because of the failure of other approaches to delineate the roles of FSH and LH in ovulation, a number of investigators have used antisera to gonadotropic hormones. It must be conceded at the outset that several problems which are inherent to the antiserum approach profoundly influence the answers obtained by their usage, (a) It is necessary to utilize acute passive, rather than active immunization, so that the antiserum effects on ovulation itself are not confounded with effects on follicular maturation and the estrogen secretion necessary for inducing an endogenous gonadotropin surge (15,50). (b) Heterologous antisera may act against homo logous pituitary hormones when tested in a standard bioassay system, where both the antiserum and antigen are exogenously injected, but may not combine with endogenously secreted hormone, or, if combination occurs, may form a soluble complex which is still biologically active (13, Anderson et al. unpublished data). (c) Antisera to FSH usually have a lower binding affinity when compared to antisera to LH (51). (d) The active site of the test hormone involved in ovulation may not necessarily be the one that is actually measured by the standard bioassays used usually for testing antiserum potencies.

B. Effects of antisera on ovulation induced by endogenous gonadotropin

Several laboratories have demonstrated that, in the absence of other treatments, several different antisera to ovine LH (AOLH) block ovulation when administered before the time of proestrus critical period (16,52,53). The efficacy of the treatment is dependent on the dose of antiserum used and on the time of administration, and is not abolished by absorbing with sheep FSH (16). In order to prevent ovulation brought about by endogenous stimulus in the rat, it is necessary to inject enough antiserum to block the equivalent of about 15 μg of rat LH, as assayed against LH by OAAD; the injection must be carried out within two hours of the onset (1400 hrs) of the critical period. Ovine antiserum is equipotent on OAAD blockade against ovine or rat LH (15); and it is not surprising that rat pituitary or serum LH can be measured so effectively with the ovine-ovine radioimmunoassay (54,55).

Similar experiments have been conducted with antiserum to ovine FSH, with no success in blocking ovulation (13) (Table 1). Antiserum R#86 was tested for its ability to prevent the effects of mouse (56) or of rat pituitary extract in the Steelman-Pohley hCG-augmentation test for FSH. While the potency was lower against rat LH, than against sheep LH, it was still effective, and a dose which failed to block ovulation (0.6 ml) (13) should have blocked all of the FSH released during the critical period (38). Two more antisera to ovine FSH (AOFSH) have now been tested and also found ineffective in blocking ovulation (Table 1). All three AOFSH indicated in Table 1 showed the ability to bind iodinated rat FSH of the NIAMDD kit, as did the AOLH. The binding was apparent in the serum harvested at estrus from rats injected earlier with AOFSH. Also, Rao and Moudgal (57), using yet another AO-FSH, could block the biological effects of rat pituitary extract. All of these data indicate the potential, at least, of formation of an antigen-antibody complex between rodent FSH and antiserum to ovine FSH. It should not be considered, however, that AOFSH has no effects, since observations later than the morning of estrus (i.e., by next cycle) show that AOFSH #86, reduces ovarian and uterine weights (13). From these data we concluded that the FSH surge in the rat probably does not play an obligatory role in ovulation induction (13). In the hamster, Goldman & Mahesh (58) showed that a non-specific, unabsorbed antiserum to gonadotropin blocked ovulation, but failed to do so after absorption with FSH. The potencies of the unabsorbed or absorbed antiserum against LH and FSH in standard bioassays were, however, not described.

C. Effects of antisera on ovulation produced by exogenous gonadotropins

Antisera to ovine LH or hCG can block ovulation induced by ovine LH or hCG in immature, PMSG-primed rats (59,60). Yang and Papkoff (45) have tested the effects of antisera administered on the day of proestrus to hamsters hypophysectomized early on that day, in order to avoid endogenous release. They report that an antiserum to oLH can block the effects of hCG, but not that of oFSH on ovulation; with an antiserum to FSH, doing the converse. They have not reported whether either of the two antisera block ovulation brought about by endogenous hormones.

Table 1. Effects of four different antisera to ovine FSH or LH on ovulation.

A/S*	Dose (ml)	Cross-reactivity of the A/S with		Effect on ¶ spontaneous ovulation	In presence of PB §		
		oLH** (μg)	oFSH*** (μg)		Overcomes high uter. H_2O	Ovulation blockade on treatment with	
						FSH 40 μg	LH 25 μg
AOFSH (R#122)	0.6	18	375	No block	Partly	Yes	Yes
AOFSH (R#86)	0.6	10	260	No block	Partly	No	No
AOFSH (R#134)	0.6	1.5	188	No block	Partly	Yes	No
AOLH (R#103)	0.3	30	N. T	Block	Completely	Yes	Yes

* Antiserum from four different rabbits immunized against NIH-FSH (R# 122, 86, 134) or NIH-LH R# 103. ** Antiserum potency (at dose shown) against LH in OAAD test; for AOFSH also correlates negatively with the amount of LH which needs to be added to the antiserum to prevent it from blocking effects of FSH on hCG-augmentation test. *** Antiserum potency (at dose shown) against FSH on hCG-augmentation. N. T. = non-testable because of cross-reaction with hCG. ¶ when injected into an otherwise untreated rat before critical period of proestrus. § PB (pentobarbital) and antiserum given at proestrus; autopsy on next morning. Reference: 4, 13, 16, 61, 62.

We have reported preliminary observations of a study of different design (4, 61, 62). The endogenous surge of gonadotropins was blocked by pentobarbital treatment at 1345 hr in 4-day cycling rats on the day of proestrus. At 1430 hr, the animals received an injection of saline, or one of the four antisera shown in Table 1, followed at 1500 hr by saline, NIH-FSH-S4 (40 μg) or NIH-LH-S14 (25 μg). Ovulation was checked the next morning (expected estrus). The dose of AOLH used was shown to be adequate in previous tests (16) to block ovulation. As can be seen from Table 1, it blocked the ovulatory effects of injected ovine LH or FSH.

In spite of rather similar potencies against ovine FSH, each one capable of neutralizing more than the injected dose of 40 μg of FSH, the three AOFSH sera gave different results when LH or FSH was tested for their effects on ovulation (Table 1). R#122 blocked both hormones; R#86 did neither, in agreement with its relative weakness in blocking LH in the OAAD test. However, R#134 blocked the ovulatory effects of FSH, without blocking LH; thus, this antiserum was the only one amongst the ones listed in the table, which blocked ovulation without possessing significant cross-reactivity with LH.

OTHER EVENTS ACCOMPANYING OVULATION

A. Completion of meiotic division of the ovum: Luteinization

Before drawing conclusions about the relative roles of FSH and LH in ovulation, other variables which normally always accompany ovulation will be examined, since they are potentially useful in deciding the issue.

During the process of preovulatory growth and follicular rupture following gonadotropin surge, the oocyte within the follicle completes the first meiotic division. During the afternoon of proestrus in the rat, resumption of meiosis occurs shortly after onset of LH release, perhaps before FSH release (63). *In vitro*, either of the hormones (NIH preparations) will induce meiosis (64), FSH doing so at doses which do not necessarily suggest that LH contamination is responsible. In a further *in vitro* study, Tsafriri and co-workers (65) have shown that LH induces both ovum maturation and progesterone secretion; however, inhibition of RNA synthesis could block the progesterone synthesis but not the maturation; FSH was not tried in this system.

One inevitable consequence of ovulation is luteinization of the granulosa cells of the follicle; while ovulation appears not to occur in the absence of luteinization, luteinization may occur in the absence of ovulation. At least two sets of circumstances can be defined in which the latter occurs: (a) when an abnormal FSH-LH ratio is produced near the time of expected ovulation (15, 16); (b) when the oocyte and granulosa cells are physically separated (66). Whether the common factor linking these observations is that it is necessary to have a normal oocyte in meiotic diapause in contact with the granulosa cells to prevent luteinization, is not certain at this point.

B. Steroid secretion and intralumenal water dissipation or retention

After the onset of the gonadotropin surge(s) but before ovulation in the rat, estrogen levels may temporarily increase over the existing high levels and later decrease, whereas progesterone levels rise from baseline followed by a decline later (36,67-69 and unpublished results). LH, but not FSH, can restore the progesterone secretion which is blocked by pentobarbital (36,70). Other studies also support the concept that LH rather than FSH is necessary for progesterone secretion (69). With respect to estrogen secretion rates, it should be noted that net levels of estrogen are falling during proestrus. Several studies have shown that LH can bring about an increase in estrogen secretion by matured follicle cells (68,71,72). However, only two groups (42,68) were able to observe with FSH, an increase in estrogen secretion.

A number of studies on the estrous cycle of rat including the present one (Table 1), have shown that intralumenal fluid accumulation and release could be used as another variable which shows some useful treatment-induced differences, probably related principally to steroid levels. Our information about the hormonal control of this variable has come from data on immature, treated animals from the laboratory of Armstrong (73-75). Briefly it can be summarized as follows: (a) estrogen is necessary for accumulation of water; (b) progesterone administered simultaneously with estrogen can prevent water accumulation; (c) estrogen is more successful at causing prolonged water accumulation in the absence of the pituitary than in its presence; (d) prolactin, in the absence of both ovary and pituitary, can enhance water loss in the continuing presence of estrogen. We have confirmed the essential role of estrogen in inducing water accumulation in the cyclic proestrus rat (15, 31, 32).

At the time when the treatments (Table 1) are initiated on the day of proestrus water accumulation is already present (23); this water normally would disappear by the following morning, when fresh ova are present (estrus). The treatments (shown in Table 1) altered this normal course of events; for this reason we need to summarize factors which can cause dissipation of the accumulated water. In immature animals, Armstrong and co-workers (73-75) showed that accumulated water disappears from the uterus when estrogen treatment ceases (presumably because some of the water dissipates continuously), or by administration of prolactin or progesterone. The latter two hormones work by inducing relaxation of the uterine cervix.

During the normal cycle, intralumenal water disappears very abruptly sometime between proestrus and estrus, this occurring later in the rats with 4-day cycles than in the 5-day cyclic rats. (67 and unpublished observations). The abruptness of the disappearance, as confirmed by the work of Ferin et al. (33) using progesterone antibodies, suggests that this is due to the normal secretion of progesterone on the afternoon of proestrus; however, the role of rising prolactin and the falling estrogen levels cannot be ruled out completely in this process. Pentobarbital administration virtually always prevents the accumulated water from disappearing by the next morning (31, 35, 39); the most likely interpretation of this is that the blockade of the LH surge led to a block of the progesterone surge, thus preventing cervix relaxation. Pentobarbital does not prevent the tonic secretion of LH apparently necessary for estrogen secretion (35, 37). In contrast to pentobarbital, administration of antiserum to LH blocks the retention of the uterine water as well as ovulation (16, 53); these data have been interpreted to indicate that the antiserum to LH terminates the estrogen secretion necessary for maintenance of the already accumulated water (16).

In the present experiment, (Table 1), in the absence of pentobarbital, no rat treated with any of the antisera showed maintenance of uterine fluid on autopsy at estrus, with AOFSH permitting ovulation, and AOLH blocking it. Pentobarbital alone permitted uterine ballooning the next day; treatment with either LH or FSH in the doses in Table 1 dissipated the water. Goldman & Mahesh

(46) were able to cause ovulation in the immature, PMSG-primed rat by either FSH or LH, but uterine ballooning (intralumenal water $\geq$ 100 mg) disappeared only with LH injection. The apparent difference between the effects of FSH and LH in adult and immature animals in inducing water loss may be related to a difference in adult and immature ovaries, or could simply represent a differential in thresholds of FSH and LH for the end points of ovulation and uterine water loss.

In the presence of both pentobarbital and antiserum (Table 1), AOLH completely blocked the retention of water seen with pentobarbital alone; AOFSH, however, blocked water retention only in some of the animals. This partial effect of AOFSH could reflect the small amount of anti-LH activity, which may have been adequate to reduce residual tonic LH secretion in some of the pentobarbital-treated rats. Interestingly, when LH is superimposed on treatment with pentobarbital and AOLH, although ovulation is still blocked (Table 1), water retention is restored, suggesting that a smaller amount of LH needs to be present for the estrogen secretion (necessary for water retention), than for ovulation (16). FSH injected into the rats treated with pentobarbital and AOLH does not induce water retention, confirming that FSH, in the presence of AOLH, cannot cause estrogen secretion (71, 72).

CONCLUSIONS REGARDING THE RELATIVE ROLES OF FSH AND LH IN THE INDUCTION OF OVULATION

The observations reviewed in this paper argue for an obligatory role for LH as the ovulating hormone, at least in the rat. Antiserum to LH, but not to FSH, blocks endogenous ovulation. Some species lack FSH surge, at least some times. LH, but not FSH, can induce progesterone secretion, causing ovulation as well. On the day of proestrus in the rat, tonic (not surge) levels of LH are adequate to maintain estrogen secretion; higher levels of LH are necessary to induce progesterone secretion and ovulation. In a recent communication by Proudfit and Schwartz (39) it has been shown that cardiac puncture can overcome pentobarbital blockade at proestrus; amongst the treated animals, a large proportion showed loss of uterine fluid on the day of estrus, than those showing ovulation, suggesting that the LH threshold for progesterone secretion is lower than for ovulation.

The FSH data suggest that the FSH surge is necessary for maturation of a different group of follicles than those ovulating at the time of the surge (13, 14). However, the observations that FSH can cause ovulation need to be kept in mind. Frequently it is said that FSH causes ovulation only because of contamination with LH. The data of Harrington et al. using chymotrypsin treated FSH (48) argue against this, since OAAD activity was lost without destroying the ovulatory ability of FSH. (What is not clear is whether LH itself loses its ovulating ability after chymotrypsin digestion – Reichert) (49).

Furthermore, ovine FSH could be blocked (Table 1) from inducing ovulation by one antiserum (R#134) which did not block LH in OAAD; R#134 also did not prevent ovulation induced by exogenous LH; similarly Yang and Papkoff (45) have reported an antiserum to FSH which blocks the ovulatory ability of FSH, but not that of LH. These data argue for the possibility that a site on the FSH molecule which is immunologically different from that on the LH molecule causes ovulation, and that this site is not the one responsible for OAAD.

Further, it can be observed from these data that for the antiserum to FSH (#86), the dose necessary to block FSH in the hCG-augmentation test is far greater than that necessary to cause ovulation in its presence (Table 1). The standard bioassay for FSH, perhaps involves a site on FSH which is not the one involved in ovulation; on the other hand, the data might also mean that AOFSH #86 impeded that part of the FSH molecule necessary for its persistence in circulation. This could reduce its potency in a chronic test like ovarian or uterine weight, but not necessarily in an acute test like ovulation.

These data appear to rule out an obligatory role for FSH in ovulation, but rise interesting questions about the validity of standard bioassays for FSH and LH for predicting the effects of FSH and LH on yet another bioassay - the ovulation of ripe follicles.

ACKNOWLEDGEMENTS

Published and unpublished work cited in this review was supported by PHS HD 07504 (Schwartz), HD-004471 (Ely), and by a grant from the Rockefeller Foundation to Dr. Oscar Hechter. We would like to thank Julian Alvarez, Brigitte Mann, William Talley and Shirley Snerling for excellent technical assistance.

The LH radioimmunoassay was made possible through supplies of immunoassay grade antiserum (ovine) from Dr. Gordon Niswender, ovine hormone for iodination from Dr. Leo Reichert, Jr., and NIH-LH-S14 used as standard from NIAMDD; for the FSH assay, the kit provided by NIAMDD was utilized.

REFERENCES

1. Hellema, M.J.C. (1971). J. Endocr. 49, 393.
2. Hisaw, F.L. (1947). Physiol. Rev. 27, 95.
3. Schwartz, N.B. and McCormack, C.E. (1972). Ann. Rev. Physiol. 34, 425.
4. Schwartz, N.B. (1974). Biol. Reprod. (in press).
5. Albert, A. (1961). In "Human Pituitary Gonadotropins", A. Albert (Ed). p. 271, Charles C. Thomas, Springfield, Illinois.
6. Igarashi, M., and McCann, S.M. (1964). Endocrinology 74, 440.
7. Steelman, S.L., and Pohley, F.M. (1953). Endocrinology 53, 604.
8. Pederson, T. (1972). In "Oogenesis", J.D. Biggers & A.W. Schuetz (Eds) p. 361, University Park Press, Baltimore, Md.
9. Carter, F., Woods, M.C., and Simpson, M.E. (1961). In "Control of ovulation", C.A. Villee (Ed.) p. 1, Pergamon Press, New York.
10. Lostroh, A.J., and Johnson, R.E. (1966) Endocrinology 79, 991.
11. Schwartz, N.B., and Hoffmann, J.C. (1972). In "Reproductive Biology", H. Balin and S. Glasser (Eds), p. 438, Excerpta Medica, Amsterdam.
12. Schwartz, N.B. (1973). In "Female Reproductive System", R.O. Greep (Ed). Handbook of Physiology, Endocrinology Vol II Part I, p. 125, Am. Physiological Society, Bethesda.
13. Schwartz, N.B., Krone, K., Talley, W.L., and Ely, C.A. (1973). Endocrinology 92, 1165.
14. Welschen, R. (1973). Acta Endocrinol. 72, 137.
15. Schwartz, N.B., and Ely, C.A. (1970). Endocrinology 86, 1420.
16. Ely, C.A., and Schwartz, N.B. (1971). Endocrinology 89, 1103.
17. Talbert, G.B., Meyer, R.K., and McShan, W.H. (1951). Endocrinology 49, 687.
18. Sasamoto, S., and Kennan, A.L. (1972). Endocrinology 91,350.
19. Holsinger, J.W., Jr., and Everett, J.W. (1970) Endocrinology 80, 257.

20. Ying, S. Y., and Greep, R. O. (1971). Endocrinology 89, 294.
21. Ross, G. T., Cargille, C. M., Lipsett, M. B., Rayford, P. L., Marshall, J. R., Strott, C. A., and Rodbard, D. (1970). Rec. Prog. Horm. Res. 26, 1.
22. Jochle. W. (1973). Contraception 7, 523.
23. Schwartz, N. B. (1969). Rec. Prog. Horm. Res. 25, 1.
24. Everett, J. W. (1961). In "Sex and Internal Secretions", W. C. Young (Ed). Vol. 1, p 497, Williams & Wilkins Co., Baltimore
25. Rodgers, C. H., and Schwartz, N. B. (1972). Endocrinology 90, 461.
26. Dufy-Barbe, L., Franchimont, P., and Faure, J. M. A. (1973) Endocrinology 92, 1318.
27. Kovacic, N., and Parlow, A. F. (1972). Endocrinology 91, 910.
28. Phemister, R. D., Holst, P. A., Spanco, J. S., and Hopwood, M. L. (1973). Biol. Reprod. 8, 74.
29. Norman, R. L., and Greenwald, G. S. (1972). Anat. Rec. 173, 95.
30. Freeman, M. E., Reichert, L. E., Jr., and Neill, J. D. (1972). Endocrinology 90, 232.
31. Schwartz, N. B. (1964). Am. J. Physiol. 207, 1251.
32. Shirley, B., Wolinsky, J., and Schwartz, N. B. (1968). Endocrinology 82, 959.
33. Ferin, M., Tempone, A., Zimmering, P. E., and Vande Wiele, R. L., (1969). Endocrinology 85, 1070.
34. McClintock, J. A., and Schwartz, N. B. (1968). Endocrinology 83, 433.
35. Beattie, C. W., and Schwartz, N. B. (1973). Proc. Soc. Exp. Biol. Med. 142, 933.
36. Barraclough, C. A., Collu, R., Massa, R., and Martini, L. (1971). Endocrinology 88, 1437.
37. Nequin, L. G., Talley, W. L., Mann, B. G., and Schwartz, N. B. (1974) Neuroendocrinology (in press).
38. Daane, T. A., and Parlow, A. F. (1971). Endocrinology 88, 653.
39. Proudfit, C. M., and Schwartz, N. B. (1974). Endocrinology (in press).
40. Harrington, F. E., and Bex, F. J. (1970). Endocrinol. Japan 17, 387.
41. Labhsetwar, A. P. (1970). J. Reprod. Fert. 23, 517.
42. Nuti, L. G., McShan, W. H., and Meyer, R. K. (1973). Prog. 55th Meeting of the Endocrine Society, p. A-114.

43. Parlow, A.F. (1972). Endocrinology 91, 1109.
44. Parlow, A.F., Bhalla, R.C., and Kovacic, N. (1972). Endocrinology 91, 711.
45. Yang, W.H., and Papkoff, H. (1974). Fert. & Ster (in press).
46. Goldman, B.D., and Mahesh, V.B. (1968). Endocrinology. 83, 97.
47. Yang, W.H., Sairam, M.R., Papkoff, H., and Li, C.H. (1972). Science 175, 637.
48. Harrington, F.E., Bex, F.J., Elton, R.L., and Roach, J.B. (1970). Acta. Endocrinol. 65, 222.
49. Reichert, L, E., Jr. (1967). J. Clin. Endo. Metab. 27, 1065.
50. Laurence, K.A., (1971). Bibliog. Reprod. 18, 325 & 491.
51. Odell, W.D., Abraham, G., Rander Raud, H., Swerdloff, R. S., and Fisher, D. (1969). In "Immunoassay of Gonadotropins" p. 54, Karolinska Symposia, Suppl. 142, Acta Endocrinologica.
52. Kelley, W.A., Robertson, H.A., and Stansfield, D.A. (1963) J. Endocrinol. 27, 127.
53. Schwartz, N.B., and Gold, J.J. (1967). Anat. Rec. 157, 137.
54. Niswender, G.D., Midgley, A.R., Monroe, S.E., and Reichert, L.E. (1968). Proc. Soc. Exp. Biol. Med. 128, 807.
55. Bogdanove, E.M., Schwartz, N.B., Reichert, L.E., and Midgley, A.R. (1971). Endocrinology 88, 644.
56. Ely, C.A., and Tallberg, T. (1964). Endocrinology 74, 314.
57. Rao, A.J., and Moudgal, N.R. (1970). Arch. Biochem. Biophys. 138, 189.
58. Goldman, B.D., and Mahesh, V.B. (1969). Endocrinology 84, 236.
59. Madhwa Raj, H.G., and Moudgal, N.R. (1970). Nature 227, 1344.
60. Sasamoto, S. (1969). J. Reprod. Fert. 20, 271.
61. Cobbs, S.B., Schwartz, N.B., and Ely, C.A. (1972). Biol. Reprod. 7, 137.
62. Schwartz, N.B., Cobbs, S.B., and Ely, C.A (1973). Proc. IVth Int. Cong. Endocrinology, Excerpts Medica (in press).
63. Ayalon, D., Tsafriri, A., Lindner, H.R., Cordova, T., and Harell, H.R. (1972). J. Reprod. Fert. 31, 51.
64. Tsafriri, A., Lindner, H.R., Zor, U., and Lamprecht, S.A. (1972). J. Reprod. Fert. 31, 39.
65. Tsafriri, A., Lieberman, M.E., Barnea, A., Bauminger, S., and Lindner, H.R. (1973). Endocrinology 93, 1378.

66. Nalbandov, A. V., (1972). In "Oogenesis", J. O. Biggers, and A. W. Schuetz (Eds). p. 513, University Park Press, Baltimore, Md.
67. Nequin, L. G., and Schwartz, N. B. (1973). Biol. Reprod. 9, 75.
68. Hori, T., Ide, M., and Miyake, T. (1968). Endocrinol. Japan 15, 215.
69. Uchida, K., Kadowaki, M., and Miyake, T. (1969). Endocrinol. Japan. 16, 239.
70. Ichikawa, S., Morioka, H., and Sawada, T. (1972). Endocrinology 90, 1356.
71. Liu, T. C., and Gorski, J., (1971). Endocrinology 88, 419.
72. Mills, T. M., Davies, P. J. A., and Savard, K. (1971). Endocrinology 88, 857.
73. Armstrong, D. T., and Kennedy, T. G. (1972). Am. J. Physiol 214, 764.
74. Armstrong, D. T., and Kennedy, T. G. (1972). Am. Zool. 12, 245.
75. Kennedy, T. G., and Armstrong, D. T. (1972). Endocrinology 90, 1503.

EFFECT OF ANTI-GONADOTROPIN SERUM ON OVULATION IN MICE

Shuji Sasamoto

INTRODUCTION

Gonadotropins are essential for follicular development and ovulation. The amount of gonadotropin required for the maintenance of mature follicles in an ovulable state is only one tenth of the amount required for the initial stimulation of follicular growth (1). When these small amounts of circulating gonadotropins are neutralized, follicles once developed to an ovulable state begin to degenerate within 3 hr and completely lose the ability to ovulate within 9 hr of neutralization (2).

Though the interval between the release of ovulating hormone and ovulation in mice and rats is about 12 hr, the need for gonadotropins in bringing about ovulation is thought to be of transient nature. Recent results of plasma LH determination by radioimmunoassay during the preovulatory period has revealed that the LH surge is a sudden event (3,4).

In the present experiments, the minimum period required for the ovulating hormone to bring about maximum ovulation has been determined using antigonadotropin sera.

RESULTS AND DISCUSSION

A. Induction of ovulation by a single injection of hCG

Immature mice, aged 20 to 25 days and weighing 7.0-9.5 g were allotted to treatment groups at random, and were given a priming sc injection of 2.5 IU of PMSG at 0900 - 1000 hr, followed by varying amounts of hCG in a single sc or iv injection 54 hr later. All injections were given in a total volume of 0.1 ml of 0.9 % NaCl. At 20-24 hr after hCG, the animals were killed and oviducts were examined for ova by the method of Burdick and Whitney (5).

The dose-response relationship for hCG in bringing about ovulation in mice is illustrated in Fig 1. The percentage of mice ovulating were transformed to probits and the results were

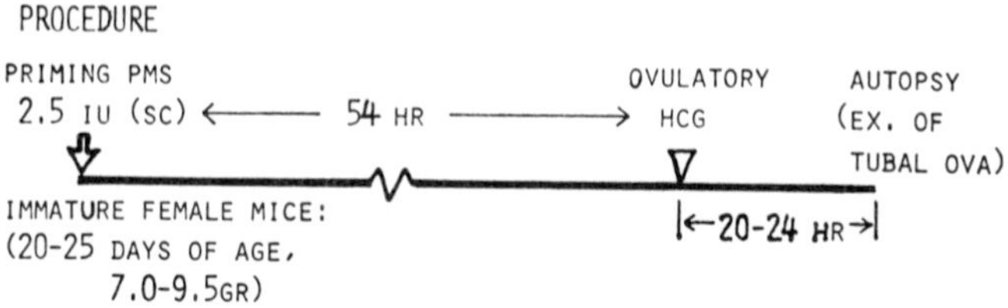

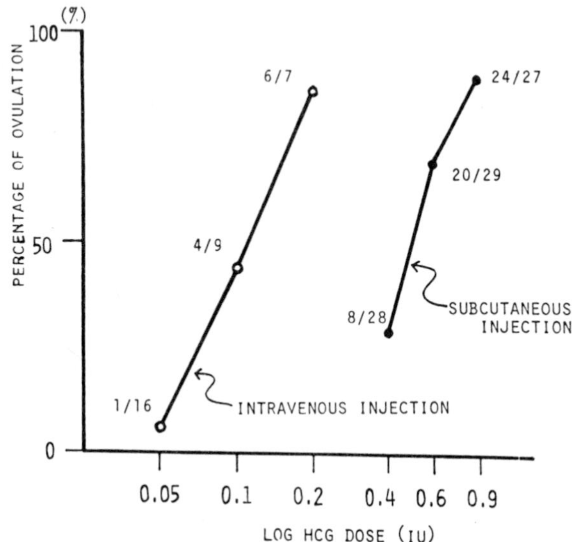

FIG 1. Log dose-response lines for induction of ovulation in immature mice pretreated with PMS -[from Sasamoto (10)].

computed as a parallel line assay. These results gave a potency of 4.6 for the iv injection relative to the sc injection with fiducial limits ($p = 0.95$) of 3.1 to 6.1.

B. HCG levels in plasma following a single injection into mice

Adult female mice, weighing 20 to 25 g, were ovariectomized and 2 weeks later the animals were given either a single iv or sc injection of 50 IU of hCG in 0.5 ml of 0.9 % NaCl. At varying time intervals after this, groups of mice ($n = 5$) were killed, blood was pooled and plasma obtained. Each plasma sample was

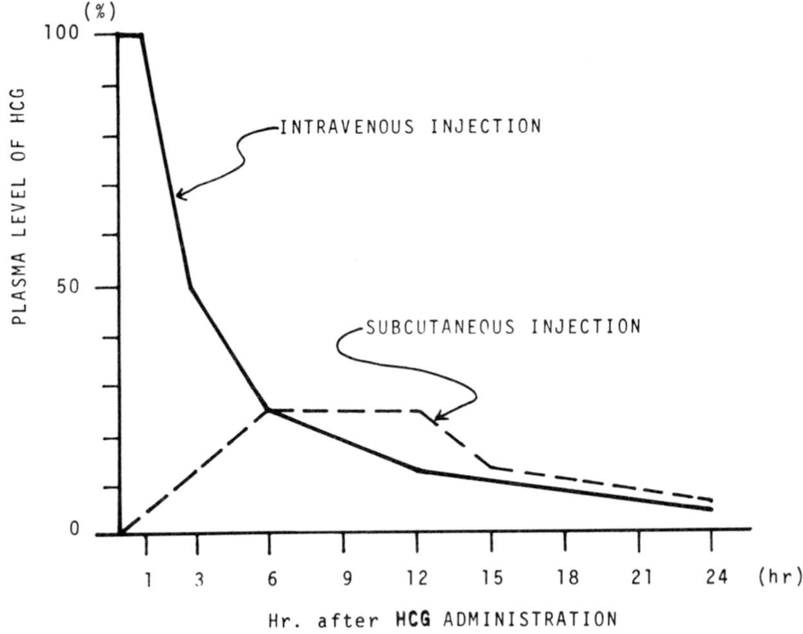

FIG 2. Plasma levels of hCG after a single injection into mice - [from Sasamoto (11)].

immediately assayed for hCG activity using immature mice pre-treated with PMSG. The activity immediately after an iv injection was defined as 100 % and hCG activity in plasma obtained at each time interval was expressed as a percentage of the initial activity (Fig 2).

The half-life of hCG after an injection was shown to be 3 hr in the mouse; after a sc injection, the plasma level of hCG reached a plateau by 6 hr and was maintained till 12 hr, but the level at the plateau was 25 % as compared to the initial level seen after an iv injection. Six hr after the subcutaneous injection, however, plasma levels were higher than those seen with iv administration.

The greater effectiveness of the iv injection compared to the sc injection of hCG in induction of ovulation is probably due to its greater concentrations in plasma during the initial period.

C. Preparation of anti-hCG serum (ACS) and the activity of ACS

Rabbits were immunized with hCG given once a week over a period of 10 weeks, emulsified in Freund's complete adjuvant. The rabbits were bled by heart puncture 1 week after the last injection. Serum was pooled and diluted tenfold with 0.9 % NaCl and stored in small aliquots at -20°.

The amount of antiserum given s c required to abolish the activity of 2 IU hCG was determined (ACS and hCG were given at different sites).

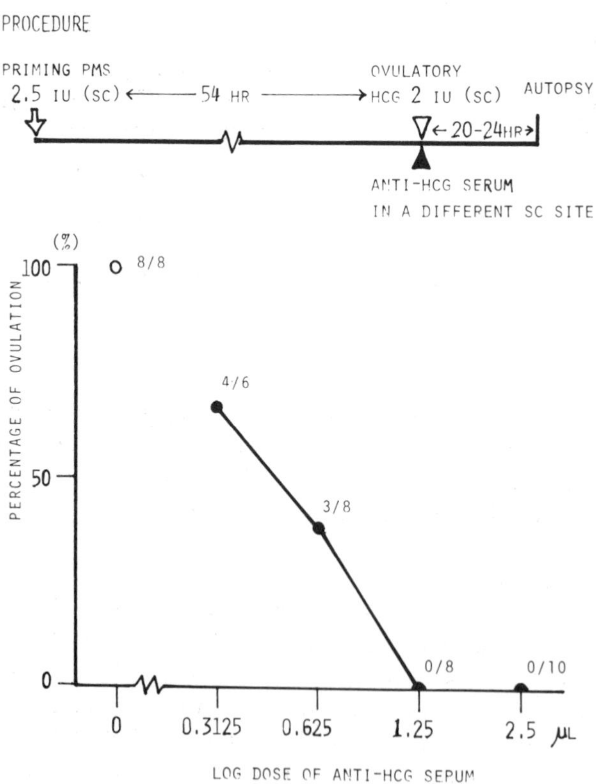

FIG 3. The activity of anti-hCG serum (ACS) to prevent hCG induced ovulation in immature mice pretreated with PMS -[from Sasamoto (10)].

The results (Fig 3) indicate that the activity of hCG was inhibited in direct proportion to the amount of the serum administered. For complete inhibition, the amount of the serum required was 1.25 μl, which was defined as 2 units (1 ml ≡ 1600 units).

D. <u>Effect of time of administration of ACS on the inhibition of ovulation</u>

The minimum time necessary for hCG to be present in the circulation to induce ovulation was determined as follows: Groups of

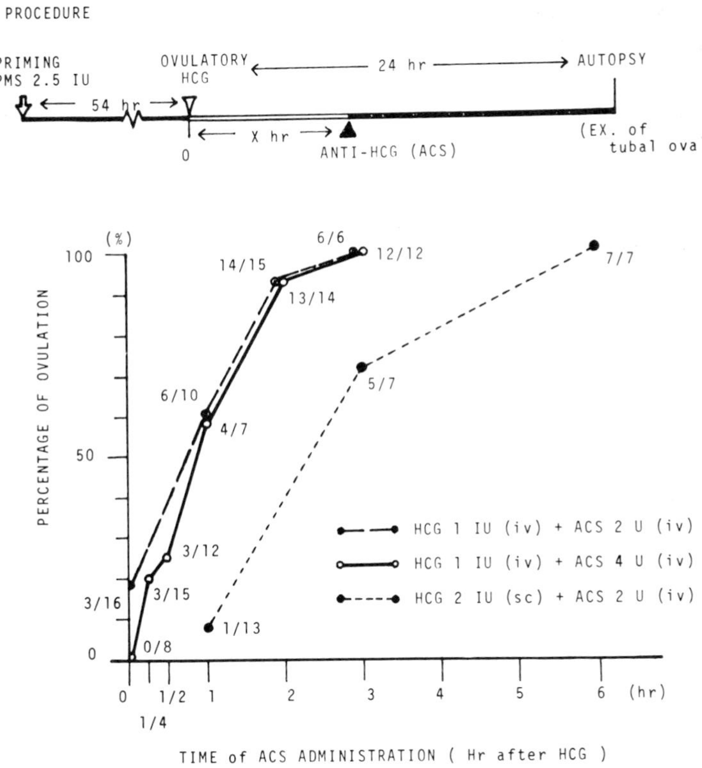

FIG 4. Effect on ovulation of anti-hCG serum (ACS) given at varying time intervals after hCG administration in immature mice pretreated with PMS - [from Sasamoto (10)].

mice, pretreated with PMSG, were injected with 1 or 2 IU of hCG given iv or sc respectively. Following this, the animals were injected iv at various time intervals with ACS in order to effect an instantaneous neutralization of circulating hCG. The effective time of hCG action in circulation is represented by the interval elapsing between the injection of the hormone and its antiserum.

When an amount of hCG sufficient to produce a maximum response was given sc and followed by ACS 1 hr later, only one out of 13 mice ovulated (Fig 4). The inhibitory effect of ACS was still observed when ACS was given 3 hr after hCG. When ACS administration was delayed until 6 hr after hCG given sc, all the animals ovulated.

On the other hand, when hCG was given iv, the inhibitory effect of ACS was observed only if given within 1 hr of hCG. When ACS administration was delayed by 2 hr, 93 % of the animals ovulated which was similar to the controls given no ACS (22/23 mice). Thus, the inhibitory effect of ACS was no longer observed when hCG was inactivated 2 hr after the iv injection. No difference was observed in results obtained with 2 and 4 units of ACS.

From these experiments it is apparent that for inducing maximal ovulation, hCG needs to be present for only 2 hr if given intravenously, or for 6 hr if given subcutaneously. This is because after an sc injection, it takes 6 hr for hCG in blood to reach the threshold for triggering ovulation.

Table 1. Effect of anti-PMSG serum (APS) on ovulation in immature mice pretreated with PMSG and given an ovulatory dose of PMSG.

Time after PMSG injection	0	1-3 min	2 hr		3 hr
Amount of anti-PMSG serum (U)	0	3	3	12	3
Proportion of mice ovulating	10/10	0/9	17/17	16/16	9/9
Percentage of ovulation	100	0	100	100	100

Similar experiments were undertaken using PMSG as an ovulating hormone and anti-PMSG serum (APS) as the inhibiting agent. Immature mice were injected i v with 3 IU of PMSG 54 hr after pretreatment with PMSG, followed by an i v injection of 3 to 12 units of APS at varying time intervals after the ovulating dose of PMSG. The results, given in Table 1, were similar to those observed in the experiment using hCG and ACS. APS completely blocked ovulation when given simultaneously with PMSG but when APS administration was delayed for 2 hr after PMSG, all the animals ovulated even though an excess amount of APS was injected. Raj and Moudgal (6) also obtained similar results using LH and anti-LH serum in immature rats pretreated with PMSG.

From these experiments, it is concluded that a 2-hr existence in circulation is sufficient for the ovulating gonadotropin to induce maximum ovulation. Any gonadotropin present in circulation after that time may not be involved in the completion of the process. Ovulating gonadotropin may play a role as an initial stimulus leading to an activation of the enzymes required for the rupture of mature follicular walls, as suggested by Rondell (7, 8) and Lipner and Greep (9).

ACKNOWLEDGEMENTS

These investigations were partially supported by grants from the Ministry of Education of Japan and Sankyo Zoki Co. (Tokyo).

REFERENCES

1. Sasamoto, S., Sato, K. and Naito, H. (1972). J. Reprod. Fert. 30, 371.
2. Sasamoto, S. and Kennen, A. L. (1972). Endocrinology 91, 350.
3. Gay, V. L., Midgley, A. R. and Niswender, G. (1970). Federation Proceedings 29, 1880.
4. Daane, T. A. and Parlow, A. F. (1971). Endocrinology 88, 653.
5. Burdick, H. O. and Whitney, R. (1941) Am. J. Physiol. 132, 405.
6. Raj, H. G. M. and Moudgal, N. R. (1970). Nature 227, 1344.
7. Rondell, P. (1970). Biol. Reprod. 2, Suppl. 2, 64.
8. Rondell, P. (1970). Federation Proceedings 29, 1875.
9. Lipner, H. and Greep, R. O. (1971). Endocrinology 88, 602.
10. Sasamoto, S. (1969). J. Reprod. Fer. 20, 271.
11. Sasamoto, S. (1965). Japan J. Animal. Reprod. 11, 65.

LUTEOTROPIC COMPLEX IN LACTATING RATS

K. Yoshinaga and J.J. Ford

INTRODUCTION

In primates and domestic animals, corpora lutea of the estrous cycle secrete sufficient amount of progesterone to prepare the uterus for implantation of fertilized ova, regardless of mating. Therefore, the luteal phase of the cycle is under the influence of functional corpora lutea. On the other hand, small laboratory animals i.e., rat, mouse and hamster, have short estrous cycles. The corpora lutea of the cycle in these animals do not secrete enough progesterone to prepare the uterus. Thus, the cycle lacks the true luteal phase and the corpora lutea are "non-functional". Mating, or equivalent stimuli applied to the vaginal-uterine cervical area, changes the cyclic function of the hypothalamo-pituitary-ovarian axis to the pregnancy type. The resulting pituitary hormone secretion converts the corpora lutea from a non-functional state to functional. Our definition of the luteotropic complex is a combination of extra-luteal hormones which participate in this conversion resulting in maintenance of the structure of corpora lutea and stimulation of progesterone secretion required to prepare the uterus for implantation.

This paper deals with the luteotropic complex during lactation in the rat with special emphasis on the relationship between ovarian progesterone secretion and its controlling factors, namely suckling stimulus, LH and prolactin.

In the rat, postpartum ovulation occurs within 24 hr of parturition. Since corpora lutea of pregnancy do not regress by this time there are two sets of corpora lutea during lactation: one,corpora lutea of pregnancy and the other, corpora lutea of lactation. The corpora lutea of pregnancy gradually degenerate, but the corpora lutea of lactation increase in size during lactation. Progesterone secretion into the ovarian venous effluent increases gradually to peak on day 12 (day 1 = day of parturition) and falls rapidly by day 16. Secretion of 20α-dihydroprogesterone (20α-OH-P) exhibits a reciprocal relationship with progesterone. On day 4 of lactation, 20α-OH-P level is higher than progesterone, but is at minimal level on day 12 when progesterone is at its peak. Similarly on day 16, the 20α-OH-P secretion is very high compared to the minimal level of progesterone (1). Similar observation has been reported by Tomogane et al. (2).

EFFECT OF NURSING LITTER SIZE ON PROGESTIN SECRETION

Increase in suckling stimulus produced an enhancement in progesterone secretion in lactating rats. Progesterone secretion rate on day 8 of lactation in rats nursing 8 pups was compared with those nursing 2. Blood was collected from either the right or the left ovarian vein, extracted with diethyl ether, progestins separated on thin-layer plates and determined by gas-liquid chromatography. Progesterone secretion rate was significantly higher in rats nursing 8 pups (8.8 $\pm$ 1.6 μg/15 min) than in those nursing 2 pups (4.6 $\pm$ 0.4). On the other hand, there was no significant difference in 20α-OH-P secretion rate between these two groups (1.7 $\pm$ 0.3 vs 2.5 $\pm$ 0.5). Similar differences in progesterone secretion have been observed in rats nursing 6 pups and 2 pups (1,3).

In another series of experiments, we compared the ovarian venous plasma concentration of progestins in rats nursing 3, 6 or 12 pups. Petroleum ether extract of plasma samples was subjected to LH-20 column chromatography for separation of progesterone and 20α-OH-P. 20α-OH-P was oxidized by Jones' reagent and progesterone was measured by radioimmunoassay. The results showed that the plasma progesterone concentration had a direct relationship to the number of pups suckling (3 pups : 1.2 $\pm$ 0.2; 6 pups : 1.6 $\pm$ 0.2; 12 pups : 2.3 $\pm$ 0.4 μg/ml); concentration of 20α-OH-P ranging between 0.54 and 0.90 μg/ml, had no direct relationship to litter size. These results suggest that suckling stimulus quantitatively influences the secretion of hormone(s) by the pituitary. Serum prolactin levels are elevated as the suckling stimulus increases (4), strongly supporting the concept that progesterone secretion during lactation is directly related to the level of prolactin. Furthermore, serum FSH and LH levels are progressively diminished as litter size increases (5).

PROGESTIN SECRETION RHYTHM DURING LACTATION

During the early stage of lactation, we observed that there is a diurnal rhythmic secretion of progestin by the ovary. From day 4 to 7 of lactation, ovarian venous blood was collected at 0900 hr and

1800 hr from rats nursing 8 or 2 pups. Plasma levels of both progesterone and 20α-OH-P were found to be significantly higher in the evening than in the morning on days 4 and 6 of lactation. This diurnal fluctuation was much less on day 5 and there was no statistical difference between the morning and evening samples in rats nursing 8 pups and 2 pups. While progesterone secretion increased from days 4 to 7, 20α-OH-P secretion decreased. It is interesting to note that progesterone/20α-OH-P ratio changed between the evening of day 4 and the morning of day 5 regardless of the number of pups suckling. A temporal loss of diurnal fluctuation on day 5 of lactation may be due to the alteration of luteal function, or may be a reflection of a change in gonadotropin secretion which is expected to occur prior to ova-implantation, if the rats had become pregnant at post-partum ovulation.

An explanation for the difference in the morning and evening progesterone secretion rates is a possible difference in the suckling stimulus during day and night. Although we have not measured the difference in suckling intensity, it is likely that the mother nurses her young more intensively during the day. Since rat is a nocturnal animal which seeks food at night, the low, morning progestin levels may be due to the low suckling stimulus during the night and the high, evening values may be due to suckling stimulus applied during the day. Bischof et al. (6) have observed a circadian rhythm of progesterone secretion on day 7 of pseudopregnancy and suggest that this may result from the nocturnal release of prolactin.

INVOLVEMENT OF LH IN THE LUTEOTROPIC COMPLEX

It has been reported that LH in various species of animals stimulates progesterone biosynthesis or secretion by the luteal tissue or the luteinized ovary (7, 8). Biosynthesis of progesterone in the human luteal tissue was stimulated by human pituitary LH (9), and a similar effect of LH was shown in the bovine corpus luteum (10-12). Injection of LH to rabbits increased progesterone, 20α-OH-P and estrogen in ovarian venous plasma (13, 14) and LH has been shown to maintain the corpora lutea in hypophysectomized rabbits. It can extend the functional life of the corpus luteum of cow (15), but in sheep, i v injection of LH on days 9 and 15 of the estrous cycle is shown to cause only a slight transitory increase in progesterone secretion (16). Carlson et al (17) on the other hand, claimed that s c injection of LH to intact and hysterectomized heifers significantly increased plasma progesterone concentration. In sheep, in situ perfusion of the luteinized ovary with LH or prolactin increased progesterone secretion (18).

In the rat, in vitro studies have shown that LH can increase progesterone synthesis in the luteinized ovarian tissue (19,20). Injection of LH either at early proestrus or at diestrus increased ovarian venous progesterone secretion (21,22). But in pseudopregnant rats where functional corpora lutea are present, LH did not increase progesterone secretion (21,22). It thus appears that stimulation of steroidogenesis by LH can be seen when the corpora lutea are not functional, and that LH cannot stimulate steroidogenesis over the functional level.

Recent studies using antiserum to LH have provided a different approach for understanding the functional role of LH. Madhwa Raj and Moudgal (24) showed that LH antiserum terminated pregnancy and that LH plays an important role in the maintenance of luteal function during the first half of pregnancy in the rat. Using this technique, the luteotropic complex in lactating rats was studied. When rats nursing 6 pups were treated with LH antiserum on days 6 and 7 of lactation, progesterone secretion was reduced by 42 % on day 8 compared with the control (7.9 $\pm$ 3.2 vs 12.5 $\pm$ 4.1 μg/30 min). Similarly, secretion of 20α-OH-P was reduced by LH antiserum. The level of progesterone in rats nursing 6 pups was reduced by LH antiserum treatment to a level similar to that observed in rats nursing 2 pups. Treatment of the latter group of rats with LH antiserum did not alter the secretion rate of progesterone (1). Injection of LH to rats nursing 2 pups increased the rate of progesterone secretion to the level seen in those nursing 6 pups. These results suggest that LH may be involved in progesterone secretion in rats nursing 6 pups, but not in those nursing 2 pups.

Although LH antiserum reduced progesterone secretion in rats nursing 6 pups, the reduction observed (42 %) was much less than that found in antiserum-treated pregnant rats. Moudgal et al. (25) showed that ovarian secretion rate of progesterone declined by 80 % 24 hr after s c injection of LH antiserum. Our recent observations confirmed their data. LH antiserum injected i v on day 8 of pregnancy terminated pregnancy within 24 hr and the progestin concentration in ovarian venous blood declined by 93 %; 20α-OH-P increased to approximately 400 % of that found in control pregnant rats.

Termination of pregnancy on day 8 and the concomitant drastic reduction in progesterone secretion following treatment with LH antiserum clearly shows that luteal function at this stage of pregnancy is largely dependent upon LH. Compared to its effect in rats on day 8 of pregnancy, LH antiserum treatment reduced progesterone secretion to a much less extent in lactating rats and particularly in rats nursing 2 pups, the reduction was negligible.

We also examined the effect of LH antiserum on maintenance of pregnancy in lactating rats. LH antiserum sufficient to terminate pregnancy in normal rats on day 8 was injected sc to pregnant-lactating rats on day 8. Resorption of embryos was observed in only 1 of 7 pregnant rats nursing 2 pups, and in 2 of 10 rats nursing 6 pups; rats were treated concomitantly with small doses of estradiol to prevent delay in implantation and to maintain pregnancy (26). LH antiserum treatment of pregnant-lactating rats nursing 6 pups resulted in a 54 % reduction in progesterone concentration and no change in the concentration of 20α-OH-P. Thus, the luteotropic complex of the pregnant lactating rat is of an intermediate type when compared with that of the normal pregnant (day 8) and the non-pregnant lactating rat, as far as the LH component required for progesterone secretion and pregnancy maintenance is concerned.

INVOLVEMENT OF PROLACTIN IN THE LUTEOTROPIC COMPLEX

The observations that serum prolactin levels increased with an increase in suckling stimulus and that the greater the number of suckling young, the higher the secretion of progesterone, suggest that prolactin directly influences progesterone secretion in lactating rats. However, in vivo and in vitro studies in the rat have shown that prolactin has no acute steroidogenic effect (20,21,27, 28). Injection of prolactin (2.5 mg twice daily for 2 days) to rats nursing 2 pups did not increase progesterone secretion (1). The following sections will deal with results obtained by elimination or stimulation of endogenous prolactin by prolactin antiserum, ergocryptine and perphenazine.

A. Effect of prolactin antiserum on progestin secretion

The direct effect of antiserum to rat prolactin on ovarian steroidogenesis was examined in vivo in lactating rats. Antiserum to rat prolactin (NIAMDD) was injected into a space between the ovary and the periovarian bursa on day 7 of lactation. Ovarian venous blood collected for 15 min, 24 hr after injection was analysed for progestin content by gas-liquid chromatography. Control groups consisted of untreated rats and those injected with normal rabbit serum (NRS). Progesterone secretion rate was significantly lower in the antiserum-treated rats (4.4 ± 0.6 μg/15 min) compared to NRS-treated rats (8.1 ± 1.2), the rats in both the groups nursing 8 pups each. Secretion rate of 20 α-OH-P was not influenced by this treatment. Similar, but less marked reduction in progesterone secretion was observed on antiserum treatment to rats, nursing 2 pups. Intrabursal injection of rat prolactin to rats nursing 2 pups, however, did not increase progesterone secretion in 24 hrs (29).

Reduction of progesterone secretion on treatment with prolactin antiserum indicates that prolactin plays an important role in lactating rats; however, the ineffectiveness of exogenous prolactin in increasing progesterone secretion is consistent with previous observations. Although endogenous secretion of prolactin in pseudopregnant rats has been reported to occur in daily nocturnal surges which start on the day after proestrus (30), progesterone secretion is not significantly elevated by day 4 (31). Further study is necessary for elucidation of mechanisms involved in the latent action of prolactin on progesterone secretion.

B. Effect of ergocryptine on progesterone secretion

Shelesnyak (32) showed that a single injection of ergotoxine terminates pseudopregnancy and pregnancy. Treatment of pseudopregnant rats with ergocornine reduced ovarian content of progesterone and increased that of 20α-OH-P (33). Concurrent with this alteration of steroidogenesis, is the increased 20α-hydroxysteroid dehydrogenase activity in the corpora lutea (34, 35) and these ovarian changes are apparently the direct result of diminished prolactin secretion which occurs after ergocornine treatment (36,37). Ergot alkaloids also reduce prolactin secretion, litter weight gains and mammary gland weights in lactating rats (38, 39).

In our study, ergocryptine was used to inhibit endogenous secretion of prolactin. Firstly, ergocryptine (1 mg) was injected sc to rats nursing 6 pups on day 7 or 10 of lactation. One day after injection, there was a decline in milk secretion, which was indicated by a marked decrease in body weight gain of suckling young. Ovarian venous progesterone concentration was not significantly decreased 24 hr after ergocryptine treatment, but by 48 hr there was a significant reduction (control group — 2.28 ± 0.33 μg/ml vs ergocryptine group — 0.17 ± 0.13 on day 9; and control group — 2.08 ± 0.41 vs ergocryptine group — 0.14 ± 0.06 on day 12).

Secondly, the effect of ergocryptine on pregnancy maintenance was studied in normal pregnant and pregnant-lactating rats. In pregnant-lactating rats, the number of suckling young was adjusted to 6 and estrogen was administered to prevent delay in implantation and later to prevent termination of pregnancy due to the lack of estrogen. Injection of 1 mg ergocryptine sc on day 6 of pregnancy to both normal and pregnant-lactating rats, resulted in termination of pregnancy. Treatment of normal pregnant rats with ergocryptine on day 9, on the other hand, did not terminate pregnancy while this same treatment resulted in abortion in 7 of 11 pregnant lactating rats. These results again indicate that the luteal function in pregnant-lactating rats is more dependent on prolactin than in normal pregnant rats.

C. Effect of perphenazine on progestin secretion

Perphenazine, a phenothiazine derivative, has been shown to increase prolactin secretion in the rat (40,41); hence, we examined if this compound would increase ovarian progesterone secretion rate in rats nursing a small litter.

Rats in groups I and II nursing 2 and 8 pups respectively, received an ip injection of 0.5 ml of 0.03 N HCl on days 6 and 7 of lactation; the rats in group III nursing 2 pups received 1 mg perphenazine in 0.5 ml 0.03 N HCl ip on days 6 and 7. Ovarian venous blood was collected on day 8 of lactation from all rats and progesterone and 20α-OH-P content was determined (Table 1). Progesterone secretion in rats nursing 2 pups was increased by perphenazine to a level found in rats nursing 8 pups. Although measurement of prolactin and LH levels in the perphenazine-treated lactating rats is necessary for final conclusion on the effect of this drug, it is likely that the increased progesterone secretion is due to the increased prolactin secretion, because this compound has been reported to inhibit FSH and LH secretion by the pituitary (42).

Table 1. Effect of perphenazine on ovarian progestin secretion in lactating rats.

Group	No. of pups	Treatment	No. of rats	Steroid secretion rate (μg/15 min)	
				Progesterone	20α-OH-P
I	2	Vehicle	5	2.72±0.45	2.14±0.72
II	8	Vehicle	10	4.44±0.33	2.89±0.36
III	2	Perphenazine	9	4.56±0.56	2.72±0.38

CONCLUSION

Lactation has a stimulatory effect on luteal function in the rat. Lactation converts the non-functional corpora lutea formed at post-partum ovulation into functional ones and maintains progesterone secretion for approximately 2 weeks. The higher the suckling stimulus applied, the greater is the amount of progesterone secreted. An increase in endogenous prolactin brought about by the suckling stimulus appears to be one of the factors involved in elevating the progesterone secretion. Progesterone secretion during early pregnancy (day 8) is more dependent on LH than on prolactin; concurrent lactation, shifts this dependency toward less LH and more prolactin. Therefore, the luteotropic complex can be of variable types which maintain progesterone secretion within a comparable range: "early pregnancy type" composed of more LH than prolactin; "pregnancy-lactation type" having a larger proportion of prolactin; and "lactation type" dominated by prolactin. The observation that the elevation of progesterone secretion is brought about by suckling stimulus, but not by exogenous prolactin suggests that further studies are required to elucidate the mechanisms involved in the luteotropic action of prolactin. Further, one can speculate that other factors also could be involved in the luteotropic complex and the role of these factors, for example, ACTH and oxytocin, in the complex remains to be elucidated by future work.

ACKNOWLEDGEMENTS

This work is supported by NIH grants HD-06467, 06047, 53973 and by a grant from The Population Council, New York.

The authors express their gratitude to NIH, NIAMD, The National Pituitary Agency, and NIAMDD rat pituitary hormone distribution program for generous gifts of ovine LH, rat prolactin and antiserum to rat prolactin (prepared by Dr. A. F. Parlow). They are also thankful to Dr. A. Watnick of Schering Corporation, New Jersey, for the gift of perphenazine, and to Dr. S. S. Wahrman of Sandos Pharmaceuticals, New Jersey, for the gift of ergocryptine. Grateful thanks are due to Dr. Roy O. Greep for reviewing the manuscript and for his guggestions and continuous support of this work. Technical assistance by Misses L. J. Gasset and J. A. Mandelbaum, Mrs. C. D. Wheeler and Mr. T. W. Flanagan and the typing of the manuscript by Mrs. S. Nieland are appreciated.

REFERENCES

1. Yoshinaga, K., Moudgal, N. R. and Greep, R. O. (1971). Endocrinology 88, 1126.
2. Tomogane, H., Ota, K., and Yokoyama, A. (1969). J. Endocr. 44, 101.
3. Eto, T., Masuda, H., Suzuki, Y., and Hosi, T. (1962). Jap. J. Animal. Reprod. 8, 34.
4. Amenomori, Y., Chen, C. L., and Meites, J. (1970). Endocrinology 86, 506.
5. Ford, J. J., and Melampy, R. M. (1973). Endocrinology 93, 540.
6. Bischof, P., Krahenbuhl, C., and Desaullies, P. A. (1973). Experientia 29, 615.
7. Savard, K., Marsh, J. M., and Rice, B. F. (1965). Rec. Prog. Horm. Res. 21, 285.
8. Armstrong, D. T. (1968). Rec. Prog. Horm. Res. 24, 255.
9. Rice, B. F., Hammerstein, J., and Savard, K. (1964). K. Clin. Endo. Metab. 24, 606.
10. Mason, N. R., Marsh, J. M., and Savard, K. (1962). J. Biol. Chem. 237, 1801.
11. Moody, E. L., and Hansell, W. (1969). Endocrinology 84, 451.
12. Hall, P. F., and Koritz, S. B. (1965). Biochemistry 4, 1037.
13. Eaton, L. W., and Hilliard, J. (1971). Endocrinology 89, 105.
14. Kilpatrick, R., Armstrong, D. T. and Greep, R. O. (1964). Endocrinology 74, 453.

15. Donaldson, L.E., and Hansel, W. (1965). J. Dairy Sci. 48, 903.
16. Short, R.V., McDonald, M.F., and Rowson, L.E.A. (1963). J. Endocr. 26, 155.
17. Carlson, J.C., Kazama, N., and Hansel, W., (1971). Endocrinology 89, 1530.
18. Domanski, E., Skrzeczkowski, L., Stupnicka, E., Fitko, R. and Dobrowolski, W. (1967). J. Reprod. Fert. 14, 365.
19. Armstrong, D.T., O'Brien, J., and Greep, R.O. (1964). Endocrinology 75, 488.
20. Channing, C.P., and Villee, C.A. (1966). Biochem. Biophys. Acta. 127, 1.
21. Yoshinaga, K., Grieves, S.A. and Short, R.V. (1967). J. Endocr. 38, 423.
22. Marsh, J.M., Telegdy, G., and Savard, K. (1966). Nature (London). 212, 950.
23. Behrman, H.R., Yoshinaga, K., and Greep, R.O. (1971). Ann. N.Y. Acad. Sci. 180, 426.
24. Madhwa Raj, H.G., and Moudgal, N.R. (1970). Endocrinology 86, 874.
25. Moudgal, N.R., Behrman, H.R. and Greep, R.O. (1972). J. Endocr. 52, 413.
26. Yoshinaga, K. (1971). Endocrinology 88, A-270.
27. Armstrong, D.T. and Greep, R.O. (1962) Endocrinology 70, 701.
28. Huang, W.Y. and Pearlman, W.H. (1962). J. Biol. Chem 237, 1060.
29. Yoshinaga, K. (1973). Endocrinology 92, A-284.
30. Freeman, M.E. and Neill, J.D. (1972). Endocrinology 90, 1292
31. Hashimoto, I., Henricks, D.M., Anderson, L.L. and Melampy, R.M. (1968). Endocrinology 82, 333.
32. Shelesnyak, M.C. (1955). Am. J. Physiol. 180, 47.
33. Lindner, H. and Shelesnyak, M.C. (1967). Acta Endocr. 56, 27.
34. Turolla, E., Baldratti, G., Scrascia, E. and Ricevuti, G. (1969). Experientia 25, 415.
35. Lamprecht, S.A., Lindner, H.R. and Strauss, J.F., III (1969). Biochem. Biophys. Acta. 178, 133.
36. Nagasawa, H. and Meites, J. (1970). Proc. Soc. Exp. Biol. Med. 135, 469.
37. Wuttke, W., Cassell, E. and Meites, J. (1971). Endocrinology 88, 737.

38. Zeilmaker, G.H. and Carlson, R.A. (1962). Acta Endocr. 41, 321.
39. Shaar, C.J. and Clemens, J.A. (1972). Endocrinology 90, 285.
40. Damon, A., Dikstein, S. and Sulman, F.G. (1963). Proc. Soc. Exp. Biol. Med. 114, 366.
41. Ben-David, M. (1968). Endocrinology 83, 1217.
42. Sulman, F.G. and Winnik, H.Z. (1956). Lancet 270, 161.

ROLE OF LUTEINIZING HORMONE AND PROLACTIN IN THE LUTEOTROPIC PROCESS

H. G. Madhwa Raj, G. J. Macdonald and R. O. Greep

INTRODUCTION

The corpus luteum of the three species commonly used in the laboratory viz. rat, mouse and hamster, has been the subject of extensive investigations over the years and yet the results remain controversial and confusing. The early and pioneering work of Astwood, Lyons, Simpson and Evans - to name a few - established a luteotropic role for hypophyseal prolactin in pregnant rats (1). While, this led to the proposition of prolactin being the sole luteotropin in the rat (2), Greenwald (3, 4) concluded that in the pregnant hamster, prolactin with FSH constitutes the minimal "luteotropic complex". With the advances in the immunochemistry of gonadotropins, another approach to the study of this problem became available. Thus, using specific antibodies to FSH and LH, the latter hormone was shown to be obligatory for maintenance of gestation in the intact pregnant rat (5, 6) and hamster (7), and for the production of progesterone in the corpus luteum of the rat (8, 9). As a result of these studies, the idea of LH being a component of the luteotropic complex is gaining ground (1). We describe here some of our recent studies in an attempt to delineate the possible roles of LH and prolactin in this complex.

EXPERIMENTAL

A. Studies using anti-prolactin serum

A specific and potent antiserum (a/s) to rat prolactin was prepared in rabbits using an immunization schedule described earlier (6). After absorption with normal rat serum, the anti-prolactin serum showed a single precipitin band against purified rat prolactin and this totally cross-reacted with rat pituitary extract. It did not react with both ovine and rat FSH or LH, sheep prolactin and serum or placental extracts from day 12 pregnant rats (Fig 1). In the quantitative precipitin test, the a/s showed a titer of 2.24 mg antibody per ml, capable of combining with 400 μg rat

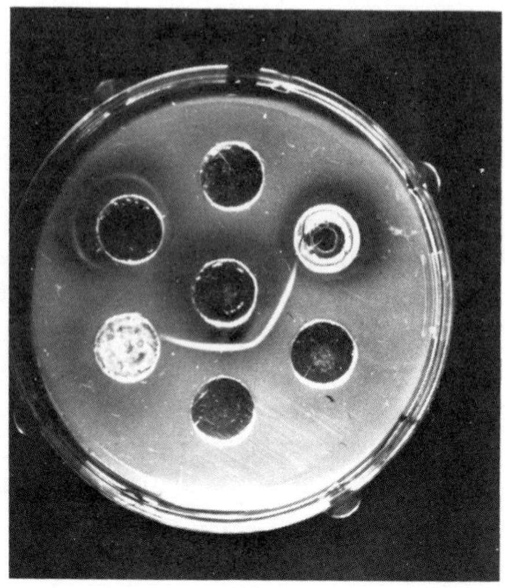

FIG 1. Immunologic reactions of prolactin antiserum in agar gel. Central well : anti-rat prolactin serum. Peripheral wells contain clockwise from top, purified rat LH (10 μg), normal rat serum, rat pituitary extract (1 pituitary eq.), rat prolactin 10 μg, extract from placenta of 12 day pregnant rat and rat pituitary FSH (50 μg).

prolactin. In a systemic pigeon crop-sac assay when prolactin (0.25 mg/day) and a/s (0.8 mg antibody/day) were given intramuscularly at separate sites for 4 days, it was observed at autopsy on the 5th day that the a/s inhibited the proliferation of the crop sac cells and reduced the crop sac weight significantly (from 1753.8 $\pm$ 112.8 mg to 778 $\pm$ 36.6 mg). However, the a/s when administered from days 1 to 9 failed to inhibit the trauma-induced decidual cell reaction in intact or hypophysectomized rats bearing pituitary transplants (Table 1). This was puzzling in view of the known luteotropic action of prolactin in this species. Hence the acute effects of the a/s on progesterone production was studied by injecting the a/s (1 ml) between days 8-10 of lactation to rats nursing 8 pups; the controls received 1 ml of normal rabbit serum. A significant reduction in the peripheral plasma progesterone levels

Table 1. Effect of prolactin antiserum on decidual cell reaction in rats.

Gr.	Daily treatment from days 1-9	Volume injected	Traumatized uterine horn weight, mg ± SD
I	Normal rabbit serum	0.5 ml	1428.0 ± 224.0
II	Anti-prolactin	0.5 ml	1375.0 ± 223.0
III	Normal rabbit serum	0.5 ml	1256.0 ± 78.0
IV	Anti-LH serum	0.5 ml	1121.0 ± 66.0
V	Anti-prolactin	1.0 ml	1410.0 ± 75.0

Pseudopregnancy was induced by cervical stimulation at estrus (day 1) and uterus traumatized on day 5. Groups I & II : intact rats; Groups III-V : hypophysectomized on day 5; 1 pituitary homotransplanted on day 2.

was observed in the a/s treated group (77.5 ± 4.1 vs 55.3 ± 5.7 ng/ml, $p < 0.05$).

B. Studies on maintenance of pregnancy in the hamster

In hamsters hypophysectomized on day 4 of gestation, pregnancy can be maintained up to day 8 with a combination of FSH and prolactin (3,4). However, in the intact pregnant hamster, administration of LH a/s between days 6 - 11 terminates gestation (7) and these effects are reversible by progesterone, indicating the requirement of LH for luteal function during this period. Studies were undertaken to compare the effects of a/s with those of hypophysectomy and replacement therapy during this period of pregnancy, as no such data were available. Hypophysectomy or treatment with LH a/s on day 8 of pregnancy resulted in vaginal bleeding within 48 hr followed by resorption of embryos. Supplementation with 5 or 10 µg of LH given sc in sesame oil - 5 % bees wax, did not reverse these effects. But a dose of 25 µg delayed the onset of external bleeding, and at 50 µg level, an excellent rate of fetal survival was noted (Table 2). Higher doses of LH were again deleterious. When combination of gonadotropins was used in replacement therapy, it was noted that while 200 µg FSH with 2 mg prolactin brought about a fetal survival of 31 %,

Table 2. Involvement of LH in the maintenance of early pregnancy in the hamster.

Treatment days 8 - 11	Ovaries mg ± SE	NS/N	Avg. No. of live sites/animal
Non-operated control	55.5 ± 1.6	10/10	12.3 ± 0.7
Anti-LH*	29.6 ± 2.4	0/6	0
HPX control	17.2 ± 1.3	0/4	0
HPX + 10 µg LH	21.5 ± 0.5	0/4	0
HPX + 25 µg LH	19.2 ± 0.6	0/6	0**
HPX + 50 µg LH	48.2 ± 3.2	7/7	10.4 ± 1.4
HPX + 100 µg LH	47.3 ± 2.8	5/6	5.8 ± 1.7

HPX = hypophysectomy on day 8; N = Total number of hamsters used; NS = Number of animals with sites; * 0.5 ml on day 8 only
** delayed vaginal bleeding on days 11 and 12.

Table 3. Maintenance of pregnancy in hypophysectomized hamsters using combination therapy.

Daily treatment days 8 - 11	Ovaries mg ± SE	NS/N	Avg. No. of live sites/animal
10 µg LH + 2 mg prolactin	16.1 ± 1.2	0/5	0
25 µg LH + 2 mg prolactin	38.9 ± 3.3	10/10	9.1 ± 0.7
200 µg FSH + 2 mg prolactin	24.2 ± 1.6	4/15	3.8 ± 1.7

LH and FSH were administered once daily in sesame oil-bees wax; Prolactin was given as two injections daily in saline. N = Total number of hamsters used; NS = Number of animals with sites.

2 mg prolactin (NIH-P-S10, 25.6 IU/mg), given with 25 μg LH promoted the survival rate to 78 % (Table 3).

The termination of pregnancy observed in the non-supplemented groups was invariably accompanied by involution and total disappearance of corpora lutea and degeneration of interstitium by day 14. Supplementation with 50 μg LH alone, or 25 μg LH with 2 mg prolactin was effective in preventing this luteolysis and the corpora lutea were similar to controls in size and degree of luteinization (Figure 2).

Hypophysectomy on day 12 did not result in abortion in all animals, 6 out of 9 hamsters retaining live fetuses as seen on day 15. The other 3 animals showed resorption or expulsion of fetuses.

Thus, the above experiments bring out the fact that LH is an essential requirement for maintaining the structural and functional integrity of the corpus luteum and confirm the previous observation of Jagannadha Rao et al. (7). Further, in previous investigations where LH was able to induce implantation (10) or maintain pregnancy (11) in hypophysectomized animals, this hormone was administered in sesame oil- bees wax or 16 % gelatin as delay vehicles. Conversly, all the studies using saline injections of LH have failed to demonstrate such an effect, even when given as multiple daily injections. Thus, it was of interest to study the release patterns of LH given in various vehicles. Rats hypophysectomized 48 hr prior to experimentation were given 50 μg LH s c in saline or one of the 3 delay vehicles viz., sesame oil - bees wax, 16 % gelatin, 75 % polyvinyl pyrrolidone. Blood samples were obtained at various time intervals after the injection and plasma was analysed for LH content using a radioimmunoassay. Following injection in saline, the plasma level of LH was high at 10 min, and increased to peak levels (about 10-fold) at 1 hr. However, by 8 hr, the level had returned to control values. In contrast, plasma levels from groups treated with LH in delay vehicles exhibited a gradual increase and the peaks were less in magnitude (4-6 fold less). Such increased levels were sustained up to 16 hr and the levels were still significantly higher than saline controls at 24 hr (Table 4). These observations indicate that even multiple injections of LH in saline does not result in a continuous and gradual exposure of ovaries over a prolonged period of time.

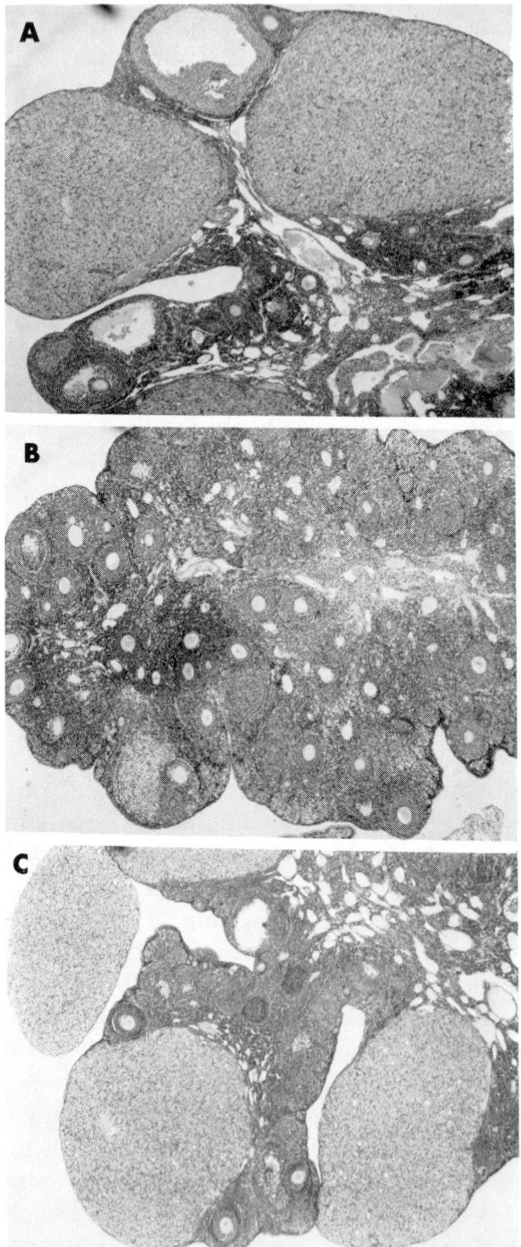

Figure 2 : Histologic appearance of ovaries from pregnant hamsters (all x 40). A. normal pregnant hamster, day 12; B. pregnant hamster hypophysectomized on day 8, autopsied on day 12; C. pregnant hamster hypophysectomized on day 8 and treated with 50 ug LH daily; autopsy on day 12.

Table 4. Plasma LH release patterns after a single injection of LH in various vehicles.

Vehicle	Plasma LH levels (ng/ml, mean ± SE) at various time intervals							
	0 min	10 min	1 hr	2 hr	8 hr	16 hr	24 hr	48 hr
Saline	6.6±1.2	40.4±10.9	66.0±10.9	48.8±3.6	8.0±0.5**	8.0±0.5**	9.0±0.6**	7.6±0.8
Sesame oil-bees wax	6.6±0.9	17.2±2.5	23.8±2.8	23.2±5.1	26.6±2.4	15.0±0.7	11.8±1.2*	10.4±0.9
75% polyvinyl pyrrolidone	5.5±0.6	12.6±1.8	28.8±1.6	33.4±1.8	35.6±1.6	21.0±0.6	19.8±1.9*	17.8±1.6
16% gelatin	5.7±0.3	14.0±1.7	26.0±3.4	29.0±2.8	23.4±1.2	11.2±1.1	11.2±0.6	8.8±0.5

Rats were used 48 hr after hypophysectomy. 50 µg NIH-LH-S 17 injected subcutaneously in 0.2 ml of vehicle.
*Significantly higher than value at 0 time. **Not significant from 0 time value.

DISCUSSION

In the foregoing experiments, evidence has been presented in support of the fact that LH,or LH and prolactin can reverse the effects of hypophysectomy on the corpus luteum in day 8 pregnant hamsters. While neutralizing antibodies to prolactin could not affect decidual reaction in pseudopregnant rats, they were able to reduce progesterone secretion in lactating rats. Recently McLean and Nikitovich-Winer (12) have demonstrated that antiprolactin-serum is effective only when given on proestrus day and on that basis, postulated a critical period for activation of the corpus luteum by prolactin, after which this hormone is not necessary for luteal maintenance. The alkaloid drugs, ergocornine and ergocry-ptine have been extensively used to inhibit prolactin secretion and in such investigations pseudopregnancy, decidual reaction and pre-implantation stages of pregnancy have been found to be affected. However, at these dose levels, ergocornine significantly inhibits LH release also (13). At higher doses it completely inhibits LH secretion and ovulation (14). Hence the results obtained with such drugs should be interpreted with caution. Recently Wuttke and Meites (15) observed that pseudopregnancy in rats was maintained for 10 days even upon treatment with 50 µg ergocornine. Doehler and Wuttke (16) have further shown that two daily injections of ergocryptine to rats did not interfere with mating, implantation and normal gestation, and concluded from this that pseudopregnancy and pregnancy (but not lactation) can be maintained without a rise in serum prolactin. Conversly, injections of LH in delay vehicle does not maintain vaginal diestrus of hypophysectomized rats treated with estradiol (17), and anti-LH serum does not affect progesterone secretion induced by pituitary autografts (18), or affect decidual reaction in graft-bearing rats, as demonstrated above.

Thus it is evident that ovarian progesterone secretion can be sustained to different degrees by either LH or prolactin alone, depending on the model system used. While low to moderate levels of net progesterone output can be supported by prolactin alone, LH is obligatory in situations requiring high progesterone. Further, in any model system using intact animals, the tonic levels of LH and prolactin can be visualised to be synergistic in bringing about optimal progesterone production. Thus, in the intact pseudopregnant rat, withdrawal of LH stimulus inhibits decidual reaction (19) and is reversible with progesterone and estrogen, but not estrogen alone.

This brings us back to the issue of controversy - the luteotropic activity *per se* of LH or prolactin. While both can increase net progesterone output, it would be illogical to conclude that one can replace the other at the molecular level, as the two hormones have entirely different amino acid sequences, tertiary structure and exclusive physiologic actions. The principal locus of action of LH in stimulating progesterone synthesis seems to be in promoting cholesterol ester hydrolysis by activating cholesterol esterase (20). Also it stimulates the incorporation of acetate carbon to cholesterol (21) and conversion of cholesterol to pregnenolone (22). Prolactin has been shown to activate the sterol acyl-transferase involved in mobilization of precursor pools of cholesterol required for sustained progesterone output (23). It also inhibits 20 α - hydroxy steroid dehydrogenase activity (24), and hence increases net progesterone secretion by reducing conversion to its catabolite. Thus, neutralization of LH or prolactin could reduce net progesterone secretion by two different mechanisms and acting at different loci in the steroid biosynthetic machinery. The ability of corpus luteum to secrete progesterone during a steady-state is a net result of an integrated action of prolactin and LH in the normal intact animals of these species.

ACKNOWLEDGEMENTS

The gift of rat prolactin NIAMD rat prolactin RP-1, and the ovine hormones NIH-FSH-S9, NIH-LH-S17 and S18, NIH-P-S10 by the Endocrine Study Section, Bethesda, are gratefully acknowledged.

Supported by grants from NIH-03736, The Ford Foundation and the Bing Fund.

REFERENCES

1. Nalbandov, A. V. (1973). In "Handbook of Physiology", R. O. Greep and E. B. Astwood (Eds). Section 7, Vol II, Part I, pp 153.
2. Greenwald, G. S. and Johnson, D. C. (1968). Endocrinology 83, 1052.
3. Greenwald, G. S. (1967). Endocrinology 80, 118.
4. Greenwald, G. S. (1973). Endocrinology 92, 235.
5. Madhwa Raj, H. G., Sairam, M. R. and Moudgal, N. R. (1968). J. Reprod. Fert. 17, 335.
6. Madhwa Raj, H. G. and Moudgal, N. R. (1970). Endocrinology 86, 874.
7. Jagannadha Rao, A., Madhwa Raj, H. G. and Moudgal, N. R. (1972). J. Reprod. Fert. 29, 239.
8. Moudgal, N. R., Behrman, H. R. and Greep, R. O. (1972). J. Endocr. 52, 413.
9. Behrman, H. R., Moudgal, N. R. and Greep, R. O. (1972). J. Endocr. 52, 419.
10. Macdonald, G. J., Armstrong, D. T. and Greep, R. O. (1967) Endocrinology 80, 172.
11. Moudgal, N. R. (1969). Nature 222, 289.
12. McLean, B. K. and Nikitovich-Winer, M. B. (1973). Endocrinology 93, 316.
13. Wuttke, W., Cassel, E. and Meites, J. (1971). Endocrinology 88, 737.
14. Madhwa Raj, H. G., and Greep, R. O. (1973). Proc. Soc. Exp. Biol. Med. (in press).
15. Wuttke, W. and Meites, J. (1972). Endocrinology 90, 438.
16. Doehler, K. D. and Wuttke, W. (1973). Acta Endocr. (Kobenhaven). Suppl 173, pp 45.

17. Macdonald, G. J. and Greep, R. O. (1970). Proc. Soc. Exp. Biol. Med. 134, 936.
18. Macdonald, G. J., Moudgal, N. R., Madhwa Raj, H. G. and Greep, R. O. (1973). Proc. Soc. Exp. Biol. Med. (in press).
19. Maneckjee, R., Madhwa Raj, H. G. and Moudgal, N. R. (1973). Biol. Reprod. 8, 43.
20. Behrman, H. R. and Armstrong, D. T. (1969). Endocrinology 85, 474.
21. Armstrong, D. T. (1968). Rec. Prog. Horm. Res. 24, 255.
22. Hall, P. F. and Koritz, K. (1965). Biochemistry 4, 1037.
23. Behrman, H. R., Orczyk, G. P., Macdonald, G. J. and Greep, R. O. (1970). Endocrinology 87, 1251.
24. Wiest, W. G., Kidwell, W. R. and Balough, K., Jr., (1968). Endocrinology 82, 844.

ULTRASTRUCTURAL CHANGES IN THE CORPUS LUTEUM OF PREGNANCY IN THE GOLDEN HAMSTER FOLLOWING LH DEPRIVAL

Mukku Venkatramaiah, T. C. Anand Kumar, Kamala Kumar, A. Jagannadha Rao and N. R. Moudgal

INTRODUCTION

The work of Greenwald and collaborators (1,2) has suggested that the corpus luteum of the pregnant hamster is regulated by a luteotropic complex consisting principally of FSH and prolactin, and that LH in small amounts, has a salutary effect. Our recent studies using an immunological approach, however, have indicated that LH has a major role in maintaining luteal function during pregnancy in the hamster and that lack of LH leads to structural and functional luteolysis (3). The dependence on LH appears to be acute since deprivation of it even for 2 hours has been shown to cause abortion (4). Preliminary results (4) have indicated that corpora lutea from pregnant hamsters (on day 7) which were deprived of endogenous LH support for 12 hours, fail to respond to LH stimulus in vitro. These findings prompted us to examine the early ultrastructural changes that may have occured in the corpus luteum of the pregnant hamster following LH-deprival.

MATERIALS AND METHODS

Methods to produce and characterize antisera to oLH (LH a/s) have been described in detail elsewhere (5). Cycling female golden hamsters (Mesocricetus auratus) of our colony were kept for mating with males of proven fertility. The day on which sperms were seen in the vagina was considered as day 1 of pregnancy and exploratory laporatomy was performed on day 6 to confirm pregnancy. On day 7, these were given intracardiac injections of 0.1 ml of LH a/s . Control animals did not receive any treatment. Animals were killed by ether anaesthesia followed by cervical dislocation at 30 min, 1,2,4 and 8 hr after the a/s injection.

Corpora lutea excised from the ovaries were immediately fixed by immersion either in 6 % glutaraldehyde containing 0.01 %

picric acid and buffered with 0.1 mM solution of sodium cacodylate, pH 7.4 or in Dalton's fluid (6) for 2-4 hr. The tissues fixed in glutaraldehyde were washed in buffer, post-fixed in 1 % OsO_4 (buffered to pH 7.4 with sodium cacodylate) for 1-2 hr, washed again, dehydrated through ascending series of ethanol, and embedded in Araldite; the tissues fixed in Dalton's fluid were similarly processed, but without post-fixation. Sections were cut on a Reichert OMU_3 ultramicrotome using glass knives. Thick sections (1-2 μ) were mounted on glass slides and stained with toluidine blue for optical microscopy. Thin sections showing silver to light golden interference colours were mounted on coated copper grids, stained with uranyl acetate, followed by lead citrate staining and viewed in a Philips EM 300 electron microscope.

OBSERVATIONS

The granulosa-lutein cell of an untreated pregnant hamster is shown in Plate 1A. The peripherally occuring electron-dense nuclear heterochromatin is less than the centrally occuring euchromatin. Three types of lipid droplets can be distinguished in the cytoplasm: the first variety is uniformly grey and it is surrounded by a system of cytoplasmic whorls comprised of annular membranes (Plate 2A). The second variety has a thin granular "shell" around it which is found frequently in close association with mitochondria. The third category (Plate 3A) of lipid droplets is larger in size than those of the first two and they have a relatively more electron-lucent content and are surrounded by a granular shell. The cytoplasmic whorls in the latter two categories of lipid droplets are not as extensively developed as in the first category. It must be pointed out, however, that this classification is purely arbitrary and is based on certain clearly discernable ultrastructural features; the functional significance of these types of lipid droplets is not clear at present. The mitochondria are of various sizes and their cristae are electron-dense (Plate 4A).

In the corpus luteum of LH a/s treated hamsters most of the changes observed in the granulosa-lutein cells at short intervals are progressively exaggerated with time. Comparison of a control luteal cell (Plate 1A) with that deprived of LH for 30 min (Plate 1B) shows a striking change in the nucleus; the electron-dense nuclear chromatin is increased in almost all the cells of

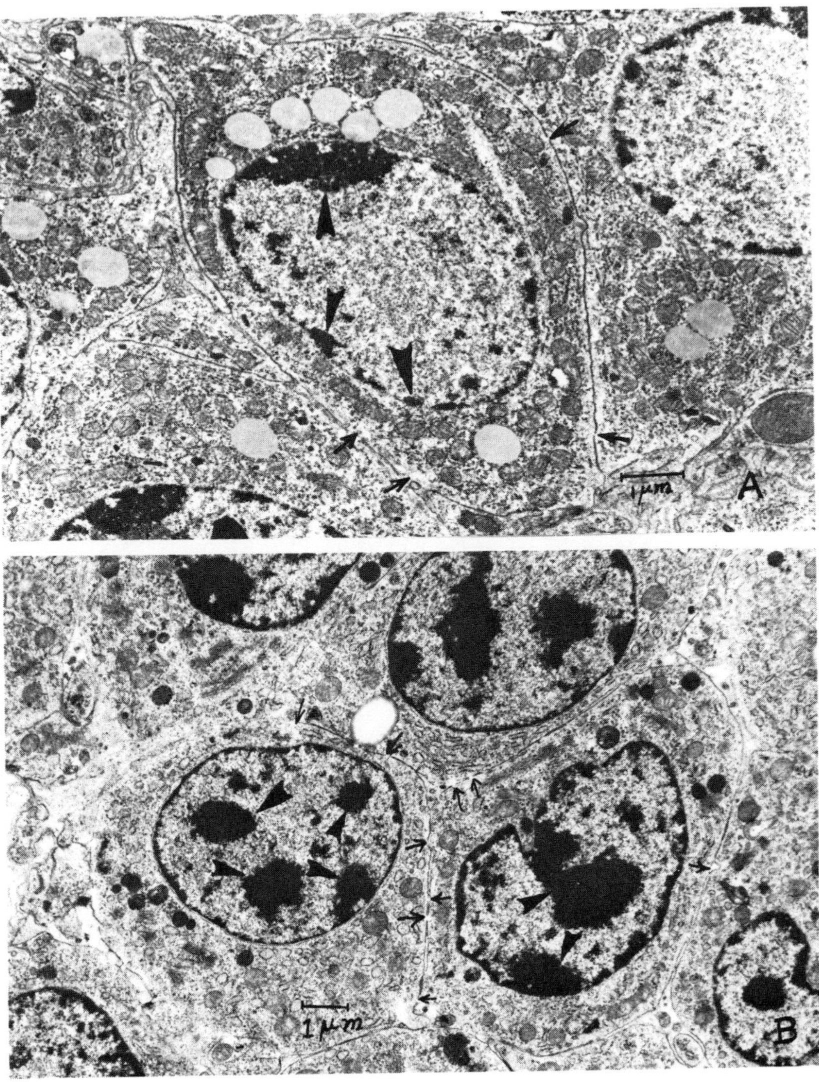

Plate 1. Comparison of a granulosa luteal cell of an untreated pregnant hamster (A) with the luteal cell of a hamster deprived of LH for 30 min (B). Heterochromatin (arrow heads) is increased over the euchromatin in the latter. Gaps (arrows) occur in the plasma membrane of both the cells, but relatively more in B.

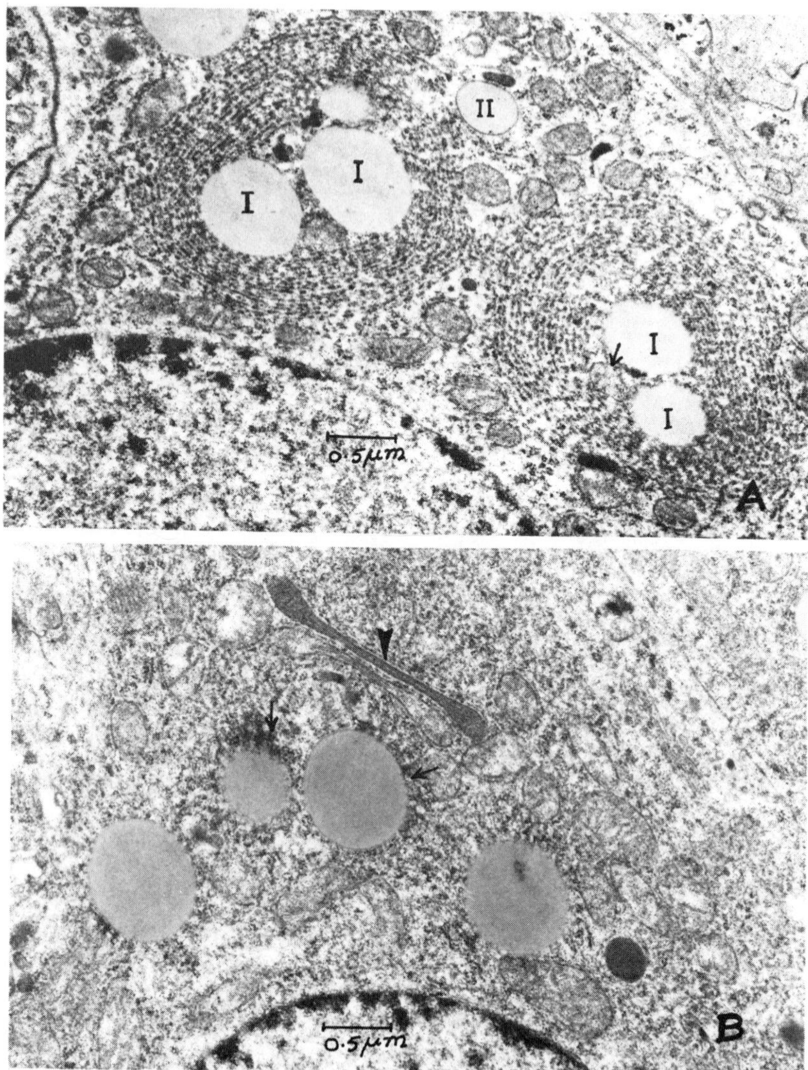

Plate 2: Luteal cell of a control (A) and LH A/S treated (for 1 hr) hamster (B). Note the different kinds of lipid droplets (I & II) and their close association with mitochondria (arrow). In B there is a reduction in the cytoplasmic whorls and in the area surrounding some of the lipid droplets(I)show an increase in electron density. Also note the pleiomorphic nature of a mitochondria in B.

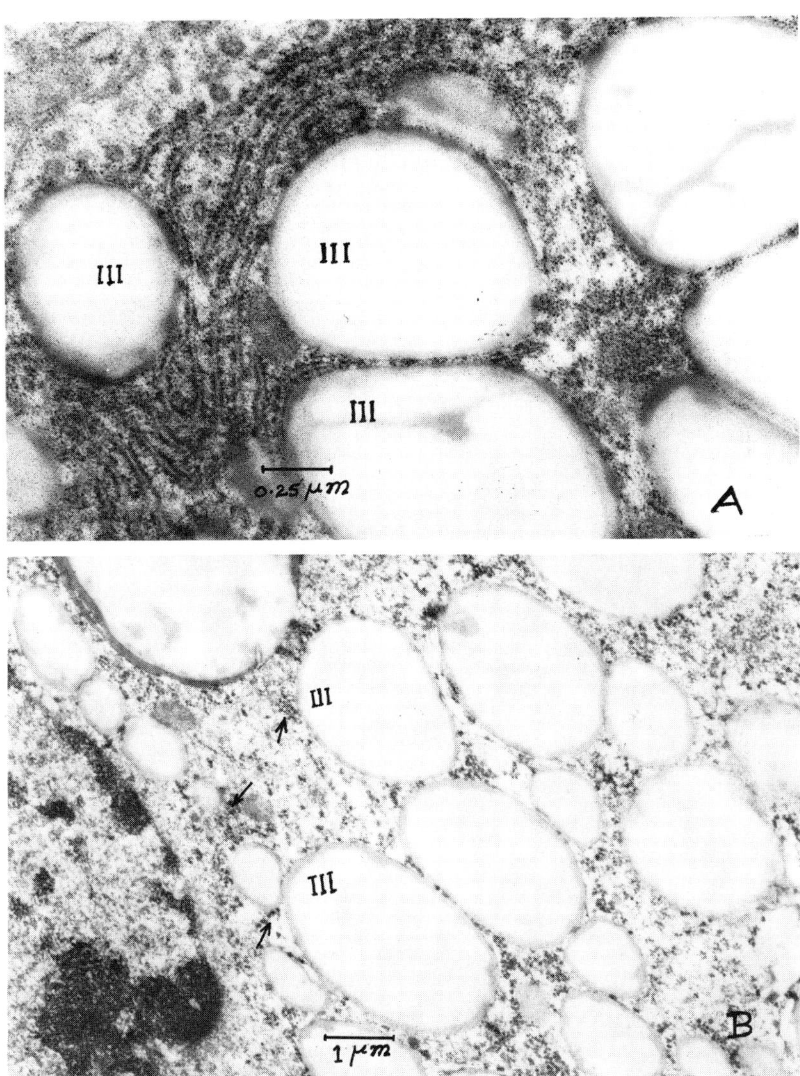

Plate 3. Depicts the lipids of category III (III) present in the luteal cell of control (A) and that of LH-deprived (for 8 hrs) hamster (B). Note the relative absence of whorls surrounding lipid droplets, and the abundance of free-ribosome-like bodies (arrows) in B.

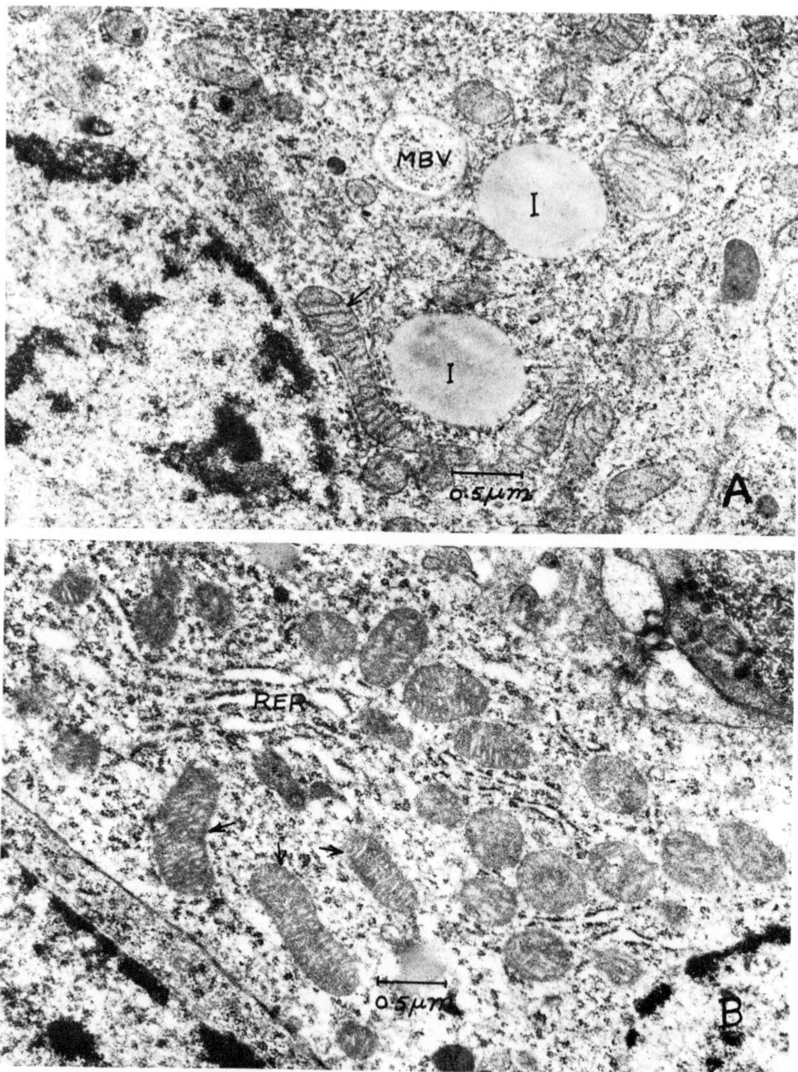

Plate 4. Mitochondria (arrows) in the luteal cell of an untreated (A) and LH-deprived (8 hrs) Hamster (B). Note the reduction in the electron density of the mitochondrial matrix giving rise to 'empty' spaces and relative abundance of rough endoplasmic reticulum (RER) in B. Characteristic membrane-bound cytoplasmic vesicles (MBV) can be seen in A.

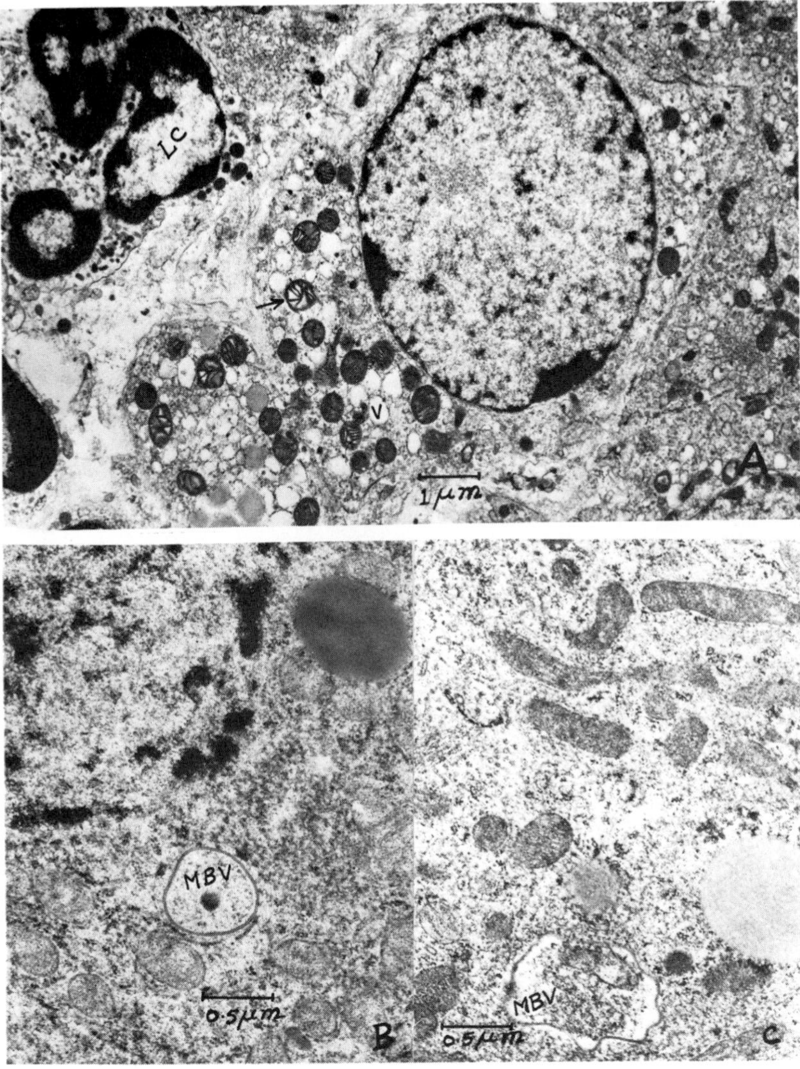

Plate 5. (A) A luteal cell of hamster deprived of LH for 8 hr showing infiltration of leucocytes (LC), presence of vacuoles (V) and mitochondria (arrow) with electron-lucent matrix. (B) & (C) Effect of LH-deprival (4 hr) on membrane bound cytoplasmic vesicles (MBV). Note the distorted MBV in treated luteal cell (C) compared to the control (B).

TABLE I. EFFECT OF LH A/S ON THE GRANULOSA-LUTEIN CELL OF PREGNANCY IN THE HAMSTER

LH DEPRIVAL	HETERO-CHROMATIN[1]	L-I	L-II	L-III	MITOCHONDRIA	MBV[2]	PLASMA MEMBR.	OTHER OBSERVATIONS
NIL	LESS	+++	++	+	ELECTRON-DENSE MATRIX	CONTENTS EVENLY DISPERSED	MOSTLY INTACT	VERY LITTLE RER[3]
30 MIN	MORE	+++	++	+	NO CHANGE	NO CHANGE	BROKEN AT MANY PLACES	NO CHANGE
1 HR	MORE	+++	++	+	FEW AFFECTED[4]	NO CHANGE	''''	GRANULOCYTES
2 HR	MORE	++	++	+	MAJORITY AFFECTED	DISTORTED	''''	''''
4 HR	MORE	++	++	+	''''	''''	''''	''''
8 HR	MORE	+	+	+++	ALL AFFECTED	''''	''''	IN ADDITION TO GRANULOCYTES, MORE RER THAN SER[5].

NUMBERS IN SUPERSCRIPT INDICATE THE FOLLOWING :
1. RELATIVE ABUNDANCE OVER EUCHROMATIN; 2. MEMBRANE-BOUND CYTOPLASMIC VESICLES; 3. ROUGH ENDOPLASMIC RETICULUM; 4. MATRIX BECOMES ELECTRON-LUCENT; 5. SMOOTH ENDOPLASMIC RETICULUM;
L-I, L-II & L-III REFER TO LIPID DROPLETS OF CATEGORY I, II & III.

the treated corpus luteum. Breakages in the plasma membranes appear to occur more frequently following a/s treatment. In the luteal cells that are exposed to a/s for 1 hr the lipids of category I become more electron-dense, and in contrast to the controls, the cytoplasmic whorls around them are greatly reduced (Plate 2B). Eight hours treatment with LH a/s brings about an increase in the number of lipid droplets of category III. The cytoplasmic whorls around these droplets are not seen, instead free-ribosome-like bodies can be observed (Plate 3B). The mitochondria start becoming pleiomorphic as early as 30 min after a/s treatment (Plate 2B). Eight hours following LH a/s treatment all the mitochondria are affected and their matrix becomes relatively electron lucent giving them an 'empty' appearance (Plate 4B). At this stage, the cytoplasm contains a relatively high amount of rough endoplasmic reticulum (RER). Leucocyte (granulocyte) infiltration into the corpus luteum and appearance of cytoplasmic vacuoles could be seen in the luteal cells as early as 1 hr after LH a/s injection; both these phenomena are exaggerated with increase in time (Plate 5A).

The membrane-bound cytoplasmic vesicles (MBV), which appear to be characteristic of a functional luteal cell in the hamster, become distorted following LH deprival (Plate 5B & 5C). All the ultrastructural changes described above are summarized in Table 1.

DISCUSSION

The process of luteolysis, as visualised by light microscopy in the corpus luteum of the cycling hamster, involves characteristic leucotyte infiltration, pycnosis of the nuclei and vacuolation of the cytoplasm (8). Electron microscopic studies (7) have confirmed these observations and have also shown that the mitochondria become pleiomorphic and that there is an increase in the RER. Okamura et al. (9) have confirmed that $PGF_{2\alpha}$ in pregnant rats brings about similar ultrastructural changes in the luteal cells.

The different categories of lipid droplets, the gaps in the plasma membrane, and the membrane-bound cytoplasmic vesicles are some of the interesting features of the granulosa lutein cells of the control hamsters. In the absence of information on the ultrastructural changes associated with the process of intracellular steroid synthesis and metabolism, it is difficult to adduce any meaning to the different categories of lipids seen in the electron-micrographs. Further studies are needed to determine whether these different categories represent sequential stages in steroid metabolism.

Though both the control and LH-deprived luteal cells show gaps in plasma membrane, they are present to a greater degree in the latter. While the possibility that these gaps are artifacts cannot entirely be ruled out, it is interesting to note that such gaps are evident in tissues fixed in two different fluids. Further, these gaps occur only in the plasma membrane of the luteal cell and not in other cells like granulocytes or in the membrane-bound vesicles of the cytoplasm. The functional significance of these gaps, however, is not clear.

In addition to the observed increase in the gaps in the plasma membrane, the most striking early effects of LH-deprival pertain to an increase in the electron-dense heterochromatin material. Since both these changes were observed within 30 min of LH a/s injection, it is difficult to determine whether the primary effect of LH-deprivation is at the level of the plasma membrane or at the nucleus.

The other effects of LH deprival on the corpus luteum are : leucocytic infiltration, pycnosis of the nuclear chromatin, cytoplasmic vacuolation, distortion in shape of mitochondria and an increase in the RER. All these features are characteristic of the process of luteolysis during the normal estrous cycle of hamsters (7, 8) as well as in $PGF_{2\alpha}$ induced luteolysis in rats (9). Thus, the present investigation, in addition to providing ultrastructural evidence in support of our earlier observation (3) that LH-deprival in pregnant hamsters leads to luteolysis, furnishes a structural basis for further detailed biochemical investigations on the mechanism of luteolysis.

ACKNOWLEDGEMENTS

Part of this work was carried out at the All India Institute of Medical Sciences, New Delhi. The work was supported by individual grants made to Dr. T. C. Anand Kumar and Dr. N. R. Moudgal by the Indian Council of Medical Research, The Ford Foundation and the W. H. O.

REFERENCES

1. Greenwald, G.S. (1967). Endocrinology 80, 118.
2. Greenwald, G.S. and Rothchild, I. (1968). J. Animal. Sci. 27 (suppl) 139.
3. Rao, A.J., Madhwa Raj, H.G. and Moudgal, N.R. (1972). J. Reprod. Fert. 29, 239.
4. Moudgal, N.R., Jagannadha Rao, A., Rhoda Maneckjee, Muralidhar, K., Venkatramaiah Mukku, and Sheela Rani, C.S. (1974). Rec. Prog. Horm. Res. 30, 47.
5. Madhwa Raj, H.G. and Moudgal, N.R. (1970). Endocrinology 86, 874.
6. Dalton, A.J. (1955). Anat. Rec. 121, 281.
7. Leavitt, W.W., Rasom, C.R., Bagwell, J.N. and Blaha, G.C. (1973). Am. J. Anat. 136, 235.
8. Greenwald, G.S. (1967). Arch. D' Anat. Micro. Morph. Exper. 56, (suppl 3-4), 281.
9. Okamura, H., Sen-Lian Yang, Wright, K.H. and Ballah, E.E. (1972). Fert. Steril. 23, 475.

MECHANISM OF ACTION OF LUTEINIZING HORMONE - RELEASING HORMONE

Fernand Labrie, Georges Pelletier, Pierre Borgeat
Jacques Drouin, Muriel Savary, Jean Côté, and Louise Ferland

INTRODUCTION

Early experiments by Harris and co-workers (1-3) led to the suggestion that the central nervous system exerts its regulatory role on gonadotropin secretion through neurohumoral substances released in the median eminence area and transported by a portal blood system to the anterior pituitary gland. The first direct support for this concept was the demonstration of LH-releasing (4-7) and FSH-releasing (8, 9) activity in hypothalamic extracts of different animal species.

Recently, after more than 10 years of research in many laboratories, the neurohormone controlling gonadotropin secretion has been isolated from porcine (10-12) and ovine (13) hypothalami and characterized as a decapeptide having the following structure: (pyro) Glu-His-Trp-Ser-Tyr-Gly-Leu-Arg-Pro-Gly-NH_2 (14-16). This peptide stimulates the release of both LH and FSH under a wide variety of experimental conditions (10-13, 15-20) and has been called the LH-releasing hormone / FSH-releasing hormone (LH-RH or FSH-RH)(10), or the gonadotropin-releasing factor (20).

Although some useful information about the mechanism of action of LH-RH could be obtained from studies performed with different preparations of the purified neurohormone, the recent availability of synthetic LH-RH (21-23) and of its analogues opened new possibilities for studies on the mechanism of action of this neurohormone.

STIMULATORY EFFECT OF SYNTHETIC LH-RH ON BOTH SYNTHESIS AND RELEASE OF LH AND FSH

Out first interest was to investigate whether LH-RH stimulates both synthesis and release of LH and FSH. Chronic treatment (6 days) of adenohypophyseal cells in monolayer culture with increasing concentrations of synthetic LH-RH led to a progressive increase in the release of LH into the culture medium and to a

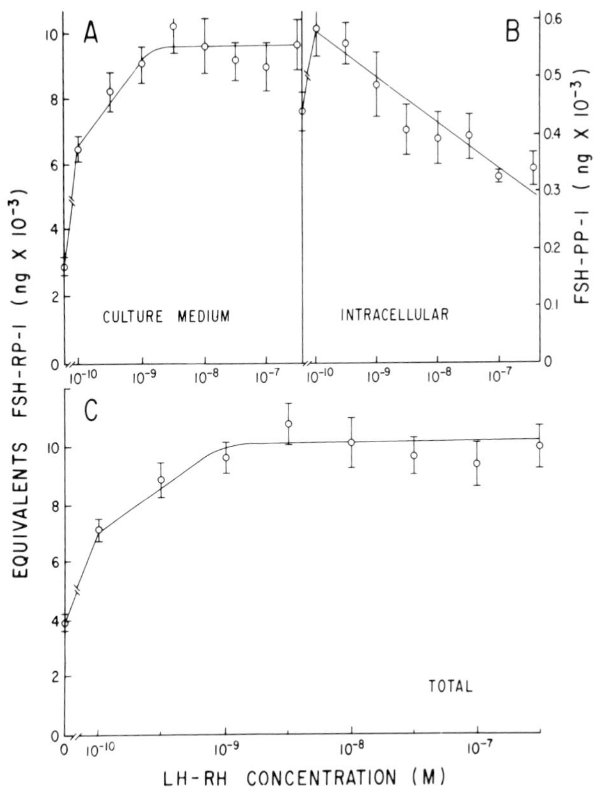

FIG 1. Effect of chronic treatment (6 days) of anterior pituitary cells in monolayer culture with increasing concentration of synthetic LH-RH on FSH release (A), intracellular content of FSH (b) and total (tissue plus culture medium) radioimmunoassayable FSH (C). Cells were cultured for 7 days before beginning the experiment. The culture medium was removed after the first 24 hr of incubation in the presence or absence of increasing concentrations of LH-RH and the new medium was left for the following 5 days. Results are presented as mean ± S. D. of data obtained from triplicate dishes. FSH content at day O was 1630 ± 60 ng – equivalents NIAMD-rat-FSH-RP-1, from Labrie et al. (24).

marked depletion of the intracellular LH content when measured at the end of the experiment (24). 3×10^{-7} M LH-RH increased the total radioimmunoassayable LH (tissue plus culture medium) by 4-fold (from 6505 $\pm$ 735 to 23,695 $\pm$ 715 ng); a 75 % increase in total LH (10,495 $\pm$ 895 ng) over the control was observed even with a dose of 1×10^{-10} M.

Since the cell content of LH at day 0 was 10,630 $\pm$ 60 ng (equivalents LH-RP-1), and 3,390 $\pm$ 570 ng of the hormone was found to be released spontaneously during the first 24 hr of incubation, we computed that under our culture conditions, approximately 20 % of the intracellular content of LH is released daily. In the presence of 10^{-6} M LH-RH, 15,870 $\pm$ 330 ng of LH was found in the culture medium during the first 24 hr, thus indicating that increased LH synthesis had already occurred during that period.

Fig. 1A shows that the release of FSH during chronic treatment with LH-RH was increased 2-fold by a dose of 10^{-10} M of the neurohormone and that it reached a plateau (3-fold stimulation) at doses of 3×10^{-9} M and above. While the intracellular concentration of LH was reduced to 17 % of the control level in the presence of 3×10^{-9} M LH-RH for 6 days, the FSH content was decreased to only 70 % of the control level (Fig. 1B) at a concentration of 3×10^{-7} M LH-RH. Fig. 1C shows that the total FSH content (tissue plus culture medium) was raised from 3910 $\pm$ 290 ng to 7110 $\pm$ 410 ng FSH at a concentration of 1×10^{-10}M LH-RH. A plateau of stimulation (approximately 10,000 ng of FSH/petri dish) was reached at a concentration of 1×10^{-9} M LH-RH.

Under our culture conditions, the daily release of FSH (1,355 $\pm$ 155 ng) represents approximately 80 % of the intracellular hormone content at day 0 (1,630 $\pm$ 60 ng). These data indicate a 4-fold higher rate of turnover of FSH than of LH. Since 4,090 $\pm$ 630 ng of FSH was released during the first 24 hours of incubation in the presence of 3×10^{-7} M LH-RH, it appears that the synthesis of FSH is also markedly stimulated during this short period of incubation with the neurohormone.

These data clearly indicate that synthetic LH-RH, besides stimulating the release of LH and FSH, also enhances the synthesis of these two hormones; this increased synthesis occurred in the first 24 hr of incubation. The increased synthesis may be a direct action of the neurohormone or may occur secondarily due to a depletion of the pituitary stores of the hormones. These results are in agreement with those of Vale et al. (25) and support data obtained using rat adenohypophysis organ cultures where purified (26,27) and synthetic (27) gonadotropin-releasing hormones have been found to stimulate both release and synthesis of LH and FSH. Kobayashi et al. (28,29) also have reported that addition of saline extracts of hypothalami to monolayer cultures of rat adenohypophysis led to an increase of total gonadotropin when measured by bioassay. Though it is evident from the above that LH-RH brings about an increase in the release as well as synthesis of the two gonadotropins, it is difficult to rule out the possibility of a decreased lysosomal or autophagic activity under the influence of the releasing hormone.

EFFECT OF CYCLIC AMP DERIVATIVES AND THEOPHYLLINE ON LH AND FSH RELEASE

Fig. 2 illustrates the stimulatory effect of 5mM N^6-monobutyryl cyclic AMP (mbcAMP), 5mM N^6, 2'-o-dibutyryl cyclic AMP or 5 mM theophylline on LH release during five successive 2-hr incubations of rat adenohypophyseal cells in monolayer culture. 5 mM mbcAMP led to a maximal 47-fold stimulation (1,900 ± 329 vs 40 ± 11 ng/ml) of LH released between 2nd and 4th hour of incubation, with a progressive decrease to a 14-fold stimulation observed between 8 and 10 hr of incubation with the cyclic AMP derivative. 5 mM dbcAMP led to an approximately constant 10- to 14-fold stimulation of LH released between the 2nd and 10th hr of incubation. The maximal effect of 5 mM theophylline is more rapid, a 18-fold stimulation of LH release being observed during the first 2 hr of incubation with a progressive decrease to basal levels after 6 hr of incubation.

A possible role of cyclic AMP in the control of FSH release was suggested by the finding that theophylline potentiates the effect of a crude preparation of FSH-releasing hormone on FSH release (30). Theophylline alone had no effect on hormone release. In the experiment described in Fig. 2, mbcAMP, dbcAMP and theophylline led to a stimulation of LH release similar to that observed for FSH.

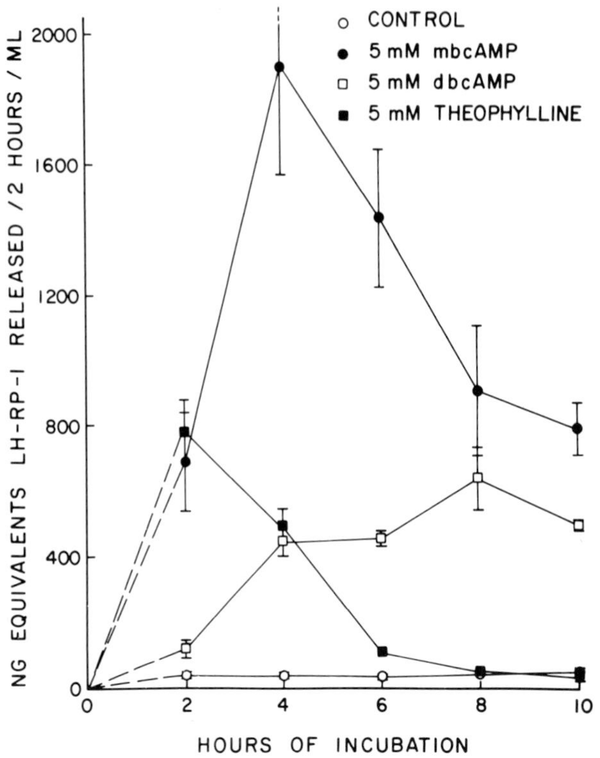

FIG 2. Effect of mbcAMP, dbcAMP and theophylline on LH release from anterior pituitary cells in monolayer culture. Cells from female rat anterior pituitaries were incubated for 5 days before beginning the experiment. Cells were then incubated in a volume of 3 ml for five successive 2-hr incubation periods in the presence or absence of 5 mM mbcAMP, 5 mM dbcAMP or 5 mM theophylline. Results are expressed as mean $\pm$ SD of data obtained from duplicate dishes. (From Drouin and Labrie).

ULTRASTRUCTURAL CHANGES ACCOMPANYING CHRONIC TREATMENT OF GONADOTROPHS IN CELL CULTURE WITH LH-RH

Chronic treatment of adenohypophyseal cells in monolayer culture with LH-RH has been shown to increase both synthesis and release of gonadotropic hormones (24). Since no data are available on the morphology of adenohypophyseal cells in monolayer culture, it seemed of importance to study at the electron microscope level, the modifications induced by LH-RH after 6 days of incubation.

In control cultures, well granulated gonadotrophs were identified on the basis of the size of their secretory granules and the presence of dilated rough endoplasmic reticulum (RER) cisternae. The other granulated cell-types were identified as somatotrophs, mammotrophs, thyrotrophs and corticotrophs. In cultures exposed to 1×10^{-8} M LH-RH for 6 days (Fig. 3), typical control gonadotrophs were replaced by markedly hypertrophied cells. These enlarged cells were classified as gonadotrophs on the basis of their dilated RER cisternae and large irregularly shaped nucleus located at the periphery of the cytoplasm (31). They contained usually a few small secretory granules or were completely degranulated while the Golgi apparatus was usually well developed. Such depletion of secretory granules agrees well with the observed decrease in FSH and LH content (Fig. 1) (24). That this depletion of secretory granules had not been observed in gonadotrophs after 6 hr of incubation of the pituitary halves in the presence of mbcAMP (32) could represent a phenomenon which occurs only after a long-term stimulation. Bundles of microfilaments dispersed in the cytoplasm were not infrequently observed.

The enlargement of gonadotrophs in tissue culture after a long-term stimulation with LH-RH agrees well with the hypertrophy of gonadotrophs observed _in vivo_ after castration (31,33). It should, however, be mentioned that the castration cells have an increased number of granules and a more dilated RER. Specificity of the stimulated effect of LH-RH has been confirmed at the morphological level by the absence of modifications in the other cell types.

PARALLEL STIMULATORY EFFECT OF LH-RH AND SOME OF ITS ANALOGUES ON CYCLIC AMP ACCUMULATION AND LH AND FSH RELEASE

Although the observation of a stimulatory effect of theophylline,

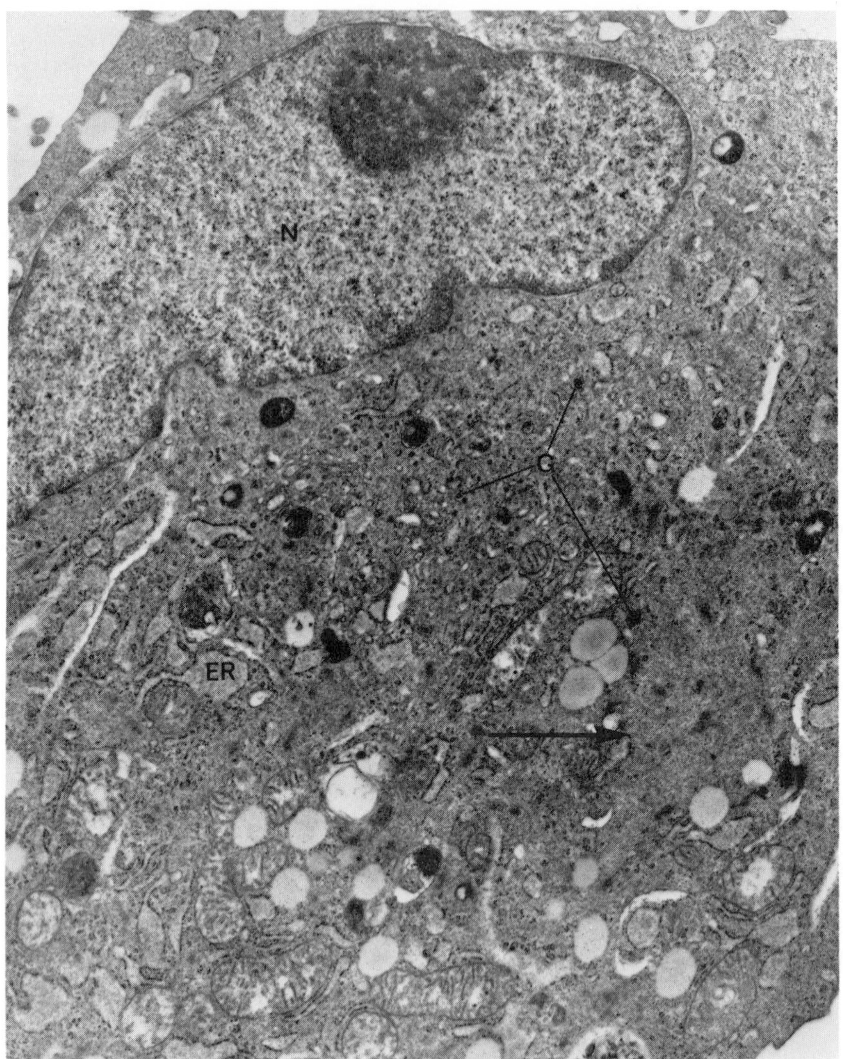

FIG 3. A gonadotroph after 6 days in monolayer culture in the presence of 1 x 10^{-8} M LH-RH. The cell is markedly hypertrophied. In the cytoplasm, the dilated cisternae of the rough endoplasmic reticulum (ER) are abundant and a few secretory granules (G) are present. The nucleus (N) is large and irregular and located at the periphery of the cell. A bundle of microfilaments (→) can be observed. x 15,000.

mbcAMP, and dbcAMP (Fig. 2) on LH release was suggestive of a role of cyclic AMP in the control of gonadotropin secretion, definitive proof of the role of the adenylate cyclase system as a mediator of the action of LH-RH could be obtained only by measurements of adenohypophyseal adenylate cyclase activity or cyclic AMP concentrations under the influence of the neurohormone.

Concentrations of synthetic LH-RH ranging from 5 to 100 ng/ml led to a 160 to 250 % increase over control of adenohypophyseal cyclic AMP concentrations (19). A close correlation was then found between the rates of LH and FSH release and changes of adenohypophyseal cyclic AMP concentrations, both as a function of time of incubation and increasing concentrations of the neurohormone. The concentration of LH-RH required for half-maximal stimulation of cyclic AMP accumulation and LH release is between 0.1 and 1 ng/ml or between 1×10^{-10} and 1×10^{-9} M (19). Kaneko et al. (50) have also recently reported that synthetic LH-RH (1 μg/ml) increased cyclic AMP levels in rat anterior pituitary _in vitro_.

The potential importance of LH-RH analogues in the control of fertility has led to the synthesis of a wide variety of analogues of the decpeptide by several laboratories. Such analogues have already provided much information on the structure-function relationships of the LH-RH molecule (34,35) and offer the opportunity of investigating the relative potency of these compounds on cyclic AMP accumulation and hormone release. Further, the finding of a close correlation between their effect on these two parameters would add strong support for the role of cyclic AMP as mediator of the intracellular effects of the releasing hormone.

The LH-RH analogues used for such a study and their relative potencies on LH release measured by different laboratories using _in vitro_ and _in vivo_ tests (34-40) are illustrated in Fig. 4. It can be seen that the biological activity of these compounds ranges from less than 0.001 % (des-His^{2}-DesGly^{10} -LH-RH-ethylamide) to 500-1,000 % (desGly^{10}-LH-RH-ethylamide) the activity of LH-RH itself. When increasing concentrations of these compounds were tested for their effect on cyclic AMP accumulation and LH and FSH release in rat hemipituitaries _in vitro_, a close correlation was consistently found amongst the values of these three parameters (41); this further provides strong evidence for the cyclic nucleotide as a mediator of LH-RH action (19,24).

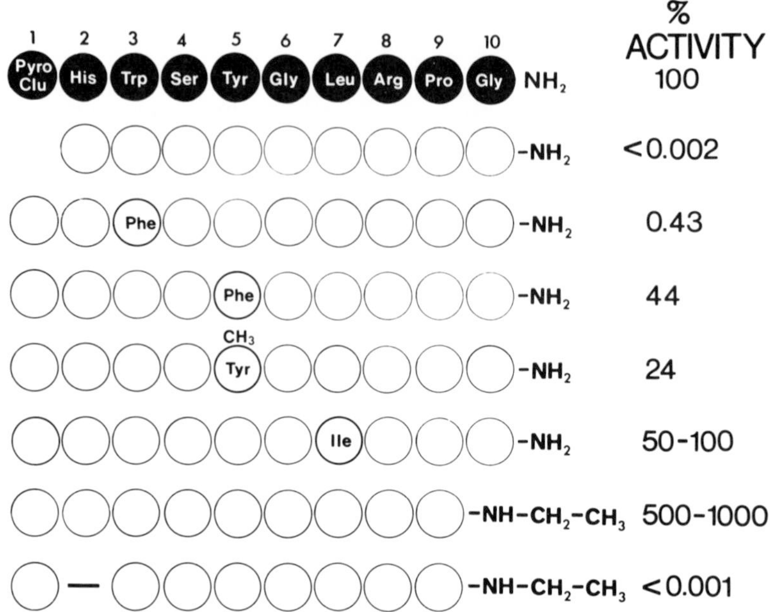

FIG 4. Relative biological activity of LH-RH and some of its analogues: des(pyro)Glu-LH-RH, (Phe^3) LH-RH, (Phe^5) LH-RH, (O-methyl-Tyr^5) LH-RH, (Ile^7) LH-RH, des-Gly^{10}-LH-RH-ethylamide and des-His^2-des-Gly^{10}-LH-RH-ethylamide. A close correlation was found between changes of intracellular levels of cyclic AMP in the presence of increasing concentrations of the various analogues and LH and FSH release in rat anterior pituitary tissue *in vitro*.

EFFECT OF PROSTAGLANDINS ON THE RELEASE OF LH AND FSH

It is well known that prostaglandins (PGs) stimulate adenylate cyclase activity in various systems (42-44) including the anterior pituitary (45), and a few studies suggest that PGs may well control intracellular cyclic AMP levels (46-49).

Fig. 5 shows that 1×10^{-7} M PGE_2 led to a ~10-fold stimulation of LH release during the first two, 2-hr incubation periods of pituitary cells in monolayer culture with a progressive decrease to a 2.5-fold stimulation of hormone release between the 8th and 10th hour of incubation. Similar findings were observed on FSH release also (data not shown).

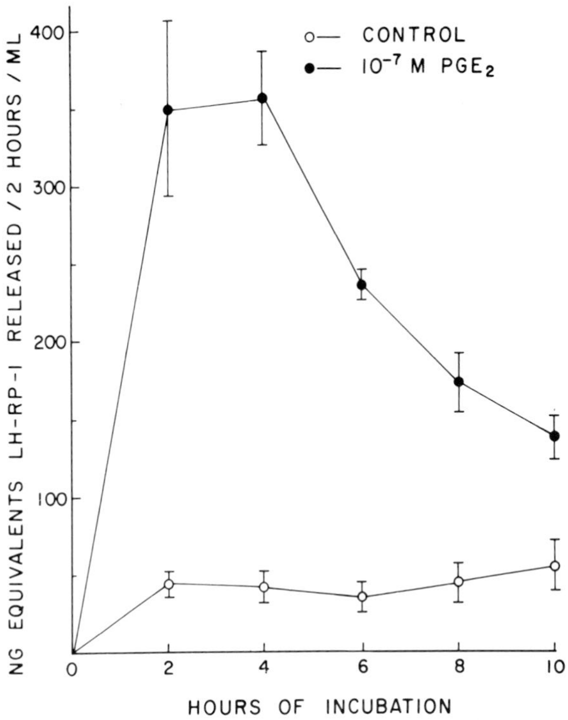

FIG 5. Effect of PGE$_2$ on LH release from anterior pituitary cells in monolayer culture. Experimental conditions were as in Fig 2. except for the presence of 1×10^{-7} M PGE$_2$ in the appropriate groups. From Drouin and Labrie (1973).

Coupled with the observation of an inhibition of LH release by indomethacin, a PG synthetase inhibitor, or by 7-oxa-13-prostynoic acid, a PG-antagonist, and the stimulatory effect of PGE$_1$ and PGE$_2$ on cyclic AMP formation in the anterior pituitary (Borgeat, Drouin and Labrie - unpublished data), the present finding of a marked stimulation of both LH and FSH release by PGE$_2$ suggests that PGs may play an important role in the action of LH-RH in the anterior pituitary gland.

REFERENCES

1. Green, J. and Harris, G.W. (1947). J. Endocr. 5, 136.
2. Harris, G.W. (1948). J. Physiol (London), 107, 418.
3. Harris, G.W. (1955). In "Neural control of the pituitary gland" Edward Arnold, London.
4. McCann, S.M., Taleisnik, S. and Friedman, H.M. (1960). Proc. Soc. Exp. Biol. Med. 104, 432.
5. Harris, G.W. (1961). In "Control of Ovulation", C.A. Villee (Ed). Pergamon, Oxford, p. 56.
6. Courrier, R., Jutisz, M. and Colonge, A. (1963). C.R. Acad. Sci. (Paris), 257, 3774.
7. Schally, A.V., Bowers, C.Y., Carter, W.H., Arimura, A., Redding, T.W. and Saito, M. (1969). Endocrinology 85, 290.
8. Igarashi, M. and McCann, S.M. (1964). Endocrinology 74, 446.
9. Kuroshima, A., Ishida, Y., Bowers, C.Y. and Schally, A.V., (1965). Endocrinology 76, 614.
10. Schally, A.V., Baba, Y., Arimura, A., Redding, T.W. and White, W.F. (1971) Biochem. Biophys. Res. Comm. 42, 50.
11. Schally, A.V., Arimura, A., Baba, Y., Nair, R.M.G., Matsuo, H., Redding, T.W. and Debeljuk, L. (1971). Biochem. Biophys. Res. Comm. 43, 393.
12. Schally, A.V., Nair, R.M.G., Redding, T.W., and Arimura, A., (1971). J. Biol. Chem. 246, 7230.
13. Amos, M., Burgus, R., Blackwell, R., Vale, W., Fellows, R., and Guillemin, R. (1971). Biochem. Biophys. Res. Comm. 44, 205.
14. Matsuo, H., Baba, Y., Nair, R.M.G., Arimura, A. and Schally, A.V. (1971). Biochem. Biophys. Res. Comm. 43, 1334.
15. Baba, Y., Matsuo, H. and Schally, A.V. (1971). Biochem. Biophys. Res. Comm. 44, 459.
16. Burgus, R., Butcher, M., Ling, N., Monahan, M., Rivier, J, Fellows, R., Amos, M., Blackwell, R., Vale, W. and Guillemin, R., (1971). C.R.Acad. Sci. 273, 1611.
17. Schally, A.V., Kastin, A.J., and Arimura, A. (1971). Fert. Steril. 22, 703.
18. Schally, A.V., Arimura, A., Kastin, A.J., Matsuo, H., Baba, Y., Redding, T.W., Nair, R.M.G., Debeljuk, L., and White, W.F. (1971). Science 173, 1036.

19. Borgeat, P., Chavancy, G., Dupont, A., Labrie, F., Arimura, A., and Schally, A.V. (1972). Proc. Natl. Acad. Sci., U.S.A. 69, 2677.
20. Guillemin, R. (1972). Contraception, 6, 1.
21. Matsuo, H., Arimura, A., Nair, R.M.G., and Schally, A.V. (1971). Biochem. Biophys. Res. Comm. 45, 822.
22. Monahan, M., Rivier, J., Burgus, R., Amos, M., Blackwell, R., Vale, W. and Guillemin, R. (1971). C.R.H. Acad. Sci. 273, 508.
23. Geiger, R., König, W., Wissmann, H., Geisen, K. and Enzman, F. (1971). Biochem. Biophys. Res. Comm. 45, 767.
24. Labrie, F., Pelletier, G., Lemay, A., Borgeat, P., Barden, N, Dupont, A., Savary, M., Côté, J. and Boucher, R. (1973) 6th Karolinska Symposium on Research Methods in Reproductive Endocrinology, E. Diczfalusy (Ed.) p. 301.
25. Vale, W., Grant, G., Amos, M., Blackwell, R. and Guillemin, R. (1972). Endocrinology 91, 562.
26. Mittler, J.C., Arimura, A. and Schally, A.V. (1970). Proc. Soc. Exp. Biol. Med. 133, 1321.
27. Redding, T.W., Schally, A.V., Arimura, A. and Matsuo, H. (1972). Endocrinology 90, 764.
28. Kobayashi, T., Kobayashi, S ., Kigawa, I., Mizuno, M. and Amenomori, Y. (1963). Endocrinol. Jap. 10, 16.
29. Kobayashi, T., Kigawa, T., Mizuno, M. and Sato, H. (1964). Gumma Symp. Endocrinol. 1, 249.
30. Jutisz, M. and De La Llosa, M.P. (1969). C.R. Acad. Sci. (Paris), 268, 1636.
31. Kurosumi, K. (1968). Arch. Histol. Japon, 29, 329.
32. Pelletier, G., Lemay, A., Beraud, G. and Labrie, F. (1972). Endocrinology 91, 1355.
33. Farquhar, M.G. (1971). Mem. Soc. Endocrinol. 19, Hellers, H. and Lederis, K. (Eds). Cambridge, University Press. 79, 124.
34. Coy, D.H., Coy, E.J. and Schally, A.V. (1973). Prog. 55th Meeting Endocr. Soc., p. A-145.
35. Schally, A.V., Arimura, A., Carter, W.H., Redding, T.W., Geiger, R., König, W., Wessman, H., Jaeger, G., Sandow, J., Yanaihara, N., Yanaihara, C., Hashimoto, T. and Sakagami, M. (1972). Biochem. Biophys. Res. Comm. 48, 366.
36. Coy, D.H., Coy, E.J. and Schally, A.V. (1973). J. Med. Chem. 16, 83.

37. Coy, D.H., Coy, E.J. and Schally, A.V. (1973). J. Med. Chem. 16, 827.
38. Fujino, M., Kobayashi, S., Obayashi, M., Shinagawa, S., Fukuda, T., Kitada, C., Nakayama, R., Yamasaki, I., White, W.F. and Rippel, R.H. (1972). Biochem. Biophys. Res. Comm. 49, 863.
39. Fujino, M., Kobayashi, S., Obayashi, M., Fukuda, T., Shinagawa, S., Yamasaki, I., Nakayama, R., White, W.F. and Rippel, R.H. (1972). Biochem. Biophys. Res. Comm. 49, 698.
40. Yanaihara, N., Hashimoto, I., Yanaihara, C., Tsuji, K., Kenmochi, Y., Ashizawa, F., Kaneko, T., Ika, H., Saito, S., Arimuro, A. and Schally, A.V. (1973). Biochem. Biophys. Res. Comm. 52, 64.
41. Borgeat, P., Labrie, F., Cote, J., Ruel, F., Schally, A.V., Coy, D.H., Coy, E.J. and Yanaihara, N. (1973). J. Mol. Cell. Endocrinology (in press).
42. Wolfe, S.M., and Shulman, N.R. (1969). Biochem. Biophys. Res. Comm. 35, 265.
43. Peery, C.V., Johnson, G.S. and Pastan, I. (1971). J. Biol. Chem. 246, 5785.
44. Sato, S., Szabo, M., Kowalski, K. and Burke, G. (1972). Endocrinology 90, 343.
45. Zor, U., Kaneko, T., Schneider, H.P.G., McCann, S.M., Lowe, I.P., Bloom, G., Borland, B. and Field, J.B. (1969) Proc. Natl. Acad. Sci., U.S.A. 63, 918.
46. Ramwell, P.W. and Shaw, J.E. (1970). Rec. Prog. Horm. Res. 26, 139.
47. Zor, U., Kaneko, T., Lowe, I.P., Bloom, G. and Field, J.B. (1969). J. Biol. Chem. 244, 5189.
48. Butcher, R.W. and Baird, C.E. (1968). J. Biol. Chem. 243, 1713.
49. Kuehl, F.A., Jr., Humes, J.L., Tarnoff, J., Cirillo, V.J., and Ham, E.A. (1970). Science 169, 883.
50. Kaneko, T., Saito, S., Oka, H., Oda, T. and Yanaihara, N., (1973). Metabolism, 22, 77.

HYPOTHALAMIC CONTENT OF LUTEINIZING HORMONE RELEASING FACTOR AND ITS MECHANISM OF ACTION ON THE RAT ANTERIOR PITUITARY

T. Makino, Michio Takahashi, K. Yoshinaga and Roy O. Greep

Both natural and synthetic luteinizing hormone releasing factors (LRF) are known to stimulate the discharge of LH and FSH from the pituitary gland both *in vivo* and *in vitro*. The effect of changing physiological and pharmacological milieu on LRF in the hypothalamic tissue and the mechanism of action of LRF on the pituitary are not clearly understood. This paper describes (i) the use of a sensitive and specific radioimmunoassay for LRF by which the hypothalamic content of LRF was analyzed and (ii) a probable intracellular mechanism of LH and FSH release from the pituitary.

The production of anti-LRF serum and radioimmunoassay for LRF have been described earlier (1). Fifty mg of synthetic LRF (Lot No. TAP-023, Takeda Chemical Industries Ltd, Japan) were deamidated without significant peptide bond cleavage by incubation in 0.5 N HCl with continuous stirring for 24 hr at 23°. The pH of the deamidated LRF was then brought to 7.0-7.3 with NaOH and lyophilized. This deamidated LRF was found to release a significant amount of LH from the rat pituitary during a 4 hr incubation *in vitro*, indicating that deamidation is not affecting the release activity. The deamidated LRF was conjugated to bovine serum albumin (BSA) using 1-ethyl-3 (3-dimethyl-aminopropyl)carbodiimide-HCl (EDC) as the coupling agent. The deamidated LRF, 40 mg of EDC and 170 mg of BSA were dissolved in 6 ml of water, the pH was adjusted to 6.5 -7.0, and incubated in the dark for 16 hr at room temperature. The conjugate was then dialyzed against phosphosaline buffer at 4° for 48 hr, and was then diluted in 0.15 M saline to a final volume of 12 ml. Five to six-months old New Zealand white female rabbits were immunized with the conjugate in Freund's complete adjuvant (Difco) by repeated multiple (10 sites) dorsal intradermal injections in a volume of 0.25 ml. Booster injections were given at 2-week intervals.

Nondeamidated LRF (5 μg) was radioiodinated by a modified chloramine-T method and applied to either Bio-Gel P-2 or Sephadex G-10 column (column size 0.9 x 17.0 cm). The specific activity of the labeled LRF was 140-160 uCi/ug. The diluted

Table 1. Displacement of ^{125}I-LRF from its antibody by different compounds.

Hormones	Relative Cross-reactivity *
Synthetic LRF (Takeda)	100.0
Rat hypothalamic extract (NIAMD-rat-HE-RP-1)	100.0**
Synthetic TRF (Beckman)	<0.01
Rat-LH (NIAMD-rat-LH-RP-1)	<0.03
Rat-FSH (NIAMD-rat FSH-RP-1)	<0.03
Substance P (Beckman)	<0.15
Lysine-Vasopressin (Sigma)	<0.02
Arginine-Vasopressin (Sigma)	<0.02
Oxytocin (Sigma)	<0.01

*Molar weight required to replace 30 % of ^{125}I-LRF is divided by the amount of LRF required to displace comparable % of level.
**Weight of pure LRF present uncertain, see text.

antiserum and ^{125}I-LRF were incubated in 0.2 M tris-acetate buffer (pH 7.3) at 4° and the antigen-antibody complex was precipitated by the addition of an excess amount of sheep anti-rabbit gamma globulin. The optimal time for the first incubation was found to be 2 to 4 hr. Synthetic TRF, rat LH and FSH, substance P, lysine and arginine Vasopressin and Oxytocin were found not to displace ^{125}I-LRF from the antibody (Table 1).

Table 2 shows the biological potency of the anti-LRF serum. Intravenous administration of the antiserum to 4-day cyclic female rats at 1300 and 1500 hr on proestrus brought about an inhibition of ovulation in 6 out of 8 animals, (one animal showed the presence of only one ovum, and another 2 ova). In contrast, the ip injection failed to inhibit ovulation. Simultaneous administration of large amounts of LRF (250 ng) reversed the effect seen with the antiserum. No significant changes in pituitary, ovarian and uterine weight were observed after treatment with the antiserum. Normal rabbit serum (NRS) treatment had no effect on ovulation.

One of the antisera showed at 1:5000 to 1:1000 dilution, about 30 to 40 percent binding with ^{125}I-LRF. The range of the

Table 2. Effect of anti-LRF serum on ovulation in normal cycling female rats.

Group	No. animals	No. ova (L)	No. ova (R)	Body wt. (g)	Ant. Pit wt. (mg)	Ovarian wt. (mg)	Uterine wt. (mg)
Control (NRS, i v)	5 (5)*	8.2±1.3	5.0±1.3	274.6±10.9	10.9±1.2	73.2±4.0	452.9±11.7
A/S (i v)	8 (2)	0.1±0.1	0.3±0.2	262.6±7.7	9.57±0.5	61.6±3.4	534.8±34.4
A/S (i p)	5 (5)	6.8±1.1	6.0±0.6	258.2±11.9	8.30±0.7	68.7±2.9	498.5±39.7
A/S+LH-RF (i v)	5 (5)	8.2±1.3	5.0±1.3	270.2±7.4	9.26±0.7	64.2±1.9	452.9±11.7

Organ weights and the number of ova are Mean ± S. E. M. *Number of animals which had ovulated are shown in parenthesis.

standard curve was from 50 to 5000 pg of LRF. The hypothalamic content of LRF measured by radioimmunoassay indicated that the content in 31-day old immature female rats is less than half of that found in mature animals (46-day old). The LRF content on diestrus and estrus was high and no significant change from this was observed on proestrus at 1000 and 1600 hr. Multiple i v injection of reserpine (5.0 - 7.5 mg/kg body weight) to regularly cycling rats on proestrus (1100, 1230, 1330 and 1430 hr) blocked ovulation the next day, lowered serum LH concentration at the critical period and reduced the hypothalamic content of LRF. On the other hand, 1.0 mg of reserpine and 2.0 to 5.0 mg of melatonin per each injection could not inhibit ovulation.

In _in vitro_ pituitary culture, 60 to 70 per cent of LRF initially added to culture medium was still detectable by radioimmunoassay after a 6-hr incubation in an atmosphere of 95 % O_2, 5 % CO_2 at 37°. Effect of synthetic LRF on pituitary cyclic AMP was studied _in vitro_ and the minimum dose of synthetic LRF required to increase cyclic AMP as measured by radioimmunoassay (2) is shown in Table 3. The time-course study on the effect of synthetic LRF and hypothalamic extract (NIAMD-HE-RP-1) on pituitary cyclic AMP level is shown in Table 4. While 1.0 - 10.0 ng of LRF brought about a marked increase in pituitary cyclic AMP content within 5 min, 0.1 ng and 20.0 ng of LRF failed to do so. The pituitary content of cyclic AMP was increased within minutes after incubation with 5.0 - 15.0 ng of LRF and the optimal LRF effect on cyclic AMP formation was obtained in 3 to 10 minutes

Table 3. Minimum dose of synthetic LRF required to increase cyclic AMP in vitro in the rat anterior pituitary *.

LRF added to treated flasks (ng)	Control			Treated		
	1	2	3	1	2	3
0.1	1.09	1.27	(CE)¶	1.15**	1.32	—
1.0	1.10	1.18	1.31	1.56	1.39	1.24
3.0	1.35	1.22	—	10.42	13.19	—
10.0	—	—	1.30	—	—	6.0
20.0	1.10	1.13	1.26	1.39	1.36	2.46

*All pituitary halves after 30 min were incubated for 5 min in Krebś-Ringer buffer with or without synthetic LRF
**The values are picomoles of cyclic AMP per mg of anterior pituitary wet weight; mean of duplicate or triplicate assays are given. ¶ CE = Cerebral cortex extract (4 mg).

of incubation (Table 4). Though some experimental variability was noted in cyclic AMP values, these data suggest that a few nanograms of LRF are sufficient to produce measurable increase in the level of cyclic AMP in the anterior pituitary.

Adenyl cyclase activity in the pituitary homogenate could be enhanced by 15 to 20 ng of LRF and 10 mg of the hypothalamic extract as shown in Table 5. Adenyl cyclase activity was measured according to the method of Krishna (3) and expressed as cpm of ^{14}C-cyclic AMP formed from ^{14}C-ATP.

Table 4. Effect of synthetic LRF and hypothalamic extract (HE) on cyclic AMP concentration of rat anterior pituitary (AP) in vitro - a time course study.

Experiment	After pre-incubation	Incubation time (min)					
		1	2	3	5	10	30
	picomoles of cyclic AMP per mg of AP						
Treated (LRF 5 ng)	2.49	2.46	--	3.66	5.28	3.24	1.20
Control	2.49	2.46	--	2.30	1.20	1.14	1.14
Treated (LRF 15 ng)	--	2.44	2.53	--	3.47	2.63	--
Control	--	1.88	2.25	--	1.72	2.00	--
Treated (HE 2 mg)	1.14	--	--	3.83	--	3.91	2.50
Control (CE* 2 mg)	1.31	--	--	1.36	--	1.33	1.56
Treated (HE 4 mg)	1.76	--	3.38	--	--	3.53	4.88
Control (CE 4 mg)	1.76	--	1.71	--	--	1.43	1.88
Treated (HE 4 mg)	0.68	3.28	3.38	--	--	3.19	6.38
Control	1.54	2.19	1.80	--	--	1.20	1.43

* CE = Cerebral cortex extract.

Table 5. Effect of LRF and rat hypothalamic extract (HE) on adenyl cyclase activity of rat anterior pituitary.*

Experimental	1 min	2min	5 min	10 min
	Adenyl cyclase activity (cpm of ^{14}C-cyclic AMP produced)			
Treated (LRF 15 ng)	936.0	2,206.7	--	4,367.5
Control (CE** 10 ng)	1,199.8	2,063.9	--	3,724.8
Treated (LRF 20 ng)	1,079.0	2,063.9	--	5,604.4
Control (CE 10 mg)	1,486.9	2,277.2	--	3,267.1
Treated (HE 10 mg)	--	1,556.9	1,721.6	2,579.1
Control (CE 10 mg)	--	1,320.1	1,507.6	1,761.3

*The values represent the mean of duplicate determinations.
**CE = Cerebral cortex extract.

Effect of exogenous dibutyryl cyclic AMP and theophylline on LH and FSH release is shown in Table 6. Theophylline (1 mM), particularly in combination with dibutyryl cyclic AMP (10 mM) brought about significant release of LH and FSH into the medium; theophylline alone increased LH release. Effects of PGE_1 and $PGF_{2\alpha}$ on pituitary cyclic AMP, FSH and LH are shown in Table 7 Large amounts of exogenous PGE_1 and $PGF_{2\alpha}$ induced a marked increase in the level of pituitary cyclic AMP, but little LH and FSH were released as compared to control; small amounts of the prostaglandins had the reverse effect, i.e., they reduced the formation of cyclic AMP and enhanced the release of LH and FSH. Where the two PG inhibitors, indomethacin and 7-oxa-13-prostynoic acid (7-oxa) (a gift from Dr. Josef Fried of the University of Chicago), were used, no change in the basal secretion pattern of LH and FSH was observed. However, 10 μg of 7-oxa reduced the LH release stimulated by LRF.

Estradiol and the nonsteroidal weak estrogenic substance, compound F6066 were tested for their ability to release LH and FSH *in vitro* (3). 100 μg of compound F6066 and 0.1 μg of estradiol benzoate increased the release of both LH and FSH (Table 8), suggesting that estrogenic substances can modulate the gonadotropin secretion without having any effect on cyclic AMP.

Table 6. Effect of dibutyryl cyclic AMP and theophylline on LH and FSH release*

Experiment	LH released in med. (ng/mg AP)	FSH released in med. (ng/mg AP)
1 mM cyclic AMP (4)	2,472.6±312.5	2,190.0±134.7
Control (4)	1,809.5±296.9	1,609.5±285.7
10 mM cyclic AMP (4)	3,190.5±234.0	2,647.6±242.4
Control (4)	2,457.1±255.3	1,695.3±780.6
10 mM cyclic AMP + 1 mM theophylline (3)	3,345.9±204.2**	2,994.4±235.8**
Control (3)	2,066.7±142.1	1,180.5±218.3
5 mM theophylline (3)	3,792.6±199.3***	3,133.3±644.2
Control (3)	3,066.7±117.6	2,688.9±288.9
10 mM theophylline (4)	3,190.5±407.5***	3,466.7±107.8***
Control (4)	1,504.8±486.2	1,523.8±304.8

* The values are the means ± S. E. and all pituitary halves were incubated in 2 ml of TC 199 for 4 hours. Reference preparation used : NIAMD-rat LH or FSH RP-1.
** $p < 0.005$; *** $p < 0.05$. No. in paranthesis indicate the number of flasks used.

Table 7. Effects of prostaglandin E_1 and $F_{2\alpha}$ in vitro on pituitary cyclic AMP, FSH and LH release

Experiment	LH released in med. (ng/mg. AP)	P value	FSH released in med. (ng/mg. AP)	P value	Cyclic AMP in ant. pit. (picomoles/ mg. AP)	P value
PGE_1 0.5 µg	3,255.7±258.7	0.01	4,847.8±467.1	0.01	6.99±0.39	0.005
Control	1,456.7±260.6		2,240.8±207.0		1.56±0.59	
PGE_1 20 µg	1,938.3±366.5	N.S	2,897.5±175.1	N.S	49.91±12.37	0.025
Control	2,169.2±182.7		2,205.0±191.6		0.77± 0.18	
$PGF_{2\alpha}$ 30 µg	2,288.6±151.8	0.05	3,502.5±322.6	N.S.	7.79± 0.25	0.001
Control	1,588.0±248.3		3,673.6±224.9		1.85± 0.10	
$PGF_{2\alpha}$ 300 µg	2,316.4±152.1	N.S.	3,486.6±592.3	N.S.	78.47± 5.57	0.005
Control	2,798.0±230.8		3,673.6±184.0		3.03± 1.43	

*All pituitary halves were incubated in 2 ml. of TC 199 with or without PG for 4 hr; 3 flasks in each group; Reference preparation NIAMD rat LH or FSH RP-1; The values are means ± S. E. AP = anterior pituitary.

In summary, the hypothalamic content of LRF, can be altered by changing the physiological and pharmacological milieu. Since endogenous prostaglandins are in low concentration in the pituitary compared to the amounts used in in vitro experiments, it is

Table 8. Effects of estradiol, F6066 and LRF *in vitro* on LH and FSH release and pituitary cyclic AMP.

Experiment	No. of flasks	Released in medium, ng/mg anterior pituitary		Pituitary cyclic AMP picomoles/mg anterior pituitary.
		LH	FSH	
F6066 100 μg	4	3,018.6±559.8*	3,049.4±306.8**	0.68±0.12 (3)
Control	4	1,307.8±272.6	1,426.8± 42.0	0.92±0.26 (3)
Estradiol 1 μg	4	2,877.5±223.1**	2,701.1±120.0**	0.98±0.11 (3)
Control	4	1,875.0± 94.2	1,400.6±217.7	1.13±0.08 (3)
LRF 15 ng	3	4,040.1±226.0**	3,657.5±303.2**	6.60±0.49 (4)***
Control	3	1,523.3±113.0	1,321.7±101.6	1.34± 0.13 (4)

* $p < 0.05$; ** $p < 0.01$; *** $p < 0.001$. Reference preparation = NIAMD rat LH or FSH RP-1.

difficult to translate the results obtained from these studies to *in vivo* system. However, it is possible that the prostaglandins may serve as one of the local regulatory agents of cell function in the release of LH and FSH. The data strongly support the hypothesis that the release of LH and presumably FSH also by LRF is mediated by the adenyl cyclase-cyclic AMP system.

ACKNOWLEDGEMENT

The authors wish to thank Miss Janet Ackley for her excellent technical assistance. This work was supported by grants from the National Institutes of Health HD-03736 and HD-06467, The Ford Foundation and the Milton Fund of Harvard University.

REFERENCES

1. Makino, T., Takahashi, M., Yoshinaga, K. and Greep, R.O. (1973). Contraception 8, 133.
2. Makino, T. (1973). Amer. J. Obst. & Gynecol. 115, 606.
3. Makino, T. and Greep, R.O. (1973). Fertil. and Steril. 24, 116.

BIOSYNTHESIS OF GONADOTROPINS AND THEIR RELEASING FACTORS

Katsumi Wakabayashi, Tadashi Asai, Takashi Higuchi
Bun-ichi Tamaoki, and Samuel M. McCann

INTRODUCTION

Since the discovery of existence of hypothalamic gonadotropin releasing factors (1-3), many studies have been conducted on their mechanism of action. Though there is a general agreement on the ability of these factors to release LH and FSH from the anterior pituitary both in vivo and in vitro, it still remains to be clarified whether these increase the de novo biosynthesis of LH or FSH. In the present paper, we have reviewed the results of the previous studies, and our recent experiments on the mechanism of action of release factors.

A BRIEF REVIEW OF THE PREVIOUS STUDIES

Both in vivo and in vitro systems have been used, but the former has a merit that it is carried out in a physiological environment; however, the amounts of hormones which are released and stored are difficult to compute. For this purpose the exact volume of the blood as well as the disappearance rates of the hormnes in individual animals have to be known; no such studies have been made in detail thus far. On the other hand, using in vitro system, the pituitary tissue can be maintained at the most for 3 to 4 hr in a seemingly physiological state. During this period, for example, carbon dioxide formation from glucose,and amino acid incorporation into protein are shown to increase linearly (4). Superfusion technique is useful for studying the mechanism of action, as this is suitable for carrying out a time course study. Tissue culture is another technique which is of great use, particularly for studying chronic effects; this could be used only if the original responsiveness of the tissue is maintained , and this, however, is questionable.

In addition to being able to compute in this system the release and storage of gonadotropins , it is also possible to obtain direct evidence of de novo biosynthesis of a hormone by following the incorporation of radioactive precursors into the isolated hormonal fraction.

Kobayashi et al. (5) were the first to show a stimulatory effect of hypothalamic extract on gonadotropin production in tissue culture. Since then, the long-term effects of hypothalamic crude extract (6), partially purified releasing factor preparations (7) and synthetic LHRF (8) have been studied in tissue culture (Table 1). It has been concluded from these studies that LHRF increases the biosynthesis of LH. A continued presence of LHRF in the medium may be responsible for this increase in LH biosynthesis. It has also been observed that following castration, the level of LH both in the pituitary and plasma increases. Our own experiments indicated that castration and immunization with LH increased the incorporation of ^{14}C-leucine into the LH fraction (4, 9, 10).

Table 1. List of representative *in vitro* investigations

System	Source of releasing factor	Assay method used	Effect	Reference No.
Tissue culture (rat AP)	HE	Bioassay	Total gonadotropins ↑	5
Tissue culture (rat AP)	HE	Autoradiography	^{3}H-Leu uptake in PAS+cell ↑	6
Incubation (OvX-EBP-(rat AP)	Purified LHRF	Bioassay	Total LH ↑	11
Incubation (rat AP)	HE		^{14}C-Leu, glucosamine into LH →	16
Incubation (rat AP)	HE	Radioimmunoassay	Total LH ↑	13
Incubation (OvX-EBP-rat AP)	Purified LHRF	Bioassay	Total LH ↑	12
Tissue culture (rat AP)	Purified LHRF & FSHRF	Radioimmuno assay	Total LH, FSH ↑	13
Incubation (male OrchX TP-treated rat AP)	Purified LHRF	Bioassay	Total LH → ^{14}C-Leu into LH →	15
Incubation (OvX-EBP rat AP)	Purified LHRF	Radioimmunoassay	Total LH ↑ ^{3}H-Leu into LH ?	20
Incubation (rat AP)	HE	Radioimmunoassay	Total LH →	17
Tissue culture (rat AP)	Synthetic LHRF	Radioimmunoassay	Total LH ↑ ^{3}H-glucosamine into LH ↑	8
Implantation (rat AP)	Purified LHRF	Bioassay	Total LH ↑	18

↑ = increase; → = no change; AP = Anterior pituitary; EBP = Estradiol benzoate, progesterone treated; TP = Testosterone propionate treated; HE = Hypothalamic extract; OvX = Ovariectomized; OrchX = Orchidectomized.

However, it is difficult to know, from this, whether this increased production of LH was caused primarily by LHRF, or secondarily due to the increased secretion. Using the short-term incubation system, Jutisz et al. (11, 12), and Midgley et al. (13) have observed with LHRF preparations, an increase in the total amount of LH. However, Jutisz et al. (12) later reported that the toal amount of LH did not change significantly on short-term incubation with LH-RF, and the use of double-antibody technique in following incorporation of ^{3}H-leucine into LH fraction gave results showing large variation and poor reproducibility. They further observed that the total amount of FSH increased not only with FSHRF, but also on addition of 60 mM K^+ or cyclic AMP into the medium; thus the production of FSH was considered not to be under the direct control of FSHRF.

We have estimated LH synthesized *de novo* in the rat anterior pituitary by incubating the pituitary with ^{14}C-amino acid and immunochemically separating the LH fraction (9). ^{14}C-leucine incorporation into both LH and protein fractions showed a time-dependent increase up to 8 hr, and this could be inhibited by puromycin at 20 μg/ml and by actinomycin D at 10 μg/ml (4, 9). Active and passive immunization of rats with ovine LH (NIH-LH preparation) caused specific increase of ^{14}C-leucine incorporation into LH fraction (9, 14). Testosterone propionate (TP) injection during the period of immunization significantly prevented this increase (10). The daily injection of 250 μg of TP alone caused a decrease in the LH biosynthesis; this amount was also effective in preventing the castration-induced increase in LH synthesis (10).

Paired hemipituitaries obtained from normal, castrated and TP-treated male rats were incubated in the media containing ^{14}C-leucine with or without partially purified ovine LHRF (15). LHRF stimulated the release of LH from the pituitaries of both normal and castrated male rats, but not from those of TP-treated rats. However, there were no significant differences in the total amount of LH in the incubation system between control and LHRF-treated groups indicating that LHRF did not stimulate LH synthesis.

The radioactivity in the protein fractions of LHRF-treated and control groups ranged from 96 to 113 %. The average radioactivity in the protein fraction and LH fractions of normal pituitaries was 102.5 $\pm$ 2.7 % and 101.9 $\pm$ 6.2 % respectively, as determined by 7 experiments. Similarly no significant differences in the biosynthesis of protein or LH fraction between control and LHRF-treated groups were observed in pituitaries of castrated or TP-treated males. Samli and Geschwind (16) have similarly observed using hypothalamic extract, ^{14}C-leucine incorporation to LH fraction.

Since bioassay such as the OAAD test for LH show a comparatively large variance, radioimmunoassay was used for more precise estimation of the total amount of LH. The pituitaries from normal male rats were incubated with varied amounts of an ultrafiltrate of hypothalamic extract (filtered through Diaflo membrane UM-10 to remove immunoreactive contaminants of LH) (17). This preparation showed a good dose-dependent stimulation of LH release in vitro, without showing any change in the total amount of LH.

The pituitary implants in the testis, which had earlier lost 99% of the originally stored LH, on LHRF infusion showed a 140% recovery of its LH content (18). It is questionable if this LH was freshly synthesized or simply reactivated in this special environment.

RECENT STUDIES WITH PITUITARIES FROM FEMALE RATS

Adult female rats were grouped according to the vaginal smear pattern, and two groups showing different stages of estrous cycle were sacrificed on the same day at 1000 or 1300 hr within 30 min. The hemipituitaries were incubated as pairs, the ones from proestrus (PE) rats serving as controls, while those from other stages of estrous cycle [estrus (E), diestrus I (DI), diestrus II (DII)] as experimentals; only the latter were incubated with synthetic LHRF. Four hemipituitaries were taken in each flask, preincubated for 30 min in Krebs-Henseleit-glucose medium, and LH and FSH in the media and in the tissue were measured by radioimmunoassay.

There was no significant difference in basal LH or FSH released from the pituitaries of rats at the four stages of the cycle and these are shown as "mean of control" in Table 2. Total amount of LH (i.e., tissue + medium) was different at these four stages, in a descending order of PE, (PE 1300 > PE 1000 hr), DII, DI and E. In the case of FSH, the values observed were not significantly different from each other except when compared to the highest value observed at 1300 hr of PE. Incubation with LHRF caused

Table 2. In vitro responses of the anterior pituitaries of female rats at various stages of estrous cycle to LH-RF

GTH measured	Groups	Gonadotropins in								
		Medium			Tissue			Total		
		Mean of control	Difference	Sig	Mean of control	Difference	Sig	Mean of control	Difference	Sig
LH	PE 13:00 (4)	84.6±10.3	506.1±14.5	***	998.7±156.2	-632.4±149.4	*	1083.3±149.9	-126.4±141.6	NS
	E 13:00 (3)	75.7± 4.1	100.0±25.6	NS	369.3± 7.4	-87.9± 5.4	***	444.9± 4.7	12.1± 29.5	NS
	PE 10:00 (4)	58.3± 6.8	233.4±14.0	***	613.1± 37.0	-250.6± 24.9	**	671.4± 31.4	- 7.0± 30.2	NS
	DI 10:00 (4)	44.0± 1.7	103.1± 6.9	***	412.5± 26.6	-104.4± 34.5	NS	456.5± 27.4	- 1.4± 40.3	NS
	PE 10:00 (4)	82.5± 7.0	231.9±13.4	***	596.9± 24.3	-212.3± 42.5	*	679.3± 25.5	17.4± 49.7	NS
	DII 10:00 (4)	64.6± 3.0	164.1±11.5	***	576.4± 16.7	-163.6± 21.5	**	641.5± 17.5	0.5± 15.2	NS
FSH	PE 13:00 (4)	1.46±0.09	2.43±0.09	***	5.55± 0.38	-1.47± 0.32	*	7.01± 0.45	0.96±0.32	NS
	E 13:00 (3)	1.47±0.11	1.48±0.51	NS	4.47± 0.18	-0.81± 0.09	**	5.94± 0.22	0.67±0.58	NS
	PE 10:00 (4)	0.96±0.05	1.52±0.08	***	3.20± 0.09	-0.83± 0.09	**	4.16± 0.08	0.69±0.07	**
	DI 10:00 (4)	0.86±0.03	1.12±0.13	**	3.60± 0.05	-1.07± 0.15	**	4.45± 0.06	0.05±0.06	NS
	PE 10:00 (4)	1.17±0.07	1.47±0.17	**	3.88± 0.21	-1.21± 0.11	**	5.04± 0.24	0.27±0.24	NS
	DII 10:00 (4)	1.10±0.06	1.68±0.10	***	4.51± 0.25	-1.12±0.28	**	5.61± 0.29	0.58±0.44	NS

The anterior pituitaries were incubated as pairs, one served as control and the other as experimental which was incubated with 250 ng LH-RF/ml. Mean of control with S. E. and mean of difference between the pairs with S. E. are shown. Groups connected with a mark [were incubated on the same day for exact comparison. LH and FSH are expressed as ng x NIH-LH-S 1 and μg x NIH-FSH-S1 per mg gland, respectively. * = $p < 0.05$; ** = $p < 0.01$; *** = $p < 0.001$; ( ) = Number of pairs; GTH = Gonadotropin.

release of fairly large amounts of LH and FSH from pituitaries of each group of rats. The differential response to LHRF in LH and FSH release of rats at PE and E were investigated by incubating hemipituitaries with 0, 2-250 ng LHRF. As shown in Figure 1, the difference in LH release from pituitaries of rats at PE and E may be due to the difference in the slopes of their dose-response curves. This in the case of FSH are almost parallel, the intercepts, or the minimum effective concentrations being different. In the case of proestrus rats, the pituitaries removed at 1000 and 1300 hr showed the maximum LH release with 50 ng and 250 ng LHRF/ml respectively.

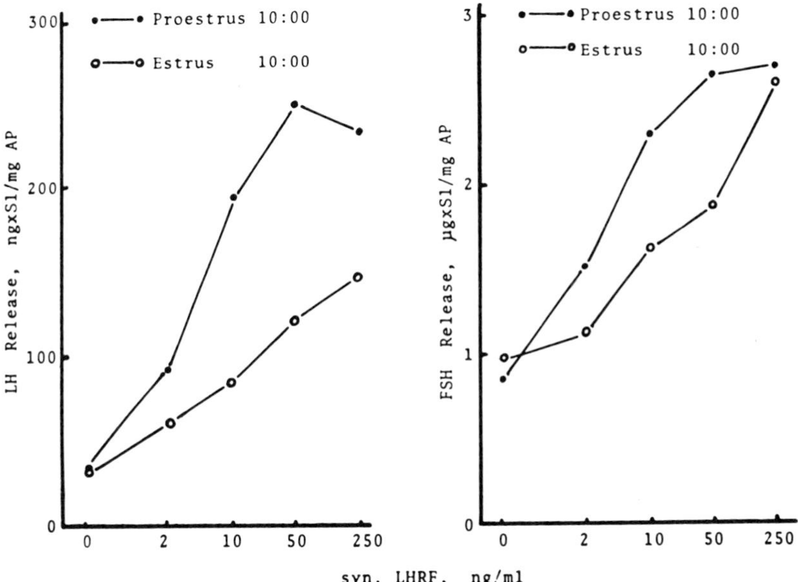

FIG 1. _In vitro_ responsiveness to synthetic LHRF of the anterior pituitaries from proestrus rats sacrificed at 1030 and 1330 hr. The hemipituitaries were randomized among 3 groups (4 halves per flask), and incubated for 3 hr after 30 min preincubation. Each point on the line is the mean of 2 flasks.

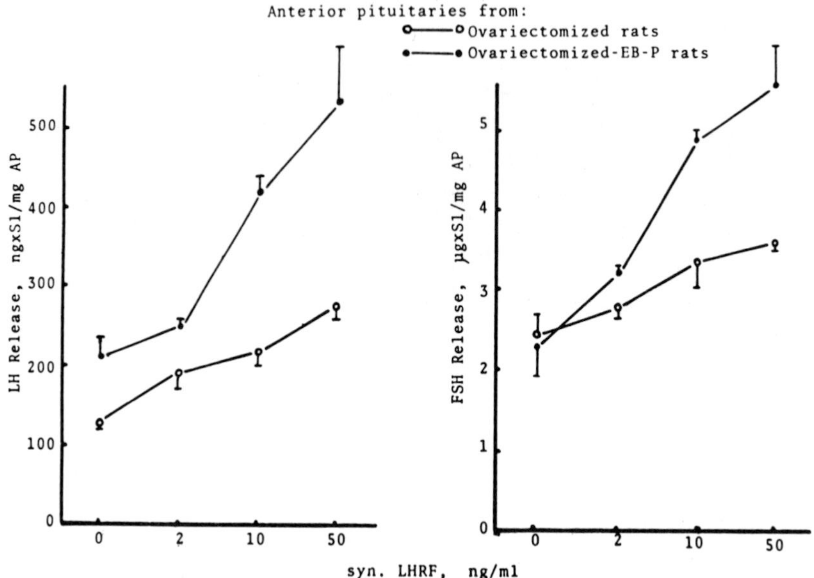

FIG 2. In vitro responsiveness to synthetic LHRF of the anterior pituitaries from ovariectomized and ovariectomized-estradiol benzoate-progesterone-treated rats. The hemipituitaries were randomized among 4 groups (3 halves per flask), and incubated for 3 hr after 30 min preincubation. Each point on the line is the mean of 4 flasks with S. E.

It is well known that pretreatment of ovariectomized rats with estradiol benzoate and progesterone (EBP) increases the responsiveness of the animals to LHRF in vivo (19). Our experiments using in vitro system have confirmed this finding (Fig. 2).

It can be seen from Table 2 that the LH released into the medium equalled that lost from the tissue on incubation with LHRF. Thus, no significant differences could be observed in the total amount of LH in the control and LHRF-treated groups at all the stages of the cycle. These results indicate that, under our experimental conditions, no stimulation of de novo biosynthesis or activation of LH is brought about by LHRF in the pituitaries from females also.

However, the total amount of FSH in the incubation system always showed a little increase with LHRF, though statistically not significant except in one case. This might suggest that LHRF causes a small increase in FSH synthesis perhaps a consequence of increased release, as was reported by Jutisz et al. (20).

CONCLUSION

The results of our in vitro experiments with both male and female rat pituitaries seem to indicate that LHRF does not cause an immediate increase in LH production, and that its primary effect is to promote LH release. We do not have any evidence against the observation that chronic treatment with LHRF leads to stimulation of LH biosynthesis. But it might be either a delayed effect which includes a long series of biochemical processes or a simple secondary effect which follows the increased LH release. The fact that, in tissue culture, the LH content of the pituitary gradually decreases if there is no stimulation by LHRF, and that the tissue LH content markedly decreases after chronic administration of steroids suggest a constant need for LHRF in the maintenance of LH content or de novo production. Our recent preliminary assay for LHRF in female hypothalami suggested a significant decrease in its level only on the afternoon of proestrus. On the other hand, the recovery of LH level after its depletion on the day of proestrus began very slowly and the content began to increase after DI (Table 2), indicating a very late effect of LHRF, or an involvement of some other factors in LH biosynthesis, which seems to occur between diestrus I and proestrus. The situation with FSH might be somewhat different in that the recovery of its pituitary content seems to be quick.

Future work on the relationship between gonadotropin releasing factor and gonadotropin biosynthesis should be focussed on these points. The clarification of the detailed biosynthetic processes of gonadotropins, would enable us to find out a step(s) which is influenced by releasing or other factors, if any.

ACKNOWLEDGEMENTS

The authors wish to express their thanks to Rat Pituitary Hormone Distribution Program, NIAMDD, for the kind supply of radioimmunoassay kits.

REFERENCES

1. McCann, S. M., Taleisnik, S. and Friedman, H. M. (1960) Proc. Soc. Exptl. Biol. Med. 104, 432.
2. Igarashi, M. and McCann, S. M. (1964) Endocrinology 74, 446.
3. Mittler, J. C. and Meites, J. (1964). Proc. Soc. Exptl. Biol. Med. 117, 309.
4. Wakabayashi, K. and Tamaoki, B. (1966). Protein Nucleic Acid and Enzyme 11, 1368.
5. Kobayashi, T., Kobayashi, T., Kigawa, T., Mizuno, M. and Amenomori, Y. (1963). Endocrinol. Japon 10, 16.
6. Kobayashi, T., Kobayashi, T., Kigawa, T., Mizuno, M., Amenomori, Y. and Watanabe, T. (1966). Endocrinol. Japon 13, 430.
7. Mittler, J. C., Arimura, A. and Schally, A. V. (1970). Proc. Soc. Exptl. Biol. Med. 133, 1321.
8. Redding, T. W., Schally, A. W., Arimura, A. and Matsuo, H. (1972). Endocrinology 90, 764.
9. Wakabayashi, K. & Tamaoki, B. (1965) Endocrinology 77, 264.
10. Wakabayashi, K. & Tamaoki, B. (1967) Endocrinology 80, 409.
11. Jutisz, M., Berault, A., Novella, M. A. and Ribot, G. (1967) Acta Endocrinol. 55, 481.
12. Jutisz, M., de la Llossa, M. P., Berault, A. and Kerdelhue, B. (1970) In "The Hypothalamus", L. Martini, M. Motta and F. Fraschini (Eds). pp 293, Academic Press, New York.
13. Midgley, A. R., Jr., Gay, V. L., Caligaris, L. C. S., Rebar, R. W., Monroe, S. E. and Niswender, G. D. (1968). In "Gonadotropins 1968", E. Rosemberg, (Ed) pp 307, Geron-X Inc., Los Altos.
14. Wakabayashi, K. & Tamaoki, B. (1966) Endocrinology 79, 477.
15. Wakabayashi, K. & McCann, S. M. (1970) Endocrinology 87, 771.
16. Samli, M. H. and Geschwind, I. I. (1967) Endocrinology 81, 835.
17. Wakabayashi, K., Antunes-Rodriques, J., Tamaoki, B. and McCann, S. M. (1972). Endocrinology 90, 690.
18. Lin, Y. C., Takahashi, M. and Suzuki, Y. (1972). Endocrinol. Japon. 19, 145.
19. Ramirez, V. D., & McCann, S. M. (1963). Endocrinology 73, 193.
20. Jutisz, M., Kerdelhue, B., Berault, A. and de la Llossa, M. P. (1972). In "Gonadotropins", B. B. Saxena, C. G. Beling, and H. M. Gandy (Eds) pp 64, Wiley-Interscience, New York.

CHORIONIC GONADOTROPIN PRODUCED FROM THE CULTIVATED TROPHOBLAST

Shimpei Tojo, Matsuto Mochizuki and Takeshi Maruo

The purpose of this investigation is to study the process of hCG biosynthesis by chorionic tissue in a short-term culture using ^{3}H-proline as a marker and to analyze the biochemical properties of hCG synthesized.

MATERIALS AND METHODS

A. Preliminary study

Human chorionic tissue obtained aseptically on therapeutic abortion in the first trimester of pregnancy was minced into fragments of about 1 mm^3 and was cultivated by the modified method of Tromwell (1), in synthetic medium - 199 containing 100 IU of penicillin and 100 μg of streptomycine per ml. No serum component was added to the medium to simplify the procedure of extraction and purification of hCG. Viability of the cultivated trophoblast was checked by radioautographic techniques (2) using ^{3}H-thymidine, ^{3}H-uridine or ^{3}H-proline. HCG in the medium and supernatant of the homogenized tissue was estimated by bioassay [ovarian weight method in immature female rat (3,4)] and radioimmunoassay (5). HCG used for this radioimmunoassay system was extracted from the human chorionic tissue (6-10). Total protein content of the cultivated tissue was measured by the method of Kjeldahl.

The culture media were pooled and filtered through a Sephadex G-100 column. The protein was determined in the effluent fractions either by the method of Lowry (11) or by recording O. D. at 280 nm; the ratio of the amount of hCG to total protein was expressed as percentage.

B. Extraction and purification of hCG

To the culture medium was added 5 μCi ^{3}H-proline per ml. Cultivation of the chorionic tissue was carried out in 10 dishes for periods of 3 - 5 days. The hCG in the medium was extracted and purified by filtering the concentrated medium on a Sephadex G-100 column (20 x 900 mm) at 4°, the column was equilibrated and eluted with 0.005 M tris-HCl buffer, pH 8.6. The radioactive protein fraction from above was chromatographed on DEAE cellulose column (20 x 150 mm), equlibrated with 0.005 M tris-HCl buffer, pH 8.6, and was eluted by using a linear gradient of 0.005 M -0.4 M tris-HCl buffer solution, pH 8.6.

C. Biochemical and immunological analysis of hCG

1. Polyacrylamide disc gel electrophoresis : After chromatography on DEAE-cellulose, the partially purified hCG fractions were subjected to polyacrylamide disc gel electrophoresis, using 3 columns for each fraction. One of the columns was stained for protein detection with amido black 10-B solution. The others were sliced into 2.4 mm segments employing the device of Chrambach. ^{3}H-radioactivity and immunoreactive hCG in each segment were measured.

2. Estimation of sialic acid content : The content of sialic acid of radioactive hCG fraction from DEAE-cellulose column was estimated by the thiobarbiturate method of Warren (12).

3. Immunological analysis : The immunological cross-reactivity of radioactive hCG fraction from DEAE-cellulose column was examined by a modification of the method of Ouchterlony (13) using specific anti-hCG serum and anti-hCFSH (human chorionic FSH) serum (6-10).

4. Test for localization of ^{3}H-proline in the chorionic tissue : The localization of ^{3}H-proline in the cultivated chorionic tissue was examined radioautographically by the dipping method (2).

RESULTS

A. Viability of the cultivated trophoblast

Radioautographs of the chorionic tissue cultivated for 3 days were prepared after 2 hr exposure to ^{3}H-thymidine, or ^{3}H-uridine or ^{3}H-proline. In all cases, the isotopic labelling was of high intensity in cytotrophoblast and stromal cell, but little in syncytiotrophoblast.

Although ^{3}H-thymidine uptake could be detected only to small extent in cytotrophoblast and stromal cell in the chorionic tissue cultivated for 7 days, ^{3}H-uridine uptake was high; no ^{3}H-proline uptake could be recognized.

B. HCG production

Both bioreactive as well as immunoreactive hCG in the chorionic tissue increased transiently from 4-8 hr after beginning of the cultivation and thereafter decreased. The protein content of the tissue also followed the same pattern, except that the increase was seen upto 16 hr, declining thereafter. In the culture medium hCG increased approximately linearly through the third day of culture and it began to reach a plateau on the fifth day (Fig 1).

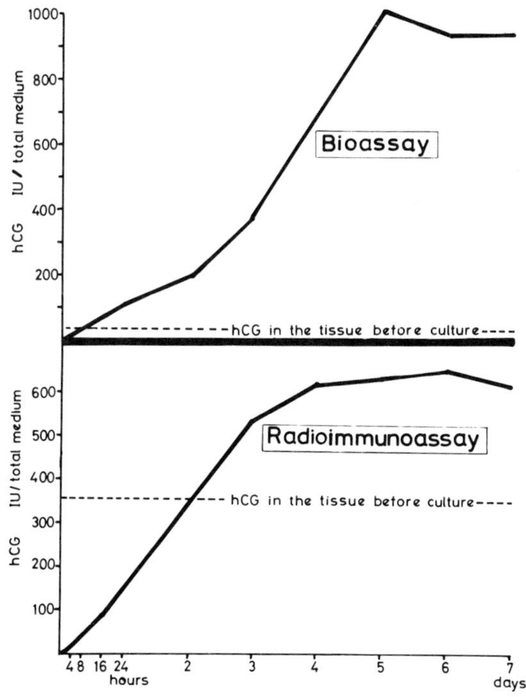

FIG 1. HCG in the medium during cultivation.

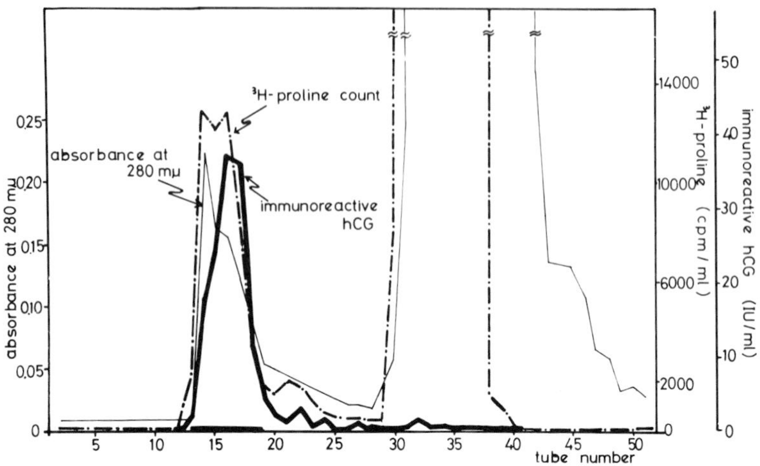

FIG 2. Gel filtration of concentrated medium on Sephadex G-100 (3 day culture)

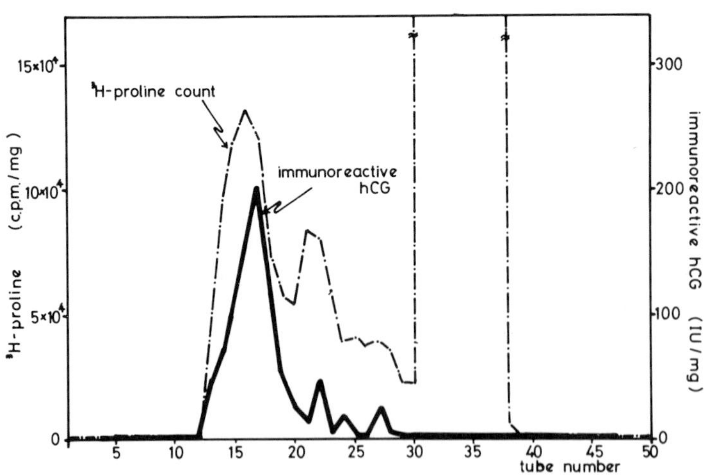

FIG 3. Elution profile of hCG (radioactive and immunoreactive) on Sephadex gel (3 day culture).

The ratio of hCG to total protein in chorionic tissue was 0.46 % on the first, 0.28 % on the second and 0.30 % on the third day of culture. On the other hand, in the culture medium, this ratio increased with time, being 3.67 % on the first, 21.38 % on the second and 59.76 % on the third day. The ratio in the whole culture system varied from 0.64 % on the first day of culture to 1.07 % on the third.

C. Isolation of labeled hCG

The pooled medium from 10 dishes cultivated over a 3-day period was concentrated to about 5 ml in a rotary evaporator. This was filtered through a Sephadex G-100 column (Fig 2) and then was separated into two fractions - tube numbers 13-18 and 29-43. The protein in the former fraction showed a close correlation with ^{3}H-radioactivity and immunoreactivity (Fig 3) suggesting that the protein synthesized in the above system is hCG-like material. The latter fraction corresponded to the elution area of free amino-acid and saline.

In order to investigate the properties of the radioactive protein corresponding to the immunoreactive hCG, this fraction was further purified on DEAE-cellulose column. The adsorbed protein was quantitatively recovered at a conductivity of $<$ 4.0 m.mho and peaks of ^{3}H-radioactivity could be seen at a conductivity 1.0-4.0 m.mho and 4.1-11.5 m.mho (Fig 4). A small and a large fraction at conductivities of $<$ 4.0 m.mho and 7.0-12.0 m.mho respectively were obtained which exhibited both immuno and bio-reactivity. In the latter fraction, immuno- and bioreactivity of hCG coincided completely with ^{3}H-radioactivity.

Essentially similar results were obtained in case of 5-day culture also (Fig 5 and 6).

D. Biochemical and immunological properties of the biosynthesized hCG

Fractions eluted at a conductivity of 4.2 - 6.5 m.mho showed on disc gel electrophoresis several bands with low migration (Fig 7). Both radioactivity and the immunoreactivity appeared as a sharp peak in segment number 7 of the polyacrylamide disc and this corresponded to the migration area of native hCG. Fraction eluting at a conductivity of 7.8 - 11.3 m.mho showed a

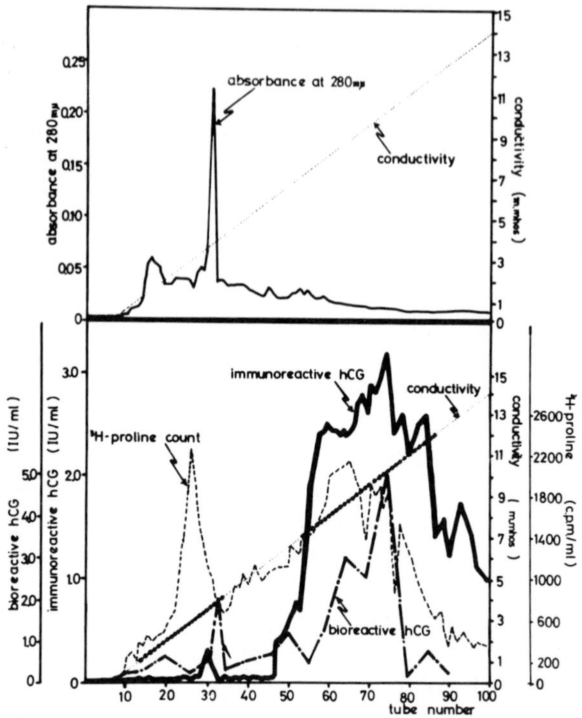

FIG 4. Elution profile on hCG (radioactive and immunoreactive) on DEAE cellulose (3 day culture).

faster migration, darker band and several faint bands with low migration. The latter corresponded to the migration area of native hCG in which the radioactivity and the immunoreactivity of synthesized hCG coincided completely.

Sialic acid content of the radioactive hCG fraction recovered from DEAE-cellulose column varied from 0.04-0.05 % (Table 1), in contrast to the native hCG which has a sialic acid content of 3.8 %.

In Ouchterlony immunodiffusion using two different types of antisera, the fraction eluting at a conductivity of 2.5 - 4.0 m.mho gave no precipitin line against either anti-hCG or anti-hCFSH sera, while the fraction eluting at a conductivity of 4.2 - 6.5 m.mho gave precipitin line only with anti-hCG serum. On the

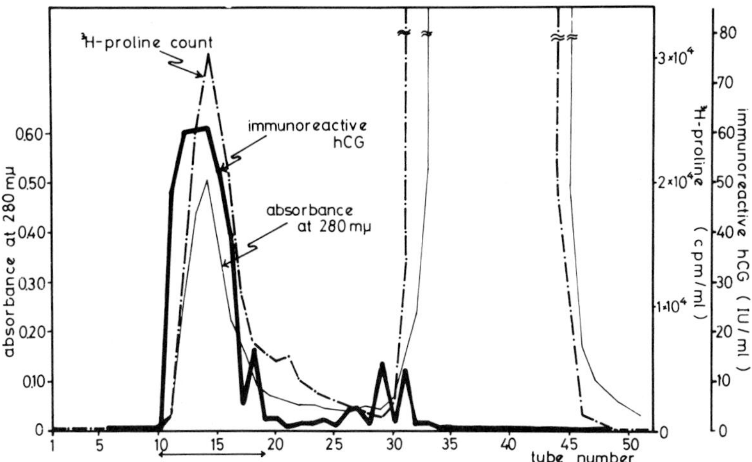

FIG 5. Gel filtration of concentrated medium on Sephadex G-100 (5 day culture).

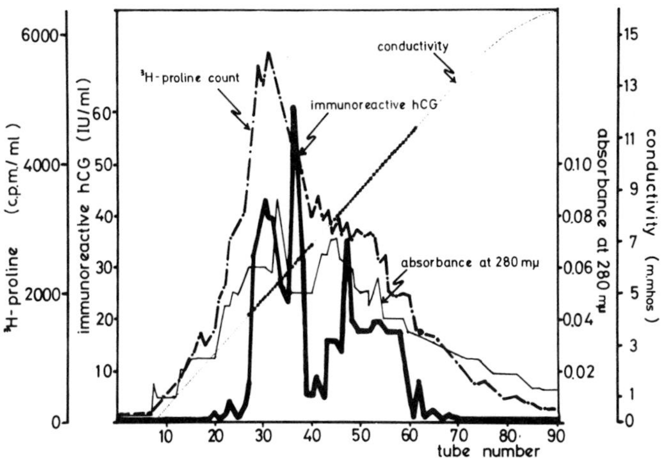

FIG 6. Elution profile of hCG (radioactive and immunoreactive) on DEAE cellulose (5 day culture).

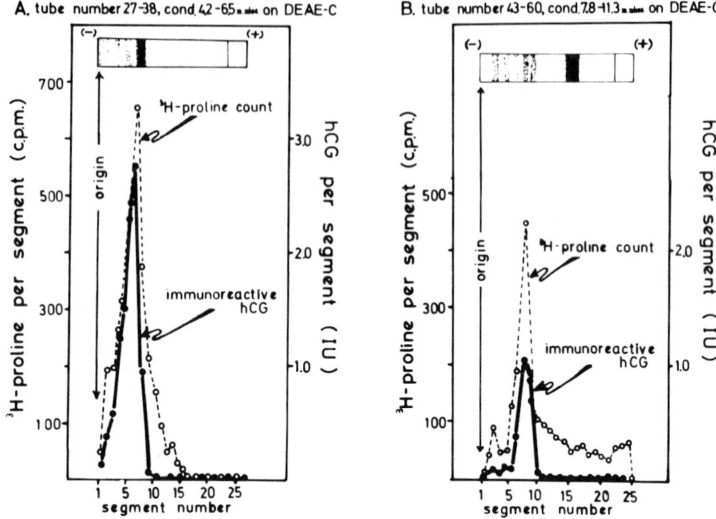

FIG 7. Polyacrylamide disc electrophoresis of hCG isolated from culture (in 7 % gels).

Table 1. Sialic acid content of biosynthesized hCG.

Tube number	20 - 26	27 - 38	43 - 60
Conductivity (m. mhos)	2.5 - 4.0	4.2 - 6.5	7.8 - 11.3
Sialic acid (%)	0.04	0.04	0.05

(Content of sialic acid of native hCG : 3.0 - 3.8 %).

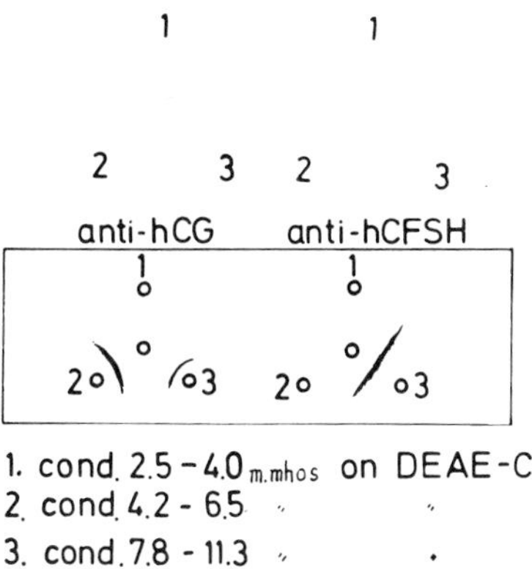

FIG 8. Immuno-diffusion pattern of biosynthesized hCG.

other hand, fraction eluting at a conductivity of 7. 8-11.3 m.mho gave precipitin lines against both the antisera (Fig 8).

In the radioautographic study of chorionic tissue cultivated over a 3 or 5 days period, silver grains of ^{3}H-proline could be seen clearly on the surface area of syncytiotrophoblast.

COMMENTS

Attempts to study the mode of production and the biochemical properties of hCG isolated from cultured chorionic tissue obtained from the first trimester of pregnancy have been successful.

Uptake of ^{3}H-thymidine, ^{3}H-uridine and ^{3}H-proline by the cultivated tissue indicated that this tissue remains viable and is capable of synthesizing protein over a 7-day period.

The total bioreactive hCG in the medium following cultivation compared to that in the chorionic tissue in situ, was found increased by 40-fold, while the increase in the immunoreactive hCG was only 4-fold. However, the ratio of the amount of hCG to total protein in the whole culture system varied from 0. 64 to 1. 07 %.

There was a transient increase in the production of hCG as well as total protein during the first 4-16 hr of culture. Since serum was excluded from the culture medium, the above results suggest that the chorionic tissue is active in synthesizing hCG even in a serum-free medium.

Using ^{3}H-proline as a marker, and a combination of Sephadex G-100 gel filtration and DEAE-cellulose chromatography, it was possible to establish a correlation of ^{3}H radioactivity with immuno- and bioreactivity of hCG in the eluted fractions suggesting that hCG labeled with ^{3}H-proline was biosynthesized in this system.

In contrast to the elution profile of native hCG on DEAE cellulose column (eluted at a conductivity of 1.5 - 4.2 m.mho), the biosynthesized hCG was eluted at a higher conductivity suggesting that the latter was more tightly bound to the anion exchanger and required a higher concentration of salt to displace it from the column at a given pH. In addition, sialic acid content of the biosynthesized hCG was much less than that of native hCG. Interestingly, however, in polyacrylamide disc-gel electrophoresis, the movement of both biosynthesized labeled hCG and the native hCG were similar.

From the results of the above study, it might be suspected that the biosynthesized labeled hCG has a structure or conformation different from that of native hCG.

Moreover, in the immunodiffusion test, the biosynthesized hCG eluted at a conductivity of 4.2-6.5 m.mho gave a precipitin line only with anti-hCG serum, while that eluted at a conductivity of 7.8-11.3 m.mho, showed a faint precipitin line with anti-hCG serum, but a clear precipitin line with anti-hCFSH serum. This suggests that hCFSH is also biosynthesized in the culture system used.

ACKNOWLEDGEMENT

This study was supported by Grant No. 757187, Japanese Ministry of Education.

REFERENCES

1. Trowell, O.A. (1959). Exp. Cell. Res. 16, 118.
2. Boyd, G.A. (1955). "Autoradiography in Biology and Medicine" Academic Press Inc., New York.
3. Sealy, J.L. and Sondern, C.W. (1940).Endocrinology 26, 813.
4. Tojo, S. (1968). Clin. Endocr. 16, 509 (in Japanese).
5. Tojo, S., Mochizuki, M., Tokura, K. and Mizusawa, T. (1969). Clin. Endocr. 17, 523, (in Japanese).

6. Ashitaka, Y. (1970). Acta Obst. et Cynec. Jap., 17, 124.
7. Ashitaka, Y., Tokura, Y., Tane, M., Mochizuki, M. and Tojo, S. (1970). Endocrinology 87, 233.
8. Ashitaka, Y., Mochizuki, M., and Tojo, S. (1972). Endocrinology 90, 609.
9. Tojo, S., Mochizuki, M., Ohga, Y., Shimura, T., Maruo, T. and Nishimoto, H. (1972). Folia Endocr. Japon., 48, 639.
10. Tojo, S., Mochizuki, M. and Ashitaka, Y. (1973). Endocrinology, Proc. of the IV International Cong. Washington D.C.,(June 1972), Excerpta Medica (in press).
11. Lowry, O.H., Rosebrough, N.J. and Randall, R.J. (1951) J. Biol. Chem. 193, 265.
12. Warren, L. (1959). J. Biol. Chem. 234, 1971.
13. Ouchterlony, O. (1953). Acta. Path. Microbiol. Scan., 32, 231.

INTERACTIONS BETWEEN PROSTAGLANDINS AND GONADOTROPINS ON CORPUS LUTEUM FUNCTION

Harold R. Behrman, T. S. Ng and Gayle R. Orczyk

INTRODUCTION

The increased availability of prostaglandins (PGs) for experimental studies and the development of very sensitive radioimmunoassay procedures for quantitating PGs has opened a new avenue of research in reproductive endocrinology. Prostaglandins have historically been associated with the reproductive system, but only in the past few years has any progress been made in elucidating the biological role of these compounds. In general, there are two mechanism of PG action that have been proposed in the reproductive as well as other endocrine systems: (a) as mediators of hormone action (1); (b) as attenuators of hormone action (2,3).

The studies of Kuehl and collaborators have delineated a possible sequence of events in which PGs are depicted as mediating the action of LH on the immature mouse ovary (1). With respect to ovulation, PGs play a fundamental role as evidenced by the ability of inhibitors of PG synthesis to block this gonadotropin-induced phenomenon (4-6) and the marked increase in follicular PG content following administration of gonadotropin to induce ovulation (7), In this gonadal event, it appears that PGs mediate a gonadotropin action. In the present discussion, emphasis is placed on the role of PGs in corpus luteum function, and in this gland the action of PG appears to belong to the second category — namely attenuation of hormone action.

There is ample evidence to permit the conclusion that the corpus luteum is dependent upon gonadotropins for progesterone secretion and it is possible that the life-span of the corpus luteum could be regulated by the rate of gonadotropin secretion from the pituitary. For example, in the human, Speroff and Vande Wiele demonstrated that a continual supply of LH is necessary to maintain the corpus luteum (8). In laboratory and farm animals, it is known that a factor is released by the uterus which actively promotes corpus luteum regression (9). Although no uterine luteolysin is evident in the human and non-human primate, it is nonetheless difficult to conclude that corpus luteum regression in these species occurs as a result of a loss of gonadotropin support, since little or no change in the circulating gonadotropin levels, albeit low, occurs either prior to or during corpus luteum regression (10). Hence, corpus luteum regression in the human may also result from a direct action of some factor(s) which may interfere with gonadotropin action on the corpus luteum, thereby inducing regression. In this respect, estrogens have been shown to produce a decrease in progesterone secretion in the primate (12, 13), and a possible mechanism of intragonadal control of corpus luteum regression may exist.

Since the first report by Pharriss (14) that PGs modified corpus luteum function, a host of publications have appeared demonstrating the luteolytic activity of $PGF_{2\alpha}$. This action of $PGF_{2\alpha}$ has been shown in virtually all laboratory and domestic animals including the rhesus monkey but, in humans, $PGF_{2\alpha}$ -induced luteolysis has not been unequivocally demonstrated. The mechanism whereby $PGF_{2\alpha}$ produces a loss in the ability of the corpus luteum to secrete progesterone remains unresolved, but several hypotheses have been forwarded. These include: (i) constriction of the ovarian vein (15); (ii) depression of ovarian blood flow (16); (iii) change in ovarian hemodynamics resulting in a decreased blood flow to the corpus luteum (17); (iv) stimulation of a pituitary luteolysin (18); and (v) antagonism of gonadotropin action (3).

Evidence will be presented to support the hypothesis that the luteolytic action of $PGF_{2\alpha}$ is expressed through an antagonism of gonadotropin action. This hypothesis does not preclude the possibility that, in part, the loss in gonadotropin action <u>in vivo</u> may occur through a depression of blood flow to the corpus luteum as a result of a change in ovarian hemodynamics by $PGF_{2\alpha}$.

RESULTS AND DISCUSSION

In 1971, we reported that the "antagonistic action of LH and $PGF_{2\alpha}$... suggests a possible mechanism of luteolysis induced by prostaglandin" (3). This conclusion was based on the observation that administration of $PGF_{2\alpha}$ to pseudopregnant rats produced a decrease in ovarian secretion of progesterone within 30 min and this effect was prevented by simultaneous administration of LH. In addition, in animals hypophysectomized 1 hr before treatment, $PGF_{2\alpha}$ produced a slight stimulation of progesterone secretion over the hypophysectomized controls and also attenuated the acute stimulation of progesterone secretion induced by LH administration. No change in the ovarian venous flow-rate occurred which ruled out the possibility that the effects of $PGF_{2\alpha}$ were due to ovarian venous constriction, and since the anterior uterine vein was ligated, the possibility that $PGF_{2\alpha}$ reduced ovarian arterial flow-rate was ruled out. Other workers have reported that the luteolytic effect of $PGF_{2\alpha}$ is not due to a net change in blood flow to the ovary (19). Recent data of Niswender (20) shows that ovarian arterial flow-rate determined by Doppler analysis is highly correlated with progesterone secretion during estrous cycle of sheep, but whether this response is $PGF_{2\alpha}$ -mediated is not known.

The action of $PGF_{2\alpha}$ in producing luteolysis is a direct gonadal effect. This conclusion was based on data obtained from hypophysectomized rats in which the corpora lutea were maintained by chronic treatment with exogenous prolactin (21). Administration of $PGF_{2\alpha}$ to these animals neutralised the luteotropic effect of prolactin and produced a marked depression in progesterone synthesis. These data were interpreted as an antagonism by $PGF_{2\alpha}$ of prolactin action. This hypothesis is supported by the recent data of Chatterjee who demonstrated that prolactin can reverse the luteolytic activity of $PGF_{2\alpha}$ in the rat (22).

Further evidence for the action of $PGF_{2\alpha}$ directly on the corpus luteum was obtained from organ culture studies reported by O'Grady et al. (23) and ourselves (24); $PGF_{2\alpha}$ was shown to reduce progesterone output in rabbit and rat corpora lutea respectively in the two laboratories. In cultured rat corpora lutea, $PGF_{2\alpha}$ not only inhibited progesterone synthesis from labelled acetate but also inhibited protein synthesis determined from the incorporation of labelled amino acids into protein. In this same study, it was found that $PGF_{2\alpha}$ was produced by corpora lutea and stimulation of luteal $PGF_{2\alpha}$ production was induced by addition of LH to the culture media; a striking stimulation of $PGF_{2\alpha}$ production by corpora lutea was observed by addition of PGE_2 to the culture media. These data raise the interesting possibility that an intraluteal mechanism for control of function may exist through endogenous $PGF_{2\alpha}$ synthesis. It is difficult to envisage a possible vascular mediation of the decrease in progesterone production induced by $PGF2\alpha$ in corpora lutea incubated *in vitro.* Nonetheless, these observations do not rule out the possibility that *in vivo*, luteolysis induced by $PGF_{2\alpha}$ occurs, in part, from a change in ovarian hemodynamics.

The hamster is very sensitive to luteolysis induced by $PGF_{2\alpha}$ (25) and the influence of the uterus on hastening an early demise of the corpus luteum is well documented (26). In Table 1 a dose-response of the effect of $PGF_{2\alpha}$ on circulating progesterone in the hamster during early pregnancy is shown. $PGF_{2\alpha}$ at a level of 25 μg in a single dose consistently results in an almost complete loss of circulating progesterone 24 hr later. At this dose and at doses up to 150 μg, there is no visible effect of the drug on the animal. $PGF_{1\alpha}$ is also effective in inducing luteolysis but is only one-fifth as active as $PGF_{2\alpha}$. PGE_2, at a dose of 100μg/animal, had little effect on circulating progesterone levels and

Table 1. Effect of prostaglandins on circulating progesterone in the pregnant hamster *

Treatment	N	Progesterone (ng/ml)
Control	19	8.2 ± 0.5
$PGF_{2\alpha}$ (μg)		
10	6	6.8 ± 0.6
12.5	2	9.4 ± 1.6
25	5	0.2 ± 0.2
50	10	1.1 ± 0.4
100	5	0.1 ± 0.1
150	8	0.1 ± 0.1
$PGF_{1\alpha}$ (μg)		
50	4	6.2 ± 1.1
100	4	1.4 ± 0.7
PGE_2 (μg)		
100	5	6.5 ± 0.7

*Adult, pregnant hamsters (day 6) were administered PG at the indicated level in a single dose, i p in sesame oil. Blood was collected 24 hr later and the implantation swellings examined. Progesterone was determined by radioimmunoassay in serum after extraction with petroleum ether.

these data indicate that at least four times more PGE_2 than $PGF_{2\alpha}$ is required as an effective dose. Labhsetwar (27) previously reported that PGE_2 was less active than $PGF_{2\alpha}$ in this respect. There is thus a clear differentiation in the structure-activity relationships between prostaglandins for induction of luteolysis in the hamster.

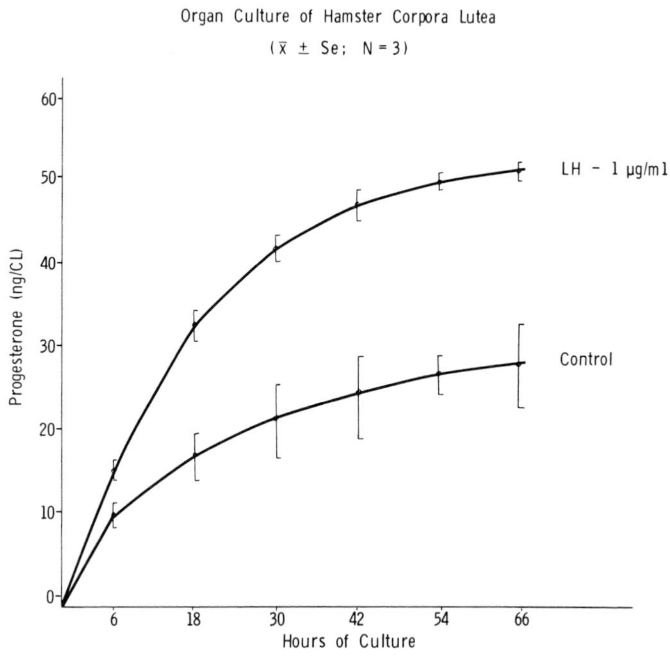

FIG 1. A time-course study of the effects of LH on progesterone secretion by hamster corpora lutea in organ culture.
Pregnant hamsters (day 8) were sacrificed and corpora lutea (CL) were dissected free. The CL (10-12 CL/culture dish) were incubated at 37° in an atmosphere of 95 % O_2, 5 % CO_2 in 1 ml of Trowell's T-8 culture media containing 5 % fetal calf serum, 100 U penicillin, 100 µg streptomycin and 0.25 µg fungizone. The incubation conditions were similar to that reported earlier (24) with the exception that the CL were placed directly on the stainless steel grid.

Due to the extreme sensitivity of the hamster to the luteolytic action of $PGF_{2\alpha}$, we initiated in vitro studies using cultured hamster corpora lutea in order to gain further information on the action of $PGF_{2\alpha}$. In Figure 1, the cumulative progesterone synthesis by hamster corpora lutea maintained in organ culture for 66 hr is shown. A release of progesterone in a burst was found to occur in the first hour of culture and therefore, all cultures were preincubated in control medium for one hour and the media then changed to include treatments [either saline (control) or NIH-LH-S14 (1 µg/ml)]. The medium was changed at intervals indicated in Figure 1. The initial release of progesterone during the preincubation

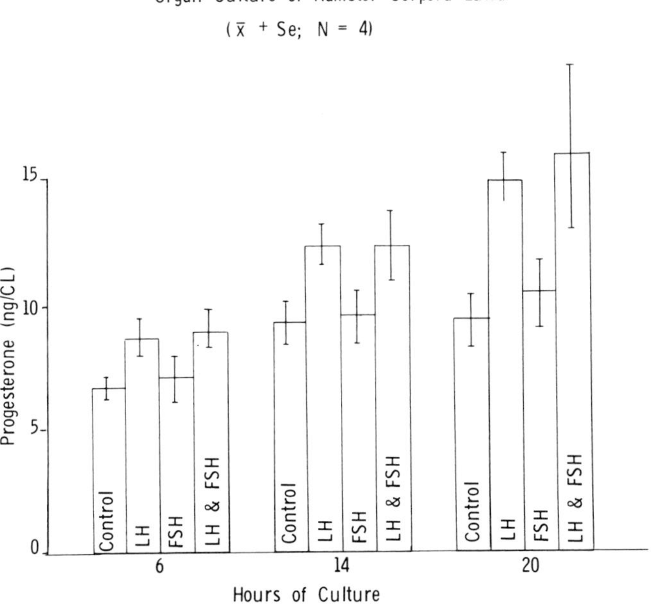

FIG 2. Effect of FSH and LH on progesterone secreted by hamster corpus luteum in organ culture.
The animals and incubation conditions were identical to that described in Figure 1. 2-3 CL were placed in each culture dish and saline, NIH-LH-S16 (0.5 µg), NIH-FSH-S9 (0.5 µg) or a combination of LH and FSH added.

period was approximately 5-10 fold greater than that which occurred during the next 24 hr. In contrast to rat corpora lutea in culture (24) where a near linear production rate of progesterone was observed for up to 96 hr, hamster corpora lutea incubated in an identical manner demonstrated a marked reduction in output after 24-30 hr in culture. Nonetheless, addition of LH to the incubation medium resulted in a marked increase in progesterone synthesis thereby supporting the conclusion that the tissue was viable and retained the ability to respond to gonadotropic stimulation.

The effect of FSH, alone or in combination with LH, on progesterone output by cultured hamster corpora lutea is shown in Figure 2. LH, or LH in combination with FSH, stimulated progesterone synthesis as early as 6 hr, showing an even greater progesterone production at 20 hr of culture. FSH alone had no effect on progesterone output and also did not modify the stimulation of progesterone output by LH. Thus it appears that FSH alone does little to maintain progesterone secretion by corpora lutea in this system. There is considerable evidence published by Greenwald (28) that FSH is a necessary luteotropin in the hamster and this action is synergistic with prolactin. This concept is presently being evaluated in cultured hamster corpora lutea, but no information is as yet available.

In Figure 3, progesterone output by hamster corpora lutea cultured in the presence of a hemipituitary, $PGF_{2\alpha}$ or their combination is shown. These studies were conducted to obtain information on luteal function using a homologous source of pituitary gonadotropins. After 30 hr of incubation it is evident that corpora lutea cultured with hemipituitary secreted a significantly greater amount of progesterone than the control corpora lutea. In contrast to earlier data with rabbits (23) and rats (24), $PGF_{2\alpha}$ alone had little or no effect on progesterone output. In other identical incubations, we have varied the concentration of $PGF_{2\alpha}$ added to the culture media (0.1, 1 or 10 μg/ml) and have found no inhibitory effect on progesterone output, but rather observed a variable degree of stimulation particularly at higher doses. Of particular significance in the present studies was the ability of $PGF_{2\alpha}$ to neutralize the luteotropic effect of the pituitary tissue. It was concluded that this luteotropic response was due to gonadotropic hormones released from the pituitary, and the action of $PGF_{2\alpha}$ was expressed as an antagonism of action of these gonadotropins. This response is identical to the effect we noted in the pseudopregnant rat (3) in vivo

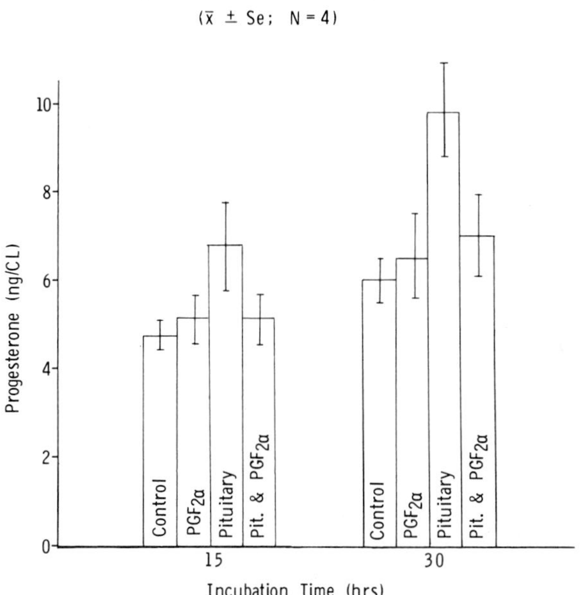

FIG 3. Effect of $PGF_{2\alpha}$ and hamster pituitary extract on progesterone secreted by hamster corpus luteum in organ culture. The animals and incubation conditions were identical to that described in Figure 1. Media, $PGF_{2\alpha}$ (10 µg/ml) made up in media, hemipituitary or a combination of $PGF_{2\alpha}$ and hemipituitary were added to each culture dish containing 2-3 CL.

where $PGF_{2\alpha}$ had a slight stimulatory effect on progesterone secretion, apparent for up to 30 min after an iv injection into animals, hypophysectomized 1 hr earlier. But when $PGF_{2\alpha}$ was administered simultaneously with LH, it prevented the stimulation of progesterone secretion.

The effect of $PGF_{2\alpha}$ on hamster corpora lutea incubated in the presence of LH or LH and prolactin is shown in Figure 4. Following either 12 or 24 hr of culture, $PGF_{2\alpha}$ produced a marked decrease in progesterone output by corpora lutea incubated with LH. This effect was not as apparent in cultures containing both LH and

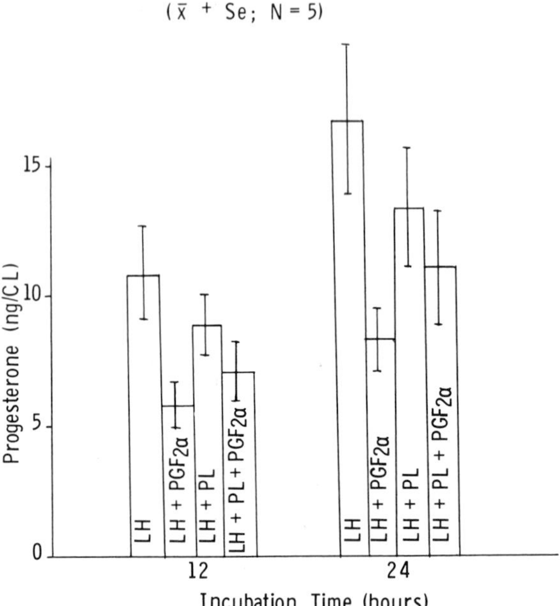

FIG 4. Effect of LH, prolactin and $PGF_{2\alpha}$ on progesterone secretion by hamster corpus luteum in organ culture.
The animals and incubation conditions were identical to that described in Figure 1. All culture dishes (2-3 CL) contained NIH-LH-S18 (1 μg/ml) to which either $PGF_{2\alpha}$ (10 μg/ml), NIH-P-S10 (5 μg/ml) or $PGF_{2\alpha}$ and prolactin were added to 2-3 CL.

prolactin. A similar action of $PGF_{2\alpha}$ was noted by Channing (29) in cultures of granulosa cells. Thus, both in vivo and in vitro the action of $PGF_{2\alpha}$ may be interpreted as an inhibition or neutralization of gonadotropin expression on the corpus luteum. In fact, as we noted earlier (3) this action of $PGF_{2\alpha}$ is not unlike the effects produced by LH neutralization with a specific antiserum in vivo and in vitro (30,31) with the exception that $PGF_{2\alpha}$, in addition to LH, also blocks prolactin action on the corpus luteum (21). It has not been established if the action of chorionic gonadotropins is blocked by $PGF_{2\alpha}$, but in one experiment where hamster corpora lutea were cultured in the presence of a hemipituitary and a portion of a hamster placenta, no depression of progesterone output was noted, although progesterone production was stimulated by the addition of these two tissues.

SUMMARY AND CONCLUSIONS

There is ample evidence that $PGF_{2\alpha}$ is an effective luteolytic agent and appears to be the natural uterine luteolysin in domestic animals (32). Corpus luteum regression in the primate does not appear to be controlled by a uterine luteolysin (33) and the factors involved in this response, other than the requirement for maintenance of function by gonadotropin (8) and the lytic action of estrogen (11, 12, 13) are unknown. Conflicting data exists whether $PGF_{2\alpha}$ causes luteolysis in the human, but recent data indicates that the time of the menstrual cycle when $PGF_{2\alpha}$ is administered may be important in order to demonstrate a luteolytic effect (34). Prostaglandins are, nonetheless, synthesized by the human corpus luteum (Orczyk, unpublished observation). Considerably more research must be done in order to understand the mechanisms involved in regression of the human corpus luteum.

The events associated with corpus luteum regression are expressed as a loss of progesterone secretion but also include leucocytic infiltration, decreased vascularity and luteal cell degeneration (28). Although the primary action of $PGF_{2\alpha}$ on the corpus luteum is interpreted as gonadotropin antagonism, the secondary actions may be a consequence of this primary action. For example, changes in ovarian hemodynamics may be a secondary event induced by a loss of action of gonadotropins, the primary event. Support for this interpretation is based on the well-documented hyperemic effect of LH on the ovary and loss of vascularity of the corpus luteum during regression (17, 28). Thus, the species differences in response to the luteolytic action of $PGF_{2\alpha}$ may be due, in part, to secondary events involved in luteolysis.

In studies examining the mechanism of luteolysis, particular attention must be devoted to the interval between treatment with $PGF_{2\alpha}$ and the measurement of changes in luteal function to determine whether the event being measured is primary or secondary in nature. The secondary events associated with luteal regression would not be expected to occur in organ culture of corpora lutea and this is probably the reason why $PGF_{2\alpha}$ alone produced either no effect or a slight stimulation of progesterone synthesis. Under organ culture conditions, a minimum amount of gonadotropin would be expected to be carried over after removal, rinsing and preincubation of the tissue, and therefore little antagonism of low residual gonadotropin activity could be expressed. In addition, because secondary events associated with luteolysis such as leucocytic invasion and decreased vasculature cannot occur in culture studies, the decrease in progesterone synthesis would not be expected to occur as rapidly in culture as in vivo where these responses, as a consequence of a loss of gonadotropin action, would augment the fall in progesterone secretion.

Although several hypotheses have been forwarded on the mechanism of $PGF_{2\alpha}$ -induced corpus luteum regression, the data gathered in this laboratory indicate that this response is due to a direct action on the gonad. In addition, $PGF_{2\alpha}$ exerts an action directly upon the corpus luteum and this response which occurs in vitro appears not to be mediated by vascular changes. With the aid of both in vivo and in vitro experimental models, the mechanism of action of $PGF_{2\alpha}$ appears to result from an antagonism of action of gonadotropins, and corpus luteum regression occurs not as a result of active luteolysis but rather indirectly through a loss of gonadotropin action. Luteal regression induced by $PGF_{2\alpha}$ can thus be interpreted as due to a loss of gonadotropin support.

ACKNOWLEDGEMENTS

The authors extend their appreciation to NIAMDD, NIH, Bethesda, Maryland, U.S.A. for the gifts of pituitary gonadotropins, to Evan Morgan and Elaine Babiarz for their skillful technical assistance, and to Drs. J. Brooks, D. Grinwich, and T. Mellin for their suggestions and counsel in the preparation of this manuscript.

REFERENCES

1. Kuehl, F.A., Humes, J.L., Tarnoff, J., Cirillo, V.J., and Ham, E.A., (1970). Science 169, 883.
2. Steinberg, D., Vaughan, M., Nestel, P.J., Strand, O. and Bergstrom. S. (1964). J. Clin. Invest. 43, 1533.
3. Behrman, H.R., Yoshinaga, K., and Greep, R.O. (1971). Ann. N.Y. Acad. Aci. 180, 426.
4. Orczyk, G.P. and Behrman, H.R. (1972) Prostaglandins 1, 3.

5. Armstrong, D. T. and Grinwich, D. L. (1972). Prostaglandins 1, 21.
6. O'Grady, J. P., Caldwell, B. V., Auletta, F. J. and Speroff, L., (1972). Prostaglandins 1, 97.
7. LeMaire, W. J., Yang, N. S. T., Behrman, H. R., and Marsh, J. M. (1973). Prostaglandins 3, 367.
8. Speroff, L., and Vandewiele, R. L. (1971). Am. J. Obstet. and Gynec. 109, 234.
9. Ginther, O. J. (1967). J. An. Sci. 26, 578.
10. Moghissi, K. S., Snyder, F. N., and T. N. Evans (1972). Am. J. Obstet. Gynec. 114, 405.
11. Johansson, E. D. B. and Gemzell, C. (1971). Acta Endocrinol. 68, 551.
12. Auletta, F. J., Caldwell, B. N., Van Wagenen, G., and Morris, J. M. (1972). Contraception 6, 411.
13. Gore, B. Z., Caldwell, B. V., and L. Speroff. (1973). J. Clin. Endocrinol. & Metab. 36, 615.
14. Pharriss, B. B., Wyngarden, L. J., and Gutknecht, G. D. (19) (1968). E. Rosemberg (Ed). Geron-x, Inc., Los Altos, Calif.
15. Pharriss, B. B. and Wyngarden, L. J. (1969). Proc. Soc. Exp. Biol. Med. 130, 92.
16. Duncan, G. W. and Pharriss, B. B. (1970). Fed. Proc. 29, 1232
17. Thorburn, G. O., and Hales, J. R. S. (1972). Proc. Aust. Physiol. Pharmacol. Soc. 3, 145.
18. Labhsetwar, A. (1973). Prostaglandins 3, 729.
19. Chamley, W. A., Buckmaster, J. M., Cain, M. D., Cerini, J., Cerini, M. E., Cumming, I. A., and Goding, J. R. (1972). J. Endocr. 55, 253.
20. Niswender, G. D., Diekman, M. A., Nett, T. M., Akbar, A. M. (1973). Biol. Reprod. 9, 87.
21. Behrman, H. R., Macdonald, G. J., and Greep, R. O. (1971). Lipids 6, 791.
22. Chatterjee, A. (1973). Prostaglandins 3, 189.
23. O'Grady, J. P., Kohorn, E. I., Glass, R. H., Caldwell, B. V., Brock, W. A., and Speroff, L. (1972). J. Reprod. Fert. 30, 153.
24. Demers, L. M., Behrman, H. R., and Greep, R. O. (1972). Advances in Biosciences 9, 701.
25. Labhsetwar, A. P. (1972). J. Endocrinol. 53, 201.
26. Caldwell, B. V., Mazer, R. S., and Wright, P. A. (1967). Endocrinology 80, 477.

27. Labhsetwar, A. P. (1972). Prostaglandins 2, 23.

28. Greenwald, G. S. and Rothchild, I. (1968). J. An. Sci. 27, Suppl. 1, 139.

29. Channing, C. P. (1972). Prostaglandins 2, 327.

30. Moudgal, N. R., Behrman, H. R., and Greep, R. O. (1972). J. Endocrinol. 52, 413.

31. Behrman, H. R., Moudgal, N. R., and Greep, R. O. (1972). J. Endocrinol. 52, 419.

32. Goding, J. R., Cumming, I. A., Chamley, W. A., Brown, J. M., Cain, M. D., Cerini, J. C., Cerini, M. E. D., Findlay, J. K., O'Shea, T. D., and Pemberton, D. H. IV Int. Seminar on Reprod. Physiol. and Sexual Endocrinology. Hormones and Antagonists, P. Hubinont, (Ed). S. Karger, Basel.

33. Neill, J. D., Johansson, E. D., and Knobil, E. (1969). Endocrinology 84, 464.

34. Wentz, A. C. and Jones, G. S. (1973). Obstet. and Gynec., 4, 172.

EVIDENCE FOR A ROLE OF OVARIAN PROSTAGLANDINS IN OVULATION

D. T. Armstrong, Y. S. Moon and J. Zamecnik

Prostaglandins (PGs) have been implicated in the mechanism by which luteinizing hormone stimulates ovarian steroidogenesis *in vitro* (1). The present study was undertaken to determine whether evidence could be obtained for the role of PGs in the mediation of LH action *in vivo.*

EXPERIMENTAL

A. Pre-ovulatory elevation of ovarian prostaglandin levels

Prostaglandins of the F series were measured in rat and rabbit ovaries by radioimmunoassay (2). As illustrated in Fig 1, a marked increase in PGF content of rat ovaries was observed to coincide with the time of the proestrus elevation of serum LH. Advancement of this increase could be brought about by i v injection of exogenous LH earlier on the day of proestrus, or on the day before proestrus (Fig 1). Similar elevations of PGF in ovarian follicles of rabbits occurred in response to either endogenous (induced by coitus) or exogenous LH (Fig 2).

B. Blockade of pre-ovulatory elevation of ovarian prostaglandins with indomethacin

Indomethacin, an established inhibitor of prostaglandin synthesis in several tissues (3), was administered i v 5 hr after LH injection in rabbits, in an attempt to prevent the pre-ovulatory elevation of follicular PGF. As shown in Table 1, no detectable rise in follicular PGF levels was observed 4 hr 30 min after indomethacin injection (i.e., 9 hr 30 min after this LH injection), indicating the effectiveness of this dosage of indomethacin in blocking ovarian PG synthesis (4).

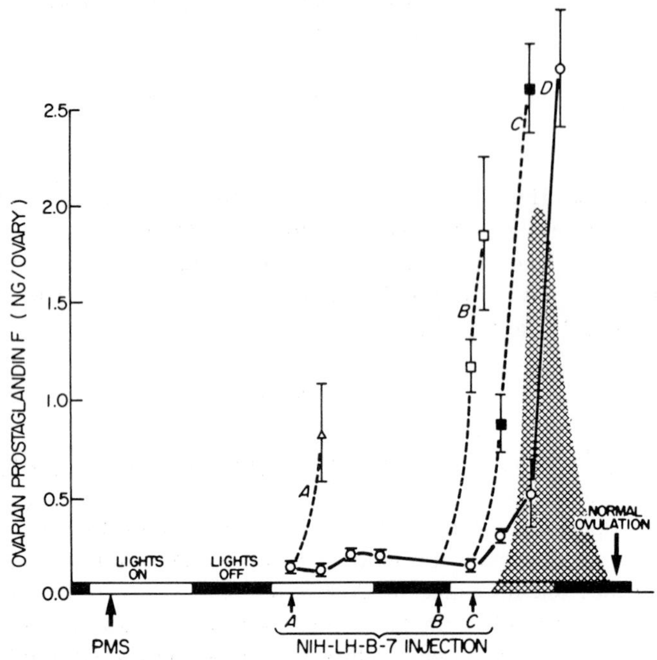

FIG 1. Pre-ovulatory elevation of ovarian PGF and its advancement by exogenous LH injection. Curves A, B and C represent ovarian PGF levels in rats which received LH (10 μg NIH-LH-B7) respectively at 10. 00 a.m. on day 1, 6. 00 a.m. on day 2, and 10. 00 a.m. on day 2 after 4 IU PMS injection on day 0. Curve D represents ovarian PGF levels in rats which received PMS but no exogenous LH. Hatched area represents normal time of endogenous LH secretion.

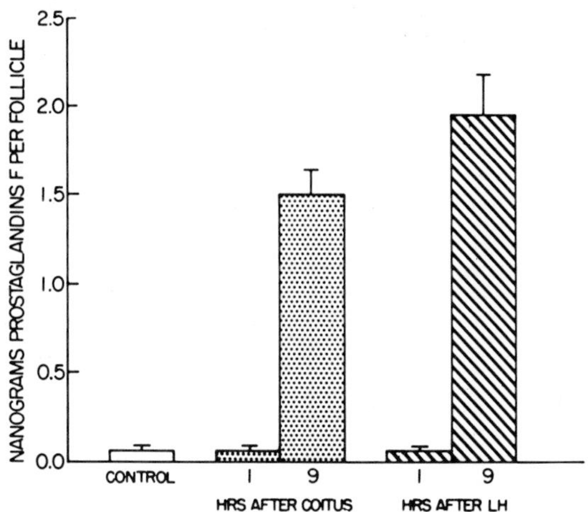

FIG 2. Elevation of PGF levels in rabbit follicles by coitus and LH injection (50 μg NIH-LH-B7).

Table 1. Elevation of follicular PGF levels 9 hr 30 min after systemic LH administration and its prevention by systemic indomethacin administration

Treatment *		Mean follicle PGF ** (pg ± S. E. per follicle.)
Hormone	Inhibitor	
none	none	< 20
LH ¶	none	742 ± 174
none	indomethacin §	< 20
LH	indomethacin	< 20

* Number of rabbits per group = 4. ** PGF measured by radioimmunoassay specific for PGs of the F series. ¶ NIH-LH-B7, 50 μg in saline, iv. § 20 mg/kg in 0.15 M phosphate buffer, pH 8.0, iv 5 hr after LH or saline injection.

Administration of indomethacin at much lower doses by intrafollicular injection was also effective in preventing the preovulatory elevation of PGF levels in injected follicles (5) (Table 2).

Table 2. Inhibition of LH-induced elevation of follicular PGF levels 9 hr 30 min after systemic LH administration by intrafollicular injection of indomethacin

Time of injection (hr after LH)	Material injected	No. of follicles.	Mean follicular PGF (pg ± S. E. per follicle)
0	none	4	1575 ± 131
0	phosphate buffer *	4	1982 ± 741
0	indomethacin **	4	262 ± 36
5	none	2	1850 ± 0
5	phosphate buffer	6	2042 ± 313
5	indomethacin	6	137 ± 29

* 1 µl of 0.15 M phosphate buffer, pH 8.0. ** 1 µl of 0.15 M phosphate buffer, pH 8.0, containing 5 µg indomethacin.

C. Blockade of ovulation by indomethacin

Follicles were examined for evidence of ovulation 24-72 hr after LH administration to rabbits which had received indomethacin by either the i v or intrafollicular route. Absence of rupture points and presence of oocytes retained within the follicles were the criteria employed to indicate blockade of ovulation. As summarized in Table 3, indomethacin (20 mg/kg) blocked ovulation when administered systemically either 30 min before or as late as 5 hr after LH injection. Similarly, intrafollicular injection of indomethacin (5 µg/follicle) prevented ovulation when administered 5 hr after LH injection (5) (Table 4).

Although ovulation was blocked by indomethacin under these conditions, luteinization of the granulosa cells of these follicles was not prevented. Figure 3 illustrates the extensive luteinization of follicles observed 72 hr after LH injection, when ovulation had been blocked by indomethacin administered either

Table 3. Blockade of ovulation in rabbits by administration of indomethacin (20 mg/kg, i v) at various times after LH injection (50 μg NIH-LH-B7, i v).

Time injected (hr after LH)	No. ovulating/No. injected
30 min before	11/12 *
30 min before	0/14
0	0/4
5	0/6
8	2/2

* Received vehicle (control).

Table 4. Effects of intrafollicular injection of indomethacin and of anti-prostaglandin serum 5 hr after i v injection of LH on ovulation in rabbits.

Intrafollicular treatment	No. of rabbits	No. of follicles ovulating/ No. of follicles injected
Phosphate buffer	5	14/16
Normal rabbit serum	1	6/7
Indomethacin	12	0/22
Anti-PGF-serum	6	1/25
Anti-PGE-serum	4	8/14

intravenously or intrafollicularly (6)

D. Failure of indomethacin to prevent LH-induced steroidogenesis

Peripheral serum levels of progesterone and 20 α-hydroxy-pregn-4-en-3-one were measured before and 1 hr after LH treatment in rabbits which had received 20 mg/kg indomethacin or the phosphate buffer vehicle 30 min before the LH injections.

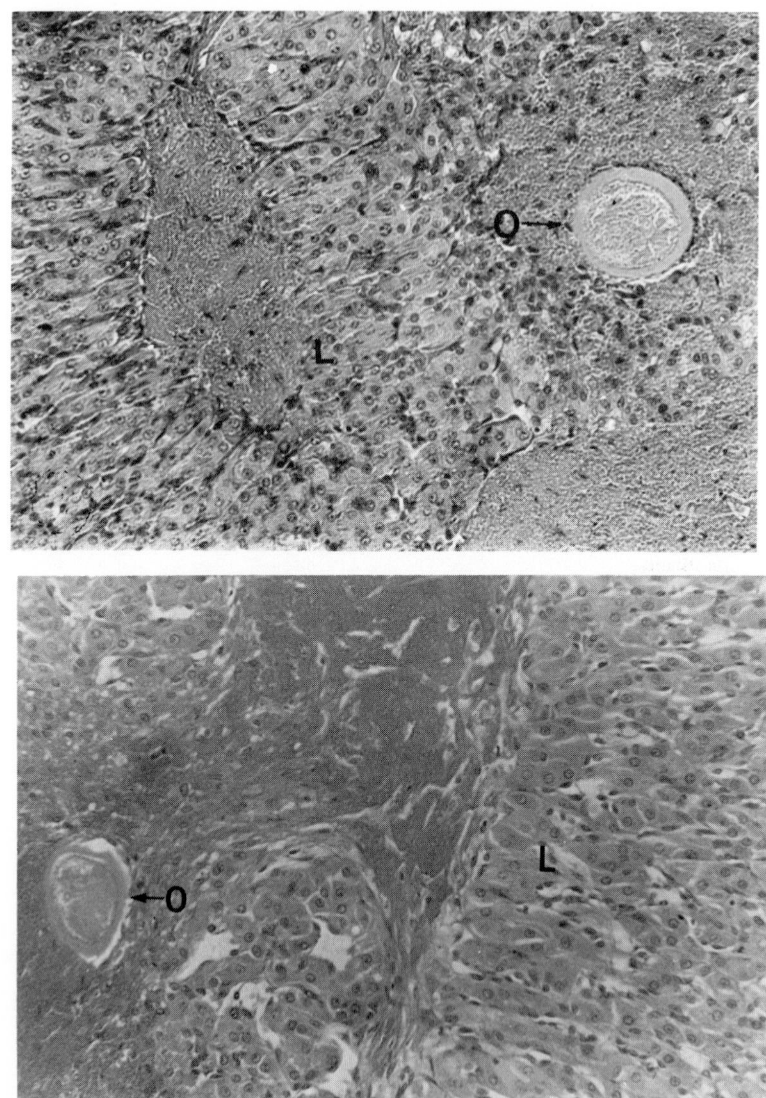

FIG 3. Follicle of rabbit 3 days after i v injection of LH; upper: administered 30 min after i v injection of indomethacin, 20 mg/kg; lower: administered 5 hr before intrafollicular injection of indomethacin, 5 μg, in 1 μl phosphate buffer. O = oocyte retained within the follicle. (x 155) (see reference 6).

Table 5. Effects of indomethacin on the ability of LH to increase peripheral plasma concentration of progesterone and 20α-hydroxypregn-4-en-3-one (20α-OH-P).

Inhibitor	Mean ± S.E. increase* in peripheral plasma concentration (ng/ml) of		Adjusted** mean increase in peripheral plasma concentration (ng/ml) of	
	Progesterone	20α-OH-P	Progesterone	20α-OH-P
None	5.35 ± 1.48	26.0 ± 11.6	5.85	71.6
Indomethacin	5.60 ± 4.47	100.6 ± 37.1	8.50	83.2

* Difference in steroid concentration in samples taken by cardiac puncture immediately before and 1 hr after LH (50 μg) administration. ** Adjusted by covariance analysis, with ovarian interstitial tissue weight as the covariate.

As summarized in Table 5, indomethacin failed to prevent the increment induced by LH in serum level of either steroid (7).

E. Blockade of ovulation by intrafollicular injection of $PGF_{2\alpha}$ antisera

Antisera prepared against either PGE_2 or $PGF_{2\alpha}$ were administered intrafollicularly 5 hr after an i v injection of LH. Control follicles received either phosphate buffer or normal rabbit serum (NRS). As summarised in Table 4, anti-$PGF_{2\alpha}$ was highly effective in blocking ovulation while anti-PGE_2 was partially effective. Neither phosphate buffer nor NRS had significant inhibiting effects on the ovulatory response of follicles to LH (5).

F. Induction of oocyte maturation and extrusion by intrafollicular injection of $PGF_{2\alpha}$

PGE_2 and $PGF_{2\alpha}$ (10 μg/follicle) were injected intrafollicularly to estrus rabbits in order to determine whether these compounds were able to mimic the actions of LH in inducing either oocyte maturation or ovulation. Control follicles were injected with LH (NIH-LH-B8, 200 ng/follicle) or 0.9 % NaCl (8). As shown in Table 6, LH was highly effective in inducing what appeared to be normal follicular rupture at the apices of 6 of 13

Table 6. Effects of intrafollicular injections of prostaglandins and LH on ovulation and oocyte maturation

Material injected *	Hours between injection and autopsy	No. of follicles Injected / Ovulated **	Nuclear stage of oocyte §		
			Dictyate	Metaphase I	Metaphase II
LH	24	7/9	-	-	3
LH	4	1/4	1	3	-
$PGF_{2\alpha}$	24	3/8	1	2	3
$PGF_{2\alpha}$	12	2/6	-	4	-
$PGF_{2\alpha}$	8	2/4	-	3	1
$PGF_{2\alpha}$	4	2/5	1	3	-
PGE_2	24	0/8	4	1	-
PGE_2	12	0/7	5	-	-
Saline	4	0/9	9	-	-

*200 ng of LH and 100 μg of PG was injected in each case. ** Oocytes extruded either through apical rupture point and not recovered, or extruded through point of injection and recovered within ovarian stroma (see text). § Oocytes recovered either in ovarian stroma (outside follicles) or retained within injected follicles.

injected follicles. The oocytes from 2 additional LH-injected follicles were found outside the follicles, within the ovarian stroma adjacent to the point of the micro-injection. The oocytes, as well as those recovered within the 5 non-ruptured follicles which had been injected with LH, had undergone germinal vesicle breakdown, and were in metaphase of either the first or second meiotic division.

Of the 23 follicles injected with $PGF_{2\alpha}$, 9 were observed to have extruded their oocytes through the point of rupture, in a manner similar to the latter two LH-treated follicles (Fig 4A). Eight of these extruded oocytes, as well as 8 of those still retained within the remaining $PGF_{2\alpha}$-injected follicles, had progressed to metaphase-I or beyond (Fig 4B). None of the oocytes from 15 PGE_2-injected or from 9 saline-injected follicles was extruded through the injection point on the follicle, and only one from a PGE_2-injected follicle had progressed beyond the dictyate stage of meiosis.

DISCUSSION

In the studies reviewed here, four types of evidences have been obtained which suggest a physiologic role for PGs in

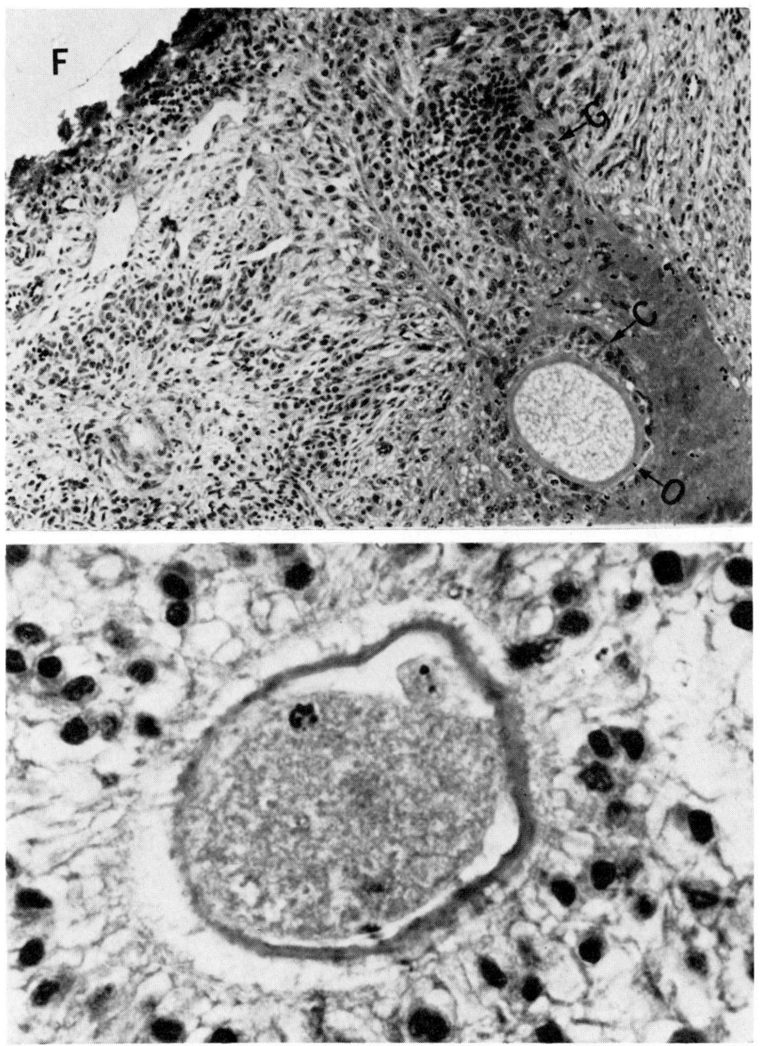

FIG 4. Rabbit follicle (F) injected 12 hr previously with $PGF_{2\alpha}$ (10 µg) intrafollicularly. A: (upper) shows oocyte (0), with surrounding cumulus cells (C), and follicular fluid with some granulosa cells (G), extruded into ovarian stroma (x 175).
B: (lower) oocyte at second meiotic division, with a polar body, retained within the follicle (x 700).

mediating the ovulatory action of LH. First, levels of immunoreactive PGF have been observed to increase markedly in both rat ovaries and rabbit ovarian follicles in response to exogenous and endogenous LH. Second, pharmacologic inhibition of the pre-ovulatory elevation of follicular PGF levels by indomethacin was associated with blockade of ovulation, whether the inhibitor was administered via systemic or intrafollicular route. Third, administration of $PGF_{2\alpha}$ -antiserum, by the intrafollicular route at doses calculated to be several-fold greater than needed to bind all PGF in the follicle, prevented ovulation. Fourth, intrafollicular injection of $PGF_{2\alpha}$ was able to cause extrusion of the oocytes from a majority of injected follicles, possibly by induction of contractions of smooth muscle cells within the theca externa, with the result that the oocyte is forced through the point of least resistence of the follicle wall. This point of least resistance in injected follicles is the point at which the follicle was punctured, whereas under normal physiologic conditions, it is the distended apical region of the follicle wall, weakened by proteolytic digestion under the influence of LH action (9).

The effectiveness of $PGF_{2\alpha}$ to induce oocyte maturation suggests that the PG may also be a mediator of this second physiologic action of LH. The time after LH injection at which follicular PGF levels have first been observed to be elevated (10) (5 hr) coincides reasonably well with the time at which resumption of meiosis began in the present study.

The other ovarian actions of LH, i.e., its ability to stimulate, acutely, the secretion of progestins from the interstitial cells, and its ability to initiate luteinization of granulosa cells, were not prevented by indomethacin treatment, suggesting that these LH responses are not mediated via PGs. Both of these are rapid responses, requiring only a few minutes of exposure to LH for their initiation (11, 12), and both appear to be mediated via cyclic AMP (13, 14). These findings offer no support for the proposal that PGs play an obligatory role in the mechanism by which LH activates ovarian adenyl cyclase (1). Elevated ovarian levels of PGF appear not to occur until well after the activation of adenyl cyclase has occurred, but seem instead to coincide more closely with the time that responsiveness of this enzyme to LH stimulation is lost (15).

From the present studies, it is not possible to draw firm conclusions concerning the mechanism(s) by which follicular PGs contribute to the ovulatory process. However, it seems clear that their participation occurs at a later stage in the series of pre-ovulatory alterations induced by LH, since ovulation could be prevented by blocking PG synthesis or action as late as 5 hr after LH treatment. By this time, many of the pre-ovulatory follicular alterations, such as follicular swelling, hyperemia, oocyte maturation, have already been initiated.

The possibility suggested previously (5) that contraction of smooth muscle within the follicle wall may contribute to the rupture process receives support from the present findings that the oocytes from a high percentage of follicles injected with $PGF_{2\alpha}$ were found to have been extruded through the point of injection, as though forced through this point of least resistance by contractions of the follicle. Additional support for such a contractile process has recently been provided by studies of P. Virutamasen and A. R. Fuchs (personal communication) who have observed pulses of elevated intra-ovarian pressure occurring with greatly increased frequency in rabbits 9-14 hr after injection of an ovulatory dosage of hCG. Intravenous injection of $PGF_{2\alpha}$ resulted in immediate occurrence of similar trains of pulses. Thus, follicular $PGF_{2\alpha}$ may serve as a trigger for ovulation by inducing contractions of ovarian (follicular) smooth muscle cells, thereby providing the final force which causes the follicular wall, weakened by proteolytic enzyme activity (16) to rupture.

ACKNOWLEDGEMENTS

Prostaglandins $F_{2\alpha}$ and E_2 antisera were generously supplied by Dr. H. R. Behrman, Merck Institute for Therapeutic Research, Rahway, New Jersey, and indomethacin, by Dr. W. D. Dorian, Merck, Sharpe & Dohme (Canada) Ltd., Montreal. This research was supported by grants from the Medical Research Council (Canada) and from the Ford Foundation.

REFERENCES

1. Kuehl, F.A., Humes, J.L., Tarnoff, J., Cirillo, V.J. and Han, E.A. (1970). Science, 169, 883.
2. Behrman, H.R. (1971). The Physiologist 14, 110.
3. Vane, V.R. (1971). Nature (New Biol). 231, 232.
4. Zamecnik, J.R. & Armstrong, D.T. (1973). Proc. Can. Fed. Biol. Soc. 16, 29.
5. Armstrong, D.T., Grinwich, D.L., Moon, Y.S. and Zamecnik, J. (1974). Life Sciences (in press).
6. Armstrong, D.T., Moon, Y.S., and Grinwich, D.L. (1973). Adv. Biosci. 9, 709.
7. Grinwich, D.L., Kennedy, T.G. and Armstrong, D.T. (1972). Prostaglandins 1, 89.
8. Moon, Y.S. and Armstrong, D.T. (1974). Fed. Proc. (in press).
9. Espey, L.L. (1967). Am. J. Physiol. 212, 1397.
10. LeMaire, W.J., Yang, N.S.T., Behrman, H.R. and Marsh, J.M. (1973). Prostaglandins 3, 367.
11. Solod, E.A., Armstrong, D.T. and Greep, R.O. (1966). Steroids 7, 606.
12. Ellsworth, L.R. and Armstrong, D.T. (1971). Endocrinology 88, 755.
13. Torrington, J.H. and Baggett, D. (1969). Endocrinology 84, 989.
14. Ellsworth, L.R. and Armstrong, D.T. (1973). Endocrinology 92, 840.
15. Marsh, J.M., Mills, T.M. and LeMaire, W.J. (1972). Biochim. Biophys. Acta. 273, 389.
16. Espey, L.L. and Rondell, P. (1968). Am. J. Physiol. 214, 326.

POSSIBLE ROLE OF PROSTAGLANDINS IN THE SECRETION OF GONADOTROPINS

A. P. Labhsetwar, H. S. Joshi and A. Zolovick

INTRODUCTION

Secretion of gonadotropins from the anterior pituitary is regulated by the hypothalamus through the elaboration of releasing factors into the portal circulation. Several types of stimuli which influence gonadotropin secretion do so, in part by modifying the secretion of the releasing factors. In recent years it has become evident that the effect of these stimuli on the hypothalamic neurons which synthesize gonadotropin releasing factors may be mediated by monoamines. Thus it has been observed that dopamine and/or norepinephrine promote gonadotropin secretion while serotonin inhibits it (1). This dual hypothalamic control over gonadotropin secretion may indeed be involved in physiological conditions such as ovulatory release of gonadotropins, at which time the balance between these contrasting influences may be in favor of the catecholaminergic (CA) system (2,3). However, the regulatory system may not be as simple and probably involves additional factors. One of these factors may be prostaglandins (PGs). It is the intention of this survey to discuss briefly the possible role of PGs and their interaction with monoamines in the regulation of gonadotropin secretion.

PROSTAGLANDINS AND CENTRAL NERVOUS SYSTEM (CNS)

One of the reasons for questioning the role of PGs in the hypothalamic control of gonadotropin secretion is the fact that PGs are endogenous to the hypothalamus. Indeed, Holmes and Horton (4) reported the presence of PGs - E_1, E_2, $F_{2\alpha}$ and $F_{1\alpha}$ in the brain of dog including hypothalamus. Brains of several other species including rats are also known to contain PG $F_{2\alpha}$ and perhaps other PGs (4). Further, PGs have been found to modulate sympathetic transmission. The convincing evidence for this was provided by Hedqvist (5) in the peripheral nervous system. He showed that stimulation of nerves to spleen or heart caused increased release of CA which could be blocked by PG E_2 or E_1, but not by PG $F_{2\alpha}$. The nerve stimulation was also associated with enhanced secretion of both E and F types of PGs, and administration of exogenous inhibitors of PG biosynthesis augmented the transmitter output (5). It thus appears that PG Es interact with CA to inhibit adrenergic transmission. What role PG Fs play in such an interaction is not known. The interaction between PG Es and CA may also be applicable to the CNS, as Siggins et al. (6) showed that decrease in activity of cerebellar Purkinje cells brought about by a local application of norepinephrine could be antagonized by PG Es but not by PG Fs. In contrast to inhibition of PG Es of CA-transmission, PG Fs were reported to potentiate CA release from adrenergic nerve terminals in the cutaneous vascular bed (7).

PROSTAGLANDINS AND GONADOTROPIN SECRETION

Evidence has accumulated to show that adrenergic transmission is essential for gonadotropin secretion, as α-adrenergic blockers and inhibitors of CA-biosynthesis can interfere with gonadotropin secretion (1) and ovulation (3, 8). In view of the above evidence that PGs are not only endogenous to hypothalamus but also may modulate adrenergic transmission, the possibility that the hypothalamic PGs may play such a role in gonadotropin secretion appears attractive and deserves exploration. We reported that administration of PG $F_{2\alpha}$ in antifertility doses to pregnant rats was associated with a several-fold rise in pituitary LH stores which was higher than the highest levels found on the day of proestrus in cyclic rats. Since PG $F_{2\alpha}$ did not interfere with ovulation, we postulated that this PG may stimulate synthesis and release of LH from the pituitary gland. The latter possibility was supported by the fact that the treated animals showed fresh ovulation (9). More recently direct evidence has been obtained to show stimulatory effects of PGs on gonadotropin secretion. Intraventricular injection of PG $F_{2\alpha}$ into bilaterally spayed rats primed with estrogen caused a several-fold increase in plasma LH within 15 min (Table 1). A similar injection of vehicle alone (phosphate buffer, pH 7.4) also caused a significant increase in LH, but the rise following PG injection was greater than that following the injection of buffer. When rats were not primed with estrogen, the rise in LH following PG injection was only marginal (Table 1). Tsafriri et al. (10) reported that exogenous administration of PG E_2 restored ovulation in rats treated with Nembutal to block ovulation, and this stimulatory effect was associated with increased release of LH (11). Intra-

Table 1. Effects of intraventricular injection of vehicle (phosphate buffer) or PG $F_{2\alpha}$ (10 µg) on plasma LH in spayed rats.

Treatment		LH (ng/ml) at various times (min) after injection		
		0	5	15
Estrogen[a] primed	Vehicle	100	512	482
	PG $F_{2\alpha}$	100	812	1555
No priming	Vehicle	100	85	85
	PG $F_{2\alpha}$	100	308	400

[a] Adult rats which had been spayed 1-3 weeks prior to use were primed with 50 µg/day of estradiol benzoate (s c) for 2 days. Intraventricular injections were given on the third day under ether anesthesia.

ventricular administration of PG E_1 but not PG E_2 or $F_{2\alpha}$ in ethanol to cyclic rats in which ovulation was blocked with Nembutal stimulated LH release and ovulation (12). On the other hand, in the bilaterally spayed rats a similar application of PG E_2 but not PGs E_1 or $F_{2\alpha}$ released LH and FSH (13). By contrast, Carlson et al. (14) reported that in sheep intracarotid infusion of PG $F_{2\alpha}$ during the luteal phase of the cycle caused a sharp increase in LH secretion. These results taken together imply that PGs stimulate LH secretion, but the kind of PG involved and the optimal endocrine conditions for the manifestation of stimulatory effect remains to be delineated.

GONADOTROPIN SECRETION AND INHIBITORS OF PROSTAGLANDIN BIOSYNTHESIS

If PGs stimulate gonadotropin secretion and endogenous PGs are not involved in LH release, then it follows that inhibitors of PG synthesis such as aspirin or indomethacin should interfere with the release of LH from the pituitary gland. This has been studied

Table 2. Effects of injection of aspirin into anterior hypothalamic area on progesterone-induced ovulation in immature rats[a].

	No. rats ovulating / No. treated	% inhibition of ovulation	Ova / ovulating rat
Control	15/15	0	10.1
Sham (vehicle)	9/10	10	10.8
Aspirin (120 µg)[b]	2/15	87	3.5
Aspirin (80 µg) (intra-pituitary[c])	4/5	20	7.5

[a] Rats received s c injection of 5 I U PMS at 11 a.m. on day 29 of age followed by a single s c injection of 1 mg progesterone 24 hr later. Material to be tested was stereotaxically injected bilaterally in a vehicle composed of propylene glycol : saline (1:1, pH 6.8) in a volume of 2 µl under ether anesthesia between 1 and 2 p.m. on day 30. Autopsy was performed on day 31 and tubal ova counted and brains examined to verify the site of injections (3).
[b] Total bilateral dose. [c] Intrapituitary injections made using trans-auricular approach.

mainly with respect to ovulation. Orczyk and Behrman (15) reported that a single subcutaneous injection of aspirin (300 mg/kg or more) a few hours before the expected LH surge in PMS-treated immature rats, blocked ovulation in a high proportion of animals. Ovulation in such rats could be restored either by i v injection of 10 µg of LH (NIH-S-16), LRF or by a combination of PG E_2 and $F_{2\alpha}$ (16). Although these results imply a central site of action of aspirin, they do not necessarily exclude the peripheral site, i.e., ovary, as the dose of LH used was well above the threshold. In adult rats, ovulation blocked by anti-estrogens (17) or Nembutal (10) can be restored by 2.5 to 5 µg of LH. The central action could involve hypothalamus and/or pituitary. We recently observed that an intrahypothalamic but not intra-pituitary injection of aspirin blocked progesterone induced ovulation in PMS-primed immature rats (Table 2). Simultaneous injection of PG $F_{2\alpha}$ with aspirin fully restored ovulation in such rats suggesting that aspirin was interfering with ovulation by specifically inhibiting PG synthesis in the hypothalamus (Table 3).

Table 3. Reversal of aspirin-blocked ovulation by PG $F_{2\alpha}$ or dopamine[a].

	No. rats ovulating / No. treated	% inhibition of ovulation	Ova / ovulating rat
Aspirin (120 µg)	2/15	87	3.5
Aspirin (120 µg) PG $F_{2\alpha}$ (1 µg)	8/10	20	9.0
Aspirin (120 µg) Dopamine (180 µg)	11/11	0	8.9

[a] PG $F_{2\alpha}$ (THAM) or dopamine was dissolved in the same aspirin solution (3).

PROSTAGLANDINS AND HYPOTHALAMUS

The fact that an intra-hypothalamic injection of aspirin can interfere with ovulation and this can be restored by simultaneous injection of PG $F_{2\alpha}$ imply that hypothalamic PGs may play a role in the release of LRF. The most plausible explanation as discussed already, appears to be the potentiation by PG $F_{2\alpha}$ of adrenergic transmission. Such a hypothesis received some support from recent experiments. It is well known that a single injection of progesterone into PMS-primed immature rats induces ovulation (18, 19). The stimulatory effect of progesterone on ovulation are transmitted through an α-adrenergic pathway in the hypothalamus, as stereotaxic injection of phenoxybenzamine, an α-adrenergic blocker, into the anterior hypothalamic area prior to the critical period can interfere with stimulatory effects of progesterone on ovulation (20). Injection of aspirin into hypothalamus interfered with progesterone-induced ovulation, but this could be restored not only by simultaneous injection of PG $F_{2\alpha}$ as stated earlier but also by dopamine (Table 3). The fact that a deficiency of PG can lead to interference with the passage of stimulatory impulses of progesterone via an α-adrenergic pathway and dopamine can overcome this interference suggests that CA and PG $F_{2\alpha}$ interact to potentiate adrenergic transmission for ovulatory release of gonadotropins (3).

CONCLUSIONS

Several lines of evidence now indicate that PGs can promote gonadotropin secretion under appropriate conditions. It seems likely that PGs do so by potentiating adrenergic transmission which is normally required for gonadotropin secretion. Thus the presence of relatively high levels of PGs in the hypothalamus may have considerable physiologic significance.

ACKNOWLEDGEMENTS

Unpublished observations in the authors' laboratory were supported in part by a grant from the Ford Foundation and by the Institutional Funds of the Worcester Foundation. Prostaglandins used were generously furnished by the Upjohn Co., Kalamazoo, Michigan, USA.

REFERENCES

1. McCann, S. M., Kalra, P. S., Kalra, S. P., Donoso, A. O., Bishop, W., Schneider, H. P. G., Fawcett, C. P. and Krulich, L. (1972). In "Gonadotropins", B. B. Saxena, C. G. Beling & H. M. Gandy (Eds), p. 49. Wiley Interscience, New York.
2. Labhsetwar, A. P. (1971). Acta Endocrinologica 68, 334.
3. Labhsetwar, A. P., and Zolovick, A. (1973). Nature New. Biol. 249, 55.
4. Holmes, S. W., and Horton, E. W. (1968). In "Prostaglandin Symposium of the Worcester Foundation for Experimental Biology", P. Ramwell and J. Shaw (Eds), p. 21, Lnterscience Publishers.
5. Hedqvist, P. (1971). Annals of New York Acad. Sci. 180, 410.
6. Siggins, G., Hoffer, B., and Bloom, F. (1971). Ann. New York Acad. Sci. 180, 302.
7. Kadowitz, P. J., Sweet, C. S., and Brody, M. J. (1972). European J. Pharmacol. 18, 189.
8. Labhsetwar, A. P. (1972). J. Endocrinology 54, 269.
9. Labhsetwar, A. P. (1970). J. Reprod. Fert. 23, 155.
10. Tsafriri, A., Lindner, H. R., Zor, U., and Lamprecht, S. A. (1972). Prostaglandins 2, 1.
11. Tsafriri, A., Koch, Y. and Lindner, H. R. (1973). Prostaglandins 3, 461.

12. Spies, H. G., and Norman, R. L. (1973). Prostaglandins 4,131.
13. Harms, P. G., Ojeda, S. R., and McCann, S. M. (1973). Science 181, 760.
14. Carlson, J., Barcikowski, B., and McCracken, J. (1973). J. Reprod. Fert. 34, 357.
15. Orczyk, G. and Behrman, H. (1972). Prostaglandins 1, 3.
16. Behrman, H. R., Orczyk, G. P., and Greep, R. O. (1972). Prostaglandins 1, 245.
17. Labhsetwar, A. P. (1970). J. Endocrinology 46, 551.
18. McMormack, C. E., and Meyer, R. K. (1973). Gen. and Comp. Endocr. 3, 300.
19. Ying, S. Y., and Meyer, R. K. (1969). Endocrinology 84, 1466.
20. Zolovick, A., and Labhsetwar, A. (1973). Nature 245, 158.

GONADOTROPINS AND CYCLIC AMP IN VARIOUS COMPARTMENTS OF THE RAT OVARY

K. Ahrén, H. Herlitz, L. Nilsson, T. Perklev, S. Rosberg and G. Selstam

INTRODUCTION

Luteinizing hormone is among the hormones which were early presumed to use cyclic AMP as an intermediate in their action according to the second-messenger theory (1). In harmony with this theory are the observations that LH increases tissue levels of cyclic AMP in bovine corpus luteum slices (2), in whole ovaries from the mouse (3) and the prepubertal rat (4-7), in isolated rat ovarian follicles (4), and in porcine granulosa cells (8). There are, however, also observations indicating that LH might have effects on its target cells, other than those mediated by cyclic AMP. While LH is reported to have a very marked effect on progesterone secretion in isolated luteinized tissue of the rat ovary (9), Mason et al. (6) have recently reported that it has only a weak and inconsistent effect on cyclic AMP levels in this tissue.

The situation for FSH is more unclear than for LH because very few in vitro effects have been unequivocally demonstrated for this gonadotropin. One of these clearly established in vitro effects is that FSH increases the rate of glycolysis in the isolated prepubertal rat ovary (10). Further, Koch et al. (11) have recently shown that FSH increases cyclic AMP content in isolated prepubertal rat ovaries and this is true even in the presence of an anti-β LH serum which completely abolishes the effect of LH.

As part of a long-term program in studies on the mechanism of action of gonadotropins, cyclic AMP has been determined in this laboratory in three types of rat ovarian preparations: 1. the whole prepubertal ovary, 2. isolated follicles from 32-day old rats injected with PMSG (on day 30), and 3. isolated corpora lutea from 33-39-day old rats injected with PMSG on day 30. Effects of gonadotropins added in vitro to the preparations or injected to the rats shortly before the extirpation of the ovaries, have been studied. In vitro effects of gonadotropins have been compared with those of prostaglandins. Special attention has been paid to the possibility that in vitro preparations of the ovary might release cyclic AMP to the incubation medium, an aspect which has not been studied before.

MATERIALS AND METHODS

Sprague-Dawley rats which show the first spontaneous ovulation at the age of 41-42 days were housed in air-conditioned quarters on a regular day and night schedule (lights between 0500 to 1900 hr). Whole ovaries, used for direct analysis of cyclic AMP content or for incubation in vitro, were taken from 23-, 24-day old animals. Thirty day old rats were injected (between 0800-0900 hr) with 10 IU of PMSG and ovarian follicles were dissected on the morning of day 32 (0900-1200 hr). It is well known that a single injection of PMSG to immature rats can produce a premature growth of ovarian follicles and an endogenous release of LH with subsequent ovulation. Under our experimental conditions, it has been established that the PMS-injected rats have an endogenous LH release in the afternoon of day 32, with ovulation occuring on the same night and show the presence of 12 $\pm$ 2 ova in the tubal ampulla on the morning of day 33, corresponding to the normal no. of ova found in the cyclic rat (12). For experiments with corpus luteum, the same "PMSG-model" was used, and the corpora lutea were dissected from 33-39-day old rats. Corpora lutea taken 6-10 hr after ovulation (from 33-day old rats) are designated as "one-day-old corpora lutea".

One ovary (weighing 5-7 mg) or 4-5 isolated follicles (each weighing around 0.2 mg) or 4-5 isolated corpora lutea (each weighing 1-1.5 mg) were incubated at 37° in Krebs bicarbonate buffer containing half the usual calcium concentration and 5.5 mM glucose. When whole ovaries were used, they were preincubated for 30-60 min in the medium without hormones followed by incubation in medium containing hormones or prostaglandins. In experiments with ovarian follicles and corpora lutea, hormones and prostaglandins were added to the same medium in which preincubation (30 min) was carried out.

Cyclic AMP was determined in the tissue and in the incubation medium by a modification of the protein binding assay of Gilman (13), expressed as pmole/mg protein, protein being determined according to Lowry et al. (14). Gonadotropin preparations used were gifts of National Institutes of Health, Bethesda, USA, and the prostaglandins (PGE_1 and PGE_2) were obtained by the courtesy of Ono Pharmaceutical Co. Ltd., Osaka, Japan. The anti-β LH serum used was the gift of Prof. H. Lindner, Israel, and was the same as that used by Koch et al. (11).

RESULTS

A. STUDIES WITH WHOLE OVARY

1. In vivo effects of LH: LH was injected i v to pentobarbital anaesthetized rats, and the ovaries were analysed after various periods of time (Fig. 1). Ovarian cyclic AMP level was significantly increased 20 sec after the start of the LH injection. Cyclic AMP increased rapidly during the first minute and continued to increase for 15 min. After this time there was a decrease in ovarian cyclic AMP level, but the values at 30 and 120 min were still significantly higher than those of the controls.

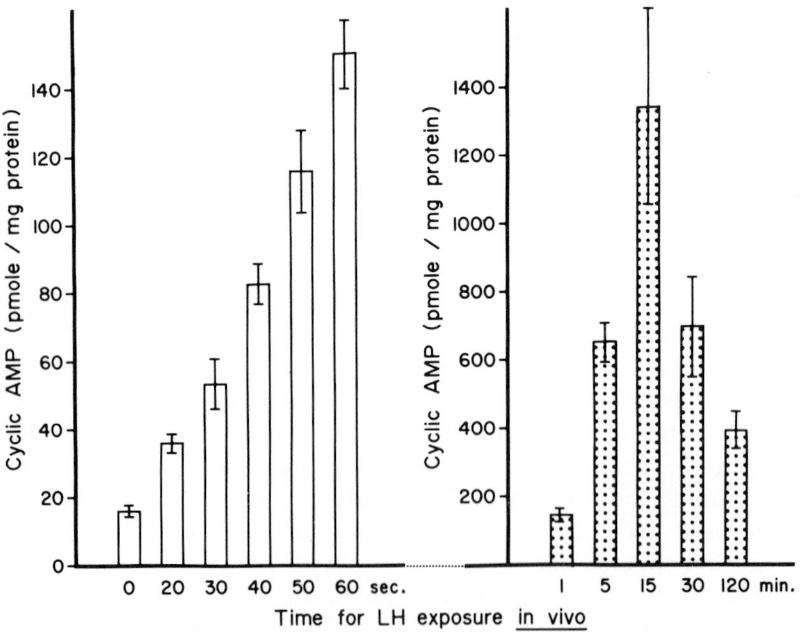

FIG 1. Effect of i v injection of LH on the cAMP level in the prepubertal rat ovary. NIH-LH-B8 (25 μg/rat) was injected in the tail vein of pentobarbital anaesthetized rats (24-25-day old, weighing 45-50 g).

2. In vitro effects of hormones and prostaglandins : It has already been reported that addition of LH to the isolated prepubertal rat ovary, both as whole ovary preparation (4,5,7) and as ovarian slices (6), increases ovarian cyclic AMP content after 1-15 min. Fig. 2 shows the time-course of an incubation experiment with a submaximal LH concentration, where ovarian and medium contents of cyclic AMP have been analysed. It can be seen that the medium and tissue contents of cyclic AMP were more or less the same at 60 min of incubation; at 120 min, the medium content was 4-5 times higher than the maximal tissue content seen

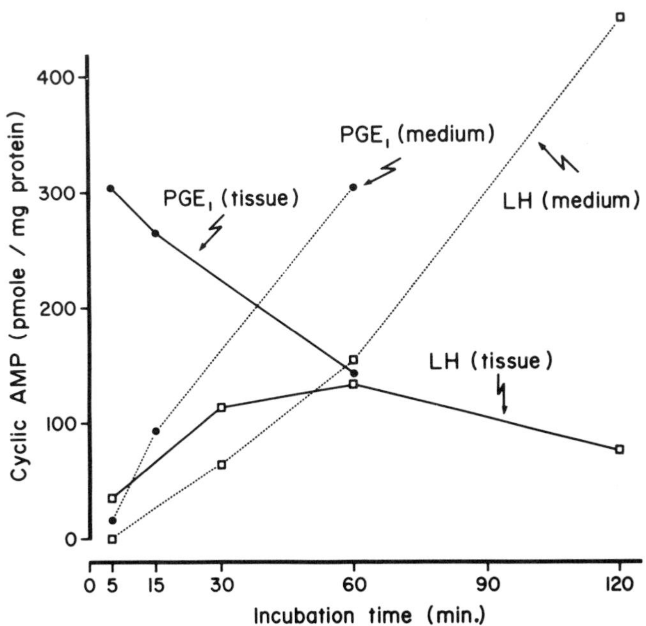

FIG 2. In vitro effects of LH and PGE$_1$ on the prepubertal rat ovary: tissue and medium contents of cyclic AMP. Whole ovaries from 24-day old rats were incubated with or without NIH-LH-B8 (1 µg/ml) and PGE$_1$ (10 µg/ml), respectively, after 60 min of pre-incubation in plain medium. Media of control ovaries (not shown in the figure) did not contain measurable amounts of cyclic AMP, and tissue level of control ovaries remained quite stable during the entire incubation period with values varying between 16 and 37 pmoles/mg protein.

at 60 min. Unstimulated ovaries (not shown in the figure) did not release significant amounts to the medium. Total amount of cyclic AMP (tissue + medium contents) increased in the LH group during the entire incubation period studied.

PGE_1 also increased the tissue as well as the medium level of cyclic AMP (Fig. 2). The time-course, however, was quite different from that seen with LH stimulation: maximal ovarian cyclic AMP content was reached within 5 min, and total amount of cyclic AMP was no longer increasing after 15 min.

Table 1. Stimulation of cyclic AMP levels in isolated ovarian follicles from PMSG injected prepubertal rats.

Group	Cyclic AMP* pmole /mg protein
Control	25.6 ± 8.3
LH : 0.1 μg/ml	40.4 ± 9.3
1.0 μg/ml	204.5 ±29.6
10 μg/ml	629.3 ±95.5
100 μg/ml	490.1 ±32.0
Prolactin : 10 ug/ml	29.0 ± 9.4
STH : 10 μg/ml	29.0 ± 5.8
FSH : 1 μg/ml	70.2 ± 7.8
10 μg/ml	186.8 ±29.6
100 μg/ml	725.0 ±79.3
TSH : 10 μg/ml	252.5 ±63.9
PGE_2 : 0.1 μg/ml	58.9 ±18.1
1.0 μg/ml	89.4 ±22.1
10 μg/ml	158.3 ±25.0

*Values represent tissue content of cyclic AMP. No significant amount of cyclic AMP was detected in the media after a short incubation period of 15 min. Each value is the mean ± S.E. of measurements of 5-6 flasks. See text for details.

B. STUDIES ON ISOLATED FOLLICLES AND CORPORA LUTEA

1. In vitro effects of hormones and prostaglandins on follicular preparations : The response of the follicles isolated from the PMSG-treated rats is probably similar to that shown by Graafian follicles dissected, on the morning of proestrus from the cyclic rat. The latter model has been used by Tsafriri et al. (15).

Table I shows that LH, FSH, TSH and PGE_2 increased cyclic AMP content in the isolated follicles. The effect of LH on the latter was more pronounced than its effect in vitro on the whole ovary. As can be seen from Fig. 3, the effect of FSH on the isolated follicle is due to an intrinsic property of the molecule itself and not due to a contamination of the FSH preparation with LH. Whether the same is true for TSH has not been tested in the present series of experiments.

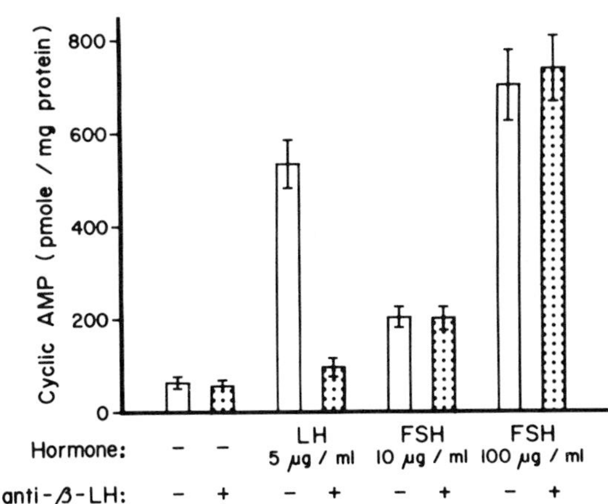

FIG 3. Ovarian follicles (4-5 in each incubation flask) from PMSG-injected prepubertal rats were preincubated for 30 min at 37° in the modified Krebs buffer. Hormones and/or anti-β LH serum (30 μl/ml medium) were then added, and the incubation continued for 15 min. Hormones and anti-serum were preincubated for 30-45 min at 37° before addition to the medium containing the ovaries.

The time-course of the effect of LH was, in principle, similar to that observed for the whole ovary. Cyclic AMP was released into the incubation medium even in this case, but a significant amount was not found until 60 min of incubation. The effect of PGE_2 (10 µg/ml) was maximal within 5 min, and decreased with longer incubation periods. The maximal effect of PGE_2 on follicular cyclic AMP levels was always less, compared to that of LH (Table 1). While PGE_1 showed an effect similar to PGE_2, high concentrations of $PGF_{2\alpha}$ were needed to obtain a measurable effect.

2. <u>In vitro effects of hormones and prostaglandins on corpora lutea:</u>
Corpora lutea were isolated from ovaries of the PMSG injected rats on different days following ovulation for 6 days. Fig 4 shows that LH increased the cyclic AMP level in the isolated corpora lutea of all ages studied, though its effect was much more on the

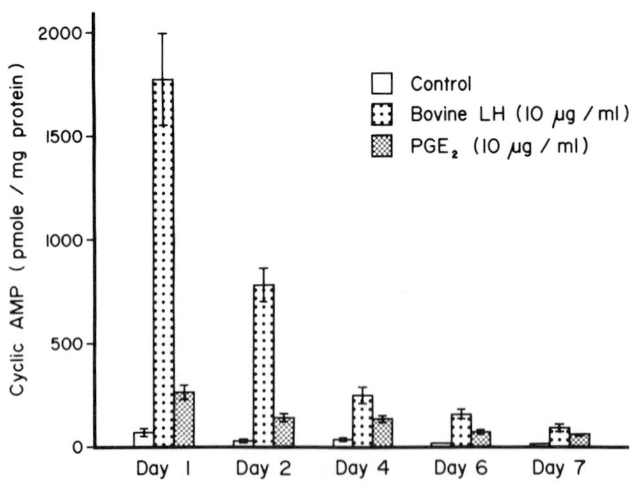

FIG. 4. Effects of LH and PGE_2 on cyclic AMP content in isolated corpora lutea of various ages. Corpora lutea of different ages (5 in each flask) were preincubated for 30 min at 37° in the modified Krebs bicarbonate buffer. LH or PGE_2, were added and incubation continued for 15 min.

younger corpus luteum. The effect on fresh corpus luteum (6-10 hr old) was, in fact, more marked than on isolated follicles. The time-course of the LH effect on the isolated corpus luteum is illustrated in Fig. 5 showing an experiment with 3-day old corpora lutea. Though the release of cyclic AMP to the incubation medium from the LH-stimulated corpora lutea was significant and had the same time-course, as observed for the whole ovary, quantitatively it was much less, as in the case of follicles.

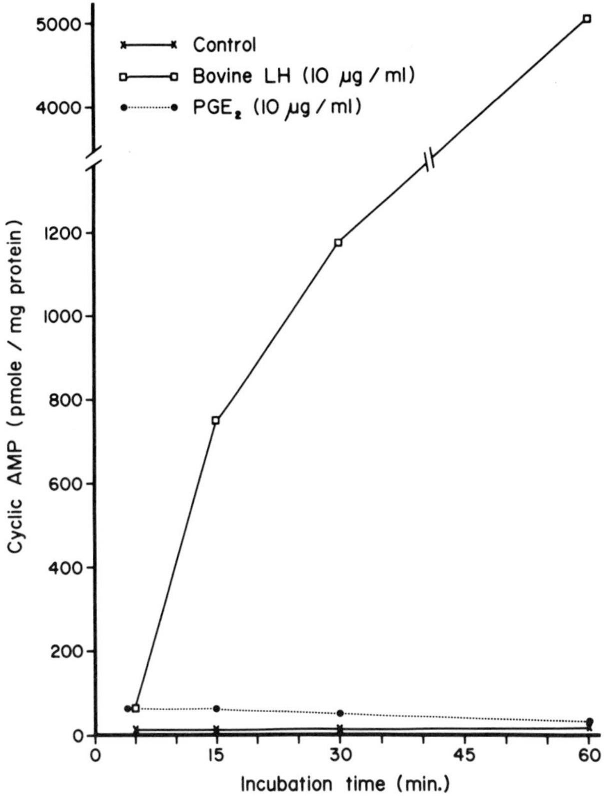

FIG 5. Effects of LH and PGE_2 on cyclic AMP levels in incubated corpora lutea — a time-course study. For experimental details see the text. Control values are very low; compared to the values with LH, those with PGE_2 are low, but are significantly different from the control values.

DISCUSSION

The rapid increase in ovarian cyclic AMP content observed after an iv injection of LH gives support to the proposal that cyclic AMP plays a decisive role in the mechanism of action of this gonadotropin. Hitherto, no metabolic effect of LH has been reported to occur with such rapidity excepting for its effect on ovarian blood flow. An increase in ovarian blood flow is known to occur 6-120 sec after iv injection of LH (16), maximal blood flow response being seen after 20 min. This is similar to the maximal increase in ovarian cyclic AMP observed in the present study (Fig. 1). The functional relationship between ovarian hyperaemia and ovarian cyclic AMP formation after LH stimulation has to be further explored.

Release of cyclic AMP into the extracellular compartment has, under various experimental conditions, been reported for erythrocytes (17), for perfused rat liver (18), for perfused cat and rat adrenals in vivo (19, 20), and for incubated rat testes (21). The present study shows that the isolated prepubertal rat ovary releases appreciable amount of cyclic AMP to the incubation medium when stimulated with LH or PGE_1. There are many important questions which ought to be further explored as a consequence of these observations. First, is cyclic AMP released from the LH stimulated ovary, even under physiological conditions ? It has been demonstrated that ACTH-stimulated adrenal, releases cyclic AMP into the adrenal venous blood under in vivo conditions in the rat and into the perfusate as shown in studies with the perfused cat adrenal. Second, is it possible that the extracellular cyclic AMP has any physiological importance, e.g. for regulation of ovarian blood flow or as a signal from one ovarian cell type to another (e.g. from granulosa cells to the oocyte), or does this phenomenon just reflect one of the routes for the stimulated cell to decrease its cyclic AMP level after acute stimulation ? Third, is the release from a cellular point of view, a "simple" diffusion of cyclic AMP to the extracellular compartment, possibly involving complex processes, e.g. binding of cyclic AMP to various proteins, compartmentalization, intricate balance between various classes of phosphodiesterase enzymes, or is it, alternatively, a specific transport mechanism involved in the release ?

The results with isolated ovarian follicles from PMSG-injected rat confirm and extend the studies of Tsafriri et al. (15), showing an increase in cyclic AMP levels after addition of LH or prostaglandins. A clear effect of FSH which cannot be explained as due to a contamination with LH was also observed (Fig. 3). In studies on isolated Graafian follicles from the rabbit, Marsh et al. (2) reported that the effect of FSH could be explained on the basis of a LH contamination in the FSH preparation. Further studies are necessary to elucidate whether there are real species differences in the reactivity to FSH or whether other differences in experimental conditions can explain these conflicting results.

The most striking feature observed from the experiments with corpus luteum is that the effect of LH markedly decreased with the age of the corpus luteum, the fresh corpus luteum showed a marked response, while LH produced only a minimal increase in cyclic AMP in the older corpora lutea (Fig. 4). These results are to a certain extent, in harmony with those of Mason et al. (6) who reported varying effects of LH _in vitro_ on isolated luteal tissue taken from the rat under various conditions. This illustrates that it is not meaningful to discuss in a general way, how _the_ corpus luteum reacts to LH, without describing the nature of the corpus luteum studied. Mason et al. (6) reported that corpora lutea from pregnant rats or slices of partially luteinized ovaries did not respond at all to LH stimulation by an increase in cyclic AMP. However, we have observed, following stimulation by LH, an increase in cyclic AMP, though small, also in the aged corpora lutea. An interesting aspect of this is whether the small effect of LH on the older corpora lutea still represents an increase in cellular content of cyclic AMP optimal for reactions regulated by this nucleotide. A final interpretation of the results presented in Fig. 4 must, in addition, take into consideration that extensive morphological changes take place during the formation of the corpus luteum, e.g. change in vascular pattern with development of sinusoidal capillaries, invasion of fibroblasts, and an increase in the proportion of completely luteinized cells (22, 23).

The fact that prostaglandins can increase cyclic AMP in the whole ovary, in isolated follicles and in isolated corpora lutea has already been reported (3, 5-7). The present study reveals, in addition, that the time-course for the _in vitro_ effects of LH and prostaglandins are quite different (Figs 2 and 5). This makes it difficult to use these types of _in vitro_ preparations not only to compare the effects of these substances quantitatively, but also to interpret experiments aimed to study the degree of additivity of the LH- and prostaglandin effects. Experiments with a perfusion preparation will probably offer a better model for such studies.

In the present study, only two compartments of the rat ovary have been analysed separately, the mature follicle and the corpus luteum. LH has been found to increase cyclic AMP in these compartments. Both these compartments are, however, rather complex structures, particularly the follicle. The results of experiments with these compartments must be correlated with similar studies on isolated cell populations and with studies which for technical reasons, have to be performed in large animals. The studies of Kolena and Channing (8) on isolated granulosa cells from the porcine ovary are of great interest in this connection. They found that granulosa cells from large ovarian follicles responded to LH with a marked elevation of cyclic AMP while granulosa cells from medium sized and small follicles showed only a very small response or no response at all. It will, therefore, be of interest to study how isolated follicles in various phases of development respond to gonadotropins _in vitro_. Such studies with rat ovarian follicles are in progress in this laboratory.

ACKNOWLEDGEMENTS

This research program is supplied by grants from the US Public Health (RO1 HD02795), the Swedish Medical Research Council (B73-03X-27-09B), the Medical Research Council of the Swedish Life Offices, and the Medical Faculty, University of Goteborg. Valuable technical assistance was given by Mrs. Ann Anderson, Mrs. Ann-Cathrine Schiott, Mrs. Anita Sjogren, and Miss. Stina Oberg.

REFERENCES

1. Robison, G.A., Butcher, R.W. and Sutherland, E.W. (1971). In "Cyclic AMP", Academic Press, New York.
2. Marsh, J.M., Mills, T.M. and LeMaire, W.J. (1972). Biochim, Biophys. Acta. _273_, 389.
3. Kuehl, F.A., Jr., Humes, J.L., Tarnoff, J., Cirillo, V.J., and Ham, E.A. (1970). Science _169_, 883.
4. Lamprecht, S.A., Zor, U., Tsafriri, A. and Lindner, H.R. (1971). Ist. J. Med. Sci. _7_, 704.

5. Lamprecht, S.A., Zor, U., Tsafriri, A. and Lindner, H.R. (1973). J. Endocrinol. 57, 217.
6. Mason, N.R., Schaffer, R.J. and Toomey, R.E. (1973). Endocrinology 93, 34.
7. Ahren, K., Hamberger, L., Herlitz, H., Hillensjo, T., Nilsson, L., Perklev, T. and Selstam, G. (1973). In "The endocrine function of the human testis", V.H.T. James, M. Serio and L. Martini (Eds). Vol. I, p 251, Academic Press New York.
8. Kolena, J. and Channing, C.P. (1972). Endocrinology 90, 1543.
9. Armstrong, D.T., O'Brien, J. and Greep, R.O. (1964). Endocrinology 75, 488.
10. Ahren, K., Hamberger, L. and Rubinstein, L. (1969). In "The Gonads", K.W. McKerns (Ed), p. 327, Appleton-Century Crofts, New York.
11. Koch, Y., Zor, U., Pomerantz, S., Chobsieng, P. and Lindner, H.R. (1973). J. Endocrinol. (in press).
12. Fuxe, K., Hokfelt, T., Sundstedt, C-D, Ahren, K. and Hamberger, L. (1972). Neuroendocrinology 10, 282.
13. Gilman, A.G. (1970). Proc. Nat. Acad. Sci. 67, 305.
14. Lowry, O.H., Rosebrough, N.J., Farr, A.L. and Randall, R.J. (1951). J. Biol. Chem. 193, 265.
15. Tsafriri, A., Lindner, H.R., Zor, U. and Lamprecht, S.A. (1972). J. Reprod. Fert. 31, 39.
16. Wurtman, R.J. (1964). Endocrinology 75, 927.
17. Davoren, P.R. and Sutherland, E.W. (1963). J. Biol. Chem. 238, 3009.
18. Broadus, A.E., Kaminsky, N.I., Northcutt, R.C., Hardman, J.G., Sutherland, E.W. and Liddle, G.W. (1970). J. Clin. Invest. 49, 2237.
19. Carchman, R.A., Jaanus, S.D. and Rubin, R.P. (1971). Molec. Pharmacol. 7, 491.
20. Peytremann, A., Nicholson, W.E., Hardman, J.G. and Liddle, G.W. (1973). Endocrinology 92, 1502.
21. Dufau, M.L., Watanabe, K. and Catt, K.J. (1973). Endocrinology 92, 6.
22. Bassett, D.L. (1943). Am. J. Anat. 73, 251.
23. Malone, T.E. (1957). J. Morphol. 100, 1.

THE ROLE OF CYCLIC AMP AND PROSTAGLANDINS IN THE ACTIONS OF LUTEINIZING HORMONE

John M. Marsh and William J. LeMaire

Luteinizing hormone has a number of effects, two of which are currently under investigation in our laboratory, namely: stimulation of steroidogenesis in the corpus luteum; initiation of the process of ovulation. In both studies,we have investigated the possible role of cyclic AMP and prostaglandins in the mechanism of action of LH, and have arrived at two distinct hypotheses.

THE ACTION OF LH ON STEROIDOGENESIS IN THE CORPUS LUTEUM

A. Early studies

The study of the effect of LH on steroidogenesis in the corpus luteum has been underway for quite some time. Our approach to the problem was to develop an *in vitro* model system in which the effects of gonadotropins and other substances could be easily measured on the steroidogenic process (1). Most of the work has been done with bovine tissue, but we have confirmed nearly all our findings with human corpora lutea as well (2). We found that if the slices of corpus luteum were incubated *in vitro* with LH,there was an increase in the synthesis of progestins (progesterone and 20β -hydroxy-pregn-4-ene-3-one), usually more than 100 % over the control level (1). This effect was specific for hormone preparations with LH activity and quite sensitive to small amounts of the hormone. The minimum effective concentration was approximately 3 x 10^{-11} M (3,4).

When we started investigation as to how LH might bring about this stimulation of steroidogenesis, we realised that our system was very similar to that used by other workers studying the mechanism of action of ACTH on the adrenal, in which the involvement of cyclic AMP was implicated (5). Thus, when exogenous cyclic AMP was added to incubating luteal slices we found that this cyclic nucleotide could mimic the effect of LH on progestin synthesis. Other nucleotides structurally related to cyclic AMP, such as 3'-AMP, 5'-AMP or ATP were ineffective (6).

This data indicated that cyclic AMP could have been a mediator of the stimulatory effect of LH. In order to test this point further, we carried out an additive type of experiment. In each study, two sets of slices from the same corpus luteum were incubated with 0.02 M and 0.04 M cyclic AMP to establish that the stimulation by cyclic AMP was maximal. A third set was incubated with the highest concentration of cyclic AMP and 10 µg/ml of LH. A fourth set was incubated alone as a control. The results are shown in Fig. 1. If LH transmitted its effect on progestin synthesis solely

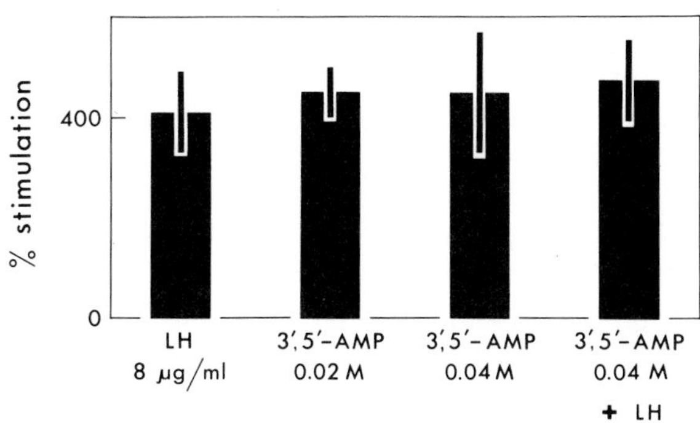

FIG 1. Effect of cyclic AMP (3',5'-AMP) plus LH on the µg of progesterone synthesized in incubating slices of bovine corpora lutea. Six sets of slices were prepared from a single corpus luteum. One set, the zero time sample, was analyzed for the mass of progesterone immediately without incubation. Another set was incubated under control conditions for 2 hours. One more set was incubated in the presence of LH 8 ug/ml. Two more sets were incubated with either 0.02 M or 0.04 M cyclic AMP, and the last set was incubated with 0.04 M cyclic AMP plus LH 8 µg/ml. The zero time and the control values were subtracted from the treated values and only the % stimulation is shown. The height of the bars represents the mean of 4 experiments and the vertical lines, the standard deviations. The preparation of the slices, the incubation and the measurement of progesterone, were described previously (6).

via cyclic AMP, then it follows that slices of corpora lutea, already maximally stimulated by saturating levels of the cyclic nucleotide, should show no further response when LH was added. The data in Fig. 1 indicate that this indeed is the case and that therefore, this nucleotide could be a mediator of this action of LH.

Further support for this hypothesis came from our findings that LH caused a striking increase in the endogenous concentration of cyclic AMP (as much as 100-fold) (7). This effect was again specific for LH and could be observed at the earliest interval examined (2.5 min after the addition of the hormone) and this was long before any effect could be seen on steroidogenesis (30 min to 1 hr). This time relationship would be expected if cyclic AMP was a mediator of LH action. An investigation was then carried out to determine if this rise in endogenous cyclic AMP was due to a stimulation of the adenyl cyclase or an inhibition of the phosphodiesterase. Assays were developed for the measurement of these two enzymes in homogenates of corpora lutea and we found that LH stimulated the adenyl cyclase, but had no effect on the phosphodiesterase (8).

B. <u>The role of prostaglandins</u>

Our next undertaking was to assess the effect of prostaglandins on adenyl cyclase. The addition of prostaglandins to incubating slices of bovine corpora lutea has been shown by others to bring about an increase in progestin synthesis (9). Whether this effect might also be mediated by cyclic AMP was studied by us. Six prostaglandins (PGE_1, PGE_2, PGB_1, PGA_2, $PGF_{1\alpha}$, and $PGF_{2\alpha}$) were tested for an effect on adenyl cyclase. PGE_1 and PGE_2 did indeed have a significant stimulatory effect, about equal in magnitude to that of a saturating level of LH. PGE_1 and PGE_2 were about equally potent and appeared to be more effective than PGB_1 and PGA_2. PGE_2 was also tested for an effect on phosphodiesterase, but, as was found for LH, no effect was observed (10).

We considered the possibility that the PGs might also be mediators of LH, acting between the receptor and its effect on adenyl cyclase. LH could presumably increase the concentration or activity of a hypothetical endogenous PG, which in turn could stimulate adenyl cyclase. To test this possibility, we carried out another additive type experiment similar to the one described previously. The maximal effective concentration of PGE_2 on adenyl cyclase was determined. In another aliquot of the same homogenate, LH was added with this saturating amount of PGE_2 to see if a greater stimulation could be achieved. If LH transmitted its effect on adenyl cyclase solely via a PG, there should have been no further response to LH, when the homogenate was already maximally stimulated by PGs. It was found, however, that LH produced a clearly additive effect with a saturating amount of PGE_2 (10). This indicated to us that the effect of LH and the effect of PGs were separate phenomena, and that PGs were probably not mediators of the action of LH. A quite different conclusion was reached by another group of investigators using a different model system and a different approach (11). They assessed the accumulation of ^{14}C labeled cyclic AMP in incubated whole mouse ovaries and found that LH, PGE_1 and PGE_2 increased this accumulation. They also considered the possibility that PGs might be mediators in the action of LH on adenyl cyclase, and they tested this possibility using a PG antagonist, 7-oxa-13-prostynoic acid. They found that this antagonist would not only competitively block the action of the PG on cyclic AMP accumulation, but also competitively block the action of LH. They concluded from this that a PG receptor functions as a necessary intermediate in the action of LH. Their results are even more intriguing in that they were also able to demonstrate an additive effect of LH and PG on ^{14}C-cyclic AMP accumulation (11). It is very difficult to reconcile the results obtained from additive experiments with those obtained with the antagonist 7-oxa-13-prostynoic acid.

Using this antagonist, which was generously given to us by Dr. Josef Fried of the University of Chicago, we attempted to block the effect of PGE_2 and LH on adenyl cyclase in homogenates of corpora lutea. However, consistent inhibition could not be observed using 7-oxa-13-prostynoic acid in this homogenate system. Using a system similar to that used by Kuehl et al. (11), in which slices of bovine corpora lutea were incubated in the presence of ^3H-labeled adenine the effect of LH and 7-oxa-13-prostynoic acid were assessed on the accumulation of ^3H-cyclic AMP.

The method of incubation used was a modification of that described by Kuo and DeRenzo (12); in this, slices of bovine corpora lutea were incubated for 1 hr in Krebs-Ringer bicarbonate buffer (KRB) (pH 7.4) containing (8-^3H) adenine, rinsed in 0.154 M NaCl, and then incubated again in the buffer alone for 30 min, as a control, or in the presence of LH, or LH plus 7-oxa-13-prostynoic acid.

Table 1. Effect of 7-oxa-13-prostynoic acid* on ^{3}H-cyclic AMP accumulation in bovine corpora lutea

Slices of (0.3-0.5 g) bovine corpora lutea were preincubated in Krebs-Ringer bicarbonate (KRB) buffer (pH 7.4) for 1 hr with 25 μCi of (8-^{3}H) adenine in an atmosphere of 95 % O_2 and 5 % CO_2. The slices were then rinsed in 0.154 M NaCl and incubated again for 30 min in KRB buffer (pH 7.4) containing 0.01 M theophylline alone, in the buffer containing LH (NIH-LH-S 11) (0.05-1.5 μg/ml), or in buffer containing LH (0.05-1.5 μg/ml) plus 7-oxa-13-prostynoic acid (50 μg/ml) in an atmosphere of 95 % O_2 and 5 % CO_2. The slices were then homogenized and the cyclic AMP isolated as described previously (14).

LH μg/ml	7-oxa 50 μg/ml	^{3}H-adenine incorporation into ^{3}H-cyclic AMP (dpm x 10^3/g)								
		Experiments								
		1	2	3	4	5	6	7	8	9
-	-	18	21	135	40	48	31	71	43	267
1.5	-	440	2110	1840	1188	572	169	4800	1380	3940
1.5	+	378	1480	1270	1270	563	115	3410	1590	2420
0.5	-	232	1060	477	649	229	118	1460	704	1320
0.5	+	113	694	472	503	174	54	1350	507	635
0.15	-	84	436	428	144	189	67	509	550	888
0.15	+	73	178	361	192	84	38	397	266	385
0.05	-	31	114	113	52	51	54	179	101	311
0.05	+	16	62	196	47	67	39	127	78	229

* A gift from Dr. J. Fried.

^{3}H -cyclic AMP was isolated by a modification of the procedure of Krishna et al. (13) and this involved an additional cellulose thin-layer chromatography to achieve radiochemical purity (14). Using this technique, we found that LH caused a marked increase in the accumulation of ^{3}H-cyclic AMP, which was very similar in magnitude to that observed previously on the accumulation of mass amounts of cyclic AMP (7).

Table 1 shows the results of 9 experiments in which we attempted to determine if 7-oxa-13 prostynoic acid had a competitive inhibitory effect on the stimulation caused by LH. LH was added at concentrations from 0.05 µg/ml to 1.5 µg/ml to duplicate sets of slices. The PG antagonist, 7-oxa-13 prostynoic acid, was added at 50 µg/ml to one of the sets of slices, and its effect on the stimulation by LH of ^{3}H-cyclic AMP accumulation was measured. We found that first there was considerable variability from one corpus luteum to the next. Secondly, 7-oxa-13 prostynoic acid did produce an inhibition of the LH stimulation of cyclic AMP accumulation, but its effect was not a totally consistent one. In 5 of the 36 cases, as shown by the underlined values in Table 1, the 7-oxa-13-prostynoic acid seemed to have a slight stimulatory effect. Most important, however, was that although we observed an inhibition of the effect of LH with this PG antagonist, we could not demonstrate that it was of the competitive type. Variability of the data obtained with 7-oxa-13-prostynoic acid was such that a Lineweaver-Burk plot could not be constructed using a computer program (15). This is obviously crucial to any interpretation of the data, since a non-competitive inhibition by 7-oxa-13-prostynoic acid could be just a general poisoning phenomenon. This is the current status of our studies on PGs with corpora lutea, and the situation still remains unsettled. We are presently attempting to measure endogenous PG levels in control and LH-treated tissue; if PGs are part of the mechanism of action of LH, there should be some change in their concentration, their location, or their physical state.

C. The fate of endogenous cyclic AMP in corpora lutea

In an attempt to determine how cyclic AMP might mediate the action of LH, we undertook an investigation to determine where the endogenous cyclic AMP was located in the cell and in what state it existed (14). As described earlier, ^{3}H-cyclic AMP was synthesized in corpus luteum slices from ^{3}H-adenine, and also LH caused a marked increase in the accumulation of ^{3}H-cyclic AMP in the incubated slices. Slices of corpora lutea which had been preincubated with (8-^{3}H) adenine and then incubated with LH were homogenized in 0.25 M sucrose containing 0.05 M tris buffer, pH 7.4, 0.04 M theophylline, and 0.02 M EDTA. The homogenate was separated by differential centrifugation, using standard techniques into the 5 fractions (1,000 g; 6,000 g; 25,000 g; 105,000 g pellets; and a 105,000 g supernatant). Each pellet was washed twice and recentrifuged. DNA measurements, marker enzyme analysis and ^{3}H-cyclic AMP measurement were carried out in each fraction. Most of the ^{3}H-cyclic AMP (85 %) was localized in the 105,000 g supernatant and only small and approximately equal amounts localized in the other fractions. From the localization of the marker enzymes, particularly the glucose-6-phosphate dehydrogenase, it was apparent that this supernatant fraction contained predominantly cytosol material (14). It was assumed that the small amount of ^{3}H-cyclic AMP in the particulate fractions was bound or present within the organelles, as it centrifuged down with the particles even after repeated washing. In the cytosol fraction, however, it was not known if the cyclic AMP was entirely in the free form or if any was bound to other molecules. To assess this, the cytosol fractions from control and LH-treated tissues were subjected to ultrafiltration in an Amicon cell using a PM-30 membrane filter, which retains a globular protein of approximately 30,000 molecular weight. The amount of bound ^{3}H-cyclic AMP was calculated from the concentration of this nucleotide in the retentate after about 80 % of the cell charge has passed through the filter. Almost all (80.9 % $\pm$ 20.7 %, mean $\pm$ SD) of the ^{3}H-cyclic AMP of the cytosol of the control sample was bound to a macromolecular component. In the cytosol of the LH-treated tissue 22 % (22.0 % $\pm$ 8.87 %, mean $\pm$ SD) of the labelled nucleotide was bound. Although the percent bound was greater in the control cytosols, the absolute amounts of bound cyclic AMP in the cytosol of the LH-treated tissue was more than 5 times that in the control cytosol (14).

Several authors have reported (16) that cyclic AMP binds to the regulatory portion of a protein kinase enzyme, and in view of this, we considered the possibility that this enzyme system might represent part of the binding macromolecular material. Protein kinase assays were carried out on homogenates and subcellular fractions of corpora lutea using histone as the substrate and a

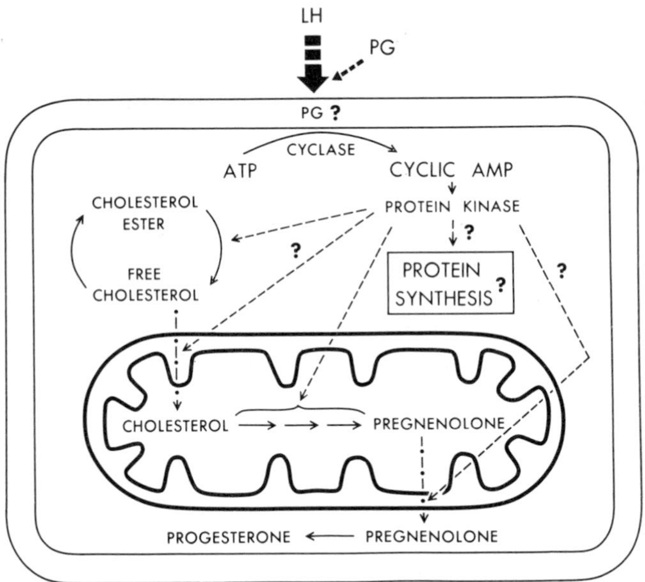

FIG 2. Current concept of LH action on steroidogenesis in the bovine corpus luteum. The abbreviation PG stands for prostaglandins. The solid arrows indicate biochemical conversions. The dashed arrows indicate stimulation. The -·-·-·-> arrows indicate transport across membranes.

minor modification of the method of Kuo et al. (17). It was found that corpora lutea did indeed contain a protein kinase and it was largely of the cyclic AMP-dependent type (14). Again the same 5 subcellular fractions were prepared as before with the exception that the homogenizing medium consisted of 0.25 M sucrose, 0.05 M tris buffer, pH 7.4, 0.25 M KCl, 0.005 M $MgCl_2$ to facilitate the assay of the enzyme. As with cyclic AMP, most of the protein kinase activity was present in the cytosol fraction (14). In addition, the enzyme activity in the cytosol was also retained by a PM-30 membrane upon ultrafiltration, indicating that protein kinase probably represents some of the macromolecular, cyclic AMP-binding material. This cyclic AMP-dependent protein kinase was then purified using standard techniques about 80-fold over that present in the cytosol (14, 18), and we have recently begun to determine, if it is involved in the action of cyclic AMP upon steroidogenesis. Preliminary data indicate that under appropriate conditions, cyclic AMP can stimulate cholesterol esterase activity (18) and cyclic AMP and protein kinase can accelerate the side-chain cleavage of cholesterol (19).

A summary of our present concept of the mechanism of LH action is illustrated in Fig. 2. We still believe that cyclic AMP is a mediator of the action of LH, but with regard to PGs, we are still uncertain of their role. Most of our data indicate that they are not involved in the action of LH, but the evidence is still inconclusive. Cyclic AMP seems to mediate the action of LH via a protein kinase and we are currently trying to establish the site of this action.

THE ACTION OF LH IN INITIATING THE PROCESS OF OVULATION

A. Preovulatory changes in steroidogenesis and cyclic AMP levels

In our studies on the action of LH on ovulation, we have used rabbit as the experimental animal, as it is a reflex ovulator and the time of ovulation can be reasonably predicted following mating or the injection of a hormone with LH activity (20,21). The first assessment of biochemical changes which occur during the process of ovulation viz. the measurement of steroidogenesis was done in our laboratory by Mills and Savard (22). Rabbits were sacrificed before and at intervals after mating. The large, mature Graafian follicles were dissected from the ovary (24), and their ability to incorporate (1 - ^{14}C) acetate into estrogens, androgens, progestins and other lipids *in vitro* was assessed. They found that follicles isolated from estrus rabbits exhibited a relatively low level of (1 - ^{14}C) acetate incorporation into all the steroids when incubated under control conditions, but showed a marked response to LH *in vitro*. Two hours after mating, both the control and LH-treated follicles showed high levels of incorporation. It appeared that at this interval the follicles were responding maximally to the high level of endogenous LH, which they were exposed to *in vivo*, and no further effect of LH could be elicited *in vitro*. At 12 hr after mating, the follicles incubated under control conditions again exhibited a low level of (1 - ^{14}C) acetate incorporation into steroids, but there was an almost total loss of the *in vitro* responsiveness to LH (22).

Thus, in the prevoulatory condition, the changes observed in _in vitro_ steroidogenesis and the LH responsiveness were very similar to the changes in the mass of estrogens and progestins in the ovarian venous blood (24) and the follicular fluid (25).

Based on our studies with the corpus luteum, we measured the accumulation of cyclic AMP in the isolated follicles on incubation, with the view of examining the possibility of this cyclic nucleotide being the mediator of this action of LH (26, 27). Graafian follicles were isolated from estrus rabbits and from rabbits at various intervals after the injection of an ovulatory dose of hCG. The isolated follicles were preincubated with (8 - ^{3}H) adenine, washed and incubated again under control conditions or in the presence of LH as described earlier. The ^{3}H-cyclic AMP was isolated and purified to radiochemical purity as described earlier in the corpus luteum studies. The follicles from estrus rabbits accumulated a low level of ^{3}H-cyclic AMP, but there was a marked increase in this accumulation when LH was included in the incubations, and this _in vitro_ stimulation was found to be specific for substances with luteinizing hormone activity. These data indicated that cyclic AMP might be a mediator of the action of LH on steroidogenesis. Following injection of hCG, there was a progressive decrease in the _in vitro_ responsiveness of these follicles to LH, until at 9 hr after hCG injection when the _in vitro_ effect of LH was no longer detectable. This loss of response to LH in terms of cyclic AMP synthesis could also be brought about by mating of the rabbit (27), and it paralleled the loss of responsiveness to LH in terms of steroidogenesis, described earlier.

B. Preovulatory changes in prostaglandin content

Since it had been proposed by other investigators that PGs might play a negative feed-back role in some tissues, it was of interest to study the involvement of PGs during the preovulatory phase in the ovarian tissue. Exogenous PGE$_1$ had been found to inhibit the rise in cyclic AMP brought about by epinephrine in adipose cells (28) and by vasopressin in kidney tissue (29). In addition, several groups of investigators (30, 31, 32) had shown that inhibitors of PG synthesis (indomethacin and aspirin) could block ovulation in rats and rabbits. This block could not be overcome by exogenous LH indicating that the inhibitors acted at the ovarian level.

In our experiments, Graafian follicles were isolated from estrus rabbits and from rabbits at various intervals after the injection of hCG. The amount of E and F prostaglandins in these follicles were measured by radioimmunoassay (30), using 2 specific antisera generously donated to us by Dr. Behrman of The Merck Institute for Therapeutic Research. We found that the follicles isolated from estrus rabbits had relatively low amounts of PGE and PGF. We have not yet determined which of the E or the F prostaglandins are present in this tissue as our radioimmunoassay does not distinguish between prostaglandins which differ only by the number of double bonds. At 1, 5 and 9 hr after the injection of hCG, there is a sharp increase in these substances and by 9 hr, the PGFs have increased 60-fold and the PGEs, 15-fold (33). The same type of rise could be brought by the injection of LH or by mating (34). Pretreatment of the rabbit with indomethacin 30 min prior to the injection of the gonadotropin completely abolished these increases (34). This finding supports the results of the radioimmunoassay and strengthens the proposal that follicular prostaglandins are directly involved in ovulation.

CONCLUSION

The preovulatory changes in steroidogenesis, cyclic AMP, prostaglandins, and the in _vitro_ responsiveness to LH just described, have led us to propose a hypothetical model on some aspects of ovulation (see Fig. 3). In this, we propose that LH acts by stimulating the adenylate cyclase and causing an increase in the accumulation of cyclic AMP, which in turn accelerates a limiting step in steroidogenesis, probably between cholesterol and pregnenolone. The evidence in support of this is that LH causes an increase in ^{3}H-cyclic AMP accumulation (29), and that exogenous cyclic AMP, in preliminary experiments, was found to increase the incorporation of (1 - ^{14}C) acetate into polar lipids, in isolated Graafian follicles (Mills, unpublished data). The steps between cholesterol and pregnenolone are the most likely site for the action of cyclic AMP, because they have been found to be the limiting steps in steroidogenesis in other steroidogenic tissues (35).

We also propose that cyclic AMP is a mediator of the action of LH which brings about a rise in PGs, on the basis of our preliminary data indicating that exogenous cyclic AMP can also cause a

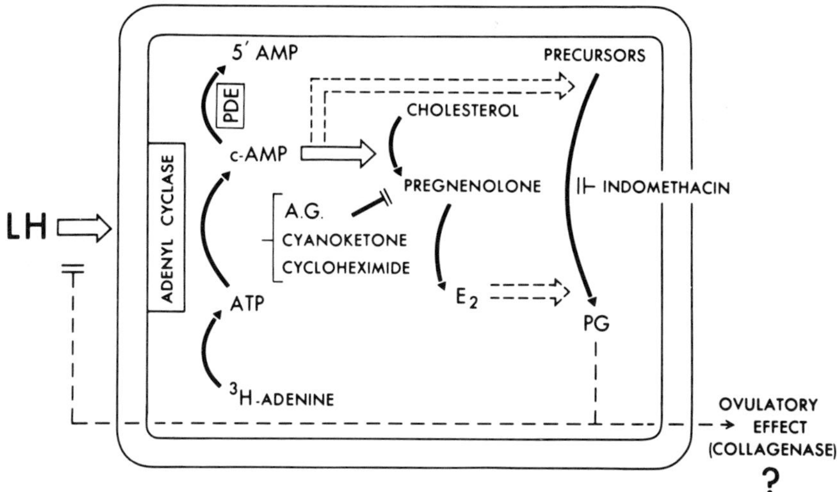

FIG 3. A hypothetical model of some aspects of ovulation. The abbreviations used are: LH = luteinizing hormone; cAMP = cyclic AMP; E_2 = estradiol; PG = prostaglandins; AG = aminoglutethimide. The solid arrows indicate biochemical conversions. The open and dashed arrows indicate stimulations. The symbol ⊤ indicates inhibition.

rise in follicular PGs in vitro. Since it is known that estrogens can increase the concentration of PGs in the uterus (36), and steroid synthesis inhibitors are known to block ovulation (37), it is possible that these steroids mediate this action of cyclic AMP. Another possibility is that cyclic AMP may activate a protein kinase, which in turn stimulates a lipase. The increased lipase activity could convert the esterified form of an unsaturated fatty acid, into its free form, which would be converted to a PG. It has been proposed that the limiting step in PG synthesis might be such a lipase-type of reaction (38); cyclic AMP has been shown to activate the hormone-sensitive triglyceride lipase of adipose tissue (39).

Finally we propose that increase in PGs results in the rupture of the follicular wall, possibly by activating a collagenase-like ovulatory enzyme. In addition, the increase in PGs is proposed to be responsible for the decreased in vitro responsiveness of the follicle to LH as the time of ovulation approaches. The reasons for these last two proposals are that: 1) Inhibitors of PG synthesis such as indomethacin block ovulation (30,32); and 2) PGE_1 has been found to inhibit the action of other hormones on cyclic AMP accumulation in their target tissues (28,29).

Some of the aspects of this hypothetical model may eventually prove to be incorrect to a greater or lesser degree, but we feel it serves a purpose in that it indicates several sites for further investigation.

REFERENCES

1. Mason, N.R., Marsh, J.M., and Savard, K., (1962). J. Biol. Chem. 237, 1801.
2. Marsh, J.M., and LeMaire, W.J., (1974). J. Clin. Endo. & & Metab. (in press).
3. Savard, K., Marsh, J.M., and Rice, B.F., (1965). Rec. Prog Horm. Res., 21, 285.
4. Marsh, J.M., and Savard, K., (1966). J. Reprod. & Fert. Suppl. 1, 113.
5. Haynes, R.C., Jr., Sutherland, E.W., and Rall, T.W., (1960) Rec. Prog. Horm. Res., 16, 121.
6. Marsh, J.M. and Savard, K., (1966). Steroids 8, 133.
7. Marsh, J.M., Butcher, R.W., Savard, K., and Sutherland, E.W., (1966). J. Biol. Chem., 241, 5436.
8. Marsh, J.M., (1970). J. Biol. Chem., 245, 1596.
9. Speroff, L. and Ramwell, P.W., (1970). J. Clin. Endo. & Metab., 30, 345.
10. Marsh, J.M. (1971). Ann. N.Y. Acad. Sci., 180, 416.
11. Kuehl, F.A., Jr., Humes, J.L., Tarnoff, J., Cirillo, V.J., and Ham, E.A., (1970). Science, 169, 883.
12. Kuo, J.F. and DeRenzo, E.C., (1967). J. Biol. Chem., 244, 2252.
13. Krishna, G., Weiss, B., and Brodie, B.B., (1968). J. Pharmacol. Expt. Ther., 163, 379.
14. Goldstein, S. and Marsh, J.M., (1973). The Fifth Annual Biochemistry-PCRI Miami Winter Symposia, Vol. 5, Protein

Phosphorylation in control mechanisms, Huijing, F. and Lee, E. Y. C., (Eds), Academic Press, New York. p. 123
15. Hanson, K.R., Ling, R., and Havir, E., (1967). Biochem. Biophys. Res. Commun., 29, 194.
16. Walsh, D.A., Brostrom, C.O., Brostrom, M.A., Chen, L., Corbin, J.D., Reiman, E., Soderling, T.R., and Krebs, E.G. (1972). Advances in Cyclic Nucleotide Research, 1, 33.
17. Kuo, J.F., Krueger, B.K., Sanes, J.R., and Greengard, P., (1970). Biochim. Biophys. Acta. 212, 79.
18. Goldstein, S., (1973). Ph.D. Dissertation, Univ. of Miami School of Medicine, Dept, of Biochemistry.
19. Caron, M.G. (1973). Ph.D. Dissertation, Univ. of Miami School of Medicine, Dept. of Biochemistry.
20. Walton, A., and Hammong, J., (1929). Brit. J. Exp. Biol., 6, 190.
21. Harper, M.J.K., (1963). J. Endocrinol. 26, 307.
22. Mills, T.M., and Savard, K., (1973). Endocrinology 92, 788.
23. Mills, T.M., Davies, P.J., and Savard, K., (1971). Endocrinology 88, 857.
24. Hilliard,J., and Eaton, L., M, (1971). Endocrinology 89, 552.
25. Younglai, E.V., (1972). J. Reprod. Fert., 30, 157.
26. Marsh, J.M., Mills, T.M., and LeMaire, W.J., (1972) Biochim. and Biophys. Acta. 273, 389.
27. Marsh, J.M., Mills, T.M., and LeMaire, W.J., (1973). Biochim. and Biophys. Acta. 304, 197.
28. Butcher, R.W. and Baird, C.E., (1968). J. Biol. Chem., 243, 1713.
29. Grantham, J.J. and Orloff, J., (1968). J. Lab. Clin. Invest., 47, 1154.
30. Orczyk, G.P. and Behrman, H.R., (1972). Prostaglandins, 1, 3.
31. Armstrong, D.T. and Grinwich, D.L., (1972). Prostaglandins 1, 21.
32. O'Grady, J.P., Caldwell, B.V., Auletta, F.J., and Speroff, L., (1972). Prostaglandins, 1, 97.
33. LeMaire, W.J., Yang, N.S.T., Behrman, H.R., and Marsh, J.M., (1973). Prostaglandins, 3, 367.
34. Yang, N.S.T., Marsh, J.M., and LeMaire, W.J., (1973). Prostaglandins (in press)
35. Hall, P.F. and Young, D.S., (1968). Endocrinology 82, 559.

36. Caldwell, B.V., Tillson, S.A., Brock, W.A., and Speroff, L., (1972). Prostaglandins, 1, 217.
37. Lipner, H. and Greep, R.O., (1971). Endocrinology 88, 602.
38. Kunze, H. and Vogt, W., (1971). Ann. N.Y. Acad. Sci., 180, 123.
39. Steinberg, D. and Huttunen, J.K., (1972). Advances in Cyclic Nucleotide Research 1, 47.

STUDIES ON THE MECHANISM OF ACTION OF LH

C. Das, G. L. Kumari and G. P. Talwar

Studies on two aspects of the action of LH are reported here and these are the synthesis of progesterone in isolated corpora lutea and the induction of ovulation in estrus rabbits.

STEROIDOGENIC ACTION

Corpora lutea of sheep respond in vitro to LH with enhanced synthesis of progesterone. 60 to 80 mg tissue was used and the progesterone formed was determined by a modification of the method of Watson et al. (1) as detailed in Figure 1. The kinetics of progesterone synthesized in the presence of LH is given in Figure 2; the effect is rapid and tends to plateau after 30 min. The dose-response curve for the action of LH is given in Figure 3. In a period of incubation of 15 min, the amount of progesterone synthesized varied with the dose of hormone, a maximum stimulation being seen beyond 0.1 μg/ml of LH.

In the next set of experiments, the requirement for continuous presence of LH for steroidogenesis was investigated. Three flasks (A, B & C) containing luteal slices were preincubated, B & C with LH (1 μg/ml), while A without LH for 5 min (Fig. 4). The tissues were washed thrice with buffer and further incubated in fresh buffer (A & B) and with 25 μl anti-LH serum (C) for 60 min. Incubation for 5 min was sufficient to stimulate production of progesterone. Anti-LH serum inhibited considerably progesterone synthesis, indicating that the hormone gets bound tightly to the tissue within 5 min and is not removed during washing; however, it is sensitive to inactivation by anti-LH.

A. Cyclic AMP and steroidogenesis

Cyclic AMP is recognised as an intracellular mediator of the actions of a number of hormones. It was found that LH stimulated the adenyl cyclase in homogenates of sheep corpora lutea (Fig 5), an observation consistent with that of others (3,4). Adenyl cyclase activity was measured by the method of Drummond

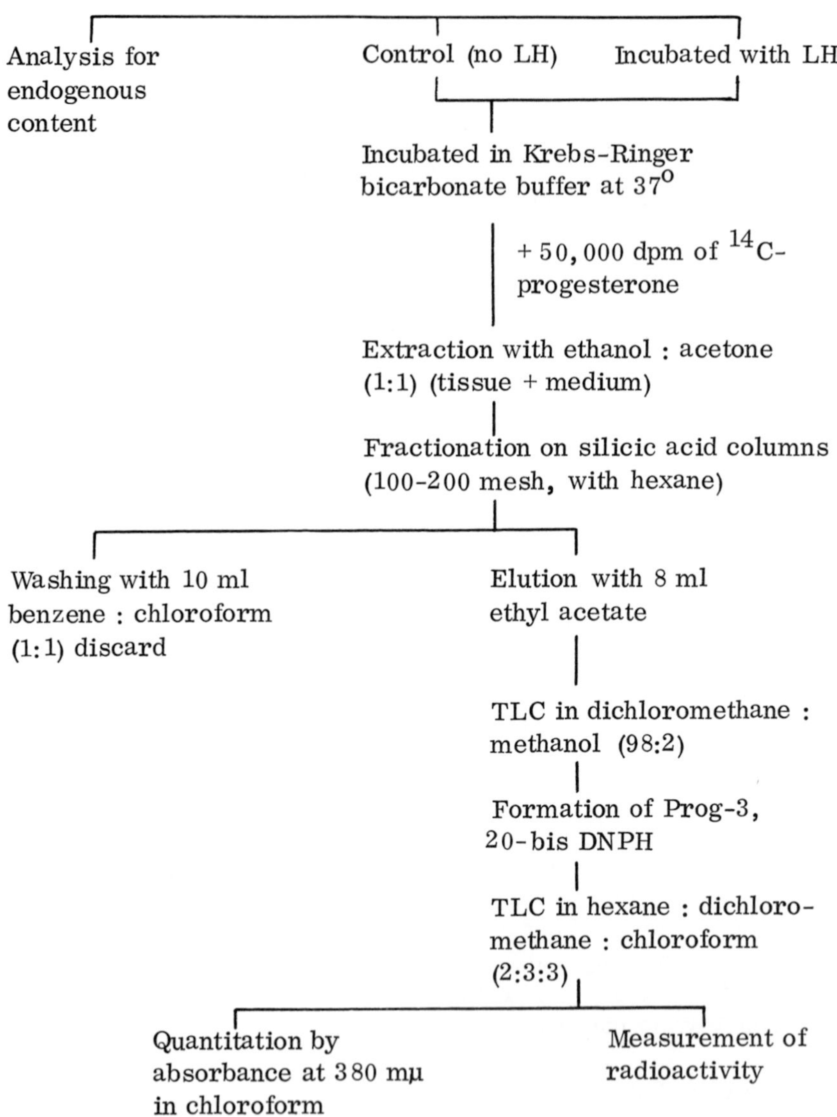

FIG 1. Procedure employed for determination of progesterone synthesized in the sheep corpus luteum slices *in vitro*.

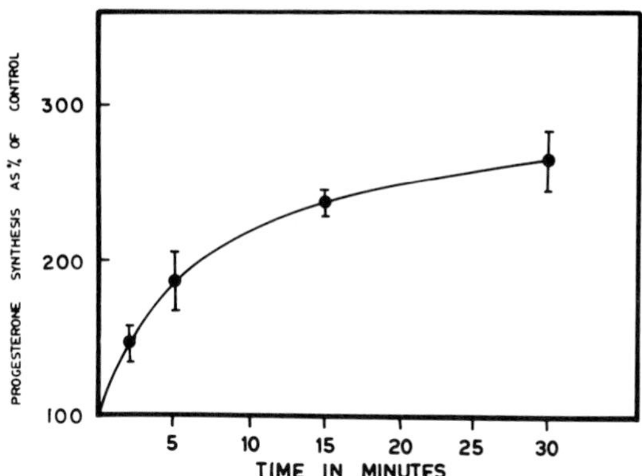

FIG 2. Kinetics of LH stimulated progesterone synthesis in sheep corpora lutea. Each point is a mean of 4 experiments ± SEM.

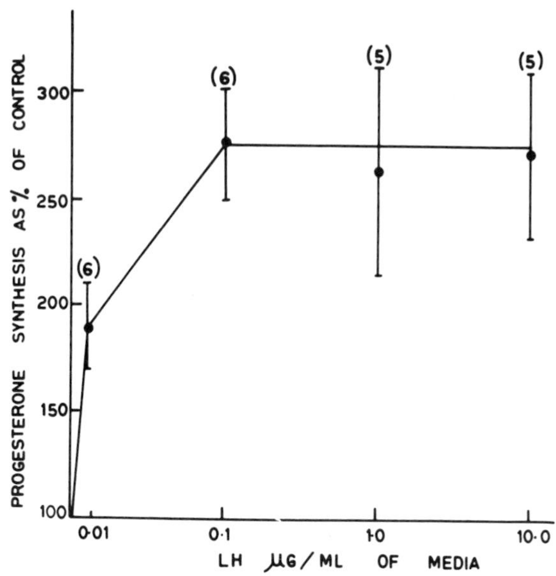

FIG 3. Dose response of LH action on the synthesis of progesterone. Figures in parenthesis denote the number of experiments. Mean ± SEM.

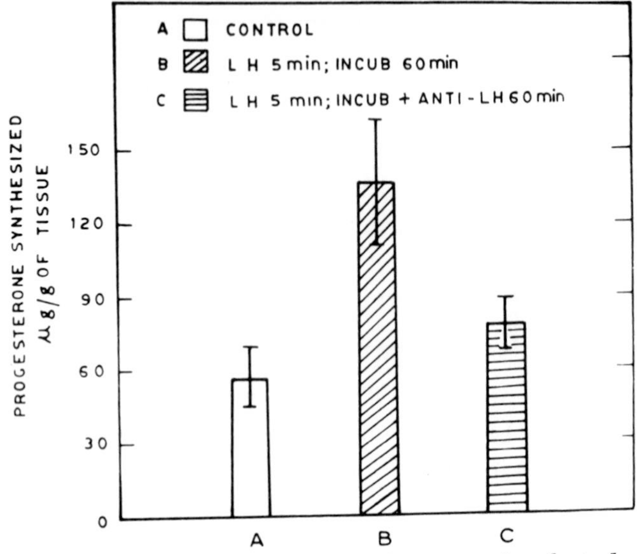

FIG 4. Effect of anti-LH on luteal slices preincubated with LH (Mean of 6 experiments ± SEM). See text for details.

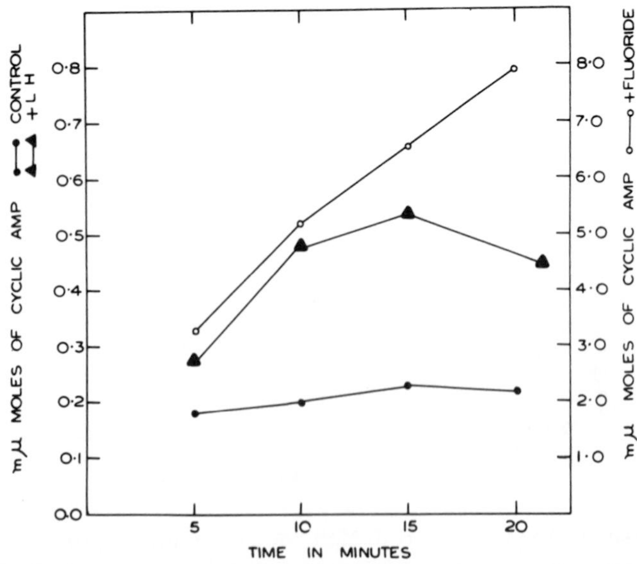

FIG 5. Action of LH on adenyl cyclase of sheep corpora lutea. Each point is mean of duplicate samples. See text for details.

and Duncan (2). Assay mixture contained in 110 µl, 40 mM Tris-HCl buffer (pH 7.5), 50 mM theophylline, 1 mM cAMP, 5.5 mM KCl, 15 mM $MgSO_4$, 20 mM phosphoenol pyruvate, 130 µg/ml of pyruvate kinase, 1 mM ATP-^{14}C (approx. 10^5 cpm) and 760 µg protein as enzyme source (luteal homogenate). The incubations were carried out in presence or absence of LH (10 µg/ml) and NaF (10 mM) at 37°.

Figures 6a and 6b show that chlorpromazine, which is known to inhibit the hormone-stimulated rise in adenyl cyclase at appropriate doses (5), does block the LH induced rise in adenyl cyclase as well as the synthesis of progesterone. Cyclic AMP when added to the incubation medium similar to LH, enhanced progesterone synthesis (Fig. 7). Thus LH action on steroidogenesis appeared to be mediated by cyclic AMP.

ROLE OF LH IN THE PROCESS OF OVULATION

While the steroidogenic action of LH is rapid, the effect of the hormone on ovulation is protracted by 10 to 12 hr. Although, there is no direct evidence available to conclude that cyclic AMP can mimic the action of LH in induction of ovulation in mammalian systems, Rondell (6) has reported that LH, cyclic AMP and progesterone have the ability to increase the distensibility of strips of follicular wall maintained in tissue culture.

To test whether cyclic AMP could initiate the process of ovulation, the nucleotide in amounts ranging from 5 to 500 µg was injected directly into one of the ovaries of rabbits using a microsyringe. No ovulation was detected in the injected or contralateral ovary in any animal. LH, if given by an identical procedure produced, however, ovulation in one or both of the ovaries depending on the dose (Table 1). Dibutyryl cyclic AMP employed at various doses (5 to 500 µg) was also found to be ineffective in induction of ovulation.

Figures 8 and 9 show that cyclic AMP injected by this route does permeate into the compartments affected by LH, as evidenced by the increase in the activities of two enzymes, alkaline phosphatase (EC 3.1.3.1) and ATPase (EC 3.6.1.3). The failure of cyclic AMP to cause ovulation under conditions in which LH induces ovulation suggests that this nucleotide is not adequate to mimic fully the actions of LH. Cyclic AMP in our experiments was injected into the stroma of the ovaries. It is not clear

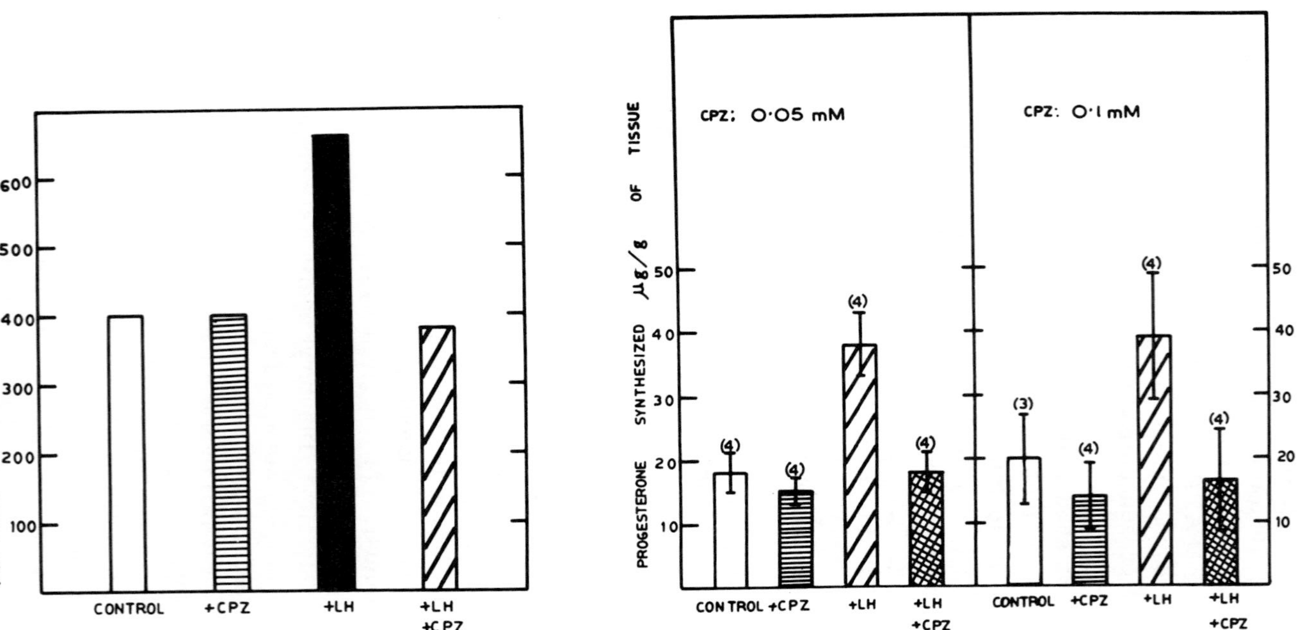

FIG 6. Effect of chlorpromazine (CPZ) on LH stimulated adenyl cyclase activity (6a, left) and progesterone synthesis (6b, right) in corpora lutea.

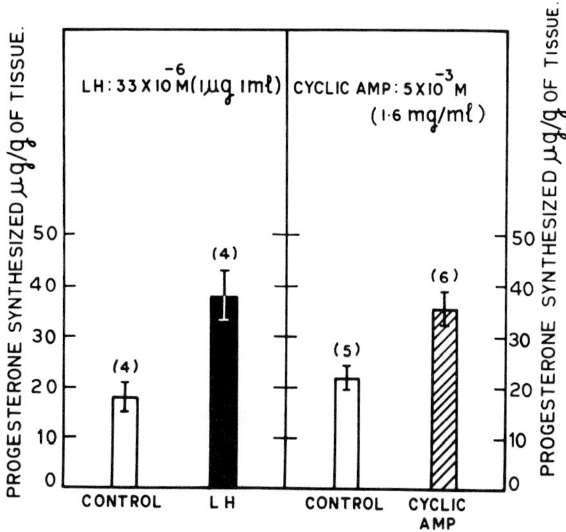

FIG 7. Stimulation of progesterone synthesis in luteal slices by cyclic AMP.

Table 1. Effect of intraovarian injection of LH, on ovulation in rabbits

Substance	Dose (µg)	No. of ovaries treated	No. of follicles ovulated in the ovaries	
			Treated	Control
	10	5	18	6
	5	6	21	7
LH	4	4	17	3
	2	5	11	0
	1	5	16	0

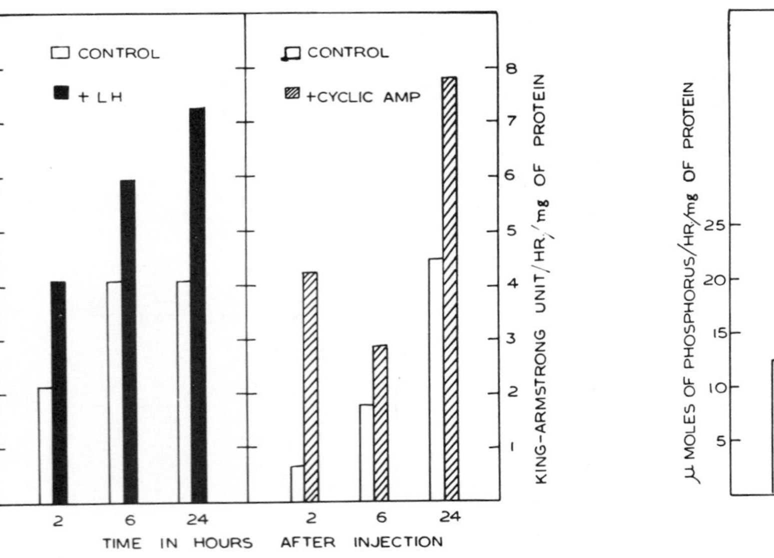

FIG 8. Effect of intraovarian injection of LH (1 µg) and cAMP (5 µg) on the alkaline phosphatase activity. Hormone or nucleotide was injected in 1 µl saline into one of the ovaries and the other received only saline. Values are mean of duplicate assays in two typical experiments (13).

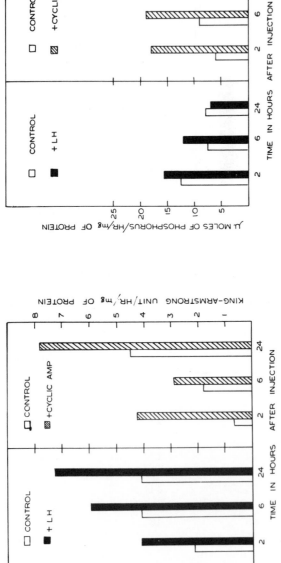

FIG 9. Effect of intraovarian injection of LH (1 µg) or cyclic AMP (5 µg) on the ATPase activity in the rabbit gonad. The experimental procedure was the same as given under Fig 8 (13).

whether the same type of cells are influenced by both cyclic AMP and LH when administered by this route as only the latter is capable of inducing ovulation. Interestingly enough, intrafollicular injection of dibutyryl cyclic AMP in chick is known to cause ovulation (7).

A. Pattern of steroid production in ovaries injected with LH or cyclic AMP

The pattern of steroids in the follicles after an intraovarian injection of LH or cyclic AMP at various time intervals has been studied. Follicles of approximately 0.5 to 1.0 mm diameter were removed from the ovaries of rabbits. They were dissected free of stromal tissue, washed with saline, placed in vials containing chilled saline and frozen at -20°C until analysis. After adding

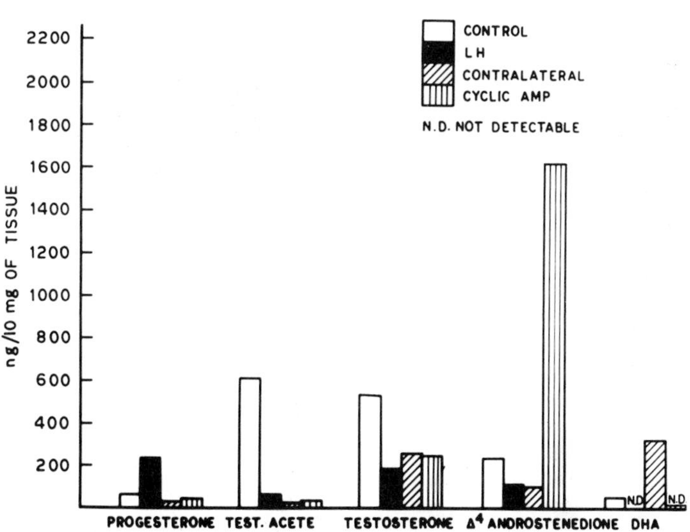

FIG 10. Steroid levels in follicles at 8 hr after intraovarian injections of LH or cyclic AMP.

3 ml of 5 N NaOH, follicles were homogenized and extracted with 3 x 20 ml ether. The dried ether extract was partitioned between benzene : petroleum ether (1:1) and 1.6 % NaOH. The former contained neutral steroids which were separated by thin layer chromatography (TLC) using chloroform : acetone (98:2) solvent system. The corresponding hormones were located by autoradiography and purified further by acetylation and TLC followed by gas-liquid chromatography.

The follicles obtained from LH treated ovaries showed preovulatory rise in progesterone and a low level of androgens before ovulation (Figures 10 and 11), whereas in the follicles of cyclic AMP-treated ovaries, progesterone level remained low while androgens were present in high amounts. The importance of steroids (6, 8-10) and other agents such as prostaglandins (11, 12) as triggers in the ovulation process has been indicated by various studies.

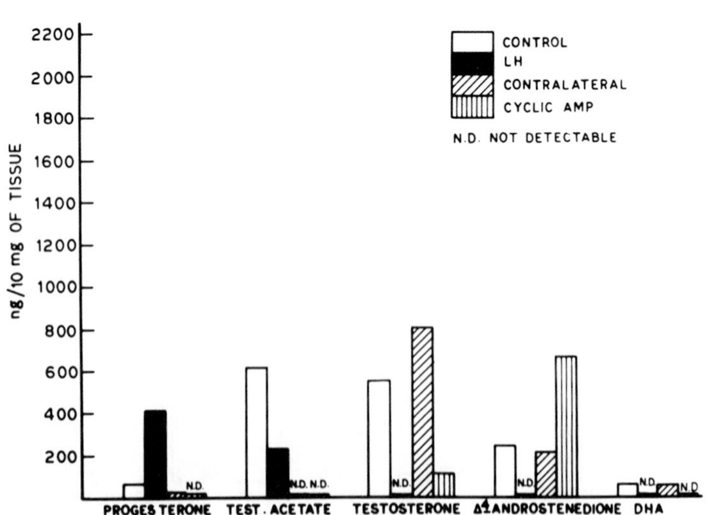

FIG 11. Steroid levels in follicles at 11 hr after intraovarian injection of LH or cAMP.

CONCLUDING REMARKS

LH stimulates the synthesis of progesterone from endogenous substrates in corpus luteum in vitro. This action is probably mediated by cyclic AMP in view of the following observations. (i) LH activates luteal adenyl cyclase; (ii) cyclic AMP added to the medium mimics the enhanced synthesis of progesterone induced by LH and (iii) inhibitors of hormone-stimulated adenyl cyclase block steroidogenesis.

Intraovarian injections of cyclic AMP or dibutyryl cyclic AMP fail to induce ovulation in estrus rabbits in conditions in which LH brings about ovulation. The cyclic nucleotide effect is discernible, however, on two ovarian enzymes - alkaline phosphatase and ATPase which are also stimulated by intraovarian injections of LH. Cyclic AMP mimics therefore, some but not all the actions of LH in the ovary. Notable differences were observed in the pattern of steroids synthesized in follicles at different time intervals after an intraovarian injection of LH or cyclic AMP.

ACKNOWLEDGEMENTS

This work was supported by research grants of The Population Council Inc., New York, the World Health Organization (Human Reproduction Division), the Council of Scientific and Industrial Research, New Delhi, and PL-480 grant No. NR 202-028 of the Office of Naval Research. Shri Sri Chand rendered valuable technical assistance.

REFERENCES

1. Watson, D.J., Romanoff, E.B., Kato, J. and Bartosik, D.B. (1967). Anal. Biochem. 20, 233.
2. Drummond, G.I. and Duncan, L. (1970). J. Biol. Chem. 245, 976.
3. Dorrington, J.M. and Bagget, B. (1969). Endocrinology 84, 989.
4. Marsh, J.M. (1970). J. Biol. Chem. 245, 1596.
5. Wolf, J. and Jones, A.B. (1970). Proc. Natl. Acad. Sci. 65, 454.
6. Rondell, P. (1970). Fed. Proc. 29, 1875.

7. Kao, L. W. L. and Nalbandov, A. V. (1972). Endocrinology 90, 1343.
8. Lipner, H. and Wendelker, L. (1971). Proc. Soc. Exptl. Biol. Med. 136, 1141.
9. Lostroh, A. J. (1971). Fed. Proc. 30, 595.
10. Lipner, H. and Greep, R. O. (1971). Endocrinology 88, 602.
11. Grinwich, D. L., Kennedy, T. G. and Armstrong, D. T. (1972). Prostaglandins 1, 89.
12. O'Grady, J. P., Caldwell, B. V., Auletta, F. J. and Speroff, L. (1972). Prostaglandins 1, 97.
13. Das, C. and Talwar, G. P. (1974). J. Reprod. Fertil (in press).

THE ROLE OF CYTOCHROME P.450 IN THE SIDE-CHAIN CLEAVAGE OF CHOLESTEROL

Peter F. Hall and Mikio Shikita

INTRODUCTION

The biosynthesis of steroid hormones in the gonads, adrenal and placenta involves the conversion of cholesterol to pregnenolone; it would appear that under normal conditions this step is obligatory for the synthesis of the steroid hormones (1). This conversion involves a side-chain cleavage of cholesterol resulting in the removal of a 6-carbon fragment in the form of isocapraldehyde (2); this has been considered the rate-determining step in the biosynthetic pathway of steroid hormones and is specifically stimulated by the tropic hormones ACTH and ICSH (3-6).

Side-chain cleavage of cholesterol occurs in the mitochondria of steroid-forming organs and requires TPNH and oxygen (7). It is known that such mitochondria and partly purified enzymes derived therefrom, are capable of converting 20 α hydroxycholesterol and 20 α , 22-dihydroxycholesterol to pregnenolone (2, 8, 9). The circumstances under which this conversion occurs suggested that side-chain cleavage may proceed according to the following pathway:

$$\text{Cholesterol} \xrightarrow{[\text{TPNH; } O_2]} 20\alpha\text{-OH-Chol} \xrightarrow{[\text{TPNH; } O_2]}$$

$$20\alpha, 22\xi\text{-diOH-Chol} \xrightarrow{[?]} \text{Pregnenolone}.$$

In spite of the inherent appeal of this proposal, evidence to the contrary has been presented (10, 11) with the result that the mechanism of side-chain cleavage remains uncertain.

It is known that hydroxylation of steroids by adrenocortical microsomes (12) and hydroxylation of various drugs by hepatic microsomes (13) require the unusual hemeprotein, cytochrome P.450. Such a hemeprotein is also required for 11 β -hydroxylation in the biosynthesis of adrenal steroids; this reaction occurs in mitochondria and can be reconstituted in vitro by mixing three purified proteins, namely a yellow flavoprotein (diaphorase), non-heme iron (adrenodoxin) and P.450 (14). When these proteins are together provided with TPNH, atmospheric (molecular) oxygen and a suitable substrate, the substrate is hydroxylated at the 11 β -position.

$$\begin{array}{ccccccccc} TPNH & & FP & & NHFe^{++} & & P_{450}\,Fe^{+++} & O_2 & Steroid \\ & \times & & \times & & \times & & \times & \\ TPN^{+} & & FPH_2 & & NHFe^{+++} & & P_{450}\,Fe^{++} & & Steroid\text{-}OH + OH^{-} \end{array}$$

These observations prompted examination of the question of whether side-chain cleavage required P.450 for the hydroxylation reactions which were proposed as part of this reaction. It was soon discovered that mitochondrial P.450 is indeed required for side-chain cleavage (15, 16); this observation was taken to support the proposed pathway involving hydroxylation at C_{20} and C_{22}.

P.450 is also required for at least two additional mitochondrial reactions involving steroid hydroxylation, namely: 18-hydroxylation in connection with the synthesis of aldosterone (17) and the side-chain cleavage of cholesterol sulfate to give pregnenolone sulfate (a reaction which occurs without cleavage of the sulfate-ester bond) (18-20). Evidence from kinetic data (20) suggested the presence of more than one species of P.450 in adrenocortical mitochondria capable of catalyzing all the above reactions and partial purification of P.450 seemed consistent with this view (21,22).

These observations clearly pointed to the need for further purification of P.450. The present studies describe the isolation, in near homogeneity, of a P.450 specific for side-chain cleavage and examine its involvement in the putative pathway by measurement of the stoichiometry of the reaction with cholesterol and hydroxycholesterols as substrates. For technical reasons these studies were performed with bovine adrenal cortex, but all that is presently known concerning side-chain cleavage suggests that this reaction proceeds by the same pathway and is subject to analogous regulatory devices in all the steroid-forming organs.

METHODS

The methods used to prepare and characterize the adrenocortical cytochrome P.450 which forms the subject of this paper, have been published in detail elsewhere (23, 24). The methods used in measuring the stoichiometry of side chain cleavage have also been published (25).

RESULTS

A. Properties of side-chain cleavage P.450.

Figure 1 shows certain important features of the adrenocortical P.450 described here. On Bio-gel A-15m, the enzyme

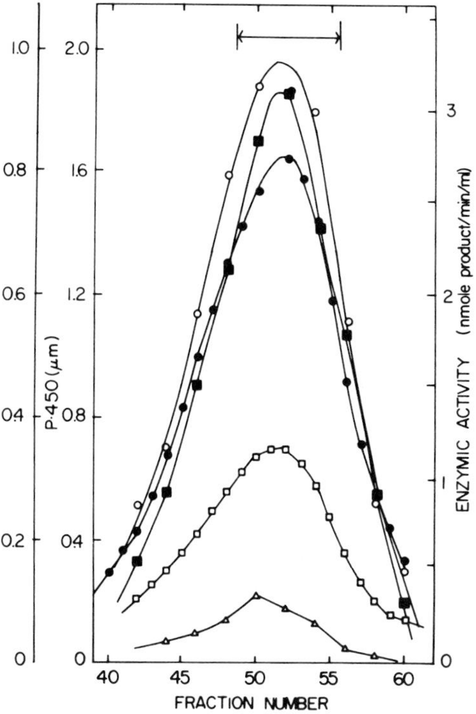

FIG 1. Chromatography of P.450 on Bio-gel A-15m. ●, A_{280}; □, A_{415}; ○, side chain cleavage; △, 11β-hydroxylase; ■, P.450 content.

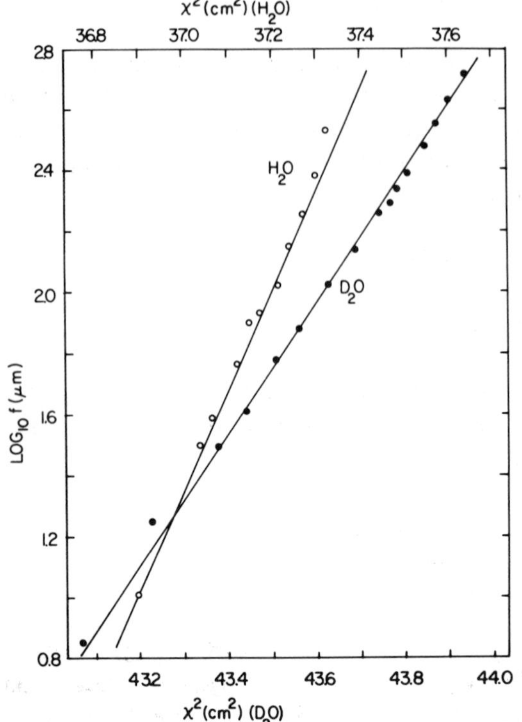

FIG 2. Analytical ultracentrifugation of cytochrome P.450.

behaves as a single peak and shows side-chain cleavage activity with minimal 11 β-hydroxylase. Moreover the enzyme is homogeneous or very nearly so, as indicated by the linear relationship observed between square of the radial distance and $\log_{10}$ recorder deflection on sedimentation equilibrium (Fig 2). The difference between the relationships observed in H_2O and D_2O provides the basis for the calculation of partial specific volume (0.765) and hence molecular weight (850,000). Sedimentation equilibrium in 6M guanidine hydrochloride (Fig 3) reveals that this P.450 is made up of 16 subunits which appear to be of the same size (MW53,000) (24); P.450 has 8 heme groups per molecule.

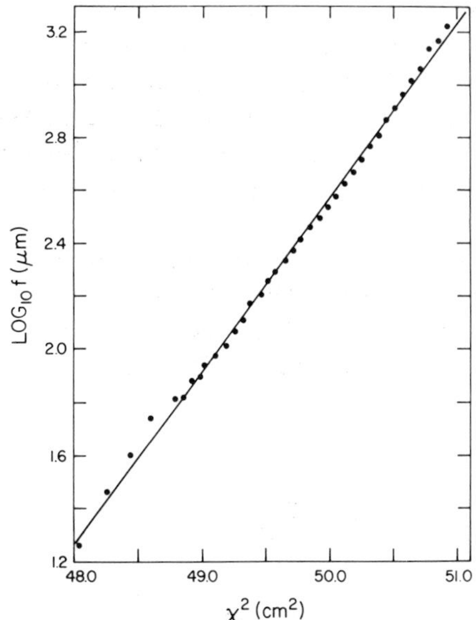

FIG 3. Sedimentation equilibrium of cytochrome P.450 performed in 6M guanidine hydrochloride. Rotor speed 30,000 rpm; temperature, 20°; protein concentration, 0.70 mg per ml.

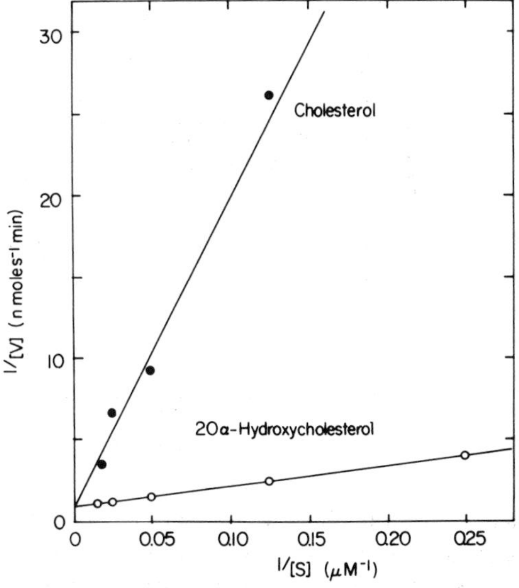

FIG 4. Lineweaver-Burk plots of side-chain cleavage with cholesterol and 20α-hydroxycholesterol as substrates.

Examination of the enzymatic activity of this P.450 reveals that it supports side-chain cleavage of cholesterol and 20 α - hydroxycholesterol with the same Vmax (20.6 nmoles/min/mg protein) but with different values for Km, namely: 0.19 mM and 0.012 mM respectively (Fig 4). The enzyme is without demonstrable 18-hydroxylase activity and shows little 11 β -hydroxylase activity (23).

Figure 5 shows certain important spectral properties of cytochrome P.450 from bovine adrenocortical mitochondria. The absolute spectrum shows five peaks (395, 412, 520, 565 and 650 nm), together with a small shoulder at 360 nm.

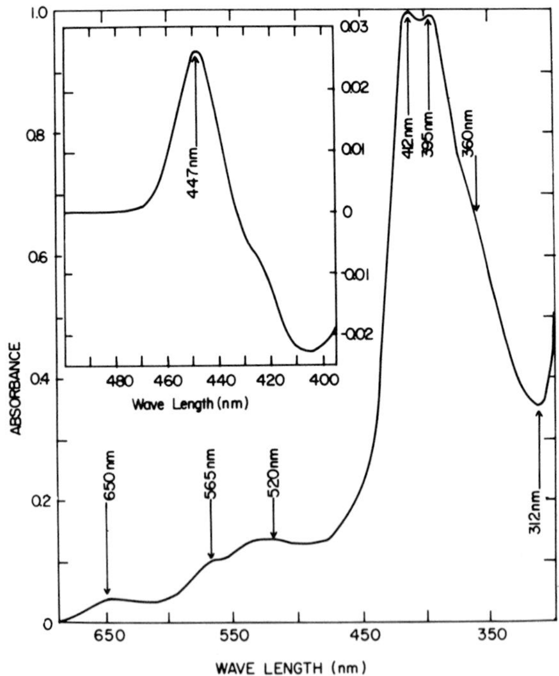

FIG 5. Absorption spectroscopy of cytochrome P.450. Full scale for absorbance with the absolute spectrum is 1.0 while that for CO-difference spectrum is 0.1.

The spectrum shows a trough at 312 nm. The carbon monoxide difference spectrum shows a peak at 447 nm and a small shoulder at 420 nm.

B. Stoichiometry of side-chain cleavage.

Figure 6 shows the side-chain cleavage of cholesterol when the oxidation of TPNH and the consumption of oxygen are measured as a function of the concentration of P.450. It can be seen that oxidation of TPNH and consumption of oxygen take place in the absence of added substrate. This background reaction is not accompanied by side-chain cleavage because of the enzyme is essentially devoid of endogenous cholesterol (23) and no pregnenolone ($<$ 0.05 nmoles/flask) is formed during this reaction. The stoichiometry, calculated as increase of oxidation of TPNH and utilization of oxygen above background (referred to here as Δ TPNH oxidation and Δ oxygen consumption), is 3:3:1 (TPNH: oxygen: side-chain cleavage) and is independent of the concentration of P.450. Nineteen determinations using three separate prepreations of P.450 revealed ratios of TPNH/side-chain cleavage of 3.0 $\pm$ 0.2 (range) and for O_2/side-chain cleavage 3.2 $\pm$ 0.4 (range).

Table 1 shows that the stoichiometry with 20 α -hydroxycholesterol is 2:2:1. In 12 determinations with 20 α -hydroxycholesterol the following values were obtained (means and ranges): TPNH oxidized/cholesterol cleaved: 1.9 $\pm$ 0.3; oxygen used/cholesterol cleaved : 2.1 $\pm$ 0.3; with 20 α , 22-dihydroxycholesterol the corresponding values were 1.0 $\pm$ 0.3 and 0.9 $\pm$ 0.4. Table 1 also shows the stoichiometry with cholesterol (3:3:1); the value shown for the stoichiometry with oxygen (3.6) is the highest value observed in these studies. Stoichiometry did not change when higher substrate concentrations were used (20.0 mM).

The consumption of hydrogen ions in relation to side-chain cleavage is shown in Table 2. It is clear that, as expected, one mole of H^+ is consumed for each mole of TPNH oxidized and hence 3 moles of H^+ are consumed per mole of cleavage with cholesterol as substrate.

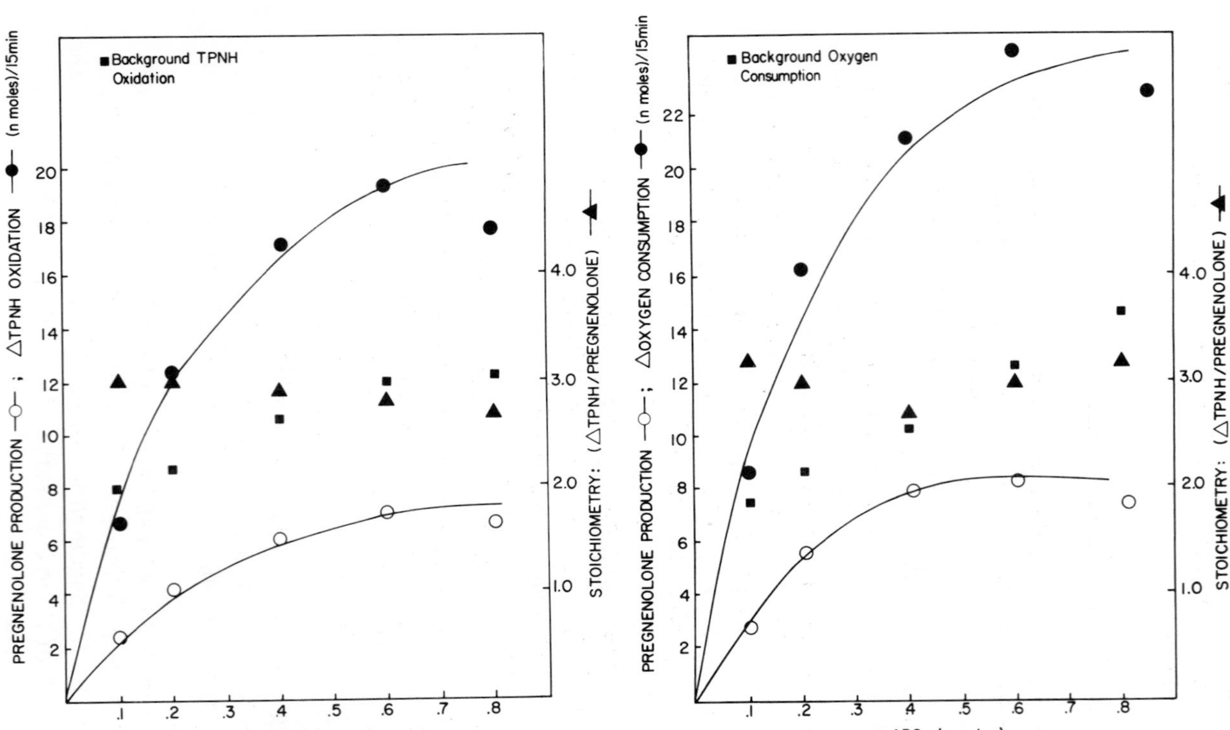

FIG 6. Utilization of TPNH (left) and oxygen (right) with and without substrate (cholesterol) as a function of concentration of P.450. The figures also show the ratios: △ TPNH/pregnenolone formed and △ oxygen/pregnenolone formed. Incubation time was 15 min.

Table 1. Stoichiometry of side-chain cleavage of cholesterol and hydroxycholesterols

Substrate	Rate of formation of pregnenolone	Rate of consumption of TPNH	$\frac{\Delta \text{TPNH}}{\text{Pregnenolone}}$	Rate of formation of pregnenolone	Rate of consumption of oxygen	$\frac{\Delta O_2}{\text{Pregnenolone}}$
	(nmoles/20 min)			(nmoles/20 min)		
Cholesterol	2.4	7.9	3.3	3.5	12.7	3.6
20α-OH-cholesterol	7.5	14.7	2.0	9.1	17.1	1.9
Di-OH-cholesterol	7.2	7.1	1.0	7.4	11.0	1.5

Table 2. Consumption of hydrogen ions during side-chain cleavage of cholesterol

Rate of formation of pregnenolone	Rate of consumption of hydrogen ions	$\frac{\Delta H^+}{\text{Pregnenolone}}$
(nmoles/20 min)		
3.2	9.7	3.03
2.1	6.5	3.0
3.7	11.4	3.10

Side-chain cleavage of cholesterol and 20 α -hydroxycholesterol was not accompanied by accumulation of reaction intermediates, so that formation of pregnenolone was accounted for by disappearance of cholesterol or 20 α -hydroxycholesterol within the limits of experimental error.

DISCUSSION

One species of cytochrome P.450 has been prepared from adrenocortical mitochondria in a state of near-homogeneity. This P.450 is a large molecule (850,000 MW) composed of 16 subunits and is specific for side-chain cleavage; it cannot be determined at this time whether the small amount of 11 β -hydroxylase activity is due to a trace contaminant or to an inherent property of the molecule itself. In keeping with studies performed with crude mitochondrial enzyme systems, our preparation catalyses cleavage of cholesterol without accumulation of hydroxycholesterols and is also capable of cleaving the side-chains of 20 α -hydroxycholesterol and 20 α , 22-dihydroxycholesterol.

When this P.450 is mixed with highly purified diaphorase and non-heme iron, together with TPNH and cholesterol, it is possible to measure production of pregnenolone, oxidation of TPNH and the consumption of oxygen and hydrogen ions. From these data, the stoichiometry of the side-chain cleavage reaction can be computed. The enzyme system is free of endogenous cholesterol so that in the absence of exogenous substrate, no pregnenolone is formed. It is not surprising, however, to find that oxidation of TPNH and consumption of oxygen take place in the absence of side-chain cleavage; presumably this represents gratuitous transport of electrons between the various components of the system. The additional oxidation of TPNH and consumption of oxygen seen when exogenous substrate was added, was used to compute the stoichiometry of the reaction. Under these conditions the stoichiometry for the side-chain cleavage of cholesterol was as follows:

Cholesterol $\pm$ 3TPNH + $3H^+$ + $3O_2$ $\rightarrow$ pregnenolone + isocapraldehyde + $3TPN^+$ + $4H_2O$.

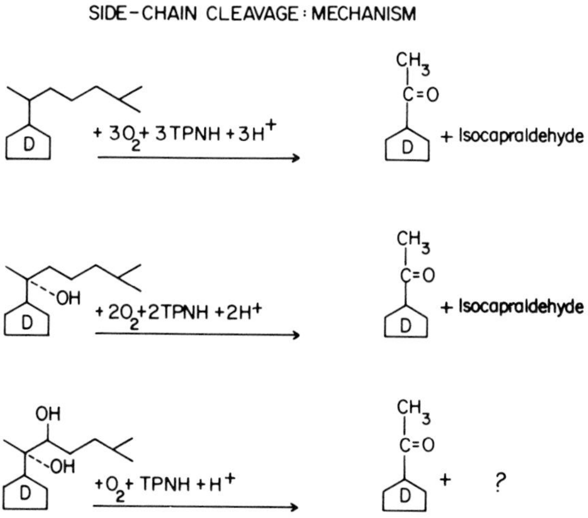

SIDE-CHAIN CLEAVAGE: MECHANISM

FIG 7. Scheme for the roles of TPNH and oxygen in the side-chain cleavage of cholesterol and hydroxycholesterols.

The stoichiometries observed with the two hydroxycholesterols (Table 1) are consistent with the scheme proposed in Fig 7; with 20 α -hydroxycholesterol as substrate, 1 mole of TPNH and 1 mole of O_2 are presumably used to hydroxylate C_{22} and as the lower line of the figure indicates, the same agents are required for the cleavage of the dihydroxy derivative accounting for the second mole of TPNH and the second mole of oxygen needed for cleavage of 20α -hydroxycholesterol. These observations are consistent with the scheme proposed in the introduction above. Moreover the studies with 20α, 22-dihydroxycholesterol as substrate confirm the report of Shimizu (26) which showed that side-chain cleavage of this substance requires TPNH and oxygen.

At least two observations in the literature appear to be inconsistent with the present findings. Firstly, Hall and Koritz (10) reported that when ^3H-cholesterol was incubated with an acetone powder of adrenocortical mitochondria, exogenous 20α-hydroxycholesterol added to the incubation medium could be isolated, following incubation, without detectable tritium. Under a variety of experimental conditions the production of pregnenolone - ^{3}H could be accounted for by disappearance of cholesterol - ^{3}H within the limits of experimental error. If 20 α -hydroxycholesterol is an intermediate in this reaction, it must be present in extremely small amounts in a form which does not permit exchange with exogenous 20 α -hydroxycholesterol.

A second discordant observation was reported by Luttrell et al. (11), who showed that an analogue of 20 α -hydroxycholesterol in which C_{22} is completely substituted by methyl groups is converted to pregnenolone by a crude enzyme system from adrenocortical mitochondria. Since one product of side-chain cleavage of the analogue, the stoichiometry and the rate of the reaction are not known, it is not possible to choose between various theoretically acceptable mechanisms for cleavage of the analogue. At this point the relevance of the cleavage of the analogue to that of cholesterol is uncertain.

It is therefore concluded that our findings appear to uphold the mechanism for side-chain cleavage postulated in earlier studies (2, 8, 9) and are difficult to reconcile with ionic and free radical mechanisms (11).

ACKNOWLEDGEMENT

The authors wish to acknowledge support under Public Health Services Grant 1 RO1 CA14638-01.

REFERENCES

1. Hall, P.F. (1970). In "The Testis", A.D. Johnson, W.R. Gomes and N.L. Vandermark (Eds). Vol. II, pp 16, Academic Press, New York.
2. Constantopoulos, G. and Tchen, T.T. (1961). J. Biol. Chem. 236, 65.
3. Karaboyas, G.C. and Koritz, S.B. (1965). Biochemistry 4, 462.
4. Hall, P.F. and Koritz, S.B. (1965). Biochemistry 4, 1037.

5. Hall, P.F. (1966). Endocrinology 78, 690.
6. Hall, P.F. and Young, D.G. (1968). Endocrinology 82, 559.
7. Halkerston, I.D.K., Eichborn, J. and Hechter, O. (1961) J. Biol. Chem. 236, 374.
8. Shimizu, K., Gut, M. and Dorfman, R.I. (1962). J. Biol. Chem. 237, 699.
9. Constantopoulos, G., Carpenter, A., Satoh, P.S. and Tchen, T.T. (1966). Biochemistry 5, 1650.
10. Hall, P.F. and Koritz, S.B. (1964). Biochim. Biophys. Acta 93, 441.
11. Luttrell, B., Hochberg, R.B., Dixon, R.W., McDonald, P.D. and Lieberman, S. (1972). J. Biol. Chem. 247, 1462.
12. Cooper, D.Y., Estabrook, R.W. and Rosenthal, O. (1963). J. Biol. Chem. 238, 1320.
13. Cooper, D.Y., Levin, S., Narasimhulu, S., Rosenthal, O. and Estabrook, R.W. (1966). Science 147, 400.
14. Omura, T., Sanders, E., Estabrook, R.W., Cooper, D.Y. and Rosenthal, O. (1966) Archives Biochem. Biophys. 117, 660.
15. Hall, P.F. (1967). Biochemistry 6, 2794.
16. Simpson, E.R. and Boyd, G.S. (1967). Eur. J. Biochem. 2, 275.
17. Greengard, P., Psychoyos, S., Tallan, H.E., Cooper, D.Y, Rosenthal, A. and Estabrook, R.W. (1967). Archives Biochem. Biophys. 121, 298.
18. Raggatt, P.R. and Whitehouse, M.W. (1966). Biochem. J. 101, 819.
19. Roberts, K.B., Bandi, L. and Lieberman, S. (1967). Biochem. Biophys. Res. Comm. 29, 741.
20. Young, D.G. and Hall, P.F. (1969). Biochemistry 8, 2989.
21. Jefcoate, C.R., Hume, R. and Boyd, G.S. (1970). FEBS Letters 9, 41.
22. Young, D.G., Holroyd, J. and Hall, P.F. (1970). Biochem. Biophys. Res. Comm. 38, 184.
23. Shikita, M. and Hall, P.F. (1973). J. Biol. Chem. 248, 5598.
24. Shikita, M. and Hall, P.F. (1973). J. Biol. Chem. 248, 5605.
25. Shikita, M. and Hall, P.F. (1973). Proc. Natl. Acad. Sci. (in press)
26. Shimizu, K. (1968). Arch. Biochem. Biophys. 125, 1016.

GONADOTROPIN-RECEPTOR ACTIVITY AND GRANULOSA-LUTEAL CELL DIFFERENTIATION

A.R. Midgley, Jr., A.J. Zeleznik, H.J. Rajaniemi, J.S. Richards and L.E. Reichert, Jr.

INTRODUCTION

It is apparent that gonadotropin-mediated ovarian responses are not only a function of concentrations of biologically active gonadotropins, but also of target cell responsiveness. Current concepts of gonadotropin action suggest that target cell responsiveness may be a function of the availability of hormone-specific receptor as well as of the efficiency by which the hormone-receptor interaction is mediated within the target cell. ("Receptor" is here used to signify a saturable, high affinity binding component which is presumed, but not necessarily proven, to be coupled to responsive systems).

In studies summarized here, attention has been focused on the changes in LH- and FSH-receptor which occur as granulosa cells differentiate and luteinize and the changes which the resulting luteal cells undergo throughout the life span of the corpus luteum. The studies have involved qualitative and quantitative binding analyses _in vivo_ and _in vitro_ using rat FSH and hCG labeled with ^{125}I. It is presumed, on the basis of published data (1-3) that the ^{125}I-hCG binds to the LH-specific receptor.

MATERIALS AND METHODS

A. Hormones

Partially purified hCG (2950 IU/mg; Roussel Corp., New York City) was further purified by chromatography on DEAE-Sephadex and gel filtration on Sephadex G-100 essentially as described by Bahl et al. (4). Details concerning the purification will be given elsewhere. The final product appeared homogeneous on electrophoresis in 7, 9 and 11 % polyacrylamide gels (95 % acrylamide, 5 % methylene bisacrylamide) at pH 8.9 in 0.01 M boric acid, 0.0032 M disodium EDTA and 0.77 M tris buffer. Bioassay (using an _in vitro_, collagenase-dissociated progesterone-synthesizing immature ovarian cell system) (5) indicated the material to have an activity of 11,550 IU/mg. Highly purified rat FSH LER-1422 (6) , had an activity 60 x NIH-FSH-S1 in ovarian augmentation assay and LH activity of 0.01 x NIH-LH-S1 in ovarian ascorbic acid assay. PMSG was obtained through the courtesy of the rat pituitary hormone program of the NIAMDD, Bethesda. Ovine FSH (LER-1654-3, 5.49 x NIH-FSH-S1 and $<$ 0.01 x NIH-LH-S1) and oLH (LER-1374 A (38-49), 2.01 x NIH-LH-S1 and $<$ 0.043 x NIH-FSH-S1) were prepared as described elsewhere (7, 8).

B. Radioiodination

Purified hCG and rFSH were each labeled with radioactive sodium (^{125}I) iodide using the low temperature (0°), short time (20 sec), minimal chloramine-T conditions described by Catt et al. (9) and Leidenberger and Reichert (10). The mass of each preparation was assessed by radioreceptor assay using ^{131}I- hormone as the labeled ligand.

C. Preparation of receptor-rich pellets

Depending on the nature of each experiment, receptor-rich pellets were prepared variously from fresh corpora lutea, residual non-luteal tissue, or frozen (-70°) whole ovaries. The tissue was gently homogenized by hand at 0° in a Kontes ground glass tissue grinder in 0.01 M phosphate buffered saline, pH 7.0, containing 0.1 % gelatin (PBS-gel) to give appropriate tissue concentrations (10-50 mg/ml). The resulting homogenate was centrifuged at 40,000 g for 20 min, the pellet resuspended in PBS-gel to a concentration of 400 µg/10 µl by gentle Teflon-glass homogenization, and dispensed into individual tubes for analysis.

D. Assessment of ^{125}I-hCG binding to receptor

Each tube received, sequentially, PBS-gel, ^{125}I-hCG, unlabeled hCG or PBS-gel, and pellet suspension. The amounts of each reactant were adjusted according to the needs of the experiment, but the final volume was kept at 120 µl. The incubations, initiated by the addition of receptor, were conducted in duplicate or triplicate at 22° for 4 hr under continuous gentle agitation. No change in specific binding has been observed with 4 hr of additional incubation. Reactions were terminated by dilution with cold buffer

(1.0 ml PBS-gel at 0°) followed by immediate centrifugation at 40,000 g for 15 min. Specificity of binding was assessed by the inclusion of more than a 1000-fold excess of unlabeled hCG in appropriate control tubes.

To determine the fraction of ^{125}I-hCG capable of binding (the "active fraction"), incubations were run with fixed amount of ^{125}I- hCG (with and without a vast excess of unlabeled hCG) and increasing amounts of receptor (obtained from homogenates of whole frozen ovaries from 35-day old rats in which pseudopregnancy had been induced by treatment with 50 IU of PMSG on day 25 and 25 IU of hCG on day 27). The amount of specifically bound ^{125}I-hCG which did not increase with addition of more receptor was considered the active fraction and generally ranged from 50 to 65 % of the total radioactivity. All binding results have been corrected to account for the distribution of the active fraction between that which was bound and that which was free.

E. Surface-binding autoradiography

To assess the distribution of binding sites within different ovarian tissues, surface-binding autoradiography was used (11, 12). In brief, this method consists of applying ^{125}I-hCG or ^{125}I-hFSH topically to frozen sections of unfixed ovaries, incubating the sections briefly, removing the unbound labeled hormone, and then localizing the bound hormone by conventional autoradiographic procedures.

F. In vivo uptake

To determine the relative ovarian uptake in vivo, 1.5-2.0μCi of ^{125}I- hCG (10-15 ng) was injected into the tail vein of ether-anesthetized rats at selected times. One hour later, the rats were decapitated, and aliquots of blood removed, the ovaries and uteri weighed and the radioactivity in all these counted.

G. Radioimmunoassay

The radioimmunoassay used to measure serum rat prolactin has been described (13). The assays for progesterone and estradiol each utilized highly specific antibodies to steroid-protein conjugates prepared at the 11-position and ^{125}I-tyrosine methyl ester conjugates of steroids prepared at the same position as the labeled ligand (14, 15).

RESULTS

A. Granulosa cell maturation

To examine further the possibility suggested by earlier surface binding autoradiographic studies (11) that follicular development might be associated with changes in LH- and FSH-receptor availability, a variety of systems were tested for their ability to initiate specific events in follicular maturation using the immature rat as a model. Systems tried included: five sc injections of FSH (LER-1422, each injection equivalent to 0.1 mg of NIH-FSH-S1), hCG (2 IU/injection), or saline (controls) at 0900 and 1800 hr begining at 0900 hr of day 25, or two sc injections of diethylstilbestrol in oil (4 mg/injection) given at 0900 hr on days 25 and 26. After two (but not one) days of FSH treatment, a marked increase in binding of ^{125}I-hCG (shown by autoradiography), as well as an increase in 3 β-hydroxysteroid dehydrogenase (3 β-HSD activity) was demonstrable in granulosa cells of most of the large, stimulated follicles. In contrast, no changes were seen in LH-binding or 3 β-HSD activity in granulosa cells of rats treated with hCG, diethylstilbestrol or saline. Likewise, no obvious changes in binding of ^{125}I-FSH were observed in granulosa cells of any rats, including those primed with FSH (16). Since these results suggested that FSH might stimulate the appearance of LH-receptor in granulosa cells, attempts were made to determine if the effects could be observed in the absence of the pituitary. For this purpose, 25-day old rats hypophysectomized on day 23 (Hormone Assay Laboratory, Chicago, Illinois) were treated as before with highly purified hFSH or saline. Following this treatment the rats were decapitated, the ovaries removed and placed in cold PBS-gel. Follicles were ruptured by pressure with a blunt probe, thereby expelling the granulosa cells into the surrounding buffer (Zeleznik, A.J., Midgley, A.R., Jr., and Reichert, L.E. Jr., - unpublished observations). As shown in Table 1, there was a much greater binding of ^{125}I-hCG to isolated granulosa cells from hypophysectomized rats treated with FSH than from similar rats treated with saline. Simultaneous incubation with 10^3- to 10^4-fold greater molar concentrations of hCG, LH and FSH indicated the binding to

Table 1. Binding in vitro of ^{125}I-hCG to granulosa cells obtained from hypophysectomized rats treated for two days with FSH or saline.

Treatment in vivo	^{125}I-hCG bound (pg/μg DNA) in presence of			
	Buffer	250 μg/ml hCG	2.91 μg/ml oLH	83 μg/ml hFSH
Saline	6.5 ± 0.1	0.7 ± 0.2	2.9 ± 0.1	8.0 ± 0.4
FSH	54.8 ± 1.0	1.3 ± 0.3	11.6 ± 0.5	54.0 ± 0.9

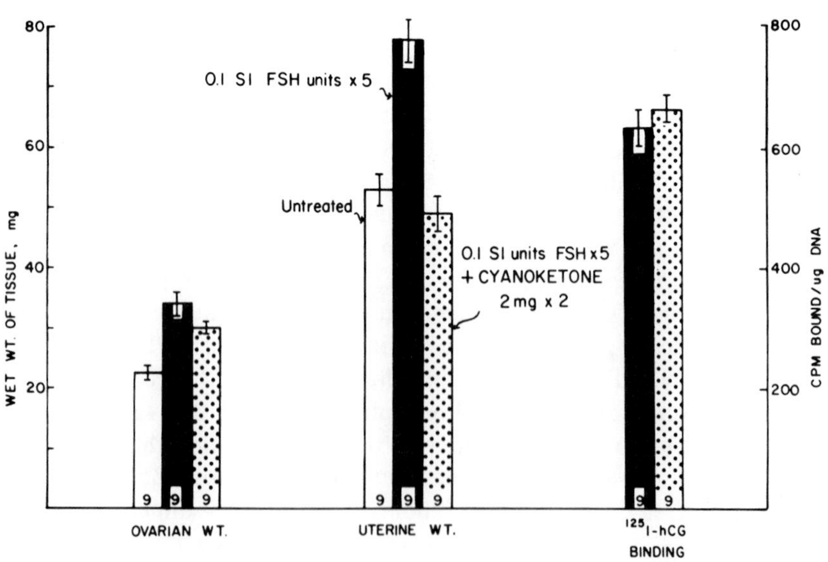

FIG 1. Effects of cyanoketone in vivo on FSH-induced stimulation of LH receptor in isolated rat granulosa cells. Nine rats per group. Vertical bars represent ± SEM.

be specific for LH and hCG.

It was observed that the uteri of the FSH-treated, hypophysectomized rats were considerably larger than those of the saline-treated controls. This suggested that the FSH, together with trace amounts of contaminating LH, had stimulated estrogen production, and raised the possibility that the FSH-induced stimulation of LH-receptor in granulosa cells might be an indirect consequence of the stimulation by estrogen. To examine this possibility, intact day 25 rats were treated as before with either saline, FSH or FSH plus cyanoketone (2 mg at 0900 hr of days 25 and 26). The latter effectively stops estrogen production by inhibiting 3 β-HSD activity (17). Comparison of uterine weights (Fig 1) reveals that cyanoketone prevented FSH-induced production of increased estrogen, but did not prevent FSH from causing increased ovarian weight or stimulating the appearance of LH-receptor.

B. Induction of granulosa cell luteinization and pseudopregnancy

To provide an in vivo model for studying changes in LH- and FSH-receptor activities in the course of differentiation of granulosa cells into luteal cells, immature rats, 25-day old, were treated with oFSH (LER-1654-3, 45 μg/injection x 5) at 0900 and 1800 hr beginning at 0900 hr of day 25, and then luteinization (and pseudopregnancy) initiated with exogenous oLH (LER 1374A (38-49), 60 μg) at 1500 hr of day 27 (Rajaniemi, H. J., Bajpai, P. K., Midgley, A. R. Jr., and Reichert, L. E., Jr. - unpublished data). FSH and LH, rather than PMSG and hCG were used since the latter hormones have exceptionally slow disappearance rates, and the continued presence of high circulating concentrations of unlabeled hormone could render changes in receptor availability difficult to ascertain. Throughout the course of this treatment, and for the following two weeks, serum concentrations of estradiol, progesterone and prolactin, weights of uteri and ovaries, and uptake of intravenous ^{125}I-hCG by these tissues were determined at approximately daily intervals. As shown in Fig 2 FSH treatment stimulated a temporary increase in serum prolactin, serum estradiol and uterine weight, and initiated a steady increase in ovarian weight. During this period no significant changes in uptake of ^{125}I-hCG by the complete ovary were observed. Administration of LH was immediately followed by a pronounced fall in serum estradiol and prolactin concentrations

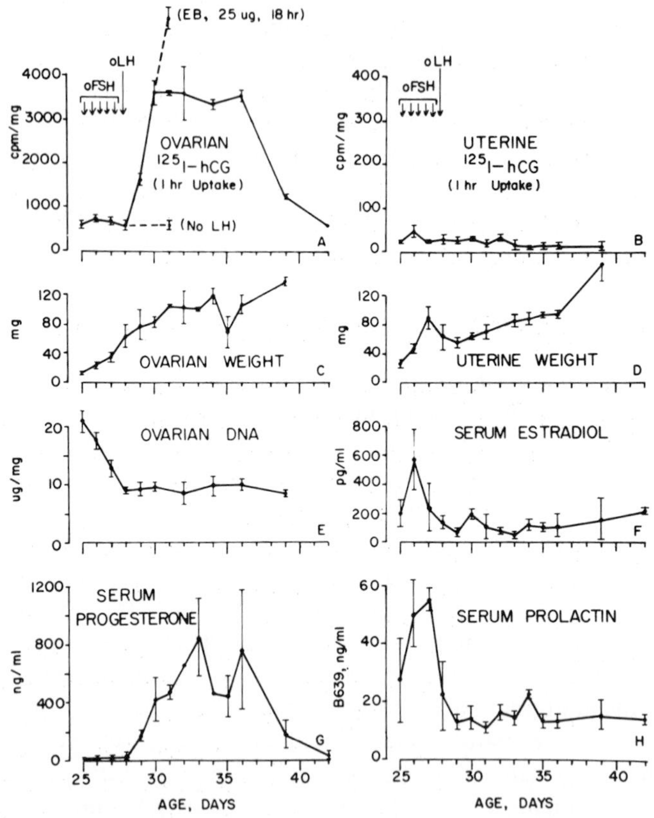

FIG 2. Effects of sequential administration of FSH and LH to immature rats on ovarian and uterine uptake of ^{125}I-hCG, ovarian and uterine weight, and serum estradiol, progesterone and prolactin. Vertical bars represent $\pm$ SEM.

and a subsequent temporary decline in uterine weight. Approximately 48 hr after LH injection, a highly significant increase in ovarian uptake of ^{125}I-hCG was found (day 29) which continued to increase for the next 24 hr reaching a maximum ($\sim$ 6.4-fold increase) on day 30. Little change in uptake was then seen for the next 6 days, but by day 39 a pronounced decline in uptake was found. The 6.4-fold increase in uptake of ^{125}I-hCG observed following LH injection was completely absent if this hormone was not administered. Subcutaneous administration of 25 μg estradiol benzoate in oil on the day when the maximal uptake was reached (day 30) resulted in a highly significant further increase when measured 18 hr later. No significant uptake of ^{125}I-hCG by uteri was observed at any time; at most times the uterine specific activity was at least 20 times less than that seen in the unstimulated ovary. Changes in progesterone concentrations were closely correlated with changes in ovarian uptake.

C. Changes in available LH-receptor throughout pregnancy

Surface-binding autoradiographic studies (11) had indicated the existence of marked binding of ^{125}I-hCG to corpora lutea of pregnant rat ovaries, a relative absence of binding to corpora lutea in ovaries obtained 2 hr after delivery, and low, persistent binding to interstitial tissue at all times. In an attempt to confirm and extend these earlier preliminary observations, corpora lutea have been carefully dissected from the remaining non-luteal tissue of ovaries obtained between 0900 and 1100 hr on almost all days of pregnancy. The two types of tissue were separately homogenized and 0.4 mg (corpora lutea, original wet weight) or 1.0 mg (non-luteal tissue) equivalents of the homogenates analyzed in vitro for their ability to bind a fixed concentration (approximately 0.5 nM) of ^{125}I-hCG (Fig 3). A steady increase in binding was observed in corpora lutea obtained over the first 10 days of pregnancy (the presence of vaginal sperm was considered to indicate day one). A further increase was seen on day 11 followed by relatively high binding until day 20. Thereafter the binding declined until values similar to those found on day 2 were present on day 23 (the day of delivery). Serum progesterone concentrations are known to change in a similar fashion throughout pregnancy (18). In contrast, although some increase in binding to non-luteal tissue may have been observed between days 2 and 4 of pregnancy, non-luteal

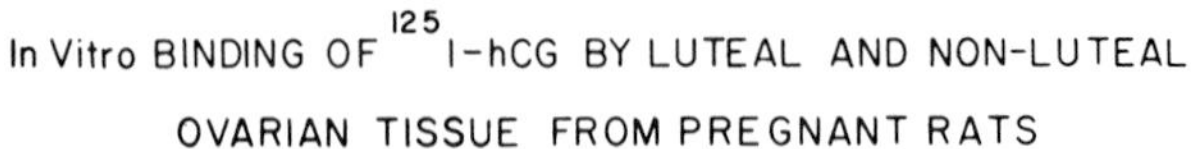

In Vitro BINDING OF 125 I-hCG BY LUTEAL AND NON-LUTEAL
OVARIAN TISSUE FROM PREGNANT RATS

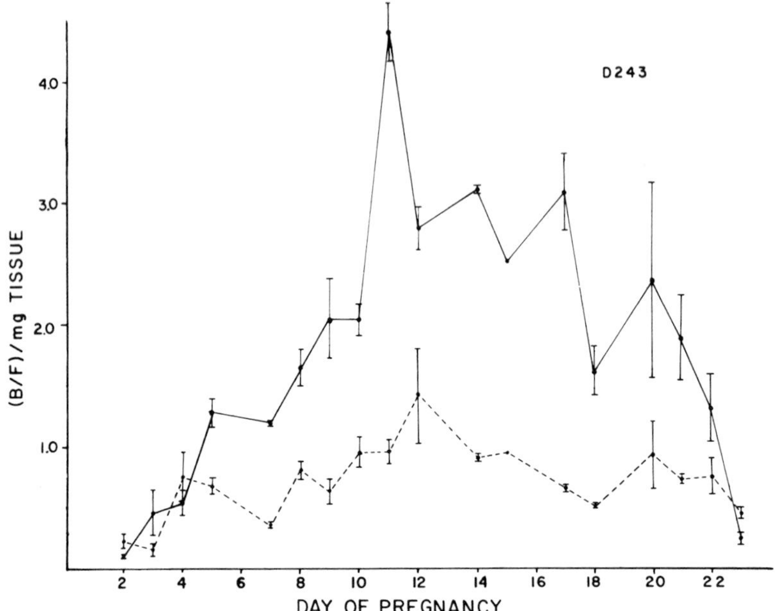

FIG 3. Binding of ^{125}I-hCG in vitro to pellets of separated luteal and non-luteal ovarian tissue from rats throughout pregnancy. Results are expressed as ratio of bound to free ^{125}I-hCG per mg tissue (wet weight). Vertical bars represent $\pm$ SEM. o———o luteal tissue o--------o non-luteal tissue.

binding remained relatively low and constant throughout pregnancy.

DISCUSSION

The results presented here strongly indicate that the life-cycle of the granulosa-luteal cell is associated with marked changes in measurable LH- and FSH-receptor activity. Changes in receptor activity must be a consequence of changes in number of available, active receptor molecules (as a consequence of changes in saturation, activation, synthesis or degradation) and/or changes in their binding affinities. Available data are insufficient to allow one to distinguish between these alternatives, but one mechanism capable of affecting the number of available active receptor molecules and worthy of attention is variable saturation by endogenous hormone. It is known that the dissociation of bound LH and FSH from receptors is extremely slow. Current data suggest, however, that receptor-saturation by endogenous hormones is not the major cause of changes in binding of exogenous hormones. Thus, surface-binding autoradiographic studies, the qualitative results of which correlate closely with in vivo uptake, in vivo autoradiographic distribution studies, and in vitro quantitative binding results, indicate markedly different yet predictable binding to granulosa cells and luteal cells within a single ovary. It might be argued that these different cell types are variably saturated due to their receiving different amounts of endogenous hormone as a consequence of differences in relative vascularity. Thus, highly vascularized, functional corpora lutea show the highest binding of exogenous ^{125}I-hCG while poorly vascularized regressing corpora lutea show the least binding. Similarly it would be difficult by the theory of variable endogenous saturation to explain why, in granulosa cells of developing follicles, FSH-receptor activity is high when LH-receptor activity is low, and vice versa. It is also noteworthy that the exogenous FSH used to stimulate follicular development and the appearance of granulosa cell LH-receptor, did not saturate FSH binding sites.

Although alternative hypotheses can be advanced, the data suggest that the appearance of LH-receptor in granulosa cells of developing follicles (medium to large size) is a consequence of the direct action of FSH. Thus it is reasonable to suppose that the site of action of a hormone is related to the distribution of its receptor, and the receptor for FSH appears to be restricted to the granulosa cell. Although action on this cell could stimulate secondary events which, after action elsewhere, indirectly act on the granulosa cell, such effects do not appear to require the presence of the pituitary gland and appear to be able to occur in the presence of effective inhibition of steroidogenesis (i.e., 3-β HSD). The results of the experiment with cyanoketone, and the lack of effect of diethylstilbestrol on inducing LH-receptor, each suggest that estrogens do not stimulate the initial appearance of LH-receptor. The possibility remains, however, the stimulation is a consequence of locally acting steroid. The role of LH (hCG) in stimulating LH-receptor appearance in developing follicles also cannot be ruled out since the possibility remains that the administered hCG stimulated the appearance of LH-receptor and then, due to a longer half-life, saturated the new sites as they formed.

On first examination, the absence of increased uptake in vivo of ^{125}I-hCG by whole ovaries during treatment with FSH (Fig 2) seems at variance with the known ability of this hormone to stimulate the appearance of LH-receptor in granulosa cells. It is likely, however, that by far the greatest total uptake of ^{125}I-hCG is a consequence of binding to interstitial and thecal tissue and the increased binding to granulosa cells in the large follicles is so diluted by the other binding as to be unrecognizable. The possibility also exists that a secondary effect of FSH action led to a decrease in binding of ^{125}I-hCG to the other tissues.

Administration of LH to a FSH-primed rat led, as expected, to massive luteinization and a striking 6.4 -fold increase in total ovarian uptake of ^{125}I-hCG. A highly significant increase in uptake was observed as early as 48 hr after the administration of LH. Earlier experiments, in which a single injection of PMSG (50 IU) was given on day 25 and a single injection of hCG (25 IU) was given on day 27, revealed a similar increase in uptake, but the initial increase was not seen until day 30. These studies suggest that, as a consequence of a longer half-life, hCG saturated the newly formed receptors resulting in an apparent 24 hr delay. From available data it is not possible to determine if the action of LH is direct or indirect, but the responding granulosa cells would have available LH-receptor at this time. It is tempting to speculate that the presence of LH- and, to a lesser extent, FSH-receptor in granulosa cells at the time of the LH and FSH surge during proestrus might account for the reported ability of both of these hormones to induce ovulation. Of some interest, the administration of LH appeared to result in a prompt fall in FSH-stimulated estradiol and prolactin concentrations and a subsequent decrease in uterine weight. The actions of estradiol at this time remain uncertain. It appears that the responding granulosa cells and resulting corpora lutea possess specific, high affinity, low capacity estradiol binding proteins (Richards, J. S. - unpublished data). Administration of estradiol on day 30, when the ^{125}I-hCG uptake had reached a maximum, resulted in a further increase in ^{125}I-hCG uptake when measured 18 hr later. The mechanisms responsible for this increase are not known.

The LH-induced, increased uptake of ^{125}I-hCG, the subsequent maintenance of high uptake, and eventual fall in uptake by corpora lutea on day 7 of pseudopregnancy were closely paralleled by similar changes in serum progesterone concentrations. The latter were characteristic of changes reported during pseudopregnancy, as induced by sterile mating and cervical stimulation (19,20). It is known that concentrations of endogenous LH remain relatively constant and low throughout pseudopregnancy (21) and yet this small amount of LH appears to be required for continued luteal function (22). The close association of available LH-receptor and serum progesterone concentrations suggests that the steady, low LH concentrations may control progesterone production according to changes in available receptor.

Similar relationships between serum progesterone concentrations and available LH-receptor in luteal (but not non-luteal) tissue appears to exist throughout pregnancy. Again luteolysis appears to be associated with a pronounced decline in receptor.

Similar relationships between serum progesterone concentrations and available LH-receptor in luteal (but not non-luteal) tissue appears to exist throughout pregnancy. Again luteolysis appears to be associated with a pronounced decline in receptor.
Of particular interest in regards to possible hormonal regulation of LH-receptor is the increase in receptor on day 11, the day at which peak concentrations of rat placental luteotropin have been reported (23,24).

ACKNOWLEDGEMENT

The authors wish to acknowledge the able assistance and contributions of Joyce Duncan in all phases of these studies.

Supported in part by a Program Project in Reproductive Endocrinology (NIH-HD-05318), a grant from The Ford Foundation, and a Population Council Fellowship (H.J.R). This is publication No. 1180 from The Division of Basic Health Sciences, Emory University, Atlanta, Georgia. One of us (A.R. Midgley) is the Career Development Awardee of The National Institute of Child Health and Human Development.

REFERENCES

1. Rajaniemi, H. J. and Vanha-Perttula, T. (1972). Endocrinology 90, 1.
2. Danzo, B. J., Midgley, A. R., Jr. and Kleinsmith, L. J. (1972). Proc. Soc. Exptl. Biol. Med. 139, 88.
3. Reichert, L. E. Jr., Leidenberger, F. and Trowbridge, C. G. (1973). Rec. Prog. Horm. Res. 29, 497.
4. Bahl, O. P. (1969). J. Biol. Chem. 244, 567.
5. Bajpai, P. K., Dash, R. J., Midgley, A. R. and Reichert, L. E. Jr., (1974). J. Clin. Endocr. (in press).
6. Reichert, L. E. Jr., and Midgley, A. R. Jr. (1968). Proc. Exptl. Biol. Med. 128, 1001.
7. Jiang, N. S. and Reichert, L. E., Jr. (1964). Biochim. Biophys Acta. 93, 436.
8. Reichert, L. E., Jr. (1974). In "Hormones and Cyclic Nucleotides", J. G. Hardman and B. W. O'Malley (Eds), (a volume of Methods in Enzymology) (in press).
9. Catt, K. J., Dufau, M. L. and Tsuruhara, T. (1972). J. Clin. Endo. 34, 123.
10. Leidenberger, F. L. and Reichert, L. E. Jr. (1972). Endocrinology. 91, 135.
11. Midgley, A. R., Jr. (1973). In "Receptors for Reproductive Hormones", B. W. O'Malley, and A. R. Means (Eds). pp 365, Plenum, New York.
12. Rajaniemi, H. J. and Midgley, A. R. Jr. (1974). In "Hormones and Cyclic Nucleotides", J. G. Hardman and B. W. O'Malley (Eds) (a volume of Methods in Enzymology - in press).
13. Niswender, G. D., Chen, C. L., Midgley, A. R., Jr., Meites, J., and Ellis, S. (1969). Proc. Soc. Exptl. Biol. Med. 130, 793.
14. Niswender, G. D. (1973) Steroids (in press).
15. England, B. G., Niswender, G. D. and Midgley, A. R. Jr., (1974). J. Clin. Endocr. (in press).
16. Zeleznik, A. J. and Midgley, A. R., Jr. (1973). Program of the 55th Annual Meeting of the Endocrine Society, A-69.
17. Goldman, A. S. (1967). J. Clin. Endocr. 27, 325.
18. Pepe, G. J. and Rothchild, I. (1973). Endocrinology 93, 1200.
19. Hashimoto, I., Hendricks, D. M., Anderson, L. L. and Melampy, R. M. (1968). Endocrinology 82, 333.
20. Bartosik, D. and Szarowski, D. H. (1973) Endocrinology 92, 949.

21. Bast, J.D. and Melampy, R.M. (1972). Endocrinology 91, 1499.
22. Moudgal, N.R., Behrman, H.R. and Greep, R.O. (1972). J. Endocr. 52, 413.
23. Linkie, D.M. and Niswender, G.D. (1972). Biol. Reprod. 8, 48.
24. Shiu, R.P.C., Kelly, P.A. and Friesen, H.G. (1973). Science 180, 968.

STUDIES ON ACTION OF LUTEINIZING HORMONE IN THE RAT

N.R. Moudgal and K. Muralidhar

INTRODUCTION

Our recent studies on the interaction of LH with its receptor in the ovary of rat and the changes in some of the ovarian functions resulting from such an interaction are described below. These include the nature of LH-receptor interaction, the biological activity of the β-subunit of LH, the physiological significance of LH binding potential of the ovary, and the ontogenicity of LH receptor.

METHODOLOGY

A. Tissue incubations

Whole ovaries or ovarian compartments or other tissues obtained from rats in different physiological states soon after autopsy were transferred to a chilled petri dish containing Krebs-Ringer bicarbonate (KRB) buffer, pH 7.4. The tissues were freed of surrounding fat, cut into pieces and amounts of 10-15 mg were incubated for 1 hr in a Dubnoff metabolic shaker at 37° in 2 ml of KRB with or without hormone. Tissue samples, after the incubation were stored frozen at -20° until further processing. The hormones used in the present study were ovine LH and their subunits (supplied by the courtesy of Drs. H. Papkoff and C.H. Li).

B. Measurement of tissue bound LH

A feature of our studies on LH action is that radioimmunoassay has been used to monitor the binding of physiologically active, unlabelled hormone to the receptors. It has been earlier shown by us that it is possible to measure the receptor-bound LH by this method (1). The production and purification of LH antiserum (a/s)(2) and the use of an assay procedure involving incubation at 37° have been described earlier (1). On the day of assay, the frozen tissue was thawed and homogenized gently with a loose fitting all-glass tissue grinder. The tissue suspension was then repeatedly washed with 4 ml aliquots of chilled 0.05 M phosphate-EDTA buffer (PBES), pH 7.4 containing 0.9 % NaCl, the tissue being suspended in the same buffer at 20 mg/ml concentration and aliquots assayed for bound hormone.

C. Cyclic AMP estimation

Tissue samples, after incubation for 1 hr with or without hormone at 37° were quickly removed and homogenized in 0.25 M $Ba(OH)_2$. It was then neutralized by adding an equivalent amount of 5 % alum. The precipitate so-formed was mixed well, homogenized with 0.4 N perchloric acid and finally the acid was neutralized with equivalent amount of 0.4 N $NaHCO_3$. This procedure for cyclic AMP extraction was based on the method of Ebadi et al. (3).

The procedure used here for the extraction of cyclic AMP binding protein was a modification of methods of Brown et al.(4) and Gilman (5). It was extracted from rabbit skeletal muscle with 0.05 M tris, pH 7.4 containing 0.005 M $MgCl_2$, 0.025 M KCl and 0.25 M sucrose (cAMP buffer-I). The homogenate was spun at 5000 g in a Sorval RC 2B centrifuge. The supernatant, dispersed into 1 ml aliquots, was stored frozen at -20°. No further purification was done.

The assay proper was essentially according to Brown et al. (4), except that Millipore filters of 0.45 μ pore size were used instead of charcoal for the separation of bound cyclic AMP from free. Filters were dissolved in 1 ml of methyl cellosolve and after addition of 5 ml of scintillation fluid (5.5 gms of Permablend in 1 litre of toluene - Packard Instrument Co.,) were counted in a Packard Spectrometer.

D. Cyclic AMP binding potential

Binding potential of rat ovarian homogenate *in vitro* to ^3H-cAMP was used as a measure of cyclic AMP binding protein concentration (considered as being inversely proportional to protein kinase activity). Ovaries pooled from rats under each of the various physiological states were homogenized with 1.5 vol of cAMP buffer-I. The 5000 g supernatant was incubated at various dilutions with 25,000 cpm of ^{3}H-cAMP (specific activity 24.1 Ci/mmole). The total volume was made up to 0.3 ml with 0.05 M tris buffer, pH 7.4 containing 0.006 M mercaptoethanol and 0.008 M theophylline (cAMP buffer-II). After 1 hr of incubation in an ice-bath, the reaction mixture was filtered over Millipore filter, washed with 50 vol of 0.01 M phosphate buffered saline, pH 7.5, and then the radioactivity on the filters counted as described above.

RESULTS

A. Nature of LH-receptor interaction

Among the tissues tested, LH binding could be observed only in the ovary (Table 1). Washing the ovarian tissue exposed to LH, repeatedly with cold PBES or normal rabbit serum failed to remove the bound hormone, thereby showing that the binding was specific. Further, it was observed that 3 washes were sufficient to remove non-specifically bound LH as demonstrated by the fact that labelled LH added to the medium before the

Table 1. Specificity of LH binding

Tissue	Hormone*	Amount bound ng/100 mg tissue
Uterus	- LH	nil
	+ LH	nil
Lung	- LH	nil
	+ LH	nil
Corpora lutea of early pregnancy	- LH	nil
	+ LH	72.50

* In all cases 10-15 mg of tissue was incubated at 37°C for 1 hr with or without 5 μg of LH/flask. For details of incubation and assay see text.

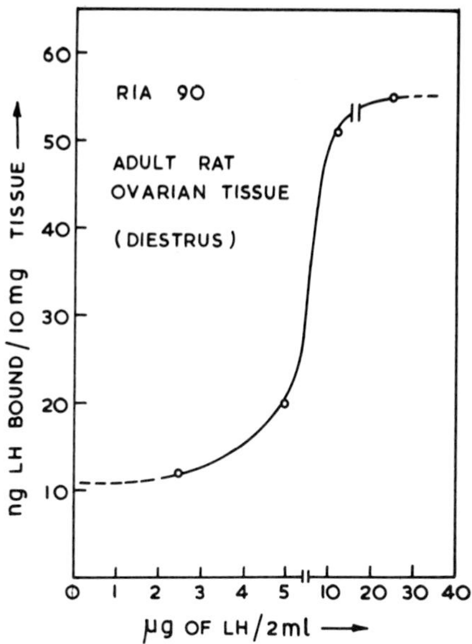

FIG 1. Dose-response curve for LH binding. Rat ovarian tissue was incubated with different amounts of LH and bound LH measured; incubation conditions and assay are described in the text. Each point represents average of two independent experiments.

start of washing could be recovered completely within 3 washes. In contrast, washing with 1:1000 diluted LH a/s resulted in the total removal of bound LH (both specific and non-specific) within the first wash itself.

Studies on LH-receptor interaction showed this interaction to be highly flexible and reversible. It exhibited a typical sigmoidal dose-response behaviour (Fig 1) similar to that observed earlier by Moudgal et al. (1) and Gospodarowicz (6) using mouse leydig tumor cells and bovine corpus luteum receptor respectively. The fact that minor changes in the concentration of LH in the medium could induce quick changes in the amount of hormone bound to the receptor was demonstrated by the following experiment. A known amount of tissue was incubated with LH and washed repeatedly with buffer to remove non-specifically bound LH. The final suspension in the buffer was then incubated at 0° in an ice bath. At different intervals of time from the start of this incubation, two equal aliquots were removed, the first consisting of suspension

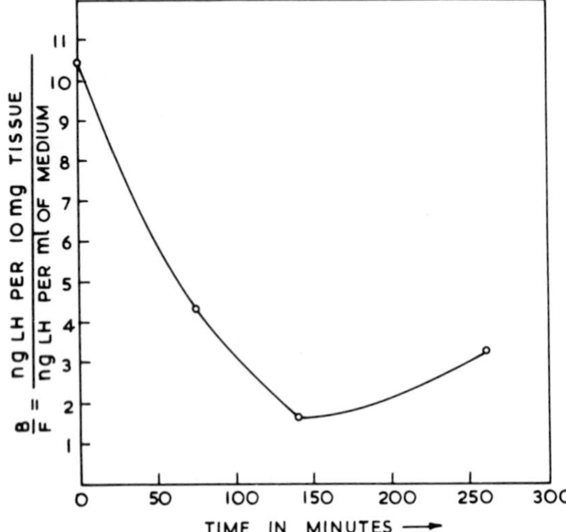

FIG 2. Figure showing the flexibility of LH-receptor interaction. The experimental details are given in the text.

(medium plus tissue) and the second, medium alone (without tissue). When these aliquots were assayed for LH content, a picture represented by Fig 2 emerged. An explanation to the observed pattern is not difficult to offer. Each time an aliquot is taken out (two aliquots of medium and one of tissue) an enrichment in the amount of LH in tissue compared to that present in the medium occurs. In otherwords, a deliberate attempt has been made here to induce the system to shift its equilibrium towards the dissociated state and the system promptly responds. But as the concentration of LH in the medium builds up to a critical point, the equilibrium reverts towards the associated state (B/F 1.6 vs 3.4, $P < 0.05$).

While the observed result, so adhering to the laws of mass action in itself is interesting, the significance of the data is much more important. Thus the result, in addition to proving the reversible nature of LH-receptor interaction, demonstrates the susceptibility of the equilibrium to modulation by changing external concentrations of LH. Further, it raises another question whether under *in vivo* conditions where fluctuations in circulating hormone levels occur, the amount of receptor bound LH does indeed change. The inability to totally displace the ^{125}I-LH bound to the receptor by the cold hormone has led to the suggestion that LH binding is "non-dischargeable" or "tight" (7). It is obvious from our retults that the very presence of excess of hormone would aid binding and not dissociation as expected. LH-receptor interaction in our opinion, is a dynamic process, where the amount and perhaps the duration of binding are highly variable, mostly dependent on the external concentration of LH. Whether there are any changes in receptor affinity itself under different physiological states is, however, not yet known. This study further suggests that at least a part of the dissociated LH is biologically active in that it is capable of reassociating with the receptor. At the present moment we are unable to account for the loss of LH in the medium; whether this loss is due to destruction of LH is yet to be ascertained.

B. Demonstration of binding of ovine LH-β subunit to rat ovarian receptor

In a variety of systems oLH-β subunit binds to rat ovaries, although its binding is not always equal to that of LH (Tables 2 & 3). As shown in Table 3, unlike LH which is capable of increasing cyclic AMP levels in the rat ovarian tissue, the β subunit is incapable by itself of doing so. This brings out the point that binding of a hormone to its target tissue may not necessarily reflect its biological activity, thus stressing on the need to correlate binding with any of the biochemical responses of the hormone. Ovine LH-β subunit has been found to be fully active in *in vivo* systems (8, 9), and partially active in some *in vitro* systems (10, 11). But attempts to demonstrate binding of ^{125}I LH-β to receptor or inhibition of ^{125}I-LH binding by unlabelled LH-β have met with little success (12-14). This has led to the general belief that the observed biological activity of LH-β in *in vitro* systems is perhaps due to contamination with whole LH. Still an explanation for the *in vivo* biological activity is hard to give, other than the fact that the system used was not free of LH. It is interesting to note that in our system, β-subunit of LH binds to luteal receptor in amounts

Table 2. Relative binding of ovine LH and its β-subunit to rat ovarian tissue

Physiological state of rat	Tissue	Hormone	Hormone concentration		LH equiv. bound ng/10 mg.
			μg	molar equiv.	
Day 7 of pregnancy	Luteal tissue	LH	5	8.3×10^{-8}	5.6
		LH-β	5	16.6×10^{-8}	6.0
		LHβ +LHα	5+2.5	16.6×10^{-8} $+3.3 \times 10^{-8}$	8.1 *
Day 16 of pregnancy	Luteal tissue	LH	3.5	5.8×10^{-8}	12.0
		LH-β	12.5	42.5×10^{-8}	48.0
Day 21 of pregnancy	Luteal tissue	LH	5	8.3×10^{-8}	4.2
		LH-β	2	6.6×10^{-8}	7.1
Immature rat on day 21	Whole ovary	LH	5	8.3×10^{-8}	< 5
		LH-β	5	16.6×10^{-8}	< 5
Adult diestrus rat	Whole ovary	LH	5	8.3×10^{-8}	20.0
		LH-β	5	16.6×10^{-8}	12.0

* The assay used here measured only whole LH or its β-subunit.

Table 3. Comparison of the biological activities of ovine LH and its β-subunit using the diestrus rat ovarian tissue.

Hormone	Hormone concentration (μg/ml)	LH equivalent bound (ng/10 mg)	% stimulation of cAMP level over control
LH	1.25	12	60
LH-β subunit	2.5	12	< 10

comparable to LH itself but without evoking a response. That the binding is not non-specific is suggested by our observation that depending on the physiological state of the animal, the binding of LH and the β subunit fluctuated in a parallel fashion (Table 2). Further work is in progress to characterize this binding of β-subunit.

C. LH binding potential of the ovary as a function of physiological status

Whether binding potential of the ovary with respect to LH varies with altered endocrine status of the animal was tested in two models. During the gestation period, binding of LH to the rat ovarian tissue does not exhibit any pattern, though an apparent but statistically insignificant increase is observed during the later stages of pregnancy (Fig 3). It is known that progesterone content of the ovary during gestation increases initially, attaining a peak on day 11, thereafter declining to minimal values by day 20 (15). It is also known that the effect of LH antiserum on ovarian progesterone production is significantly more during early pregnancy than during late pregnancy (16) suggesting a variation in dependence of the ovary on LH.

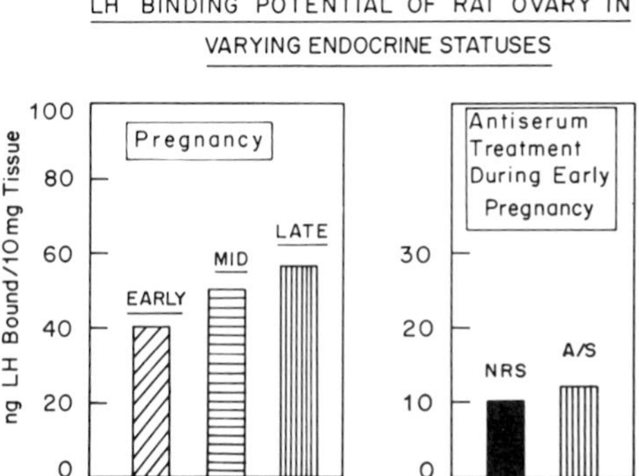

FIG 3. Variation in LH binding potential during different reproductive phases. Non-interstitial tissue comprising follicles and corpous luteum were used. For details of incubation see text. Changes during pregnancy are depicted on the left hand side of the figure, and the effect of a/s treatment on LH binding potential is shown on the right hand side of the figure. Values at each point represent a typical set of results obtained using 3 animals per point. Early = day 8; Mid = day 12; and Late = day 20 of pregnancy. Controls received NRS (normal rabbit serum).

The LH binding potential, however, does not seem to follow the above pattern. Deprival of LH from pregnant rats for 3 days (by administration of 0.2 ml LH antiserum from days 8-10) does not appear to influence binding of LH to their ovaries (Fig 3). Since the above studies on LH binding have not yet been correlated with the functional responsiveness of the ovaries, further discussion on this may be premature. Nevertheless, these results do raise the question whether binding itself could be taken as a measure of the response of ovaries under *in vivo*, and probably also under *in vitro* conditions.

D. Ontogenicity of LH receptor

When does an immature ovary start responding to LH and how it is brought about is an interesting question. The high levels of LH in circulation during the early infant stage (17) of rat in contrast to the low levels of circulating estrogen is intriguing. The neonatal rat ovary appears to be refractory to LH stimulus (K. Muralidhar and N.R. Moudgal - unpublished observation). In order to investigate whether prior exposure of the ovary to FSH is necessary for the generation of LH receptor, we tried to simulate the condition of puberty by sequential injections of PMSG and hCG at stipulated intervals to 22-day old rats. The protocol consisted of giving 50 IU PMSG on days 22 and 24, 25 IU hCG on day 26; LH binding potential was tested on days 24, 26 and 33. Ovarian tissue taken from control untreated as well as treated rats were incubated with LH and processed as described earlier; Fig 4 shows the binding pattern obtained. To our surprise, no significant difference in LH binding potential was observed between PMSG-treated and untreated rats till day 26; however, after hCG injection, a highly significant increase was obtained. Interesting as this result is, it poses several intriguing questions. For example, LH has been shown to stimulate cyclic AMP production in prepubertal rats given a single injection of PMSG, 48 hr earlier (18). On the contrary, our results show that after 2 injections of PMSG, on a day when the rats respond to hCG or LH by ovulating, the ovarian tissue does not show any

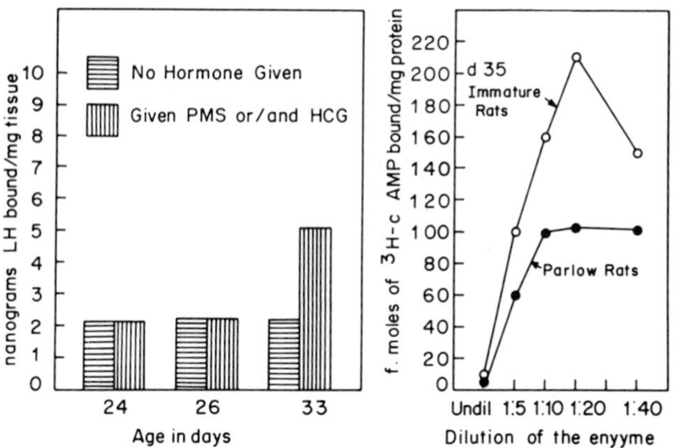

FIG 4. Ontogenicity of LH receptor. The left hand side of the figure shows the LH binding potential of rat ovary as a follow-up of PMSG and hCG injections. The right hand side depicts the difference in the in vitro cyclic AMP binding potential of ovaries from immature and immature PMSG-hCG primed rats. Details of experiment are described in the text.

significant difference in binding potential. An explanation for this could be that it need not bind more LH to exhibit the known reponses like increase in cyclic AMP or ovulation. Alternatively, the luteal tissues may have more receptors for LH than follicular tissue. Further work on the probable differences in affinities for hCG and LH depending on the predominating cell type, on the sequence of changes following a single injection of PMSG, or onset of natural puberty have to be undertaken in order to throw more light on this problem. The availability of reliable information on circulating LH levels during puberty in rats would give an insight into the overall process of the ontogenicity of LH receptors and the role of FSH in this process.

E. What is responsiveness ?

A pertinent question to be put at this juncture is what is responsiveness and how can we define this for LH ? It is realised now that structural alterations of hormones during circulation can affect their half-life and thus their in vivo biological activity (19). Mere binding to a target tissue in an in vitro system is again shown by the present work to not necessarily represent biological activity in the conventional sense. Paradoxically, neonatal rats having high circulatory levels of LH have still been categorized as non-responsive, while prepubertal rats inspite of being called immature, have been shown to respond to LH (20) in terms of cyclic AMP levels or protein kinase activity.

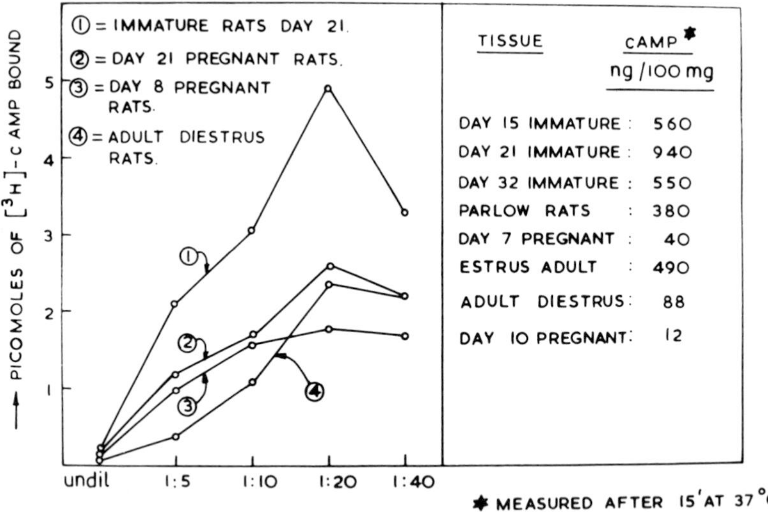

FIG 5. Figure showing changes in in vitro cyclic AMP binding potential of ovaries of rat in different physiological statuses. The X-axis represents the dilution of the crude ovarian homogenate taken as a source of cyclic AMP-receptor protein. The right side of the figure shows the absolute cyclic AMP levels in the rat ovarian tissues.

Our observations on this problem seem to bring out certain newer features of responsiveness. We have chosen for comparison 21-day old immature rat ovary as representing a relatively unresponsive tissue (it responds to a very little degree to LH in terms of increase in cyclic AMP levels), and ovaries of PMSG-hCG treated immature rats and adult rats as examples of responsive tissue (responsive in terms of steroid or cyclic AMP production). We observed in these, that parameters like LH binding potential, resting cyclic AMP levels and cyclic AMP binding potential also could contribute to responsiveness of the ovary. Compared to the non-responsive immature rat ovary, the ovary of the rat pre-treated with PMSG-hCG responds to LH much more and it is reflected by its higher LH binding potential and lower cyclic AMP-binding potential (Fig 5). In ovaries from rats differing in their degree of responsiveness (e.g., adult cycling, early and late pregnancy, immature and immature PMSG-hCG treated rats), endogenous cyclic AMP levels and cyclic AMP binding potential fluctuate in a parallel fashion. In otherwords, a tissue which has a low level cyclic AMP and a low cyclic AMP-binding potential is expected to show a higher response to LH, either in terms of cyclic AMP production and/or LH binding potential.

The high levels of cyclic AMP and the high degree of unsaturation exhibited by the cyclic AMP binding protein in the immature rat ovary bring out yet another question as to why these are not being utilized by the ovary ? Is there a compartmental separation between endogenous cyclic AMP and its binding protein (protein kinase) ? Does LH then bring about decompartmentalization ? Thus, at present we can only say that during the process of acquisition of responsiveness to LH, the protein kinase is transformed from a cyclic AMP-dependent to cyclic-AMP-independent form, consequently lowering endogenous cyclic AMP levels. In parallel, the LH binding potential also increases giving rise to possibilities of forming more cyclic AMP.

CONCLUDING REMARKS

The information that has accumulated on the LH receptor has been both valuable and intriguing. Localization of LH receptor at the tissue, cell and subcellular level for example has provided contradicting and confusing data (21,22). We do not have sufficient information on the physicochemical nature of the true receptor, thus warranting its purification. The fact that the nature and some properties of LH receptor has been shown to change with the physiological status of the animal indicates the need for a detailed investigation (especially the need to correlate with a biochemical response). In the field of biochemical actions of LH also, there does not seem to be any clear picture. The functional interrelationship between prostaglandins, cyclic AMP and LH is still not clear (23). The role of subunits in the expression of biological activity, possibility of recombination or dissociation of subunits on the receptor, the probability of other cyclic nucleotides mediating hormone action (9) are still to be investigated.

ACKNOWLEDGEMENTS

Work aided by generous grants from the Indian Council of Medical Research, New Delhi, and the Ford Foundation, New York.

REFERENCES

1. Moudgal, N.R., Moyle, W.R. and Greep, R.O. (1971). J. Biol. Chem. 246, 4983.
2. Madhwa Raj, H.G. and Moudgal, N.R. (1970) Endocrinology 86, 874.
3. Ebadi, M.S., Weiss, B. and Costa, E. (1970) J. Neurochem. 18, 183.
4. Brown, B.L., Albano, J.D.M., Ekins, R.P., Spherz, A.M. and Tampion, W. (1971). Biochem. J. 121, 561.
5. Gilman, A.G. (1970). Proc. Natl. Acad. Sci. (USA) 67, 305.
6. Gospodarowicz, D. (1973). J. Biol. Chem. 248, 5042.

7. Lee, C.Y. and Ryan, R.J. (1971). Endocrinology 89, 1515.
8. Yang, W.H., Sairam, M.R., Papkoff, H. and Li, C.H. (1972). Science 175, 637.
9. Farmer, S.W., Sairam, M.R. and Papkoff, H. (1973). Endocrinology 92, 1022.
10. Rao, Ch.V. and Carman, F. (1973). Biochem. Biophys. Res. Comm. 54, 744.
11. Gospodarowicz, D. (1971). Endocrinology 89, 669.
12. Rao, Ch.V. (March 1973). Fed. Proc. 32, Abstract No. 101.
13. Danzo.B.J.(1973). Biochem. Biophys. Acta. 304, 560.
14. Lee, C.Y. and Ryan, R.J. (1972). Proc. Natl. Acad. Sci. (USA). 69, 3520.
15. Wiest, W.G. (1970). Endocrinology 87, 43.
16. Moudgal, N.R., Behrman, H.R. and Greep, R.O. (1972). J. Endocrinol. 52, 413.
17. Goldman, B.D., Grazia, Y.R., Kamberi, I.A. and Porter, J.C. (1971). Endocrinology 88, 771.
18. Rigler, G.L. and Reidesel, M.L. (March 1973). Fed. Proc. 32, Abstract No. 15.
19. Dufau, M.L., Catt, K.J., and Tsuruhara, M.L. (1971). Biochem. Biophys. Res. Comm. 44, 1022.
20. Lamprecht, S.A., Zor, U., Tsafriri, A. and Lindner, H.R. (1973). J. Endocrinol. 57, 217.
21. Rajaneimi, H. and Vanha-Perttula, T. (1973). J. Endocrinol. 57, 199.
22. Midgley, A.R., Jr. (1971). In "Gonadotropins", B.B. Saxena, C.G. Beling and H.M. Gandy, (Eds). pp 248, Wiley-Interscience, New York.
23. Zor, U., Lamprecht, S.A., Kaneko, T., Schneider, H.P.G, McCann, S.M., Field, J.B., Tsafriri, A. and Lindner, H.R. (1972). Adv. Cycl. Nuctl. Res. 1, 503.

PURIFICATION OF THE LH-HCG RECEPTOR FROM LUTEINIZED RAT OVARIES

C. Y. Lee and R. J. Ryan

INTRODUCTION

The existence of specific, high affinity receptors for luteinizing hormone and chorionic gonadotropin has been demonstrated for rat (1) and human (2) luteal tissue, for rat Leydig cells (3,4) and mouse Leydig cell tumors (5). Binding activity has been shown to be a saturable process dependent upon time, pH, and molarity of salts (6). Binding requires the native gonadotropin molecule and neither binding nor competition for binding occurs with the subunits of LH or hCG (7). Experiments involving enzymatic digestions suggest that the receptor is lipoprotein in nature (6,7).

The present report is concerned with the purification of the LH-hCG receptors from luteinized rat ovaries.

MATERIALS AND METHODS

A. General

Holtzman rats were made pseudopregnant by priming with PMSG and hCG, and were used 6-8 days after hCG. When the binding of labeled gonadotropin is maximal, the ovaries were removed and dissected free of connective tissue and either were used immediately or were frozen on dry ice and stored at -20°F. No significant loss of binding activity has been noted after storage for one year.

Batches of ovaries and, in some instances, liver, spleen and kidneys were minced and homogenized in 10 volumes (v/w) of 40 mM tris buffer, pH 7.4. Three 30-second strokes with a motor driven Teflon-glass homogenizer were used for disruption. All solutions and tissues were kept ice-cold. The homogenate was centrifuged at 2,000 g for 15 min in a refrigerated International B20 instrument. The pellet was washed once with tris buffer and then was used for binding assays (see below) or was further purified.

B. Triton X-100 extraction

Washed 2,000 g pellets were extracted while slowly stirring, for 1 hr at 4° with 0.25 % Triton X-100 (Beckman Instrument Company) in 40 mM tris buffer, pH 7.4. Four ml of solvent was used for each gram equivalent of wet ovary. The brei was then centrifuged for 1 hr at 110,000 g in a Beckman L2-65 centrifuge. The pellet was re-extracted and re-centrifuged. The clear supernatants were combined and further purified by affinity chromatography.

C. Affinity chromatography

HCG was coupled to cyanogen bromide-treated Sepharose-4B by the method of Cuatrecasas et al.(8) as modified by Sato and Cargille (9); 200,000 IU of hCG were bound to 100 ml of Sepharose-4B. The Sepharose-hCG was washed exhaustively to remove noncovalently bound material. The Sepharose-hCG could be used repeatedly, if stored in 0.1 % sodium azide, 40mM tris buffer, pH 7.4, at 10°.

The hCG-Sepharose gel was packed in a glass column (1.2 x 7.55 cm), the bed height used depending upon the batch of ovaries to be processed. The column was run at room temperature, but the solutions applied to the column and the fractions collected were kept ice-cold. Triton extracts were allowed to run into the gel-bed, and then flow was interrupted for 15-20 min before elution continued. Similarly, when buffers were changed, flow was interrupted for 15-20 min when one column volume of buffer entered the gel.

D. Binding assays

Pellets, equivalent to 5 mg of wet ovary, were incubated at 25° with 5 ng of ^{125}I labeled hLH or hCG for 4-16 hr. The assay volume was 1 ml and the buffer consisted of 0.1 % bovine serum albumin in 40 mM tris at pH 7.4. Control tubes, to assess non-specific binding, were run in parallel and contained 200 IU/ml of unlabeled hCG. Separation of bound and free labeled gonadotropin was accomplished by millipore filtration as previously described (6). Radioactivity bound to the washed pellets was measured in an automatic gamma scintillation counter and results were expressed as specific binding (total - nonspecific).

Similarly, binding activity of soluble receptor was assessed by incubating a known amount of protein, measured by the method of Lowry et al. (10) with 5 ng of ^{125}I hCG in a volume of 1.0 ml using the assay buffer described above. Incubation was done at 25° for 30 min unless otherwise stated. Control tubes, to assess nonspecific binding, contained 200 IU /ml of hCG.

With the soluble receptor system, bound and free hormones were separated using the Carbowax-6000 technique reported by Desbuquois and Aurbach (11) to precipitate bound hormone. 0.2 ml of bovine γ globulin solution (to make a final concentration of 0.42 %) were added to each assay tube and mixed on a Vortex. 1.2 ml of 20.8 % Carbowax-6000 in 40 mM tris buffer, pH 7.4 was added. The tubes were mixed, placed in an ice bath for 20 min and then centrifuged at 2000 rpm for 10 min. The supernatant was drained and the pellet was redissolved and reprecipitated with Carbowax as described above. With only one precipitation, nonspecific binding amounted to 7-8 % of total binding and this was reduced to 2-3 % by the second precipitation.

E. Radioiodination and sources of hormones

Highly purified preparations of hLH (22870-1B, prepared in this laboratory) and hCG (a gift of Dr. Robert Canfield, Columbia University) were radioiodinated with ^{125}I. This was accomplished using the Chloramine-T method of Greenwood et al. (12) as modified by Lee and Ryan (13) to preserve biologic activity. Other hormones used were obtained from the Hormone Distribution Office, NIAMDD.

F. Preparation of antisera

Ovarian protein purified by affinity chromatography was used to immunize 5 rabbits and 2 goats. Fifty μg of protein and 1 mg of killed tubercle bacilli (Difco) were emulsified with 0.5 ml of Freund's adjuvant (Difco) and 0.5 ml of 0.9 % saline. This mixture was injected intradermally at 10-15 sites over the back. Booster injections, using the same dose of immunogen in Freund's adjuvant, were given to the rabbits at monthly intervals as a single sc injection. The same regime was employed for the goats, but the dose of immunogen was increased to 400 μg. All animals were injected im with 0.5 ml of Pertussis vaccine (Lilly) at the time of primary immunization and 1 month later. Initial bleedings were made at 6th week and continued at 1-4 week intervals. Antisera were evaluated using standard immunodiffusion techniques.

G. Miscellaneous procedures

Gel filtration on columns of Sephadex G-100 or G-200 were done as previously described (14). Amino acid analyses were done on timed acid hydrolysates using a Beckman model 121 Analyzer as previously described (15). The techniques of Ornstein (16) and Fairbanks et al. (17), with minor modifications were used for disc-gel electrophoresis.

RESULTS

A. Solubilization and affinity chromatography

Data previously published (6) indicate that the hLH-hCG binding activity contained in ovarian homogenates in 40 mM tris buffer is completely sedimentable with centrifugal forces of 2,000-4,000 g applied for 15-20 min.

Preliminary data had indicated that ^{125}I-hLH bound to 2,000 g pellets could not be extracted with 40 mM tris, pH 7.4, or 0.3 M KCl. Minimal solubilization could be achieved with sodium desoxycholate. Efficient extraction could be achieved with 0.25 % Triton X-100 (13). Similarly, 2,000 g pellet could be extracted with Triton X-100 and binding activity could be demonstrated in the soluble fraction (Fig. 1). Gel filtration revealed a void volume peak on Sephadex G-100 and this peak of radioactivity was suppressed by the addition of unlabeled hormone. Other experiments, not illustrated, indicated that the receptor-LH complex was excluded on Sephadex G-200.

Affinity chromatography of a 0.25 % Triton X-100 extract of 2,000 g ovarian pellet is illustrated in Figure 2. The bulk of the material was unadsorbed by the hCG-Sepharose gel. A small amount of material was eluted with 0.2 M NaCl - 0.005 M acetate buffer, pH 5.0, and very little with 1 M NaCl in the same buffer. A peak of protein was eluted with 3 M guanidine hydrochloride, pH 6.5. The guanidine was removed by filtration through a column of Biogel P-10. Binding activity of the various fractions is

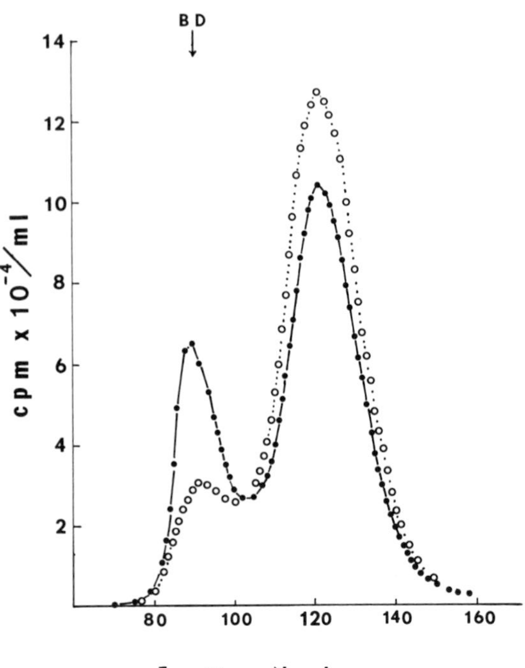

FIG 1. Gel chromatography on Sephadex G-100 of ^{125}I-hCG after incubation with a Triton X-100 extract of 2,000 x g ovarian pellet with (open circles) or without (closed circles) 200 IU/ml unlabeled hCG. BD signifies the elution position of Blue Dextran.

given in Table 1. No significant binding was found in the unadsorbed fraction and only a small amount in the NaCl eluates, but significant activity was present in the guanidine eluate. Based on the increase in binding activity, a 64-fold purification was achieved from the Triton extract. Recovery of activity from the affinity column was quantitative. Six separate experiments gave similar results.

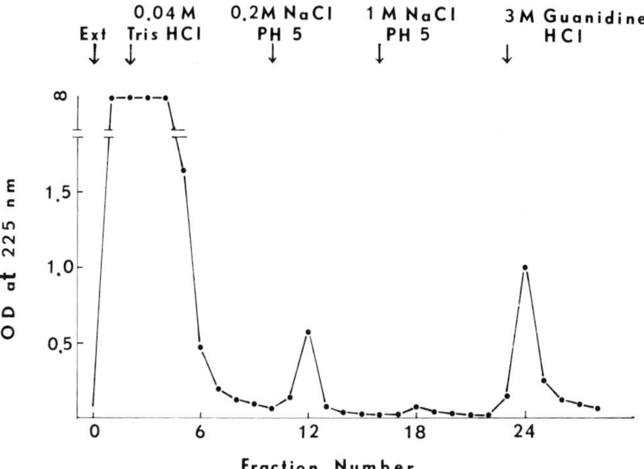

FIG 2. Affinity chromatography of Triton X-100 extract prepared from a 2,000 g pellet equivalent t0 5 g of ovaries. The hCG-Sepharose column was 1.2 x 7.2 cm. Fraction volumes were 8.0 ml.

Table 1. Purification of LH-hCG receptor by affinity chromatography*

Fraction	(^{125}) hCG bound moles x 10^{17}/µg protein	Purification fold
Crude extract	6	1
0.2 M NaCl, pH 5 eluent	22	4
1 M NaCl, pH 5 eluent	94	15
3 M guanidine HCl eluent	395	64

*HCG-Sepharose column (1.2 x 7.2 cm) was used.

B. HCG-binding characteristics of the receptor purified by affinity chromatography

Figure 3 illustrates the time-course of binding of ^{125}I-hCG to purified receptor. Equilibrium was achieved in approximately 30 min at 25^{0} in contrast to 4-5 hr using 2,000 g pellets (13). Fig 4 indicates that binding of ^{125}I-hCG was inhibited by unlabeled hCG but not by oFSH even at doses of 10 μg/ml. Data obtained by incubation of receptor with increasing concentrations of ^{125}I-hCG were analyzed by Scatchard analysis and indicated an apparent dissociation constant of 7.6×10^{-10} M.

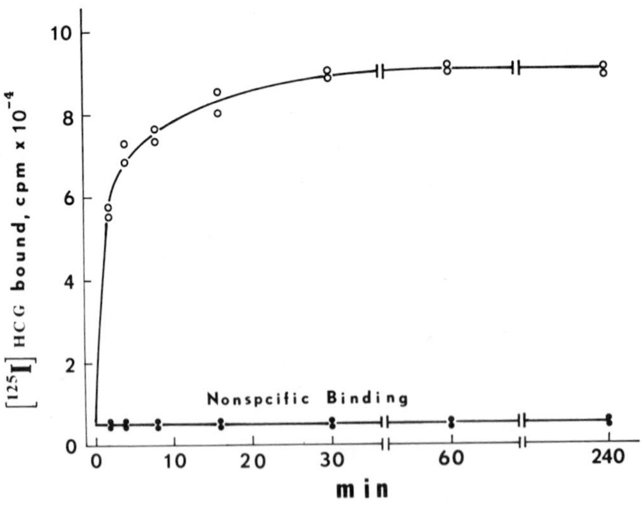

FIG 3. The time course of binding of ^{125}I-hCG to ovarian receptor purified by affinity chromatography. 42 μg of receptor protein was incubated with 6 ng of ^{125}I hCG in a total volume of 1 ml. Total binding is indicated by the open circles. Non-specific binding was determined by control tubes containing 200 IU/ml hCG.

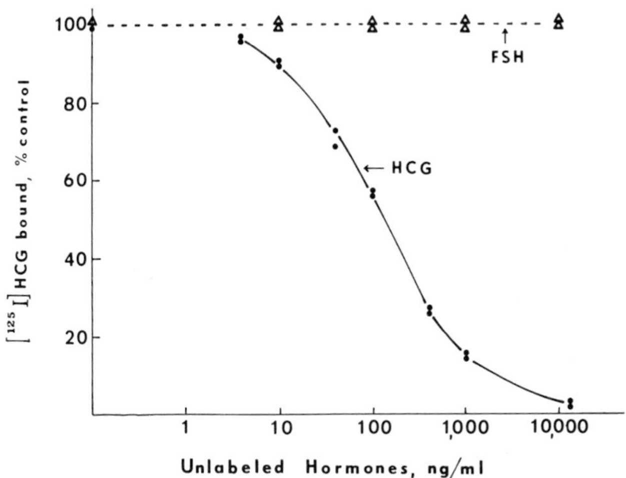

FIG 4. Specificity of ovarian receptor purified by affinity chromatography.
Receptor was incubated with 1 ng ^{125}I-hCG alone or in the presence of increasing amounts of hCG or oFSH volume of 1 ml. Incubation was at 25° for 1 hr. Binding in the absence of unlabeled gonadotropin (B_o = 34 %) was regarded as 100 %.

C. Physical and chemical characterization

Disc-gel electrophoretic patterns are illustrated in Figure 5. These patterns, and others not illustrated, indicate that the receptor purified by affinity chromatography showed only a single band in disc-gel electrophoresis in 5.6, 7.5 and 10 % SDS gels, with and without reduction by mercaptoethanol, and in 5.6 and 7.5 % alkaline gels without SDS. The mobility of the band suggested a molecular weight of approximately 70,000. No stainable material was seen when the gel was stained with Schiff reagent as described by Fairbanks et al. (17).

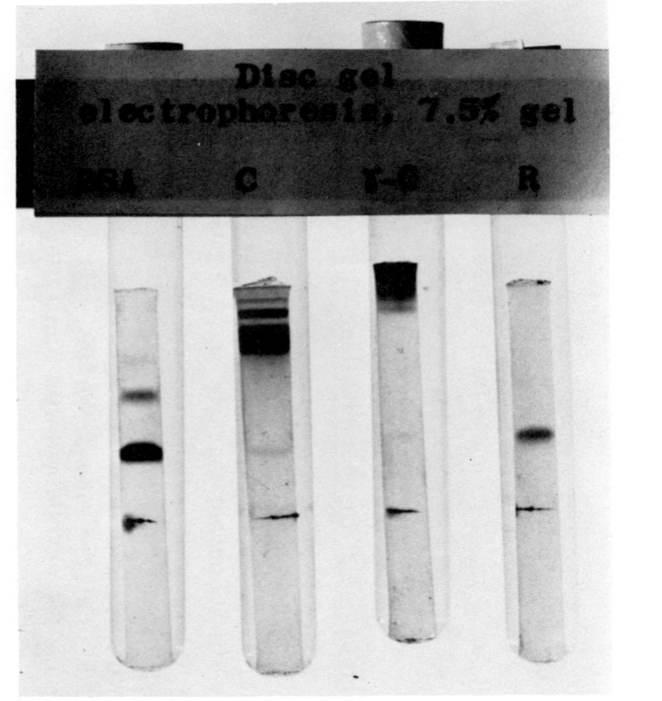

FIG 5A. Disc gel electrophoresis in 7.5 % gel-anionic system. The tubes (from left to right) represent bovine serum albumin (BSA), catalase (C), bovine γ-globulin (γ G) and purified ovarian receptor (R)

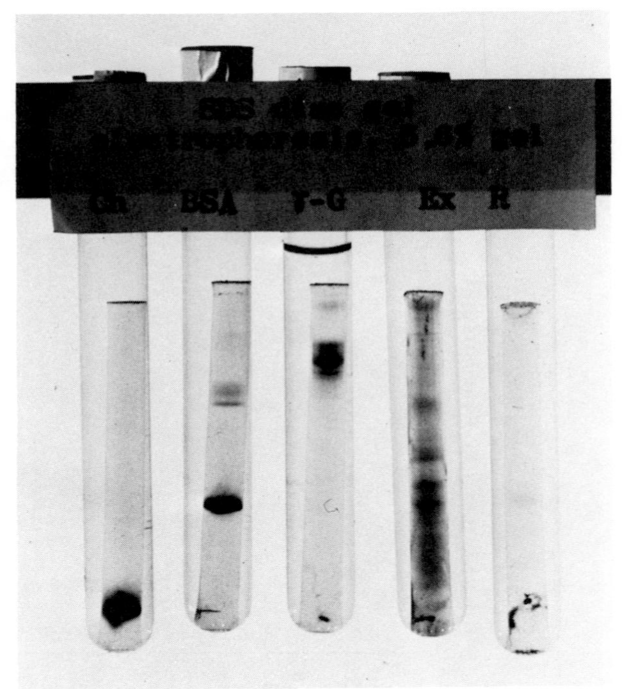

FIG 5B. SDS disc gel electrophoresis in 5.6 % gel. The tubes (from left to right) represent chymotrypsinogen (Ch), BSA, bovine γ- globulin, Triton extract of ovary (Ex) and affinity chromotography purified ovarian receptor (R).

Gel filtration of the purified receptor after incubation with ^{125}I hLH alone or with unlabeled hCG is illustrated in Figure 6. The hCG receptor complex was excluded on Sepahdex G-150. It should be noted that nonspecific binding using the purified receptor is appreciably less than seen in Figure 1 where the crude Triton extract was employed.

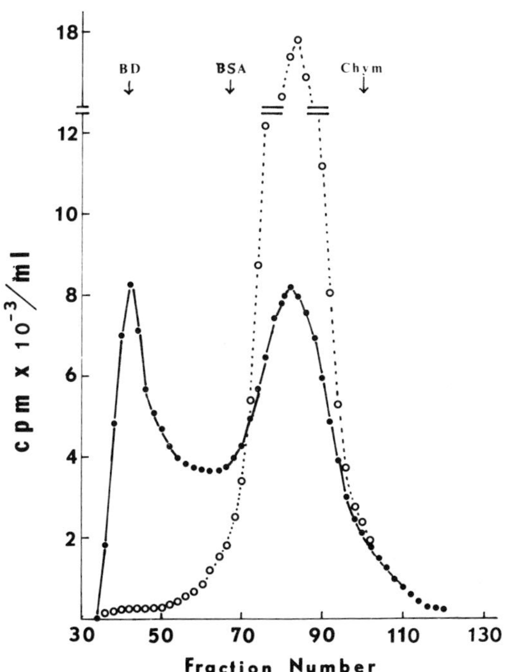

FIG 6. Gel filtration on Sephadex G-150 of purified ovarian receptor after 1 hr incubation at 25^{0} with labeled-hLH alone (closed circles) or labeled hLH plus 200 IU/ml of hCG (open circles). The elution of standard markers are indicated by BD (Blue Dextran) BSA (bovine serum albumin) and Chym (chymotrypsinogen). The column was 2.5 x 90 cm. Fractions were 3.2 ml each.

D. Receptor antibodies

Antibodies to purified receptor were raised in one goat and two rabbits. All three antisera showed only a single precipitin arc when tested at different dilutions of the antiserum and different concentrations of the antigen. No precipitin arcs were seen when the antisera were incubated with rat serum.

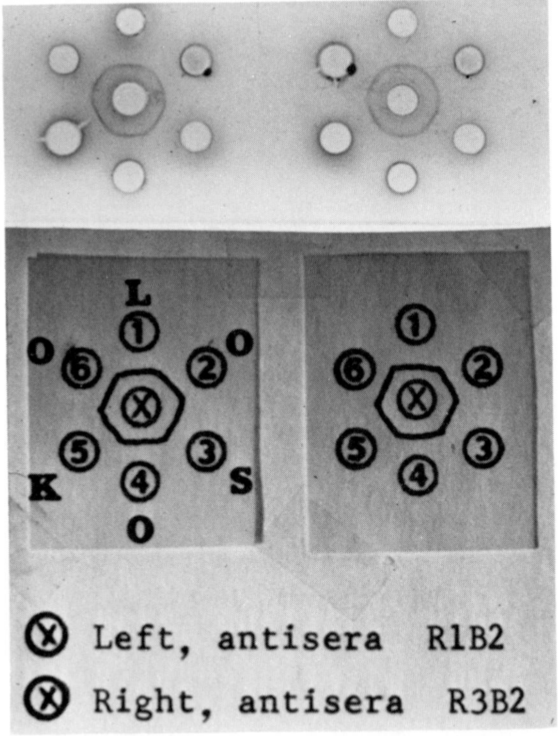

FIG 7. Immunodiffusion of antisera against affinity chromatography purified ovarian receptor and various tissue extracts.
Left: The central well contains antiserum from rabbit #1, bleeding 2. The outer wells contain Triton X-100 extracts of liver (1), ovary (2,4,6), spleen (3) and kidney (5). Right: The central well contains antiserum from rabbit #3. The peripheral wells contain Triton X-100 extracts of liver (1), spleen (3), ovary (4) and kidney (5). Affinity chromatography-purified ovarian receptor is in wells (2) and (6).

When the antisera reacted with crude Triton extracts of ovarian tissue, only a single precipitin arc was seen and this showed a reaction of identity with the purified receptor (see Figure 7). As controls for these experiments, Triton extracts of liver, spleen and kidney tissue of the same pseudopregnant rats were prepared. As shown in Figure 7, the Triton extracts of these tissues produced each a single precipitin arc against the 2 rabbit antisera. Further, this arc showed a reaction of identity with the purified ovarian receptor and the crude Triton extract of ovaries. Similar results were found with the antiserum raised in a goat.

The finding of a common antigen among purified ovarian LH receptor and crude extracts of liver, spleen and kidney was unexpected since previous data (1) had indicated that slices of liver,

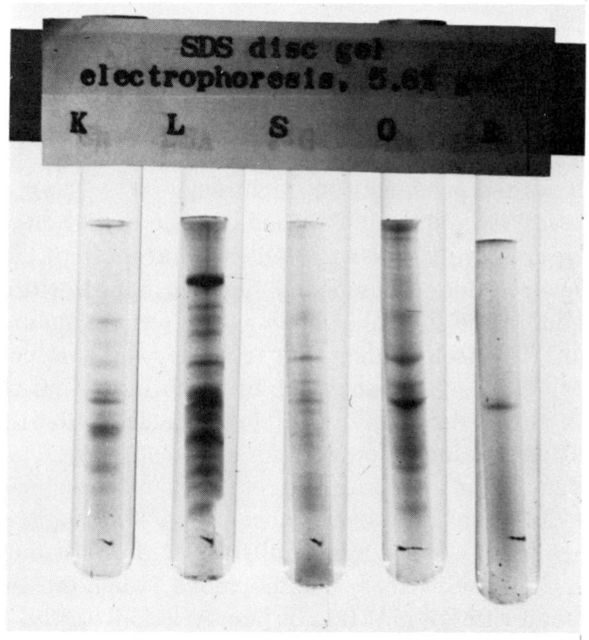

FIG 8. SDS disc gel electrophoresis, 5.6 % gel.
SDS disc gel (5.6 %) electrophoresis of Triton X-100 extracts of kidney (K), liver (L), spleen (S), ovary (O) and affinity chromatography purified ovarian receptor (R). India ink marks the tracker dye front.

spleen and kidney did not concentrate labeled-hLH during incubation. To further explore this phenomena, the disc-gel electrophoretic patterns of Triton extracts of all 4 tissues were compared with each other and with the purified LH receptor (Fig. 8). A band with the same mobility as the ovarian receptor can be seen in all the four tissues. The ovary and liver appear to contain more of this material than do the spleen and kidney.

The 2,000 g pellet from the Triton extract of liver was purified using the hCG-Sepharose affinity column and the elution schedule used for the ovarian receptor as illustrated in Fig. 2 and a similar elution profile was obtained. The guanidine eluate, after desalting, showed ability to bind ^{125}I-hCG. Furthermore, this binding was specific in that it was inhibited by unlabeled hCG, but not by FSH and analysis of a Scatchard plot indicated the dissociation constant to be 10^{-10} M, nearly identical to that found for the purified ovarian receptor.

DISCUSSION

We have several reservations about these data that we wish to discuss. The affinity chromatography used here does not seem to be as simple as the presentation might suggest. Thus, the elution of receptor activity required a rather drastic condition (3M guanidine) and this may well have affected the character of the eluted protein. Several lines of evidence suggest that alterations may have occurred. The dissociation constant for the guanidine-eluted receptor (10^{-10} M) is less than that found for the particulate receptor (10^{-11} M) (13). The behaviour of solubilized, but unpurified receptor, or purified receptor complexed to labeled-hLH or hCG, on gel filtration (exclusion on gels up to G-200) suggests that the molecular size of the receptor is greater than 70,000 daltons estimated from SDS disc-gel electrophoresis. This suggests a subunit structure and raises the possibility that this structure is altered by the elution conditions. Furthermore, when the guanidine salt is replaced with 40 mM tris buffer by gel filtration or dialysis, the guanidine-eluted protein tends to become insoluble with time.

We have had considerable difficulty in producing suitable affinity gels; in fact, we have produced only one batch that works and that is the one reported herein. We have attempted coupling by cyanogen bromide method, different ratios of LH or hCG to Sepharose at different pH values. They all have one drawback, in that they all adsorb receptor activity from Triton extracts, but the receptor cannot be eluted in a form that retains binding activity. Considerable work needs to be done to improve elution conditions and to explore other mechanisms for coupling to the solid phase.

Some of the quantitative aspects of the data, not reported here, also have presented problems. The change in dissociation constant that occurs with purification makes it difficult to calculate yields of binding activity. The yield of protein obtained in the guanidine eluted fraction, which is approximately 1.8 % of ovarian protein or 0.27 % of wet ovarian weight, is greater than that anticipated. Previous studies using a 2,000 g particulate fraction indicated that the number of binding sites was 18×10^{-15} moles/mg ovary and that one mole of receptor bound one mole of LH or hCG (13). If one assumes a molecular weight of 300,000 for the receptor (based on G-200), then calculation suggests that the yield of receptor should be 0.005 % rather than 0.27 % of wet ovarian weight. This discrepancy perhaps could be explained by the following assumptions : firstly, the bulk of the material obtained in the guanidine eluate is not receptor, but some other tissue protein. Alternatively, the estimate of the amount of receptor in the 2,000 g pellet is grossly underestimated. Perhaps some receptors may be masked or hindered while in the particulate state.

The immunodiffusion and disc-gel electrophoresis data suggest that we have a highly purified protein. We have not demonstrated, at least to our own satisfaction, that this purified protein is, in fact, the LH receptor. If, however, this purified protein, which is present in ovary, liver, spleen and kidney, is the LH receptor, then it raises a number of interesting questions and speculations.

What is the purpose of the LH receptor in liver, spleen and kidney, which are not obvious target tissues for LH or hCG ? They could be related to metabolism of the hormone or LH and hCG may have subtle biologic effects on these tissues that we do not yet appreciate. Are the receptors in these tissues capable of binding LH *in vivo* ? Failure to demonstrate concentration of labeled LH during *in vitro* incubation of slices of these tissues (1) suggest that they do not do so. This raises the possibility that target organ-specificity for this tropic hormone does not reside solely in the presence or absence of the receptor, but may also be influenced by masking or unmasking of receptors, perhaps by cell-surface glycoproteins. It is of interest that treatment of ovarian homogenates with neuraminidase enhanced LH binding (7).

Are the LH receptors in liver, spleen, and kidney "induced" by administration of PMS and hCG as appears to be the case with the ovary (1) ? We have no data on this point since we have only used tissues from primed rats.

Finally, we wonder if the process of malignant transformation might involve the expression on cell surfaces of receptors for hormones that are not tropic for the normal cell because their receptors are present, but masked, and therefore are not functional. The data of Schorr and Ney (18) concerning cyclic AMP concentrations in response to various hormones in malignant and normal rat adrenal tissues is of distinct interest in this regard. They found that malignant adrenal tissue responded to ACTH, LH, TSH, FSH, epinephrine and norepinephrine, while the normal adrenal only responded to ACTH. The appearance of lectin receptors leading to agglutination of malignant cells has been reported (19). Further, the abnormal hormonal receptors may lead to persistent stimulation of adenylate cyclase, which in the presence of limitations for the generation of ATP, may contribute to the low levels of cyclic AMP which are characteristic of malignant cells.

REFERENCES

1. Lee, C.Y. and Ryan, R.J. (1971). Endocrinology 89, 1515.
2. Lee, C.Y. and Ryan, R.J. (1973). J. Clin. Endo. & Metab. 36, 148.
3. deKrester, D.M., Catt, K.J. and Paulsen, C.A. (1971) Endocrinology 88, 332.
4. Dufau, M.L., Catt, K.J. and Tsuruhara, T. (1971). Biochem. Biophys. Res. Comm. 44, 1022.
5. Moudgal, N.R., Moyle, W.R. and Greep, R.O. (1971). J. Biol. Chem. 246, 4983.
6. Lee, C.Y. and Ryan, R.J. (1972). Proc. Natl. Acad. Sci. 69, 3520.
7. Lee, C.Y. and Ryan, R.J. (1973) in "Receptors for Reproductive Hormones", O'Malley, B.W., and Means, A.R., (Eds), Advances in Exper. Med. and Biol. Vol 36, p. 419, Plenum Press, New York.
8. Cuatrecasas, P., Wilchek, M. and Anfinsen (1968). Proc. Natl. Acad. Sci. 61, 636.
9. Sato, N. and Cargille, C.M. (1972). Endocrinology 90, 302.

10. Lowry, O. H., Rosebrough, N. J., Farr, A. L. and Randall, R. J. (1951). J. Biol. Chem. 193, 265.
11. Desbuquois, B. and Aurbach, G. D. (1971). J. Clin. Endo. & Metab. 33, 732.
12. Greenwood, F. C., Hunter, W. M. and Glover, J. S. (1963). Biochem. J. 89, 114.
13. Lee, C. Y. and Ryan, R. J. (1973). Biochemistry 12 (in press).
14. Ryan. R. J. (1969). Biochemistry 8, 495.
15. Bishop, W. H. and Ryan, R. J. (1973) Biochemistry 12, 3076.
16. Ornstein, L. (1964). Ann. N. Y. Acad. Sci. 121, 321.
17. Fairbanks, G., Steck, T. L. and Wallach, D. F. H. (1971). Biochemistry 10, 2606.
18. Schorr, I. and Ney, R. (1971). J. Clin. Investigation 50, 1295.
19. Burger, M. M. (1973). Fed. Proc. 32, 91.

THE ROLE OF CARBOHYDRATE IN THE BIOLOGICAL FUNCTION OF HUMAN CHORIONIC GONADOTROPIN

Om P. Bahl and Leopold Marz

INTRODUCTION

It is widely acknowledged that the primary site of action of a peptide hormone such as insulin (1), glucagon (2), adrenocorticotropin (3), and gonadotropins (4-6) is the plasma membranes of the target cells. All of the metabolic effects of the hormone, whether nuclear or cytoplasmic, are mediated through this initial interaction with the exterior of the cell. The physico-chemical nature of the binding and the mechanism of transduction are not yet known. Consequently, the first step in the understanding of the molecular mechanism of hormone action is to elucidate the nature of the binding to the receptors on the plasma membranes. HCG binds to the plasma membranes with an association constant of the order of 10^{10} M^{-1} (7). The glycoproteins and glycolipids which are essential components of cell surfaces, play an important role in diverse cell-surface phenomena such as interaction with macromolecules, cell recognition, cell adhesion, and contact inhibition. It is, therefore, conceivable that the carbohydrate may be involved in the interaction of the hormone with the receptor or in the various other metabolic functions including stimulation of adenyl cyclase, steroidogenesis, and last but not least, protein synthesis. Likewise, the carbohydrate may participate in the immunological activity of hCG.

HCG contains approximately 30 % carbohydrate (8, 9) which is distributed in seven carbohydrate units, four of them being linked N-glycosidically to the asparaginyl residues and the remaining three 0-glycosidically to the seryl residues (10-12). The asparagine-linked carbohydrate units are bulky, complex and multiple-branched (10) and are located at positions 52 and 78 (Fig 1) in the

---

Abbreviations used : NANA, N-acetylneuraminic acid; GluNAc, N-acetylglucosamine; GaLNAc, N-acetylgalactosamine; Man, mannose; Gal, galactose; Fuc, fucose.

```
                                           10                                   20
H-Ala-Pro-Asx-Val-Glx-Asx-Cys-Pro-Glx-Cys-Thr-Leu-Glx-Glx-Asx-Pro-Phe-Phe-Ser-Glx-Pro-Gly-Ala-

                          30                                   40
Pro-Ile-Leu-Gln-Cys-Met-Gly-Cys-Cys-Phe-Ser-Arg-Ala-Tyr-Pro-Thr-Pro-Leu-Arg-Ser-Lys-Lys-Thr-Met-

        50                                      60                                   70
Leu-Val-Gln-Lys-[Asn(CHO)]-Val-Thr-Ser-Glx-Ser-Thr-Cys-Cys-Val-Ala-Lys-Ser-Tyr-Asn-Arg-Val-Thr-Val-

                                            80                                  90
Met-Gly-Gly-Phe-Lys-Val-Glx-[Asn(CHO)]-His-Thr-Ala-Cys-His-Cys-Ser-Thr-Cys-Tyr-Tyr-His-Lys-Ser-OH
```

FIG 1. Linear amino acid sequence of hCG-α

```
                                           10                                        20
H-Ser-Lys-Gln-Pro-Leu-Arg-Pro-Arg-Cys-Arg-Pro-Ile-[Asn(CHO)]-Ala-Thr-Leu-Ala-Val-Glu-Lys-Glu-Gly-

                              30                                        40
Cys-Pro-Val-Cys-Ile-Thr-Val-[Asn(CHO)]-Thr-Thr-Ile-Cys-Ala-Gly-Tyr-Cys-Pro-Thr-Met-Thr-Arg-Val-

                      50                                   60
Leu-Gln-Gly-Val-Leu-Pro-Ala-Leu-Pro-Glx-Leu-Val-Cys-Asn-Tyr-Arg-Asp-Val-Arg-Phe-Glu-Ser-Ile-

        70                                  80                                       90
Arg-Leu-Pro-Gly-Cys-Pro-Arg-Gly-Val-Asn-Pro-Val-Val-Ser-Tyr-Ala-Val-Ala-Leu-Ser-Cys-Gln-Cys-

                                          100                                    110
Ala-Leu-Cys-Arg-(Arg)-Ser-Thr-Thr-Asp-Cys-Gly-Gly-Pro-Lys-Asp-His-Pro-Leu-Thr-Cys-Asp-Asp-

                                     120                                         130
Pro-Arg-Phe-Gln-Asp-[Ser(CHO)]-Ser-Ser-Lys-Ala-Pro-Pro-Pro-Ser-Leu-Pro-[Ser(CHO)]-Pro-[Ser(CHO)]-

                                      140
Arg-Leu-Pro-Gly-Pro-Pro-Asx-Thr-Pro-Ile-Leu-Pro-Gln-Ser-Leu-Pro-OH
```

FIG 2. Linear amino acid sequence of hCG-β .

α subunit (11) and at positions 13 and 30 (Fig 2) in the β subunit (12). The serine-linked carbohydrate units are short, linear oligosaccharide chains and are present only in the β subunit at positions 118, 129 and 131. The average monosaccharide sequence (Fig 3) in a single branch of the complex carbohydrate unit, determined by sequential removal of the monosaccharides with specific glycosidases, is NANA(Fuc)-Gal-GluNAc-Man- (9). The monosaccharide sequence (Fig 3, structure III) in a serine-linked carbohydrate unit is reported to be NANA-Gal-GalNAC- (12).

The carbohydrate moiety of hCG represents two of the limited numbers of structural patterns present in glycoproteins. The asparagine-linked carbohydrate units of hCG have similar structural features as those present in serum glycoproteins such as α_1-acid glycoprotein (13, 14) and fetuin (15), whereas the serine-linked carbohydrate units are representative of mucins (16) and blood

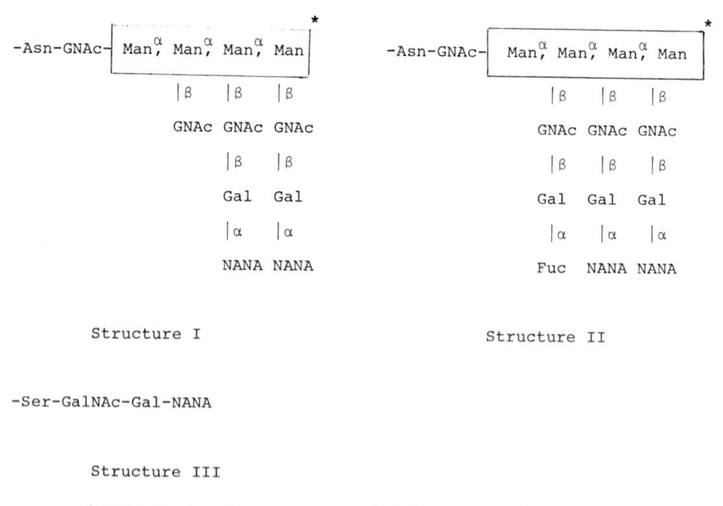

FIG 3. Structure I, sequence of the monosaccharides in the carbohydrate of the α subunit; Structure II, sequence of the monosaccharides in the asparagine-linked carbohydrate of the β subunit; Structure III, sequence of the monosaccharides in the serine-linked carbohydrate of the β subunit.

group substances (17). Evidently, hCG has two types of protein-polysaccharide linkages in the same molecule. Only a few other examples of glycoproteins of this type have been reported thus far (10).

General approach

HCG and plasma membrane receptors were both sequentially hydrolyzed with purified specific glycosidases (9). The resulting modified forms of hCG were examined for their ability to compete for binding to the membrane receptors and to the anti-hCG by using ^{125}I-labeled hCG. The rat testes homogenate (6) or a partially purified membrane preparation (18) was used in these studies. The effects of the hCG derivatives on adenyl cyclase activation and steroidogenesis were measured by using a suspension of Leydig cells (19). In order to further ascertain the role of the carbohydrate in the binding, monosaccharides, oligosaccharides, and glycoproteins were tested for their inhibitory properties in a manner analogous to the hemagglutination inhibition reaction; phytoagglutinins and blood group substances cause agglutination of red cells which can be inhibited by haptens, specific monosaccharides or oligosaccharides (20). Also, the possible involvement of the cell surface glycosyl transferases in the binding has been considered by using appropriate nucleotides as inhibitors. The effect of the inhibitors of glycosidases on the binding has been investigated. Finally, the serological activity of hCG has also been studied.

Digestions of hCG and plasma membranes with glycosidases

The following glycosidases *Vibrio cholerae* neuraminidase (9), *Aspergillus niger* β-D-galactosidase, β-N-acetylglucosaminidase (21), and α-D-mannosidase (22), free of cross-contamination and proteases, were employed. The hormone was treated sequentially with the glycosidases at 37° under nitrogen for an extended period of time. After each enzyme treatment, the sugar released was separated from the enzymic digest by dialysis and was estimated by gas chromatography (9). Each modified form of the hormone was freed of the enzyme by chromatography (Fig. 4) on DEAE-cellulose (DE-52, Whatman). Table 1 gives the percent hydrolysis of the hormone by the various enzymes.

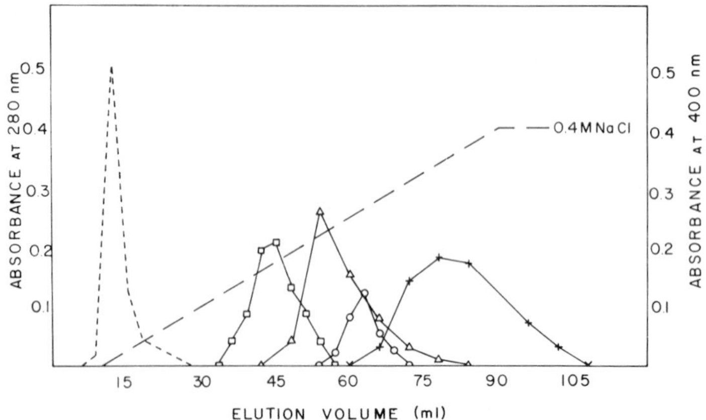

FIG 4. Separation of the hCG derivatives from glycosidases on a DEAE-cellulose column (0.7 x 18 cm), previously equilibrated with 0.05 M sodium acetate. After elution with 10 ml of the starting solution a linear salt gradient was set up between 0 and 0.4 M NaCl in 0.05 M sodium acetate (40 ml each). 3 ml fractions were collected. ------, hCG derivatives; —□—□— , neuraminidase; —Δ—Δ— β-galactosidase; x—x—x , β-N-acetylglucosaminidase; -o—o—o- , α -mannosidase.

Table 1. Percent hydrolysis of the carbohydrate of hCG by glycosidases

Sample *	% Hydrolysis
1. with neuraminidase	99
2. with β -D-galactosidase	60.0
3. with β -N-acetylglucosaminidase	52.5
4. with α -D-mannosidase	19.0

* hCG was sequentially treated with the different glycosidases listed in the order indicated (1→ 4).

The resulting modified forms of hCG-neuraminidase-(N-hCG), neuraminidase- β-galactosidase-(NG-hCG), neuraminidase- β-galactosidase- β-N-acetylglucosaminidase (NGA-hCG), and neuraminidase- β-galactosidase- β-N-acetylglucosaminidase-α mannosidase treated hCG (NGAM-hCG) - were characterized chemically by analyzing for amino acids, hexosamines, and neutral sugars. The results summarized in Table 2 indicate that there was no degradation of the polypeptide chain during the modification of the carbohydrate. Also, to ensure that the dissociation of the hormone had not occurred during the hydrolysis of the carbohydrate, the various derivatives of hCG were chromatographed on Sephadex G-100.

The plasma membranes were also treated with glycosidases in a similar manner. However, one of the problems encountered during their digestion was that the membrane receptors were partially inactivated at the pH optima of the enzymes (pH 4 to 5.5). Therefore, the duration of the hydrolysis was kept to a minimum of 5 hr, although a large excess of the enzymes was used. Under these controlled conditions only neuraminidase and β-D-galactosidase caused considerable hydrolysis as measured by the liberation of neuraminic acid and galactose.

Table 2. Amino acid[1] and hexosamine compositions of hCG and glycosidase-treated hCG

Amino acid	Neuraminidase treated	Galactosidase treated	Glucosaminidase treated	α-mannosidase treated	hCG
Lysine	10.4	11.8	12.1	11.1	12.1
Histidine	4.1	4.1	4.3	3.1	4.1
Arginine	15.2	15.6	18.7	19.5	18.8
Aspartic acid	17.7	18.0	18.0	17.2	15.5
Threonine	16.9	17.3	17.7	14.9	16.3
Serine	19.0	19.5	21.0	22.4	16.5
Glutamic acid	19.1	18.4	18.3	18.2	17.1
Proline	29.9	30.2	29.1	32.0	33.5
Glycine	13.2	14.7	14.3	18.9	13.8
Alanine	13.5	14.4	12.9	14.4	12.6
Half-cysteine	21.8	19.7	18.0	16.0	20.4
Valine	18.6	18.1	18.6	18.8	18.7
Methionine	3.9	3.4	2.9	1.3	3.2
Isoleucine	6.8	5.7	6.1	6.5	6.2
Leucine	15.3	15.2	15.1	14.7	16.6
Tyrosine	6.9	6.0	5.7	4.8	7.3
Phenylalanine	6.3	6.1	5.6	4.8	6.3
N-acetyl glucosamine	9.6%		5.2%		
N-acetyl galactosamine	1.7%		2.0%		

[1]Represents the number of residues.

Role of the carbohydrate in the immunological activity

The removal of almost all of sialic acid did not cause any significant loss in the immunological activity of hCG as determined by radioimmunoassay. In contrast to the report of Tsuruhara et al. (23) that no change in the immunological activity occured on the removal of galactose, cleavage of 60 % galactose residues resulted in a slight drop in activity; in fact, a slight decrease in the activity was observed with the cleavage of each of the monosaccharides (Table 2 and Fig 5). This may be due to the element of instability or the conformational change introduced in the molecule as a result of the degradation of the carbohydrate, since a sample of NGAM-hCG stored at -10° for several weeks, resulted in a considerable loss in the immunological activity, whereas the freshly prepared derivative invariably was found to be active. It is therefore, believed that the carbohydrate part of the molecule particularly the sialic acid, galactose, N-acetylglucosamine, and mannose residues do not act as the antigenic determinants. It would be interesting to find out if the oligosaccharides and glyco peptides fail to inhibit the hCG-anti hCG binding in the radioimmunoassay. The role of the fucose residues in the antigenicity has not been evaluated so far.

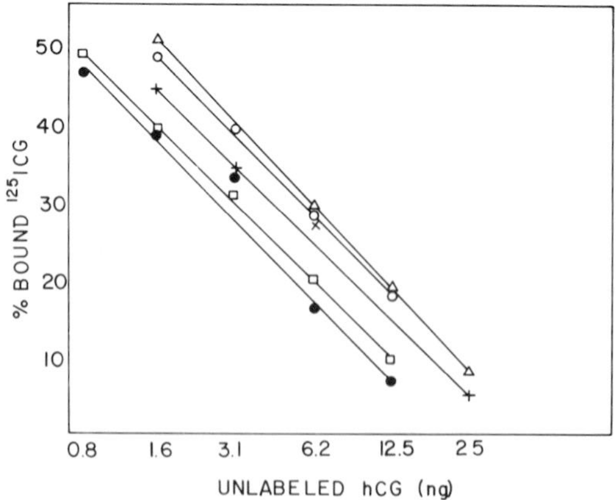

FIG 5. Radioimmunoassay of hCG derivatives: —●—●—● , native hCG; —□—□—□— , N-hCG; —△—△—△— NG-hCG; —x—x—x— , NGA-hCG; —o—o—o— , NGAM-hCG.

Table 3. Immunological and binding properties of hCG and glycosidase-treated hCG.

Sample	Immunological * activity (%)	Binding ** activity (ng).
hCG	100	17.5
Neuraminidase-treated	93 ± 10	7.5
Galactosidase-treated	78 ± 10	11.0
Glucasaminidase-treated	68 ± 10	21.0
Mannosidase-treated	71 ± 10	¶

* Determined by radioimmunoassay; values are averages of four assays.
** Amount of protein required to decrease the binding of ^{125}I-hCG by 50%.
¶ 10 ng decreased the binding of ^{125}I-hCG by 16 %, 20 ng by 19 %, and 40 ng by 25 %.

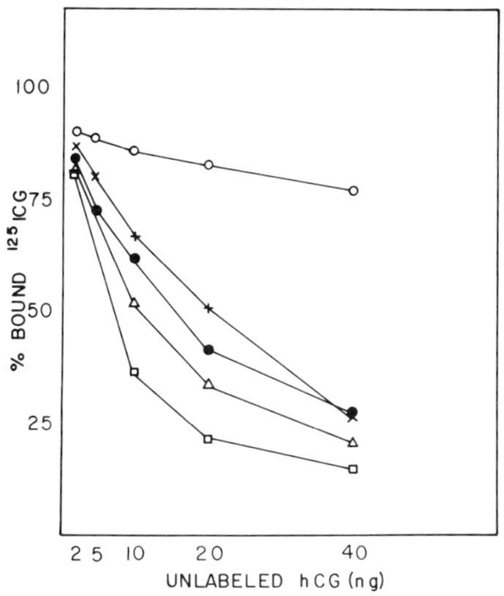

FIG 6. Competitive binding of hCG derivatives to membrane receptors using rat testes homogenate. The duration of the assay was 4 hr at 25°. —●—●—●—, native hCG; —□—□—□— , N-hCG; —△—△— NG-hCG; —x—x—x— , NGA-hCG; —o—o—o— NGAM-hCG.

Effect of carbohydrate on the binding

The removal of sialic acid resulted in a two-fold increase in the binding to the plasma membranes as evidenced by the decreased amount of desialized hCG required to displace 50 % of the ^{125}I-hCG (Table 3 and Fig 6) from the membranes. Glycoproteins in general show microheterogeneity in the carbohydrate chains particularly due to the variation in the sialic acid content. In view of the enhanced binding of the desialized hCG to the membranes, it was of interest to find out if any part of the total binding of the intact hCG to the membranes was due to the cell surface sialyl transferases. Thus, no effect on binding was observed in the competition studies using labeled intact hCG and desialyzed α_1-acid glycoprotein and fetuin indicating that all of the binding was to the specific hCG-receptors on the membranes. The nucleotides CMP, UDP, and GDP did not affect the binding of the labeled hCG to the membranes again suggesting that the transferases were not involved. However, if the membranes were preincubated for 1 hr at 30° with a large excess of the above serum

Table 4. Effect of mono- and oligosaccharides, glycoproteins, nucleotides, and lactones on the binding to the homogenate and to the membranes.

Sample	% binding homogenate	% binding Membranes
Fetuin (400 μg)	100	99
Desialized fetuin (400 μg)	81	62
α_1-acid glycoprotein (400 μg)	99	100
Desialized α_1-acid glycoprotein (400 μg)	71	38
Thyroglobulin (500 μg)	100	100
hCG-α (0.5 μg)	-	25
hCG-β (0.5 μg)	-	30
Nucleotides (CMP, UDP, GDP)	100	
Monosaccharides (Galactose, mannose, fucose, NANA)	104	
Methyl-α-D-mannopyranoside	101	
Methyl-β-D-galactopyranoside	100	
Methyl-α-D-fucopyranoside	109	
Man $\xrightarrow[1\ \alpha\ 4]{}$ GluNAc	110	
Man $\xrightarrow[1\ \alpha\ 6]{}$ GluNAc	99	
Man $\xrightarrow[1\ \alpha\ 3]{}$ GluNAc	102	
Lactofucopentose I	106	
Lactofucopentose II	100	
Lactofucopentose III	98	
2-$\underline{0}$-α-fucosyl galactose	102	
3-fucosyl lactose	98	
Sugar lactones	101	

glycoproteins, there was a 40 to 60 % loss in the binding (Table 4). This may be due to the desialized glycoproteins actually blocking the hCG sites on the membranes or causing an alteration in the overall membrane structure by binding to the membrane sialyl transferases. Since the native glycoproteins under similar conditions of preincubation did not affect the binding, the latter seems to play a predominant role.

The NG-hCG had greater binding than the native hCG, but was less active than the desialized hCG. Subsequent removal of N-acetylglucosamine residues from NG-hCG did not alter the binding significantly. Thus, the data strongly suggest that sialic acid, galactose and glucosamine are not involved in the binding; in addition, various monosaccharides and oligosaccharides failed to block the binding sites. The hydrolysis of mannose residues ($\sim$ 20 %) from NGA-hCG drastically reduced the binding. This might be due either to a drastic conformational change in hCG, or that mannose is required for the binding, because of the presence of a specific binding site on the membrane receptors. Also, the possibility of an artifact, introduced during hydrolysis of NGA-hCG by α -mannosidase, such as oxidation of methionine or cysteine residues should be considered. It is surprising, however, that the immunological activity of NGAM-hCG is not significantly different from that of NGA-hCG (Table 3, and Fig 5). This renders the possibility of a drastic conformational change or an artifact less likely. The involvement of mannose in the interaction of macromolecules to the cell surfaces and in the inter cellular interactions has been observed recently. For example, the binding site of phytoagglutinins of lentil and P. vulgaris on the red blood cell involves mannose residues (20). Similarly, Yen and Ballou (24) have recently reported the significance of mannose residues in the glycoproteins of yeast cells in the intercellular agglutination.

To test the possibility of the binding of the hormone being preceded by the hydrolysis of the carbohydrate by endogenous glycosidases, the appropriate inhibitors of the glycosidases such as sugar lactones were used in the binding assay. There was no effect of the lactones on the binding (Table 4).

The cleavage of almost all of sialic acid from the membranes resulted in a stronger binding while the hydrolysis of galactose residues, did not cause any change. It may be noted that the binding increases whether sialic acid is removed from the hormone or from the membranes.

The role of the carbohydrate in the stimulation of cyclic AMP and steroidogenesis

These studies were carried out with a suspension of Leydig cells (19). The cyclic AMP was measured by the protein binding assay (25) and testosterone by radioimmunoassay. Preliminary data indicated that the removal of sialic acid from hCG caused a considerable loss (about 80 %) in its ability to stimulate cyclic AMP formation. The NG-hCG, NGA-hCG, and NGAM-hCG exhibited even less activity. It should be pointed out that the binding does not necessarily correspond to the biological activity since all of these derivatives, with the exception of NGAM-hCG, show a considerable binding to the plasma membranes. Furthermore, all of these derivatives act as inhibitors of cyclic AMP stimulation by hCG. It is interesting to note they all stimulate steroidogenesis. Further work is in progress to study their effect on protein synthesis.

Serological activity of hCG

HCG was examined for A, B, H, and Lewis blood group activities by the hemagglutination inhibition technique (26, 27). The hormone showed detectable cross-reactivity with blood group A substance (Table 5), and this was concentrated in the α subunit; this is surprising, since the immunodominant sugar in blood group A substance is N-acetylgalactosamine and this carbohydrate is not detectable in the α-subunit. Another example of this type is an antigen, carcinoembryonic antigen (CEA) of the human digestive system, which has A-like activity but lacks N-acetylgalactosamine (28). The monosaccharide components of the antigen were sialic acid, N-acetylglucosamine, mannose and L-fucose which, with the possible exception of L-fucose, are also present in hCG-α.

Although more work is needed to determine precisely the structural components required for the A-like activity, the carbohydrate of hCG-α does seem to be associated with the serological activity. It is interesting to note that the antigenic determinants do not seem to be located in the carbohydrate portion of the molecule. Also, the carbohydrate, with the possible exception of

Table 5. Inhibition of agglutination of human anti-A serum by hCG and its subunits.

	Salivas				Porcine A substances		hCG		
	Group A_1		Group A_2		GS-009	GS-147	Intact	alpha	beta
	Se	se	Se	se					
Undiluted	-	++++	-	++++	-	-	-	-	(+)
1:2	-	++++	-	++++	-	-	(+)	-	+
1:4	-	++++	-	++++	-	-	+	-	++
1:8	-	++++	-	++++	-	-	++	-	++
1:16	-	++++	(+)	++++	-	-	++	(+)	+++
1:32	-	++++	+	++++	-	-	+++	+	+++
1:64	(+)	++++	++	++++	-	-	++++	++	++++
1:128	+	++++	+++	++++	-	-	++++	++	++++
1:256	++	++++	+++	++++	-	-	++++	+++	++++
1:512	+++	++++	++++	++++	-	-	++++	++++	++++
1:1024	+++	++++	++++	++++	-	-	++++	++++	++++
Saline	++++	++++	++++	++++	++++	++++	++++	++++	++++

Se = secretor; se = nonsecretor.

mannose, does not appear to be required for the binding. It is, however, associated with the serological activity as well as with the adenyl cyclase activation.

The precise physiological significance of the present findings is not yet clear, but it is fascinating in view of the possible role of hCG in the suppression of the lymphocyte function during the implantation of the fetus on the maternal endometrium (29). Despite the fact that at least 50 % of the fetal antigens are different from that of the mother, yet it is not rejected by the mother. It has been postulated that hCG might be involved in the suppression of the immune response of the mother by binding with maternal lymphocytes. It may be noted that hCG is the first hormone which has been found to exhibit such cross-reactivity with blood group A substance.

In conclusion, we have presented our initial studies on the role of carbohydrate of hCG in its antigenicity, binding to the membrane receptors, in the serological activity and finally in the stimulation of adenyl cyclase and steroidogenesis.

ACKNOWLEDGEMENT

The authors wish to thank Dr. W.R. Moyle for his help in the cyclic AMP and testosterone determinations. A detailed manuscript on this work is in preparation. Supported by research grants from USPHS, AM-10273, and from the Population Council of New York.

REFERENCES

1. Cuatrecasas, P. (1969). Proc. Natl. Acad. Sci. 63, 450.
2. Rodbell, M., Krans, H.M.J., Pohl, S.L. and Birnbaumer, L. (1971). J. Biol. Chem. 246, 1861.
3. Lefkowitz, R.J., Roth, J. and Pastan, I. (1970). Science, 170, 633.
4. Danzo, B.J. (1973). Biochem. Biophys. Acta 304, 560.
5. Lee, C.Y. and Ryan, R.J. (1971). Endocrinology 89, 1515.
6. Catt, K.J., Tsuruhara, T. and Dufau, M.L. (1972). Biochem. Biophys. Acta. 279, 194.
7. Saxena, B.B. and Rao, Ch. V. (1973). Biochim. Biophys. Acta. 313, 372.
8. Bahl, O.P. (1969). J. Biol. Chem. 244, 567.
9. Bahl, O.P. (1969). J. Biol. Chem. 244, 575.
10. Bahl, O.P. (1973). In "Hormonal Proteins and Peptides" C.H. Li (Ed), Academic Press, pp. 171.
11. Bellisario, R., Carlsen, R.B., and Bahl, O.P. (1973). J. Biol. Chem. 248, 6797.
12. Carlsen, R.B., Bahl, O.P., and Swaminathan, N. (1973). J. Biol. Chem. 248, 6810.
13. Eylar, E.H. and Jeanloz, R.W. (1962). J. Biol. Chem. 237, 622.
14. Wagh, P.V., Bornstein, I. and Winzler, R.J. (1969). J. Biol. Chem. 244, 658.
15. Spiro, R.G. (1964). J. Biol. Chem. 239, 567.
16. Carlson, D.M. (1968). J. Biol. Chem. 243, 616.
17. Lloyd, K.O., Beychok, S. and Kabat, E.A. (1967). Biochemistry, 6, 1448.
18. Ray, T.K. (1970). Biochim. Biophys. Acta 196, 1.
19. Moyle, W.R. and Ramachandran, J. (1973). Endocrinology 93, 127.

20. Kornfeld, S. and Kornfeld, R. (1971). In "Glycoproteins of Blood Cells and Plasma", G.A. Gameison and T.J. Greenwalt, (Eds). J.B. Lippincott Co., pp. 50.
21. Bahl, O.P. and Agrawal, K.M.L. (1969). J. Biol. Chem. 244, 2970.
22. Matta, K.L. and Bahl, O.P. (1972). J. Biol. Chem. 247, 1780.
23. Tsuruhara, T., Dufau, M.L., Hickman, J. and Catt, K.J. (1972). Endocrinology 91, 296.
24. Yen, P.S. and Ballou, C.E. (1973). J. Biol. Chem. 248, 8316.
25. Gilman, A.G. (1970). Proc. Natl. Acad. Sci. 67, 305.
26. Mohn, J.F., Cunningham, R.K., Pirkola, A., Furuhjelm, U. and Nevanlinna, H.R. (1973). Vox Sang. 24, 385.
27. Milgrom, F., Mohn, J.F. and Loza, U. (1973). Vox Sang (in press).
28. Gold, J.M., Freeman, S.O. and Gold, P. (1972). Nature New Biol. 239, 60.
29. Adcock, E.W., Teasdale, F., August, C.S., Cox, S., Meschia, G., Battaglia, F.C. and Naughton, M.A. (1973). Science 181, 845.

BIOCHEMICAL ASPECTS OF THE INTERACTION OF HUMAN CHORIONIC GONADOTROPIN WITH RAT GONADS

Yoshihiko Ashitaka and Samuel S. Koide

The biological effects of human chorionic gonadotropin on ovarian and testicular cells are considered to be similar to those of luteinizing hormone (1). Receptors for these two gonadotropins were reported to reside in the cells of the corpus luteum (2) and in the interstitial cells of the testis (3). The nature of the gonadotropin receptor has been recently demonstrated (4,5). The present study describes the fate of the hCG molecule at the target cell.

MATERIALS AND METHODS

HCG was purified from commercial preparations as described in Ashitaka et al. (6). Purified hCG was tritiated by the method described by Vaitukaitis et al. (7) and iodinated by an enzymatic method (8). The ^{3}H-hCG prepared, possessed approximately 75-80 % of the biological activity and its specific radioactivity was 5.8×10^5 dpm/µg. A representative preparation of ^{125}I-hCG retained at least 93% of the original biological activity and its specific radioactivity ranged from 66 to 74 µCi/µg.

In vivo experiments with female rats : PMS and hCG were administered to 21-day old female rats as previously described (9). ^{3}H-hCG or ^{125}I-hCG were injected into the tail vein of each rat. The rats were killed at timed intervals following injection. The radioactivity incorporated in various organs were determined and the ovaries were used for autoradiography and for receptor-hormone interaction study. Plasma membrane fraction of ovarian cells was prepared by the method of Emmelot et al. (10).

In vitro experiments with rat testes : Testes from male rats (250-350 g) were decapsulated and incubated with labeled gonadotropin in Krebs-Ringer bicarbonate (KRB) buffer for 4 hr at 37° under 95 % O_2 - 5 % CO_2. The incubated testes were washed three times with cold KRB buffer. The washed testes were divided into two groups. The testicular tissue of one group was shaken at 4° in pH 2.3 saline for 16 hr. The hormone released from the receptor sites of testes were analysed through Sephadex gel filtration, polyacrylamide disc-gel electrophoresis, and receptor-binding assay of gonadotropin by Dufau et al. (11). In addition, the released hormone was readministered to pseudopregnant rats and its uptake by the ovaries determined. The testicular tissue of the other group was re-incubated in KRB buffer containing 10mM glucose for 4 hr at 37° under 95 % O_2 - 5 % CO_2. Every hour the medium was replaced with a fresh solution. The used medium was subjected to Sephadex gel filtration and analyzed by thin layer chromatography using a developing solution of butylacetate : acetic acid : water (3:2:1).

RESULTS

As previously reported (8, 9), the ovary showed the highest uptake of ^{3}H-hCG and ^{125}I-hCG when they were injected into pseudopregnant rats via tail vein; the uptake reached a maximal level at 1.5 or 2 hr, and declined thereafter. About 20-40 % of the total radioactivity injected was concentrated in the ovaries extirpated from rats killed 2 hr later. As shown in Fig. 1, within the dose range tested (1-84 ng), the uptake in the organs assayed increased

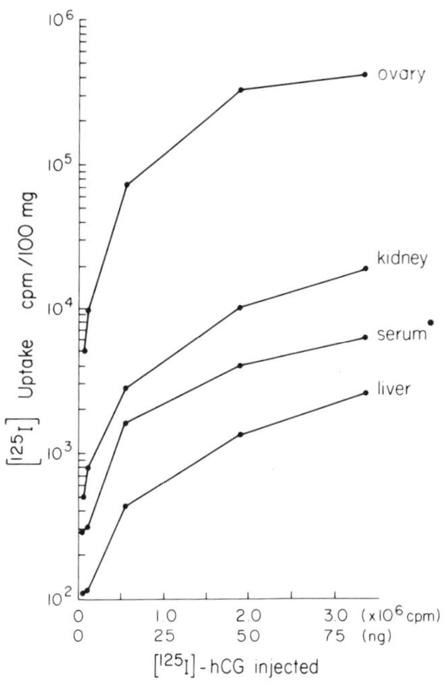

FIG 1. Uptake of ^{125}I-hCG by organs of super-ovulated rat - a dose response study. Radio-activity of each organ was determined 2 hr after administration. Each point indicates the mean of 3 values.

with increasing amounts of hCG administered. To eliminate any non-specific binding and contamination by blood, several animals were anesthetized with ether and perfused with saline via the descending thoracic aorta. The specific activity retained by the ovaries obtained from perfused rats were at least 87 % of the control value (Table 1).

Table 1. Uptake of hCG by rat ovaries 2 hr after injection.

Injected	n	cpm/100 mg	%
^{125}I-hCG*	4	3.20×10^5	100.0
^{125}I-hCG*	3**	$2.8 \times 10^5 - 3.4 \times 10^5$	87.5-106.3
^{125}I-hCG + 100 IU of cold hCG	3	4.16×10^4	13.0

* 1.9×10^6 cpm of ^{125}I-hCG; ** perfused with saline.

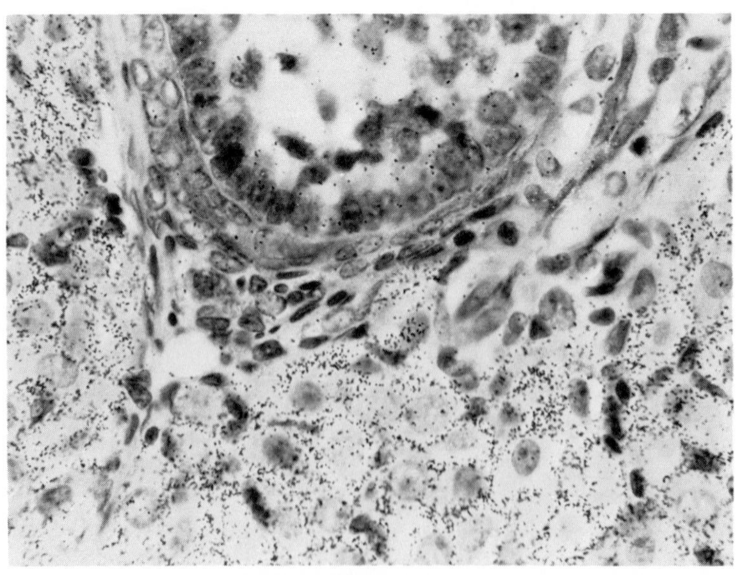

FIG 2. Autoradiograph of the ovary 2 hr after ^{3}H-hCG injection. Silver grains are concentrated around the periphery of the luteal cells (x 320).

Table 2. Interaction of ^{125}I-hCG with rat testis and receptor fraction.

	Exp. 1 (n=1)	Exp. 2 (n=8)	^{125}I-hCG**
Binding of ^{125}I-hCG* to decapsulated testis	60.0	63.1$\pm$3.6	
Bound hCG released by acid saline treatment (pH 2.3)	46.7	53.1$\pm$8.2	
HCG bound to receptor fraction of testis***	11.0	11.5$\pm$2.0	10.8$\pm$0.8

Values are mean $\pm$ SEM and expressed as percent of total radioactivity. * ^{125}I-hCG (7.5×10^5) was incubated with decapsulated testis. ** ^{125}I-hCG (8.5×10^4) was incubated with receptor fraction of testis. ***Released radioactive material was assayed by receptor-binding assay system. In each experiment 4 rats were used. In Exp. 1 ^{125}I-hCG ($8 \times 7.5 \times 10^5$ cpm) was incubated with 8 testes, and in Exp. 2 ^{125}I-hCG (7.5×10^5cpm) was incubated with a single testis each time.

Autoradiograph of ovaries following administration of ^{3}H-hCG revealed that the luteal cells accumulated the greatest of silver grains while cells of the granulosa and theca layers contained relatively few grains. The silver grains were localized at the peripheral surface of the luteal cells (Fig. 2). The present findings suggest that when hCG was administered, it was bound to the receptor sites of the luteal cell membrane, rather than being non-specifically adsorbed on the luteal cells.

When testis of rat was incubated with ^{125}I-hCG (750,000 cpm, 100 ng equivalent to about 4×10^6 cpm) in vitro, an uptake of about 60% of the total radioactivity was found (Table 2). When the incubated decapsulated testis and plasma membrane fractions of ovarian cells were treated with acid saline (pH 2.3) for 16 hr at 4°, about 50% and 70% of the bound radioactivity were extracted, respectively. On the other hand, on treatment with various solutions containing NaCl, mercaptoethanol, urea and EGTA, only 10-20 % of the radioactivity was removed. The original ^{125}I-hCG and the hormone extracted from testis showed similar binding activity.

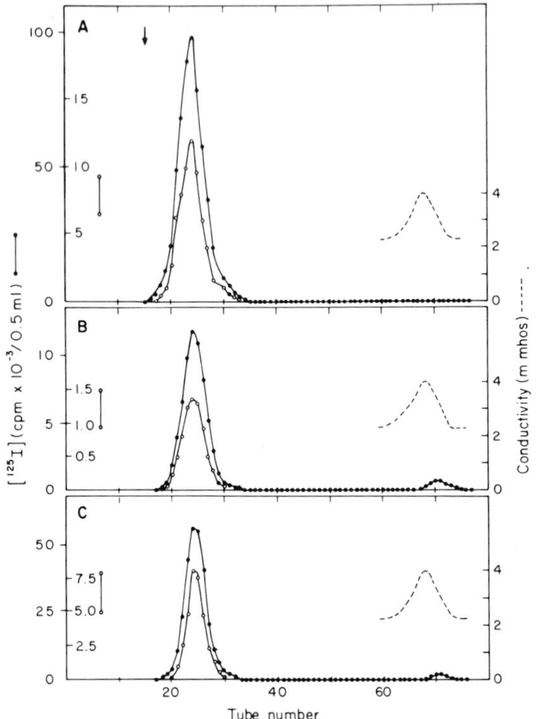

FIG 3. Gel filtration patterns and binding activity of radioactive hormone released from receptor sites of ovaries and testes. ^{125}I-hCG was injected into pseudopregnant rats i v, and membrane fraction of the luteal cells was prepared after 2 hr, or ^{125}I-hCG was incubated with decapsulated testes for 4 hr at 37°. Radioactive hormone was released from these receptor sites by treatment with acid saline (pH 2.3) at 4° for 16 hr. The extracted material was loaded on a Sephadex G-100 column (2.4 x 76 cm). The eluate of each tube of the first peak was tested for its ability to bind to the receptor fraction of testes. (A) ^{125}I-hCG; (B) radioactive hormone released from membrane fraction of the luteal cells and (C) from testicular receptor fraction. •——•, radioactivity in each tube; ∘——∘, the binding activity to the new receptor fraction of testes; (↓) indicates the void volume; --- NaCl elution.

To determine whether or not the bound hCG was altered following its interaction with the receptor, the original ^{125}I-hCG and the hormone extracted from testis and plasma membrane of ovaries were eluted on the same Sephadex G-100 column which had been equilibrated with 0.05M phosphate buffer (pH 7.5). Aliquots from each tube were incubated at 37° for 2 hr with the receptor prepared from testis. All three preparations showed similar elution pattern on gel filtration and identical binding activity with the receptor fraction of testis (Fig. 3).

The released hormone from testis was analysed by disc electrophoresis on 7.5 % polyacrylamide gel (pH 8.6) (Fig. 4). Gels

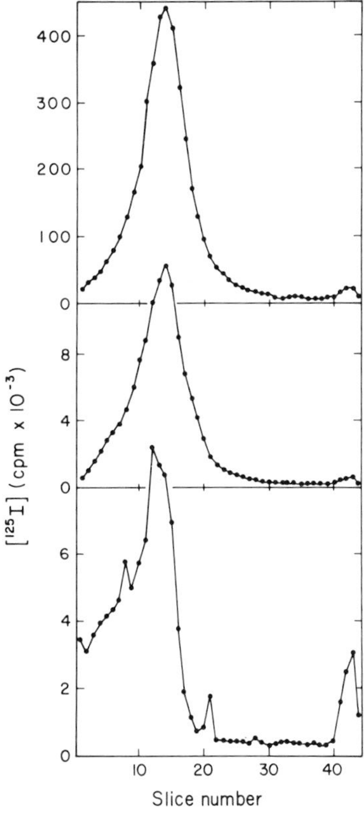

FIG 4. Electrophoresis of ^{125}I-hCG in 7.5% polyacrylamide gel at pH 8.6. Top: ^{125}I-hCG; Middle: ^{125}I-hCG treated with acid saline Bottom: ^{125}I-hCG extracted from testes by the same treatment.

were sliced transversely in 1 mm segments and the radioactivity of each segment was determined. The original ^{125}I-hCG and ^{125}I hCG treated with acid saline showed similar mobility except that the migration of the extracted hormone was slightly retarded.

The extracted hormone was injected into the tail vein of pseudopregnant rats and its distribution in various organs was examined. The uptake by the ovary showed an early peak which was observed to occur within 1/2 hr and accounted for 20 % of the radioactivity (Fig. 5). Following the initial peak, a second rise in uptake was noted at about 90 min after the first peak. This peak corresponded to the peak of radioactivity seen in the ovary following administration of the ^{125}I-hCG. The pattern of radioactive uptake by the kidney showed a maximum at one hour and this was followed by a gradual decline.

Testis was first incubated with labeled gonadotropin for 4 hr and the same tissue was incubated in KRB-glucose buffer, but without any labeled hormone. As shown in Fig. 6, the radioactivity in testes declined with incubation time. The ^{3}H-counts decreased at

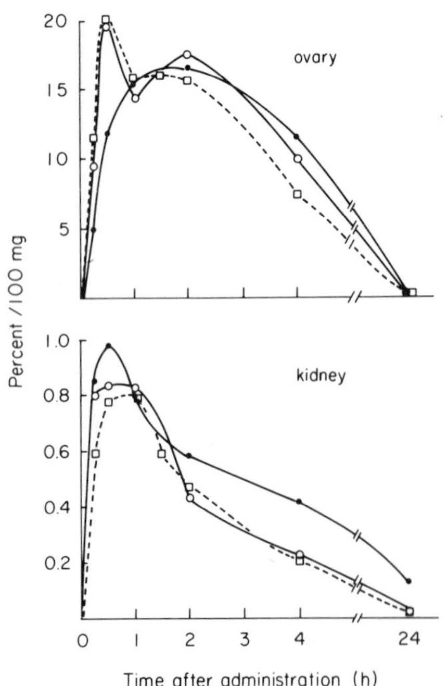

FIG 5. Uptake by ovaries and kidneys of superovulated rats following a single injection of ^{125}I-hCG and labeled hormone extracted from testis. •——• ^{125}I-hCG; ○——○ and □- - -□ radioactive hormone extracted from testes following treatment with 2.3 saline. Each point is the mean value obtained from three or four rats.

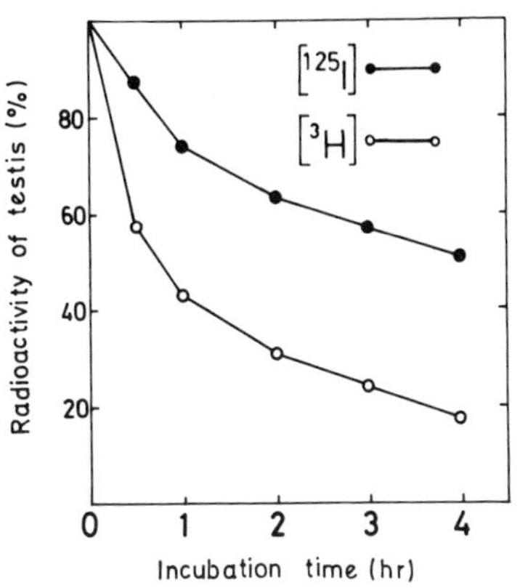

FIG 6. The radioactivity (^{125}I or ^{3}H) of testes. Testes were incubated with ^{125}I-hCG or ^{3}H-hCG in KRB buffer for 4 hr at 37°, washed three times with cold KRB and reincubated in KRB containing 10 mM glucose without labeled hCG. During the second incubation, radioactive materials were released from the testes into the incubation medium (see Fig. 7).

FIG 7. Sephadex G-50 gel filtration of tritiated material released from testes. The second incubation medium was filtered through a Sephadex G-50 column (2 x 50 cm). A high radioactive peak of ^{3}H was noted just before the position of inorganic ions.

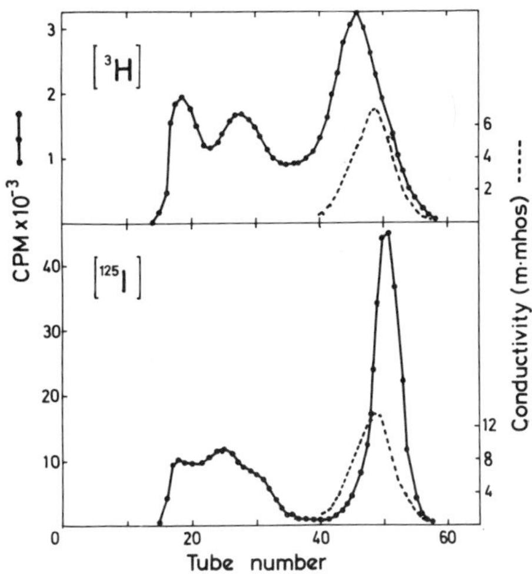

a faster rate than ^{125}I-counts. The medium after second incubation was collected, lyophilized and loaded on a Sephadex G-50 column (2 x 50 cm). A peak with relatively high radioactivity (^{3}H) appeared just before the elution of inorganic ions (Fig. 7). This peak was analysed by thin layer chromatography for sialic acid (NANA). The Rf. value of this material was slightly different from that of NANA and NAN-7. Both gave negative reaction with ninhydrin reagent. It is known that during the tritiation process NANA of hCG is reduced and tritium is placed on the position of NAN-7 (N-acetylheptulosaminic acid) (7).

DISCUSSION

The results of the present in vivo experiments and the ovarian autoradiography suggest that hCG interacts with the plasma membrane of the luteal cell and that the binding of hCG to the receptor is strong. The bound hormone could be effectively extracted only with acid-saline as reported by Dufau et al. (11).

The gel filtration pattern of the released hormone and that of original hCG were similar and these two hormones had similar binding ability to the receptor site. This finding suggests that hCG was probably carried to the target organ via the blood circulation without undergoing any modification, and that only biologically active hormone possessed the ability to interact with the cell receptor of the ovary or testis.

Although no differences were seen between the original labeled hCG and the hormone released from the receptor site as measured by the radio-ligand assay and by gel filtration pattern, it is noteworthy that the uptake by the ovary of the superovulated rats of hCG released from the receptor occurred earlier (30 min) and was relatively higher. The subsequent rapid decline in radioactivity in the ovary after the initial uptake suggested that the bound hormone was probably released rapidly from the receptor. The fact that the pattern of uptake of the 'extracted' hormone by the ovary was different from that of hCG and that the electrophoretic mobility of the former was slightly retarded suggests that the structure or the conformation of hCG might have been modified on its interaction with the receptor.

HCG bound to the receptor was not easily released by chemical treatment such as high concentration of urea, NaCl, EGTA or mercaptoethanol. The observation that the liberated ^{3}H-material behaved like a small molecular weight substance on gel- filtration on Sephadex G-50 and the fact that on thin layer chromatography, it showed an Rf slightly different from NANA or NAN-7 suggests that during interaction with the receptor, both protein as well as carbohydrate moieties of hCG are altered.

Since neuraminidase is localized in the plasma membrane of rat liver cell (12), enzymes which hydrolyze the carbohydrate portion of hCG molecule may exist in the plasma membrane of rat gonadal cells also, such that following receptor-hormone interaction, a rapid activation of adenylcyclase (13, 14) as well as an inactivation of the hormone may occur.

ACKNOWLEDGEMENTS

This work was supported by grants POIHDO 567-02 from the U.S. Public Health Service, and M-73.055C from the Population Council, the Rockefeller University, New York. We thank Miss C. Avila for technical assistance.

REFERENCES

1. Lunenfeld, B., and A. Eshkol. (1967). Vitamins and Hormones 25, 137.
2. Rajaniemi, H., and T. Vanha-Pertula. (1972). Endocrinology 90, 1.
3. Catt, K.J., M.L. Dufau, and T. Tsuruhara, (1972). J. Clin. Endocrinol. Metab. 34, 123.
4. Lee, C.Y., and R. Ryan. (1972) Proc. Nat. Acad. Sci. USA 69, 3520.
5. Rao, C.V., B.B. Saxena and H.M. Gandy. (1972) In Gonadotropins, Saxena, B.B., C.G. Beling, and H.M. Gandy (Eds). John Wiley & Sons, Inc., New York, p. 261.
6. Ashitaka, Y., M. Mochizuki and S. Tojo. (1972). Endocrinology 90, 609
7. Vaitukaitis, J., J. Hammond, and G.T. Ross. (1971) J. Clin. Endocrinol. Metab. 32, 290.
8. Ashitaka, Y., and S.S. Koide, Fertility & Sterility (in press).
9. Ashitaka, Y., Y-Y. Tsong, and S.S. Koide. (1973). Proc. Soc. Exp. Biol. Med. 142, 395.
10. Emmelot, P.C., J. Bos., E.L. Benedetti, and P.H. Rumke, (1964). Biochem. Biophys. Acta 90, 126.

11. Dufau, M. L., K. J. Catt, and T. Tsuruhara. (1972). Proc. Nat. Acad. Sci. USA. 69, 2414.
12. Schengrund, C., D. S. Jensen, and A. Rosenberg. (1972). J. Biol. Chem. 247, 2742.
13. Dorrington, J. H., and B. Baggett. (1969) Endocrinology 84, 989.
14. Kobayashi, Y. (1972). Folia Endocr. Japon 48, 412.

SOME EFFECTS OF FSH ON THE SEMINIFEROUS EPITHELIUM OF MAMMALIAN TESTIS

Anthony R. Means

Over the past several years this laboratory has been concerned with two major problems dealing with the action of FSH upon mammalian testis. The first problem has been to define in chemically precise terms the temporal sequence of events which occurs upon the initial interaction of FSH with its target cells. The second major problem is to gain a better understanding of the exact role for FSH in the initiation of spermatogenesis in mammalian testis. Whereas considerably more research is necessary before these two questions can be answered fully, we now have sufficient information to begin to construct a schematic representation of the action of FSH.

The chemistry of FSH has been eloquently reviewed in previous chapters of this volume. It is well established that this hormone is a polypeptide composed of two dissimilar subunits. Since studies with other peptide hormones such as insulin, glucagon, and ACTH had demonstrated that these hormones apparently do not enter the cells but instead bind to specific receptors present on the surface of the target cells, we wished to investigate this possibility with respect to follicle stimulating hormone and the testis. These studies were made possible by the development in the laboratories of Vaitukaitis and Ross (1) of a procedure to prepare biologically active, radio-labeled FSH. In our initial studies, binding experiments were conducted with tritiated FSH and the radioisotope was introduced into the sialic acid of the carbohydrate side chain as previously reported (1). It was demonstrated that FSH would bind specifically to testis (2). Although on a mass basis, more hormone was bound to immature tissue, demonstrable hormone binding could be found when tritiated FSH was incubated with testis from rats of all ages. Moreover, this interaction exhibited all the properties attributable to a biologically significant process. That is, it was dependent upon time and temperature of incubation as well as being a saturable process of high affinity and low capacity. Examination of the subcellular distribution of the labeled gonadotropin revealed that it was primarily associated with plasma membrane fractions. Subsequently, plasma membranes were isolated from the testis and shown to bind FSH in a specific manner. Only when membranes were prepared from seminiferous epithelium was binding demonstrable. Cells or membranes from the interstitial area of the testis exhibited absolutely no specific binding for FSH (2).

Several laboratories had reported that FSH stimulated adenylate cyclase when incubated with testis from several species of animals (3-5). If the action of this hormone were to prove similar to other peptide hormones, one would expect the interaction of FSH with its membrane binding sites to result in the activation of the adenylate cyclase. This, in fact, proved to be the case. A precise temporal correlation was shown between the binding of FSH to isolated seminiferous epithelium membranes on the one hand and activation of membrane-bound adenylate cyclase on the other hand (6, 7). Moreover, the activation of cyclase resulted in an increase in the intracellular content of cyclic AMP (8).

The next question was to determine whether the increase in cyclic AMP could be correlated with the stimulation of some intracellular event. With respect to those peptide hormones which stimulate steroidogenesis, the production of the appropriate steroid hormone proves to be an effective endpoint for the action of the hormone (9). However, available evidence suggests that FSH does not in any major way affect steroidogenesis in the testis. Therefore, we were prompted to search for other events which could serve as a marker for the action of FSH on testis cells. It has been demonstrated that certain specific enzymes, such as adipose tissue triglyceride lipase, are phosphorylated in the presence of stimulatory hormones, and this phosphorylation is mediated through the action of a cyclic AMP-dependent protein kinase (10, 11). These observations indicate a physiological role for protein kinase in the hormonal regulation of adipose tissue lipase. Likewise, this enzyme had been shown to play an important role in modulating the activity of muscle phosphorylase kinase and glycogen synthetase (12, 13). Reddi et al. (14) have shown the presence of a cyclic AMP-dependent protein kinase in testis tissue. Therefore, we decided to determine whether FSH could affect the activity of this enzyme and attempt to correlate the change in activity with binding of FSH to its receptor and activation of adenylate cyclase.

The mechanism of the activation of cyclic AMP-dependent protein kinase by cyclic AMP *in vitro* has been established using protein kinase isolated from a variety of mammalian tissues (15). This mechanism is illustrated by the following equation :

[RC] + cAMP $\rightleftharpoons$ [R x cAMP] + C. Binding of cyclic AMP to the regulatory subunit (R) of the inactive protein kinase (RC) allows dissociation of the enzyme into the regulatory subunit - cyclic AMP complex and the active catalytic subunit (C). Extrapolation of this in vitro mechanism to the regulation of cyclic AMP-dependent protein kinase in vivo would predict that hormonal modulation of the intracellular concentration of cyclic AMP would affect the protein kinase activity ratio, that is the ratio of C to RC + C. Experimental verification of this hypothesis has recently been reported by Soderling et al. (16) for the regulation of adipose tissue protein kinase by epinephrine and insulin. Therefore, we applied these techniques to a study of the regulation of protein kinase activity in testes by FSH. Incubation of seminiferous tubules isolated from testes of immature rats with FSH results in a very rapid activation of protein kinase (6-8). An effect is demonstrable as early as 3-5 minutes, and a maximal state of activation is achieved by 20 minutes at which point a three-fold enhancement of activity is observed. In addition, the increased enzyme activity can be directly and positively correlated with increased intracellular accumulation of cyclic AMP. Activation of the testicular protein kinase is specific for FSH and is dependent upon time and temperature of incubation as well as the age of the animal. Increased kinase activity in response to the continued presence of FSH exhibits a half-life of 2-4 hr. Furthermore, bound FSH can be recovered following treatment of the tissue at acid pH and this hormone retains the ability to activate protein kinase in fresh tissue suggesting that a significant portion of FSH may not be degraded while attached to testicular receptors (8).

Good correlation exists between binding of FSH and activation of testicular protein kinase. On the other hand, we have demonstrated that less FSH is necessary to maximally activate the protein kinase than is required to saturate the binding sites for this gonadotropin (8). Similar observations have been reported by Beall and Sayers (17) for the ACTH system as well as by Catt and co-workers (9, 18) for LH action upon the testis. In both these systems, less hormone seems to be required for maximal steroid production than is necessary for saturation of the receptors. It has been suggested that this may be due to the presence of spare receptors. The greater the receptor reserve, the greater the sensitivity of isolated adrenal cortical cells to ACTH. Again, similar studies have been reported for the action of glucagon on the liver by Exton et al. (19) and for TSH action upon the thyroid by Williams (20). Still another explanation for these effects of peptide hormones has been proposed by Rodbard (21). He has theorized that the receptor site may be regarded as a quantum unit so that a cell would respond in a maximal all-or-none fashion if the number of sites filled exceeds a given threshold. Mathematical treatment of this model reveals that it would be consistent with the observations made in the hCG /LH-testis system and ACTH-adrenal system. Whichever of these theories proves to be true, it is clear that for several peptide hormones including FSH, less concentration is necessary to maximally stimulate biological response than is necessary to saturate the receptor sites.

The stimulation of protein kinase by FSH was shown to be dependent upon the age of the animal (8). Similarly, FSH mediated stimulation of protein synthesis and RNA synthesis have been shown to be age-dependent (22,23). These biochemical effects of FSH apparently disappear at about the time of the first meiotic division; that is, between 21 and 26 days of age. Hypophysectomy of animals at any age results in the return of sensitivity to exogenous FSH (6-8, 24). On the other hand, we have demonstrated that seminiferous tubules of testes from mature animals contain receptor sites (2). These data suggested that during the spermatogenic process,some system or systems became active which resulted in a decreased biochemical response to exogenous FSH. In this regard Monn et al. (25) have investigated the levels of phosphodiesterase in testis during post-natal maturation. Testes of young animals were shown to have relatively low levels of phosphodiesterase. However, as the age of the animal increased, a specific isozyme of this enzyme began to appear and reached maximal levels at approximately 35 days of age. If cyclic AMP was necessary to mediate subsequent effects of FSH on the testis, it might be possible that the appearance of the phosphodiesterase isozyme would result in increased degradation of the newly synthesized cyclic AMP, thus causing a short circuit in the temporal sequence of events normally mediated by FSH. We, therefore, investigated the effect of FSH on protein kinase activity in the presence of a potent inhibitor of phosphodiesterase, 1 methyl, 3-isobutyl-xanthine (MIX). When this inhibitor is added to an incubation medium containing tubules from 16-day old rats, only a small but repeatable activation of protein kinase was observed. FSH, on the other hand produced a three-fold stimulation of enzyme activity. Moreover, when FSH and MIX were included in the incubation medium together, the activation of protein kinase appeared to be additive compared to the effect of either compound alone. When these experiments were repeated using testes from adult animals, a considerably different picture emerged. FSH resulted in no activation of protein kinase when incubated with tubules from 70-day old rats. The addition of the phosphodiesterase inhibitor resulted in a considerable activation of protein kinase in the tubule preparation. Moreover, this activation of protein kinase could again be correlated with an increase in the intracellular levels of cyclic AMP. When FSH and MIX were added together, a synergistic effect was noted with regard to the activity of protein kinase (6-8). Furthermore, Christiansen and Desautel (26) have recently reported that the specific phosphodiesterase isozyme disappears from the testis following hypophysectomy. Taken together these data offer the possibility that phosphodiesterase may play a role in the regulation of the action of FSH in mature rats. Certainly it should now be possible to directly correlate sensitivity to FSH with the activity of the specific phosphodiesterase.

Our data suggest that three of the earliest events following administration of a single dose of FSH to immature rats are the binding to receptors present on cells of seminiferous epithelium, the resulting stimulation of membrane-bound adenylate cyclase and an associated increase in the intracellular accumulation of cyclic AMP, and finally in the activation of cyclic AMP-dependent protein kinase (Fig. 1). What is now required is to elucidate the relationship of these initial events to subsequent effects of FSH on transcription and/or translation. Preliminary experiments in our laboratory show that the FSH-mediated activation of protein kinase is accompanied by an increase in the extent of phosphorylation of proteins present in various subcellular fractions. This increased protein phosphorylation precedes the stimulation of the rate of protein synthesis reported previously (22,27,28). It is now necessary to determine the specific substrates for the protein kinase and determine how phosphorylation of these proteins alters their activity or function. Studies designed to investigate this very important question are presently underway in this laboratory.

Stimulation of testicular protein biosynthesis by FSH results within 1 hr after the injection of this gonadotropin into immature or hypophysectomized animals (22,24,27-29). The increase in rate of protein synthesis appears to be of a direct nature. Two

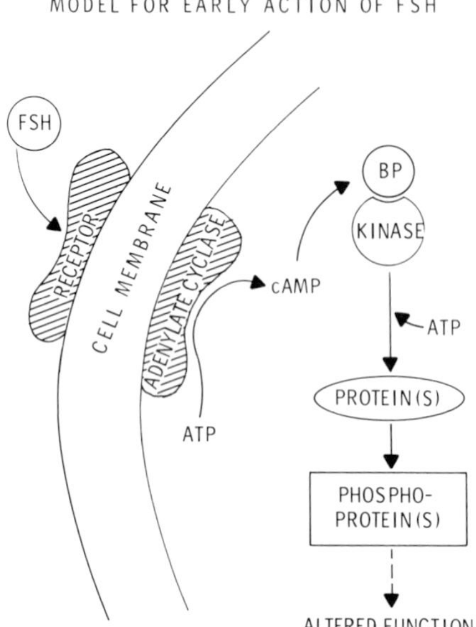

FIG 1. Schematic representation of the membrane-associated events involved in the early action of FSH upon the testis.

lines of evidence reveal that the stimulation cannot be attributed to enhanced amino acid transport into testicular cells (22). First, FSH under conditions where protein synthesis was stimulated did not increase the cellular transport of the model compound alpha amino-isobutyric acid, which is transported in a manner similar to naturally occurring amino acids but is not metabolized or incorporated to any demonstrable degree. Secondly, the stimulation by this hormone was not augmented by increasing the concentration of lysine in the incubation medium. That is, further addition of substrate did not result in increased incorporation into protein. Moreover, FSH did not increase the incorporation of radio-labeled amino acids into aminoacyl transfer RNA (22). Since FSH administration resulted in accelerated protein biosynthesis, and this hormone did not increase the transport or activation of amino acids, it was decided to investigate the effect of FSH upon the activity of testicular polyribosomes. Indeed, administration of FSH to immature rats results within 1 hr in increased testicular protein synthesis measured by either incorporation of tritiated amino acids <u>in vivo</u> or activity of isolated polyribosomes assayed in a cell-free system (27,28). On the other hand, FSH neither demonstrably influenced the proportion of testicular ribosomes appearing as polysomes, nor altered the relative proportion of various polyribosomal species. Electrophoretic analysis of soluble proteins newly synthesized in vivo or of peptides synthesized by isolated polyribosomes failed to reveal major qualitative differences (23). These results suggest that the effect of FSH on protein synthesis in seminiferous tubules must be of a general, rather than a specific nature.

Injection of actinomycin D 1 hr before injection of FSH was shown to prevent the stimulation of protein biosynthesis by testicular polysomes in vitro without demonstrably decreasing the rate of synthesis by particles from control animals (27,28). Furthermore, the synthetic messenger RNA-polyuridylic acid (poly U) increased protein synthesis in vitro by polyribosomes from treated and control animals, and incorporation was equal with polyribosomes from these two sources in the presence of excess poly U. It appears, therefore, that the capacity of polyribosomes to support peptide synthesis is the same whether these particles are isolated from hormone-treated or control animals. These observations suggested that FSH stimulates testicular protein synthesis by increasing the synthesis of RNA.

Studies were next initiated to ascertain whether FSH increased testicular RNA synthesis prior to the observed effect on protein synthesis (23,29). Specific activity of rapidly-labeled nuclear RNA was increased significantly within 15 min following a single injection of FSH. This response reached a maximum at 30 min and by 1 hr was declining rapidly towards control values. Simultaneous measurements of the acid-soluble pool of nucleotides during these experiments revealed that uptake of these compounds was not altered by FSH. Analysis of the rapidly-labeled nuclear RNA on polyacrylamide-agarose gels did not reveal major qualitative differences due to FSH. However, the base composition of the nuclear material changed markedly becoming more adenine-uridine rich, and these changes persisted after the effect on the rate of synthesis had diminished. The rapid stimulation of incorporation of rapidly-labeled nucleotides into heterogeneous nuclear RNA was shown to be paralleled by an increase in the activity of RNA polymerase II measured in isolated nuclei (30). These effects preceded stimulation of chromatin template activity, first demonstrable 30 min after FSH injection or enhancement in the activity of RNA polymerase I, which is responsible for the synthesis of ribosomal RNA at 60-90 min of FSH action. The increase in the activity of RNA polymerase I is followed by the appearance in the cytoplasm of newly synthesized ribosomal RNA within 4 hr following hormone injection (Means, unpublished observations). Thus, FSH stimulates transcription measured by a variety of techniques, and this increase in nuclear activity appears to be necessary for the subsequent stimulation of protein biosynthesis. Therefore, RNA and protein synthesis also seem to be important events in the early actions of FSH upon the biosynthetic activity of testes.

The results of the biochemical studies outlined in preceding paragraphs of this chapter offer little evidence as to the physiologic role of FSH in the male. Furthermore, if this role is involved in spermatogenesis it is still uncertain which stages of the process require FSH. It has been known for some time that chronic injections of FSH to immature rats result in an increase in the size of the gonads. Accompanying the increase in size are stimulations of both wet and dry weight, increases of the diameter of the seminiferous tubules and an apparent increase in the number of primary pachytene spermatocytes per tubular cross section (31, 32). We were able to confirm the report of Greep et al. (31) which demonstrated an increased number of primary spermatocytes per tubule when FSH was administered for 5 days to immature male rats beginning at 16 days of age (33). This increase in primary spermatocytes suggested to us that FSH might cause a stimulation of mitotic activity in cell types occurring prior to the primary spermatocyte. Indeed, this appeared to be the case when the mitotic activity of the seminiferous epithelium was examined at various times following a single injection of FSH to 15-day old rats. This gonadotropin induced a significant stimulation of the number of mitoses per tubule within 9 hr following a single injection (33). Stimulation reached a maximum of 200-300% of control at 12 hr, and by 18 hr the mitotic activity was again approaching control levels.

A well-accepted corollary of spermatogenesis is that the rate of this process cannot be altered without severely damaging the testis. Therefore, the burden of proof was upon us to demonstrate the possible significance of this apparent increase in mitotic activity. These studies were undertaken in collaboration with Dr. Claire Huckins. The first question was to determine which cell-types were apparently affected by FSH administration. Six successive generations of spermatogonia have been described in rat testis by Huckins (34) (A_1, A_2, A_3, A_4, In and B). During the initiation of spermatogenesis in immature rats, all classes of spermatogonia have appeared by 16 days, and spermatogenesis has progressed to pachytene primary spermatocytes. Huckins (35) has refined and modified a technique first described by Roosen-Runge (36) to examine germ cells, which uses pieces of tubules histologically mounted in their entirety. In such preparations, the intact spermatogonial nuclei in the peripheral layer of seminiferous epithelium are clearly visible. Perfection of this technique, therefore, has enabled the scientist to examine accurately the kinetics of spermatogonial maturation and differentiation. During spermatogonial maturation, large clusters of cells develop together and divide synchronously to form successive generations of more differentiated spermatogonia (37). The reasons for this synchronous behavior have recently been elucidated and spermatogonia are shown to be connected by intracellular bridges to form cytoplasmic syncytia. These syncytia can be best demonstrated using the whole-mount method of histological examination. Characteristically during the initial waves of spermatogenesis in immature testes, there is extensive degeneration within the various populations of differentiating spermatogonia (37). Whereas degeneration is less in the adult, it is still a normal occurrence and remains particularly noticeable in the A_2 and to a lesser degree in the A_3 spermatogonial types. Huckins (37) has shown that degeneration is readily visualized as large clusters of cells which are dying simultaneously. The reasons for degeneration among specific types of differentiating spermatogonia are unknown, but this event could provide an interesting mechanism by which the number of cells able to complete spermatogenesis can be regulated.

Huckins has examined the degeneration process with regard to the cell cycle of the differentiating spermatogonia. Her studies reveal that the degenerative process occurs at the junction of S and G_2 in the cell cycle (37). Since the degeneration occurs prior to mitosis, a decrease in the number of cells degenerating at any one time should be observed subsequently as an increase in the number of spermatogonial mitoses. Therefore, we investigated the effects of FSH on this process in testes of 16-day old rats (6, 7, 38). For the first 3 hr following a single injection of FSH, degenerating spermatogonia were shown to be abundant and not changed dramatically from control values. However, by 7 hr the incidence of degeneration had strikingly decreased to 25% of control values, and at 9 hr only a minimal number of degenerating spermatogonia were seen. These degenerating figures began to reappear by 14 hr after FSH injection and had returned to control levels by 19 hr. Comparable experiments with LH, estrogen, and testosterone demonstrated that this diminution of spermatogonial degeneration was hormone-specific. The most marked effect on spermatogonial degeneration occurs between the A_4 and intermediate cell types. In fact, almost no degeneration occurs 9 hr after FSH in this particular cell division. It is interesting to note that there is a 3-4 hr lag between maximal effects on spermatogonial degeneration on the one hand and on the increase in spermatogonial mitotic figures on the other. As mentioned above, studies using tritiated thymidine in normal immature rats demonstrated that spermatogonial degeneration occurs at the end of the DNA synthetic phase of the cell cycle. Huckins (37) has demonstrated that in 16-day old rats the length of the G_2 phase of the cell cycle, (i.e. the phase between the DNA synthetic phase and mitosis), is approximately 3 hr and this corresponds to the difference seen between the effect of FSH on degeneration and on mitotic activity. Thus, prevention of degeneration by FSH not only increases the number of viable cells which divide, but also profoundly affect the number of spermatogonia which continue to differentiate. These data provide the first evidence for a rapid and direct effect of FSH on the proliferating spermatogonial population and suggest the possibility that this hormone may have a beneficial action on DNA synthesis in such a manner as to avert the usual incidence of degeneration. Studies are now in progress to determine what relationships exist between the biochemical effects attributable to FSH action and the apparent diminution of spermatogonial degeneration. Elucidation of such relationships would provide strong evidence that FSH does have an important role in the initiation and possibly regulation of the spermatogenic process in rat testes.

The types of cells in the seminiferous epithelium that constitute the targets for the initial actions of FSH have yet to be determined. Our studies concerning the effect of FSH on spermatogonial degeneration suggest that at least one of the physiologic effects of this hormone may be manifest at the level of the type A spermatogonium. However, Dym and Fawcett (39) have demonstrated that Sertoli cell membranes surround all of the germinal components of the testis and tight junctions between adjacent Sertoli cells constitute a blood-testis barrier. Thus, the Sertoli cell may well be the most logical candidate for the primary target cell for FSH.

Several reports have appeared which suggest that the Sertoli cell is affected by FSH. Murphy (40) has reported that injection of this gonadotropin into rats results in a change in the morphology of the Sertoli cell. Studies of Castro et al. (41) suggested that FSH labeled with electron-dense substances such as ferritin was localized in or on the Sertoli cells and also in peritubular elements of the testis. The fact that the blood-testis barrier might prevent substances from reaching other sites within the germinal epithelium makes it difficult to draw conclusion from these studies. Nevertheless, these results together with our own show that the action of FSH in the immature testis must be manifest in the Sertoli cells or in the spermatogonial population. These are the only cells which are present in the germinal epithelium of the immature rat that respond to this hormone. The only definitive way of localizing the target cells for FSH is to obtain a preparation enriched in these cells and demonstrate the same temporal sequence of events that occur on administration of FSH to the normal intact animal.

We have recently begum to investigate various preparations that are enriched in Sertoli cells. These have included long-term hypophysectomized animals, animals rendered cryptorchid for long periods of time, and adult animals exposed to x-irradiation. Indeed, these animal models appear to respond to FSH. However, all of these systems suffer from one drawback, that is, they represent situations in which the germinal epithelium has been damaged in order to provide an enrichment in Sertoli cells. We now believe we have a system in which it will be valid to examine the biochemical effects of FSH in the absence of germ cells.

By using a gentle procedure (to be published elsewhere), we have been successful in destroying the gonocyte population in embryonic testis. The animals are delivered normally and develop with no apparent abnormalities except for the absence of all germ cells. The blood-testis barrier forms at about the normal time, the Sertoli cells divide until approximately 16 days of age and mature on schedule. Tubules have been prepared from testes of these animals and incubated in the presence of FSH. It binds to membranes, stimulates adenylate cyclase, increases the intracellular content of cyclic AMP, and activates the protein kinase. Thus it seems certain that at least these effects of FSH can be attributed to its action on the Sertoli cell. It is still not possible, however, to conclusively state that this biochemical sequence of events initiated by FSH is responsible for the demonstrated effects on the degeneration of the spermatogonial population. Moreover, it has not yet been possible to directly link the effects of FSH on transcription with the early membrane-associated events involving cyclic AMP. If the Sertoli cell mediates all the subsequent biochemical and physiological effects attributable to FSH, this poses a very intriguing question as to how the information generated in one cell type become transmitted to a second, and what is the chemical nature of this information-transfer process ?

Unfortunately, the information provided in this review is not sufficient to answer either question posed at the outset. These questions concerning the biochemical sequence of events which constitute the mechanism of action of FSH in the testis and the precise role played by FSH in the spermatogenic process still remain to be elucidated. However, we can begin to construct a logical sequence of events for the action of FSH in testes of immature rats. These events are listed in Table 1. We would suggest that FSH in

Table 1. Proposed temporal sequence of biochemical events initiated in mammalian testis in response to FSH.

Events	Time
Binding to plasma membrane	< 5 min
Activation of adenylate cyclase	< 5 min
Intracellular accumulation of cyclic AMP	5 min
Activation of protein kinase	5 min
Phosphorylation of proteins	15-30 min
Transcription	
Rapidly-labeled nuclear RNA	15-30 min
Stimulation of RNA polymerase II	15-30 min
Increased chromatin template activity	30 min
Stimulation of RNA polymerase I	60 min
Protein synthesis	1-2 hr
Wet weight	2-4 hr
Cytoplasmic accumulation of ribosomal RNA	3-6 hr
Dry weight	3-6 hr
Mitotic activity	6-9 hr
Decreased spermatogonial degeneration	9-12hr

its initial action on the testis binds to membrane receptors resulting in a stimulation of adenylate cyclase and increased intracellular accumulation of cyclic AMP. This cyclic AMP then interacts with a protein kinase which catalyses the phosphorylation of one or more species of protein.

The next event which can be demonstrated is the stimulation of transcription. Various methods have been utilized to show the stimulation. They include an increase in the rate of synthesis of rapidly-labeled heterogeneous nuclear RNA, a stimulation in the activity of RNA polymerase II, a transient increase in chromatin template activity, and a more prolonged enhancement of ribosomal RNA polymerase I. Subsequent to these events, protein synthesis is stimulated. The stimulation of both RNA and protein appear to be of a general,rather than of a specific nature. If our hypothesis concerning the effect of FSH on the degeneration of spermatogonial cells proves correct, this would explain the reason for a general effect on cell metabolism. Thus, since the overall effect would be to increase the number of the same cell type, one would assume that the total compliment of RNA and protein would remain constant. What is now necessary is to design experiments which will link these seemingly unassociated events in a logical manner and in so doing define the mechanism by which FSH affects the testis.

REFERENCES

1. Vaitukaitis, J.L., Sherins, R., Ross, G.T., Hickman, J., and Ashwell, G. (1971). Endocrinology 89, 1356.
2. Means, A.R., and Vaitukaitis, J.L. (1972). Endocrinology 90, 39.
3. Murad, F., Strauch, S., and Vaughn, M. (1969). Biochem. Biophys. Acta. 177, 591.
4. Kuehl, F.A., Patenelli, D.J., Tarnoff, J., and Humes, J.S. (1970). Biol. Reprod. 2, 154.
5. Dorrington, J.H., Vernon, R.G., and Fritz, I.B. (1972) Biochem. Biophys. Res. Comm. 46, 1523.
6. Means, A.R. (1973). Adv. Exp. Med. Biol. 36, 431.
7. Means, A.R. (1973). Proc. Internatl. Symp. Male Fert. Ster., Milan, (in press).
8. Means, A.R., MacDougall, E., Soderling, T.R., and Corbin, J.D. (1974). J. Biol. Chem. (in press).
9. Catt, K.J., and Dufau, M.L. (1973). Adv. Exp. Med. Biol. 36, 379.

10. Corbin, J.D., Reimann, E.M., Walsh, D.A., and Krebs, E.G. (1970). J. Biol. Chem. 245, 4849.
11. Corbin, J.D., Brostrom, C.O., Alexander, R.L., and Krebs, E.G. (1972). J. Biol. Chem. 247, 3736.
12. Walsh, D.A., Perkins, J.P., Brostrom, C.O., Ho, E.S., Krebs, E.G. (1971). J. Biol. Chem. 246, 1968.
13. Soderling, T.R., Hickenbottom, J.P., Reimann, E.M., Hunkeler, F.L., Walsh, D.A., and Krebs, E.G. (1970). J. Biol. Chem. 245, 6317.
14. Reddi, A.H., Ewing, L.L., and Williams-Ashman, H.G. (1971). Biochem. J. 122, 333.
15. Krebs, E.G. (1972). 'Current Topics in Cellular Regulation' 5, 99 B.L. Horecker & E.R. Stadtman (Eds), Academic Press, New York & London.
16. Soderling, T.R., Corbin, J.D., and Park, C.R. (1973). J. Biol. Chem. 248, 1822.
17. Beall, R.G., and Sayers, G. (1972). Arch. Biochem. Biophys. 148, 70.
18. Dufau, M.L., Watanabe, K., and Catt, K.J. (1973). Endocrinology 92, 6.
19. Exton, J.H., Lewis, S.B., Ho, R.J., Robison, G.A., and Park, C.R. (1971). Ann. N.Y. Acad. Sci. 185, 85.
20. Williams, J.A. (1972). Endocrinology 91, 1411.
21. Rodbard, D. (1973). Adv. Exp. Med. Biol. 36, 342.
22. Means, A.R., and Hall, P.F. (1967). Endocrinology 81, 1151.
23. Means, A.R. (1971). Endocrinology 89, 981.
24. Means, A.R., and Hall, P.F. (1968). Endocrinology 82, 597.
25. Monn, E., Desautel, M., and Christiansen, R.O. (1972). Endocrinology 91, 716.
26. Christiansen, R.O., and Desautel, M. (1973). Endocrinology 92, A-100.
27. Means, A.R., and Hall, P.F. (1969). Biochemistry 8, 4293.
28. Means, A.R., and Hall, P.F. (1971). Cytobios. 3, 17.
29. Means, A.R. (1970). Adv. Exp. Med. Biol. 10, 301.
30. Beale, E., Mills, N.C., and Means, A.R. (1972). Endocrinology 90, A-154.
31. Greep, R.O., van Dyke, H.B., and Chow, B.F. (1942). Endocrinology 36, 35.
32. Simpson, M.E., Li, C.H., and Evans, H.M. (1951). Endocrinology 48, 370.
33. Mills, N.C. and Means, A.R. (1972). Endocrinology 91, 147.

34. Huckins, C. (1965). Ph.D. Thesis, McGill University, Montreal, Canada.
35. Huckins, C. (1971). Cell Tissue Kin 4, 139.
36. Roosen-Runge, E.C. (1955). Z. Zellforsch. 41, 221.
37. Huckins, C. (1972). Proc. III Pan American Congr. Anat., New Orleans, p. 395.
38. Huckins, C., Mills, N.C., Besch, P., and Means, A.R. (1973). Endocrinology 92, A-95.
39. Dym, M. and Fawcett, D.W. (1970). Biol. Reprod. 3, 308.
40. Murphy, H.D. (1965). Proc. Soc. Exp. Biol. Med. 118, 1202.
41. Castro, A.E., Seiguer, A.C., and Mancini, R.E. (1970). Proc. Soc. Exp. Biol. Med. 133, 582.

CELL TYPES INFLUENCED BY FSH IN THE RAT TESTIS

Jennifer H. Dorrington and Irving B. Fritz

INTRODUCTION

Follicle stimulating hormone, together with either luteinizing hormone or testosterone, is required for the initiation of spermatogenesis in the immature rat (1). Restoration of spermatogenesis in the hypophysectomized rat also depends upon the presence of FSH and LH (2-4). Intriguingly, however, the administration of testosterone alone (5) or dihydrotestosterone (6) immediately after hypophysectomy will maintain spermatogenesis qualitatively, even though there is a decrease in the numbers of germinal cells (5).

Experiments to be reported here were designed to determine which cell types in the testes are responsive to FSH, as evidenced by an increase in cyclic AMP accumulation. It was known from previous studies that both FSH and LH stimulated adenylate cyclase activity in homogenates of dog testes (7) and in preparations from rat testes (8), but no attempt was made to identify the FSH-responsive cells. In this communication, we shall present evidence indicating that FSH does not elicit an increase in adenylate cyclase activity of interstitial cells and germinal cells, but that Sertoli cells are FSH-responsive.

HORMONAL CONTROL OF CYCLIC AMP LEVELS IN PREPARATIONS FROM THE RAT TESTIS.

Lymphatic sinusoids exist between the interstitial tissue and the seminiferous tubules in the rat testis (9). Because of this natural separation it is possible to isolate the seminiferous tubules from the interstitial tissue by careful dissection as described by Christensen and Mason (10). The isolated testicular preparations were washed in buffer and examined under the dissection microscope for remnants of contaminating tissue. The washed tissue, approximately 30 mg wet wt. of tubules or 10 mg wet wt. of interstitial tissue, was incubated for 20 min in 1 ml Krebs-Ringer bicarbonate (KRB) buffer, pH 7.4, containing 1 mg glucose per ml at 32° with constant shaking, in an atmosphere of 95 % O_2 and 5 % CO_2. The cyclic AMP was extracted as described by

Dorrington and Fritz (11) and assayed by the method of Gilman (12).

A. Interstitial tissue

Interstitial tissue incubated in the presence of 10 mM theophylline responded to LH (NIH-LH-S16) with an increase in cyclic AMP. In addition, a highly purified preparation of LH (G3-222B), having an activity 2.8 x NIH-LH-S1, stimulated cyclic AMP accumulation in interstitial cell preparations. A preparation of partially purified FSH (LER-866-3) together with LH (G3-222B) did not produce a synergistic effect on cyclic AMP accumulation (Table 1).

The ability of LH, but not FSH, to increase cyclic AMP levels in preparations of isolated interstitial tissue confirms the findings of Cooke et al. (13) and Moyle and Ramachandran (14). In accord with these observations, interstitial tissue has been shown to bind LH but not FSH (15). LH and cyclic AMP stimulated androgen synthesis by the testis *in vitro* (16-18). Ovine FSH had no effect on testosterone production, and there was no apparent synergism when added simultaneously with LH (19). Recently, however, Holt et al. (20) have reported an effect of rat FSH on the synthesis of androgens in rat testis. This may indicate a requirement by

Table 1. *In vitro* effects of partially purified LH and FSH on the cyclic AMP levels of interstitial cell preparations.

Additions*	Cyclic AMP** (pmoles/mg protein)
None	17.8 ± 3.2
0.05 μg LH (NIH-LH-S16)	118.2 ± 9.8
0.025 μg LH (G3-222B)	109.0 ± 5.4
1.0 μg FSH (LER-886-3)	22.2 ± 3.8
0.025 μg LH (G3-222B) + 1.0 μg FSH (LER-886-3)	104.2 ± 7.3

* Incubations were carried out in KRB buffer containing 10 mM theophylline. ** Each value is the mean ± S.E.M. of three experiments. From Dorrington and Fritz (11).

interstitial tissue for a species-specific FSH, and warrants further investigations. In experiments to be described, we have observed that oFSH increases the level of cyclic AMP in tubules isolated from the rat testis. These results demonstrate an absence of species-specificity with respect to the responsiveness of rat seminiferous tubules to FSH.

B. Seminiferous tubules

1. Normal adult rats : The level of cyclic AMP in seminiferous tubules isolated from testes of normal adult rats (body weight, 225-235 g) was unchanged by the addition of 10 µg FSH/ml (21). The addition of theophylline (10 mM) alone elevated cyclic AMP levels, and FSH in the presence of theophylline elicited a further increase in cyclic AMP accumulation (Table 2). Under similar conditions, LH did not influence cyclic AMP production by isolated tubules (Table 2).

Table 2 *In vitro* effects of LH (NIH-LH-S16) and FSH (NIH-FSH-S9) on the cyclic AMP levels of isolated seminiferous tubules from normal adult rat testis.

Additions*	Cyclic AMP** pmoles/mg protein/20 min incubation
None	13.2 ± 1.4
LH	15.9 ± 6.5
FSH	14.9 ± 1.5
Theophylline	31.2 ± 2.0
Theophylline + LH	34.1 ± 1.2
Theophylline + FSH	66.8 ± 6.0

*LH or FSH added : 10 µg; Theophylline 10 mM.
**Each value is the mean ± S. E. M. of three experiments, each of which was performed in triplicate. From Dorrington and Fritz (1974).

2. Immature rats : As a first step in our attempts to identify the cells sensitive to FSH, we investigated the response to FSH of tubules isolated from immature rats at times when the first wave of spermatogenesis was proceeding. Tubules from 26-day old animals, (rich in Sertoli Cells, spermatogonia and spermatocytes) responded dramatically to FSH in the presence of theophylline (Fig. 1). Subsequent development during the period from 26 days to 75 days of age results in an increase in the relative numbers of spermatids (22). In tubules prepared from the more mature testes, the response to FSH progressively decreased.

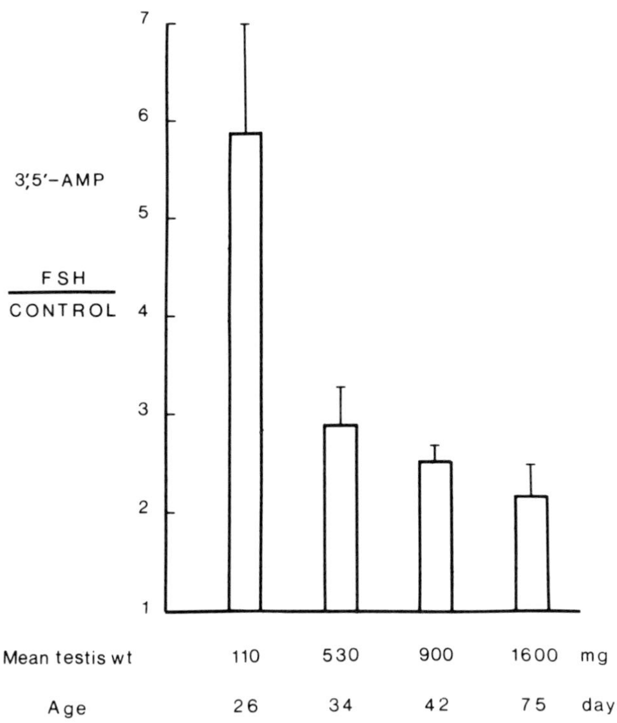

FIG 1. Ratios of the cyclic AMP levels after the addition of FSH (10 μg/ml) in vitro to that obtained in the absence of exogenous FSH, in tubules isolated at various stages during the development of the rat testis. All incubations were carried out in 10 mM theophylline.

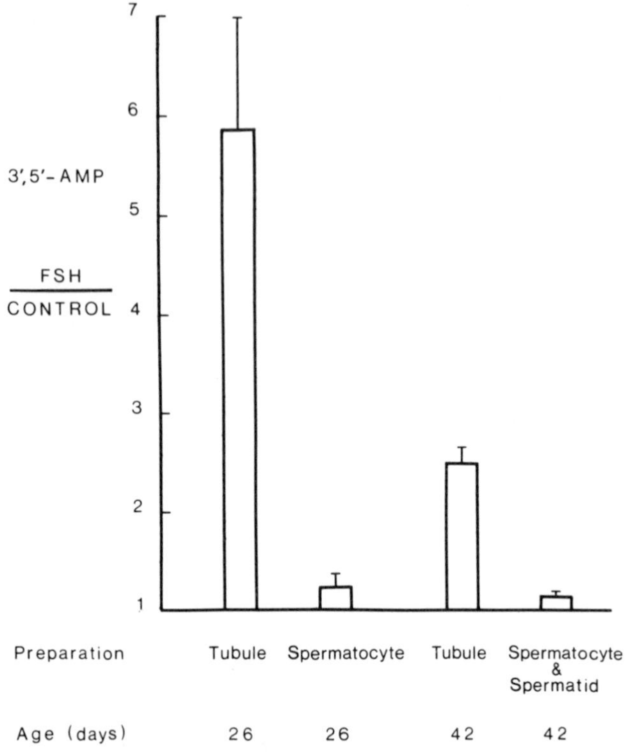

FIG 2. Ratios of the cyclic AMP level after the addition of FSH (10 μg/ml) to that obtained in the absence of exogenous FSH, in isolated tubules and in cell suspensions. All incubations were carried out in 10 mM theophylline. The cell counts from three separate spermatocyte-enriched preparations from 26-day old rats indicated that they consisted of approximately 86 % spermatocytes, at the leptotene stage of prophase or at a more advanced stage, 6 % immature spermatids, 6 % spermatogonia or preleptotene spermatocytes and 2 % Sertoli cells. The spermatid-spermatocyte preparations obtained from the 42-day old rat consisted of approximately 65 % spermatids, 28 % spermatocytes, 5 % spermatogonia or preleptotene spermatocytes and 2 % Sertoli Cells.

Tubules from 26-day old rats were employed to prepare spermatocyte-enriched suspensions, as described by Dorrington and Fritz (23). FSH addition had no effect on cyclic AMP levels of the spermatocyte preparations incubated in the presence or absence of 5 mM or 10 mM theophylline (Fig. 2).

Figure 1 showed that the response to FSH was relatively reduced in tubules from more mature testes which contained spermatids. To investigate this further, a cell suspension of spermatids and spermatocytes was prepared from tubules of 42-day old rats (23). FSH addition elicited no increase in cyclic AMP levels in the presence or absence of 5 mM or 10 mM theophylline (Fig. 2).

The above data supported the view that the FSH-responsive cells in tubules from immature rats were neither spermatocytes nor spermatids. By elimination, it appeared likely that either Sertoli cells or spermatogonia were the cells responsive to FSH. This hypothesis was strengthened by observations on preparations containing relatively large numbers of these cell types, i.e. tubules from regressed testes of hypophysectomized or cryptorchid rats.

3. Hypophysectomized rats: There is a progressive degeneration of all classes of germinal cells up to 30-35 days after hypophysectomy of adult rats, after which time the proportions remain fairly constant (Fig. 3) (24). The number of type A spermatogonia per testis is reduced to a lesser extent than any other class of germinal epithelial cells, and the number of Sertoli cells per testis remain unchanged after hypophysectomy. The mean testis weight in adult rats was 1.5 g and this fell to 300 mg, 36 days after hypophysectomy.

Addition of FSH in the absence of theophylline stimulated cyclic AMP accumulation by isolated tubules obtained from testes of adult rats killed at various times after hypophysectomy. The ratio of cyclic AMP produced in the presence of FSH relative to those observed in control tubules, increased with time after hypophysectomy (21). Thus, the stimulation of cyclic AMP production elicited by FSH is increasing during a time when the relative numbers of spermatids and pachytene spermatocytes are diminishing.

Tubules from fully regressed testes (i.e., 34-36 days after hypophysectomy) contained Sertoli cells, spermatogonia, resting spermatocytes and a small number of spermatids (Fig. 3). As shown in Table 3, 1.0 µg and 10 ug FSH/ml consistently elevated

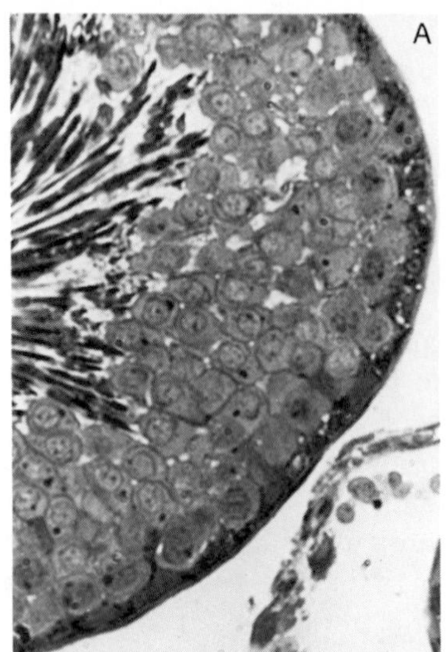

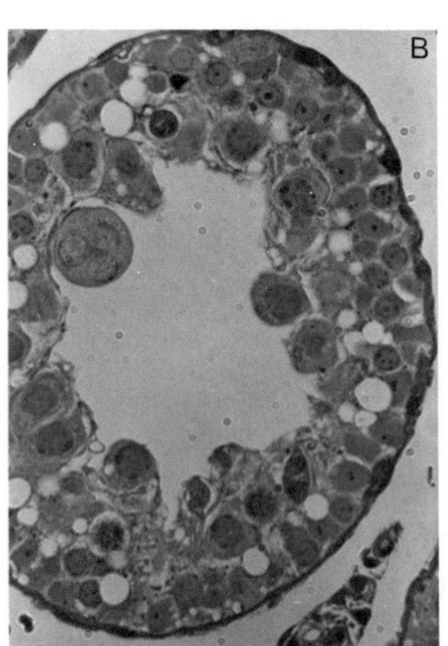

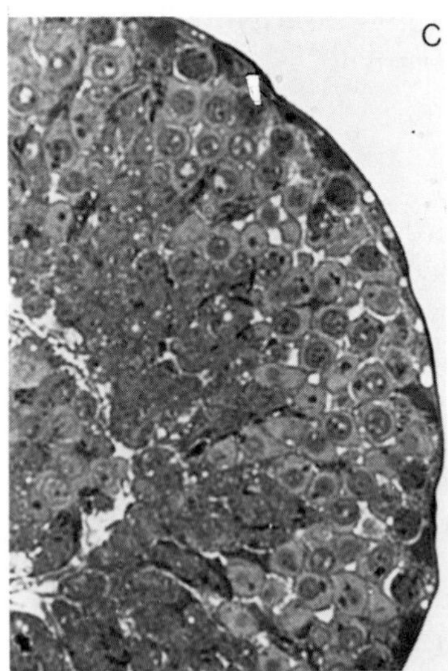

FIG 3. Microphotographs of sections of testes from the normal adult rat (A), from a rat 36 days after hypophysectomy (B) and from a rat which had been exposed to irradiation (300 rads) 8 days previously (C). Sections were fixed in 3 % glutaraldehyde in 0.2 M phosphate buffer, embedded in Epon, and 2 μ sections were washed in sodium hydroxide and stained with hematoxylin (x 525).

Table 3. The effects of theophylline and various concentrations of FSH (NIH-FSH-S9) on the levels of cyclic AMP in tubules from hypophysectomized rats *.

Additions	Cyclic AMP** pmoles/mg protein
None	9.0 ± 5.0
Theophylline (10 mM)	19.4 ± 6.3
FSH (0.1 μg)	18.8 ± 6.5
FSH (0.1 μg) + theophylline (10 mM)	41.2 ±10.0
FSH (1.0 μg)	31.4 ±15.0
FSH (1.0 μg) + theophylline (10 mM)	115.2 ±36.0
FSH (10.0 μg)	73.7 ±20.0
FSH (10.0 μg) + theophylline (10 mM)	305.1 ±45.0

*Tubules were obtained from testes allowed to regress for 29-34 days after hypophysectomy. ** Each value is a mean ± S. E. M. of 3 experiments.

cyclic AMP levels in these tubules. The addition of theophylline (10 mM) alone caused an increase in the content of cyclic AMP. Furthermore, theophylline (10 mM) enhanced the responsiveness to FSH at concentrations employed (Table 3).

4. Cryptorchid rats : Cryptorchidism was surgically induced in adult rats as described previously (11). Following cryptorchidism, the rate of regression of germinal cells is more rapid than that following hypophysectomy. Tubules of rats rendered cryptorchid for 14 days consisted mainly of Sertoli cells and spermatogonia. No spermatids and spermatozoa were evident but some primary spermatocytes remained (25). FSH increased cyclic AMP in isolated tubules from cryptorchid testes in the presence and absence of theophylline (Table 4).

5. Irradiated rats : From the above observations, it appeared likely that the FSH-responsive cells were either Sertoli cells, spermatogonia or both. To differentiate among these possibilities we have exploited the observation made by Oakberg (26) and Dym and Clermont (27) that the most radiosensitive cells in the testis

Table 4. Effects of FSH (NIH-FSH-S9) on cyclic AMP levels in seminiferous tubules from cryptorchid testes*

Additions	Cyclic AMP ** (pmoles/mg protein/20 min incubation)
None	4.9 ± 2.0
FSH (10 μg/ml)	16.0 ± 4.3
Theophylline (10 mM)	32.3 ± 6.1
Theophylline (10 mM) and FSH (10 μg/ml)	119.5 ± 10.9

* Tubules were obtained from testes allowed to regress for 14 days after surgically-induced cryptorchidism. ** Each value is the mean ± S.E.M. of 5 experiments.

are the spermatogonia.

Adult rats were anesthetized with Nembutal, and the right testis was gently manipulated through the inguinal canal into the abdomen. The animals were protected with a lead shield (4 mm thick) having a single aperture through which the left testis was exposed to 300 rads (11). Following irradiation of the left testis, the right testis was immediately returned to the scrotum. The effect of irradiation was to produce decreased numbers of spermatogonia. This was apparent five days after exposure and was most marked on the eighth day (Fig. 3c). These results confirm observations reported by Dym and Clermont (27) on the rat testis.

Tubules isolated from irradiated and non-irradiated testes were incubated in the presence of theophylline (10 mM), with and without FSH (10 μg/ml). Even though very few spermatogonia remained 8-9 days after exposure to irradiation, addition of FSH resulted in an increase in cyclic AMP accumulation comparable to that observed in tubules from the non-irradiated testes of the same animals (Table 5). The degree of stimulation of cyclic AMP production in tubules from irradiated testes was equivalent to that obtained in tubules from normal adult non-irradiated rats (Table 2).

Table 5. *In vitro* effects of FSH (NIH-FSH-S9) on cyclic AMP levels in tubule preparations from irradiated and non-irradiated testes of adult rats at varying periods after irradiation.

Time after exposure to 300 rads	Cyclic AMP (pmoles/mg protein) in tubules from			
	non-irradiated testis		irradiated testis	
	Control	FSH	Control	FSH
0 days	26.5	44.2	23.1	43.4
5 days	20.0	45.8	23.0	49.4
8 days	14.9	36.7	10.0	64.0
9 days	23.1	43.0	19.5	47.8

All incubations were carried out in Krebs-Ringer bicarbonate buffer containing 10 mM theophylline. Each value shown is the average of triplicate determinations of cyclic AMP levels in tubule preparations from a single animal in which one testis had been irradiated and one testis had been protected. From Dorrington and Fritz (11).

DISCUSSION

Our results suggest that the interstitial cells and the Sertoli cells constitute the principal cell-types within the testis which respond to LH and FSH respectively, with an increase in cyclic AMP. These observations are consonant with studies on the binding of labeled gonadotropins to testicular preparations (15, 28-30).

It is possible that the FSH stimulation of adenylate cyclase activity in Sertoli cells is related to the FSH requirement for the initiation and restoration of spermatogenesis; however, this relationship remains to be determined. The Sertoli cells support the germinal cells within the tubule, and it is possible that they provide nutrients required for the differentiation of the germinal cells. Specialized junctions called 'tight junctions' serve as attachment sites between adjacent Sertoli cells, thereby forming a continuous layer around the periphery of the tubule (9). There is a correlation between the formation of these junctions and the initiation of the secretion of tubular fluid, thus establishing the environment in which the more advanced germinal cells differentiate (31). These events take place at a time when the FSH levels increase in the immature rat (32); whether this is a purely temporal relationship or related casually is one of the fascinating problems which remains to be resolved in the field of spermatogenesis.

ACKNOWLEDGEMENTS

This study was supported by grants from the Medical Research Council of Canada and the Banting Research Foundation. We would like to thank Heather McKeracher for excellent technical assistance, and Nick Roller and Ernest Whitter for preparing the histological sections.

REFERENCES

1. Steinberger, E. (1971). Physiol. Rev. 51, 1.
2. Greep, R.O. and Fevold, H.L. (1937). Endocrinology 21, 611.
3. Lostroh, A.J. (1963). Acta Endocr. 43, 592.
4. Go, V.L.W., Vernon, R.G. and Fritz, I.B. (1971). Can. J. Biochem. 49, 768.
5. Clermont, Y. and Harvey, S.C. (1967). Ciba Found. Colloq. Endocrinol. 16, 173.
6. Ahmad, N., Haltmeyer, G.C. and Eik-Nes, K.B. (1973). Biol. Reprod. 8, 411.
7. Murad, F., Strauch, B.S. and Vaughan, M. (1969). Biochem. Biophys. Acta. 177, 591.
8. Kuehl, F.A., Patanelli, D.J., Tarnoff, J. and Humes, J.L. (1970). Biol. Reprod. 2, 154.
9. Fawcett, D.W., Leak, L.V. and Heidger, P.M. (1970). J. Reprod. Fert. Suppl. 10, 105.
10. Christensen, A.K. and Mason, N.R. (1965). Endocrinology 76, 646.
11. Dorrington, J.H. and Fritz, I.B. (1974). Endocrinology (in press).
12. Gilman, A.G. (1970). Proc. Nat. Acad. Sci. 67, 305.
13. Cooke, B.A., van Beurden, W.M.O., Rommerts, F.F.G. and van der Molen, H.J. (1972). FEBS Letters 25, 83.
14. Moyle, W.R. and Ramachandran, J. (1973). Endocrinology 93, 127.

15. de Kretser, D.M., Catt, K.J. and Paulsen, C.A. (1971). Endocrinology 80, 332.
16. Sandler, R. and Hall, P.F. (1966). Endocrinology 79, 647.
17. Rommerts, F.F.G., Cooke, B.A., van der Kemp, J.W.C.M. and van der Molen, H.J. (1972). FEBS Letters, 24, 251.
18. Dufau, M.L., Catt, K.J. and Tsuruhara, T. (1972). Endocrinology 90, 1032.
19. Dufau, M.L., Watanabe, K. and Catt, K.J. (1973). Endocrinology, 92, 6.
20. Holt, J.A., Kelch, R.P. and Payne, A.H. (1973). Proc. Soc. for the Study of Reprod., Athens, Georgia, p. 58.
21. Dorrington, J.H., Vernon, R.G. and Fritz, I.B. (1972). Biochem. Biophys. Res. Comm. 46, 1523.
22. Clermont, Y. and Perey, B. (1957). Am. J. Anat. 100, 241.
23. Dorrington, J.H. and Fritz, I.B. (1973). Biochem. Biophys. Res. Comm. 54, 1425.
24. Clermont, Y. and Morgentaler, H. (1955). Endocrinology 57, 369.
25. Davis, J.R. (1969). Biol. Reprod. 1, 93.
26. Oakberg, E.F. (1955). J. Morphol. 97, 39.
27. Dym, M. and Clermont, Y. (1970). Am. J. Anat. 128, 265.
28. Castro, A.E., Seiguer, A.C. and Mancini, R.E. (1970). Proc. Soc. Exp. Biol. Med. 133, 582.
29. Castro, A.E., Alonso, A. and Mancini, R.E. (1972). J. Endocr. 52, 129.
30. Means, A.R. and Vaitukaitis, J. (1972). Endocrinology 90, 39.
31. Setchell, B.P. (1970). In "The Testis", A.D. Johnson, W.R. Gomes and N.L. Vandermark (Eds). Vol. 1, p. 101. Academic Press, New York.
32. Negro-Vilar, A., Krulich, L., and McCann, S.M. (1973). Endocrinology 93, 660.

INDUCTION OF OVULATION WITH GONADOTROPINS : PREVENTION OF OVARIAN HYPERSTIMULATION

Melvin L. Taymor, Merle J. Berger and Irwin E. Thompson

Induction of ovulation with human gonadotropins of pituitary or urinary origin has been of tremendous benefit to the relatively small group of women suffering from infertility due to anovulation. One cannot help but wonder, in this era of increasing awareness of the problems of population over-expansion, if the time, effort and money expended for these few pregnancies is justifiable. However, the desire of an individual couple to experience parenthood is one that no individual physician can deny. Certainly, then, the minimum requirement should be that the quality of the pregnancy and of the offspring be optimum. That is why we hold no brief for those physicians who state that if one desires a pregnancy one must accept a high rate of triplet or more pregnancies as well as a high rate of ovarian over stimulation. Such multiple pregnancies are known to be accompanied by a high incidence of toxemia, miscarriage with hemorrhage and morbidity on the part of the mother and prematurity with all its dangers on the part of the offspring. We believe that these are complications that must and can be avoided, or must at least be kept at a minimum.

RESULTS OF THERAPY

Gonadotropin therapy is usually given in the form of daily injections of the FSH-rich material until there is evidence of follicular maturation, and then ovulation is triggered by the administration of hCG, usually in a single injection, so as to imitate the mid-cycle surge of LH. Table 1 summarizes the results of this efficient therapy in 92 patients treated at the Peter Bent Brigham Hospital, Boston, from 1964 to 1973. The vast majority of these patients had been previously treated with clomiphene citrate without success. In this selected group of patients 79 % of the cycles were ovulatory and there was a 54 % conception rate. Other groups reported pregnancy rates varying from 40-70 % (1,2) Of the 50 pregnancies recorded (Table 1), there were two cases of triplet or more pregnancy and four cases of severe hyperstimulation syndrome, that is, markedly enlarged ovaries with ascites.

Table 1. Therapy results at Peter Bent Brigham Hospital (1964-1973).

	Number	Percentage
Patients	92	
Cycles	221	
Ovulatory cycles	175	79
Conceptions	50	54
Multiple	15	30
Triplet or more	2	
Ovarian enlargement	27	12
Ascites	4	
Abortion	9	18

Similar complications have been reported by Gemzell and Roos (3), Vande Weile and Turksoy (2), and by a number of other workers (4). It is these two complications, particularly multiple pregnancies and marked enlargement of the ovaries that must be prevented, if this is to be an acceptable form of therapy.

CAUSES OF HYPERSTIMULATION

Table 2 lists a classification for hyperstimulation of the ovary. Some degree of ovarian enlargement should be expected in most cases. However, moderate and severe degrees of enlargement, particularly accompanied by ascites, should be considered a complication and must be eliminated. The primary reason that

Table 2. Classification of ovarian overstimulation

Mild	--	Ovarian enlargement, less than 7 cm.
Moderate	--	Ovarian enlargement, 7-10 cm.
Severe	--	(Hyperstimulation syndrome) - Ovarian enlargement greater than 10 cm. with or without ascites.

hyperstimulation occurs is because of the marked difference in responsiveness to gonadotropin therapy from patient to patient and even from cycle to cycle in the same patient. While treating our first 19 patients with gonadotropins (5), we found that the number of days of therapy at a level of 150 IU daily to promote 3 plus, or total ferning of the cervical mucus varied from 4 to 14 days (Fig 1). It was obvious, then, that a fixed dosage schedule would result in both under and over-stimulation. It is true that general categories of patients require more or less gonadotropins to achieve ovulatory cycles than others. Patients with low-gonadotropin amenorrhea require more ampules per day and more days of therapy than subjects with normal endogenous gonadotropin levels, but within these groups there is extreme variability and overlapping.

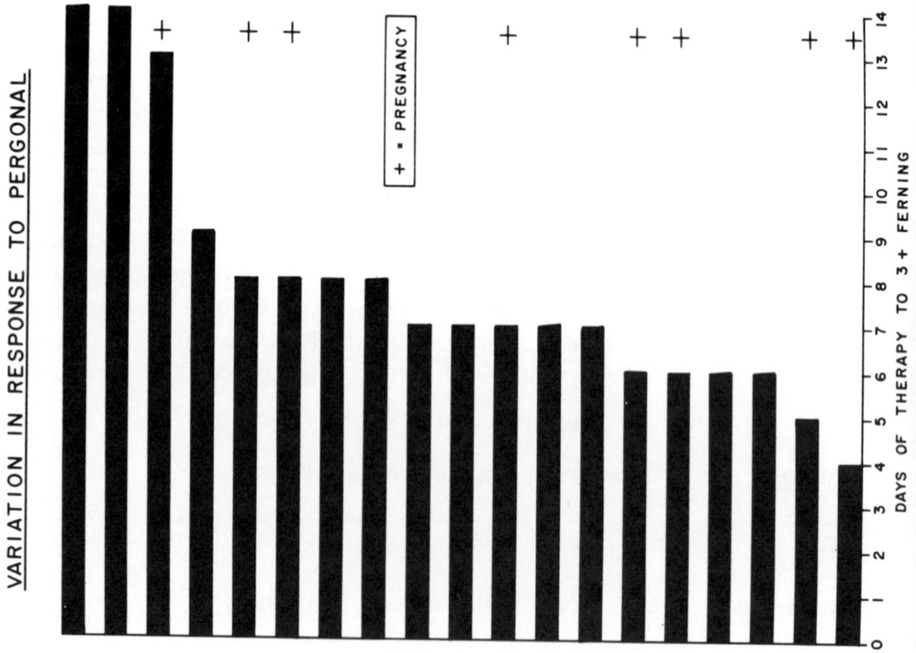

FIG 1. Variability and length of therapy to bring out 3+ ferning of cervical mucus [from Taymor et al. (5)].

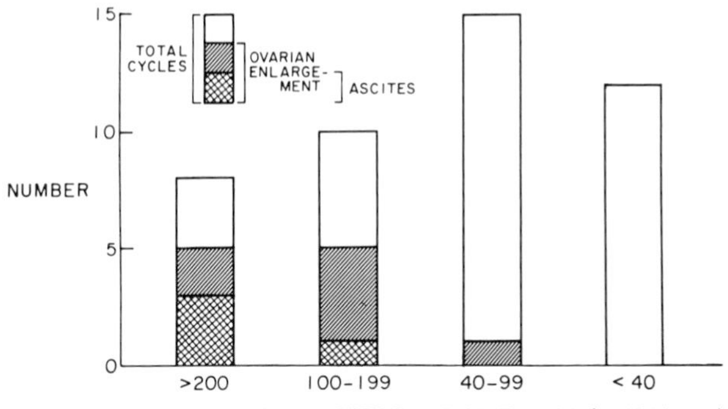

FIG 2. Relation of multiple pregnancy to level of total estrogen excretion from the day of hCG administration. Triplet or more pregnancies occurs only when estrogen excretion was over 200 µg per 24 hr [from Taymor (6)].

The work reported in this volume by Greenwald in hamsters showing that the number of mature follicles persisting in the late follicular phase is related to the amount of FSH stimulation is consistent with our concept that high and prolonged stimulation with FSH causes the ripening of too many follicles. When hCG is administered superovulation occurs which obviously results in multiple pregnancies and multiple corpora lutea formation which enlarges the ovary. The accompanying high estrogen levels may well disturb capillary permeability, which along with sodium retention may be the cause of further ovarian swelling as well as ascites.

In a search for a common denominator between multiple pregnancies and ovarian hyperstimulation, we analyzed the estrogen excretion levels in our initial series of patients (6). In this group of patients the time of hCG administration had been selected by following cervical mucus pattern and the estrogen excretion levels were available only for later analysis. There were five cases of moderate to severe ovarian enlargement and three cases of ascites, when the total estrogen levels during the 24 hr prior to hCG administration were over 200 µg and there were five cases

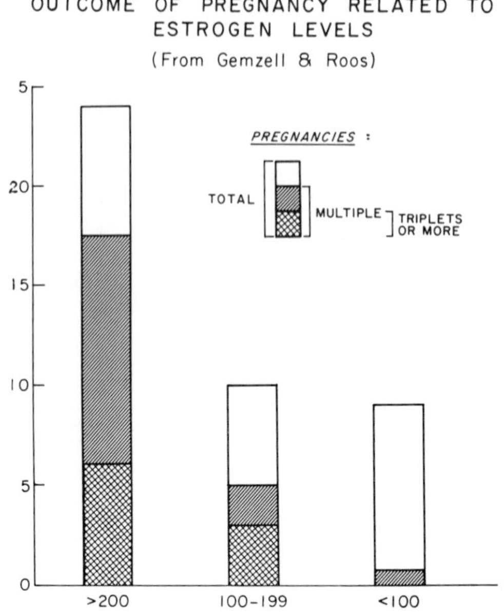

FIG 3. Relationship of ovarian enlargement and ascites to estrogen excretion levels at the time of hCG injection. Ascites occured only when estrogen excretion levels were over 200 μg/24 hr [from Taymor (6)].

of moderate to severe ovarian enlargement, but only one case with ascites, when it was between 100 to 200 μg/24 hr (Fig 2). In addition, when the levels were between 40 and 99, there was only one case of moderate ovarian enlargement and no ascites. It seemed apparent, then, that if the estrogen excretion levels could be kept below 100 μg/24 hr the incidence of severe ovarian enlargement with ascites could be kept at a minimum.

We did not have enough multiple pregnancies to analyze in a similar fashion, but we were able to take individual data reported by Gemzell and Roos (3) and make a similar evaluation in terms of estrogen excretion levels (Fig 3). Thus a parallelism was observed between the urinary estrogen levels and occurance of multiple pregnancies, the latter being more when the estrogen levels were > 200 μg/24 hr, and the incidence being minimum when the levels were below 100 μg/24 hr.

PLAN OF THERAPY

Therefore, since 1968 we have recommended that gonadotropin therapy be monitored according to the excretion of estrogen by the stimulated ovaries (6); similar recommendations have been made by other workers (7). A rapid method for the determination of total estrogen excretion is utilized (8) and Figure 4 outlines our plan of therapy. The patients are started on 2 or 3 ampules (150-225 IU) of gonadotropin daily. The initial treatment cycle is usually with two ampules. If the patient is a slow responder, three ampules (225 IU) are given as the initial dose. If the patient does not seem to be responding to two ampules daily till the fifth day, the dosage can be increased to 3 ampules daily. In occasional cases one may go as high as four ampules daily. This therapy is continued until 3 plus or total ferning of cervical mucus occurs. At this point further gonadotropin therapy is given depending upon the daily estrogen excretion. If total estrogens are between 50 and 100 µg/24 hr the dosage is dropped to 1 or 2 ampules for 2 more days, and then hCG is given. If, however,

150-225 IU of HMG daily through first day of 3+ ferning of cervical mucus.

Then daily estrogen excretion by rapid (6-8 hr.) method and maintain therapy for 1 to 3 days.

If no ferning of cervical mucus appears after 5 days, increase dosage by 1 more ampule.

After 3+ ferning, continue HMG for 2 more days according to total estrogen excretion levels.

> If less than 50 mcg/24 hr. maintain 150-225 IU level
>
> If 50-100 mcg/24 hr. drop down to 75-150 for 2 days.
>
> Whenever estrogens are over 100 mcg/24 hr. give 8000 IU HCG on that day.
>
> No HCG if estrogens go over 200 mcg/24 hr.

FIG 4. Flow sheet for administration of HMG utilizing a combination of ferning and estrogen monitoring.

the levels remain below 50, the higher dose is maintained for 2 more days, and then hCG is administered. Whenever estrogen excretion levels exceed 100 μg the hCG is given without additional HMG. The important point is not to give hCG if estrogen levels inadvertently rise over 200 μg/24 hr.

RESULTS WITH ESTROGEN MONITORING

Table 3 compares two groups of patients. The first category lists the initial 35 patients treated by our group, at which time therapy was being monitored by the fern test alone. The second group is made up of the last 57 patients of our total experience, in which therapy was monitored by measuring total estrogen excretion in the last 3 or 4 days of therapy. There was a slight diminution in the percentage of ovulatory cycles in the latter group, but the pregnancy rate was well maintained. There was a marked diminution in the incidence of multiple pregnancies, none of these being triplet or more when estrogen excretion was monitored. There was a moderate decline in the incidence of ovarian enlargement with estrogen monitoring, but of more importance, no cases of ascites were observed.

Table 3. Ovulation induction monitored by daily fern test or by daily total estrogen excretion

	By fern test		By estrogen excretion	
	No.	%	No.	%
Patients	35		57	
Cycles	81		143	
Ovulatory	76	94	102	71
Conceptions	20	57	30	53
Multiple	8	40	7	23
Triplet or more	2		0	
Ovarian enlargement	11	14 % of cycles	16	9 % of cycles
Ascites	4		0	

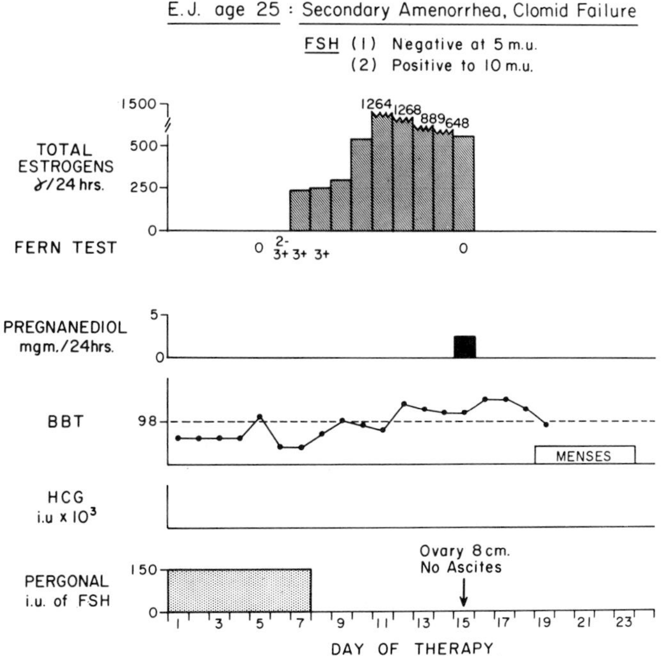

FIG 5. Shows a subject in whom estrogen excretion levels inadvertently reached 240 μg/24 hr.

Figure 5 demonstrated a case in which the estrogen levels inadvertently rose above 200 μg/24 hr, and hence hCG was not given. Estrogen excretion levels continued to increase beyond 1200 μg/24 hr. The ovaries became moderately enlarged, but neither ascites nor pregnancy occurred. We believe that if hCG had been given, we might well have had in this case an experience similar to the one recently reported in the United States, wherein sextuplets were born following gonadotropin therapy. In the latter, hCG was administered, despite knowing that the estrogen excretion levels had reached 800 μg.

ESTROGEN EXCRETION PATTERNS

More recently, in analyzing our results we have found that the rate of increase in estrogen excretion levels can also be related to the results in terms of ovulation, ovulatory cycles, anovulatory

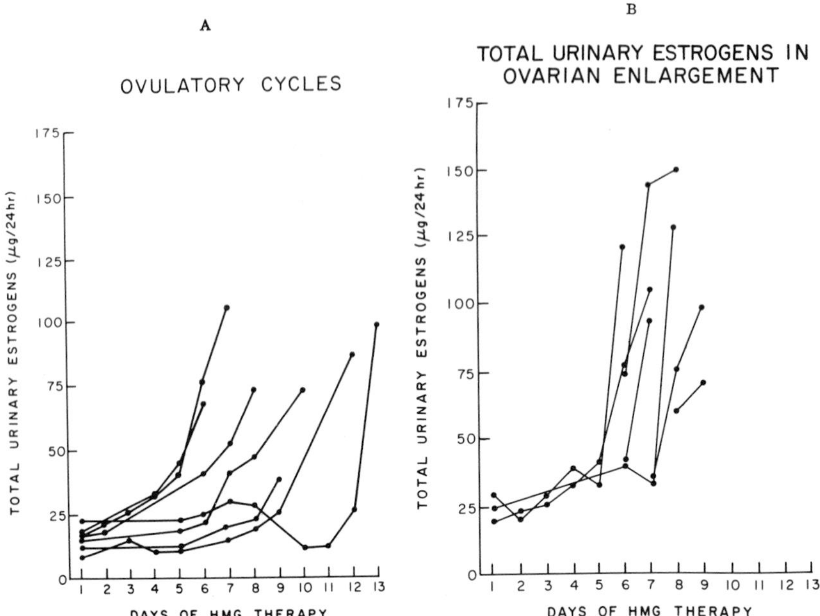

FIG 6. Total urinary estrogen excretion pattern (A) in 7 ovulatory cycles selected at random from 132 ovulatory cycles; (B) in 7 cycles where ovarian enlargement had occured [from Karam et al (9)].

cycles and cycles accompanied by hyperstimulation of the ovaries (9). Figure 6A illustrated the estrogen excretion patterns in 7 ovulatory cycles randomly selected from a large group of 132 ovulatory cycles that had been monitored by estrogen excretion. In these estrogen excretion generally rose slowly during the first 4 or 5 days of therapy, and then relatively sharply, 2 or 3 days before hCG was given. Cases in which ovarian hyperstimulation occured (Figure 6B) estrogen excretion levels rose quite sharply from the beginning of therapy. It would appear that the course of therapy that results in an estrogen excretion pattern that closely resembles the pattern of the normal ovulatory cycle is the one most likely to result in ovulation without bringing about ovarian hyperstimulation and multiple pregnancies greater than twins. Thus ovarian hyperstimulation and triplet or more pregnancies with their inherent dangers are unacceptable complications of gonadotropin therapy. Estrogen monitoring at the present time presents the best method of minimizing or completely eliminating these complications.

In conclusion, in this era, where unlimited population growth presents such a potential danger, where 30 % of the children of the world go to bed hungry, it is of the utmost importance that when there is a method available to induce ovulation and thereby pregnancy, every effort should be made to insure the highest quality of that pregnancy and of that offspring.

REFERENCES

1. Gemzell, C. (1970). Int. J. Obst. Gynec. 8, 593.
2. Vande Weile, R. L. and Turksoy, R. N. (1965). J. Clin. Endocr. 25, 369.
3. Gemzell, C. and Roos, P. (1966). Amer. J. Obst. Gynec. 94, 490.
4. Bettendorf, G. and Insler, V. (Eds) 1970. Clinical application of human gonadotropins, G. Thieme Verlag, Stuhgart.
5. Taymor, M. L., Stugis, S. H., Lieberman, B. L. and Goldstein, D. P. (1966). Fertil. & Steril. 17, 731.
6. Taymor, M. L. (1968). J. Amer. Med. Ass. 203, 362.
7. Jewelewicz, R., Dyrenfurth, I., Warren, M. P. and Vande Wiele. (1973). in "Female Infertility" E. Rosemberg (Ed.) Excerpta Medica, Amsterdam.
8. Taymor, M. L., Yussman, M.A. and Gminski, D. (1970) Fertil. & Steril. 21, 759.
9. Karam, K., Taymor, M. L. and Berger, M. J. (1972). Amer. J. Obst. Gynec. 114, 445.

USE OF URINARY ESTRONE AND OTHER PARAMETERS IN MONITORING GONADOTROPIN THERAPY

Shanti M. Shahani, P.G. Natrajan and P.C. Merchant

INTRODUCTION

The success of gonadotropin therapy for induction of ovulation and conception depends to a great extent on the accuracy and reliability of parameters used for monitoring this therapeutic regime. Chemical estimation of ovarian steriods, though feasible and commonly employed in most developed countries, is still not widely used in India. The changes in the end organs such as cervix, vaginal epithelium and endometrium, and basal body temperature (BBT) are commonly used to assess the follicular response to gonadotropins. The object of this study was to establish patterns of urinary estrone in normally menstruating women with special emphasis on the ranges during pre-ovulatory phase and evaluate its use along with other parameters in monitoring follicular responsiveness to gonadotropins.

MATERIALS AND METHODS

Serial urinary estrone estimations were carried out in 16 women with normal ovulatory cycles. These women were asked to keep their BBT records and were repeatedly called for vaginal smear cytology and cervical mucus fern and Spinnbarkeit tests. Urinary estrone was estimated by Brown's method (1). It was possible to complete the estimation within 5-6 hr, so that decision on therapy could be made by the evening of the same day.

RESULTS

A total of 195 urine samples of normal women were assayed. The means and ranges of estrone values found during normal menstrual cycle are shown in Figure 1. The mean values are low during the first week (about 5.35 μg on day 7) and rise to a peak around day 14 (17.48 ± 1.28 μg), and thereafter the values fall gradually (2). The estrone curve appears to parallel the Karyopyknotic Index (KPI) curve of vaginal smears (Figure 2),

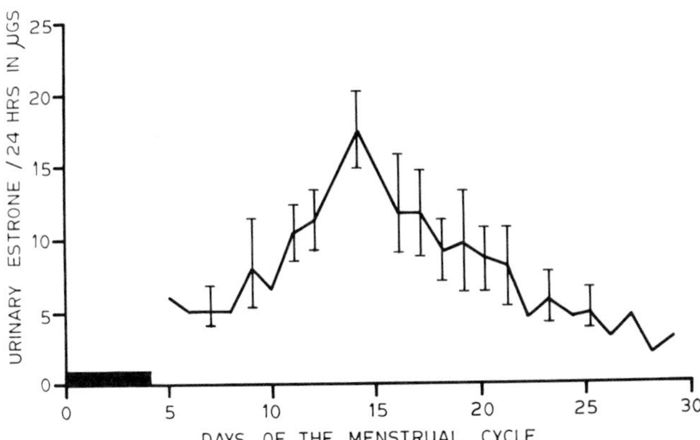

FIG 1. Shows the mean values of the urinary estrone on different days of the cycle. The vertical bars indicate the 95 % confidence limits (mean ± 2 S. E. M).

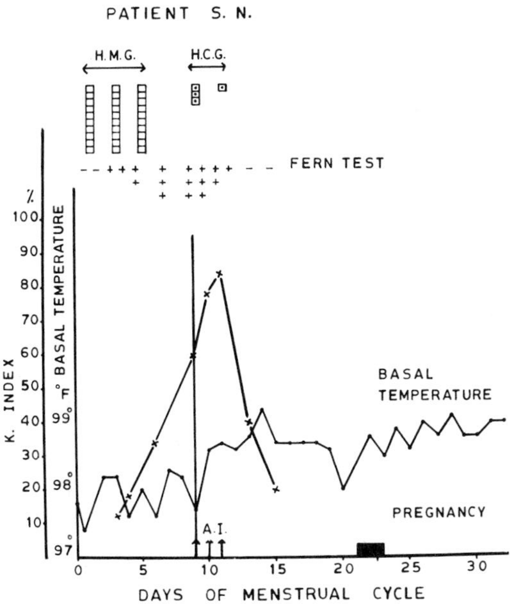

FIG 2. Shows patient S. N. a case of primary amenorrhea on gonadotropin therapy. x———x KPI; o———o BBT.

the difference being that the urinary estrone value during the pre-ovulatory period fall within a narrow range (10-20 µg) while the KPI in normal women have a wide range (40-80 %).

The relationship between the estrone peak and other mid-cyclic events in 16 normal cycles was studied. There appeared to be a good correlation of the day of estrone peak with BBT (12/13 cycles, 92 %), with KPI (11/16 cycles, 69 %), and with cervical mucus (8/9 cycles, 88 %); only in 31 % of cycles, did the KPI peak precede the estrone peak. In cases where typical pre-ovulatory or ovulatory smear patterns are obtained, this finding can be very useful in timing the fertile period.

Selected cases with amennorrhea (primary and secondary) having an infertility problem were treated with gonadotropins for induction of ovulation. Ten patients, of whom 4 had primary amenorrhea, and 6 had secondary amenorrhea were treated for 20 cycles. HMG followed by hCG was given in 12 cycles, HMG alone in 3 cycles and clomiphene citrate (clomid) followed by hCG in 5 cycles.

The parameters used for monitoring the dosage of HMG therapy were KPI, BBT, cervical mucus and urinary estrone patterns. The first 3 parameters were followed for 19 cycles, while the estrone level was monitored only for 8 cycles. In addition urinary pregnanediol was determined during the second half of the cycle to assess the luteal function.

Figure 2 shows a patient of primary amenorrhea monitored by KPI and cervical mucus. It took five days for the cervical mucus to change from + to +++ and KPI was 60 % when hCG was given. This was the sixth treated cycle and in this conception occurred and pregnancy ended in a full-term normal delivery. Eventhough this patient had implantation bleeding on day 21 and 22, a persistence of thermogenic response indicated a positive test for pregnancy.

Figure 3 shows the results of gonadotropin therapy in a patient with secondary amenorrhea. She was being monitored by serial vaginal smears, cervical mucus and urinary estrone. Unfortunately urinary estrone values were not available immediately and one had to depend mostly on KPI and cervical mucus changes. Neither the KPI, nor the cervical mucus increased satisfactorily with HMG (Pergonal) therapy. The timing of hCG (Pregnyl) was thus delayed, resulting in ovulatory cycle (confirmed by secretory endometrium), but no conception. Actually the BBT dip could be

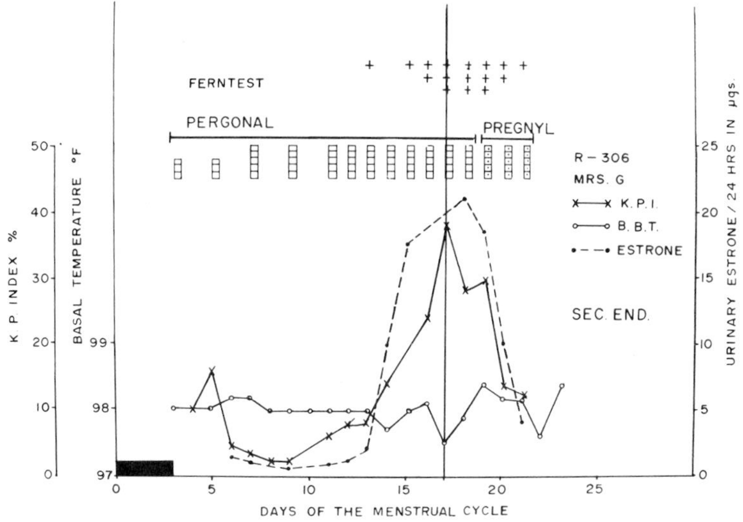

FIG 3. Shows patient T.G. a case of secondary amenorrhea on gonadotropin therapy.

observed even before hCG was given indicating ovulation occurance on HMG alone. Perhaps urinary estrone values if available in time, could have indicated the optimum timing of hCG administration.

Two cases of primary amenorrhea when treated with large amounts of HMG (2000 to 3375 IU) failed to show a stimulation of ovarian follicular activity as evidenced by KPI. One of them, later showed high urinary gonadotropins. The second case showed a lowering of KPI inspite of continued treatment and hence the treatment was stopped.

Monitoring the events during the pre-ovulatory phase is essential for a successful therapy with HMG. It is also well recognized that physical changes in cervical mucus and KPI can be used as semi-quantitative indicators of estrogenic activity. Thus theoretically the optimum time for inducing ovulation by HMG administration should be the day when estrogen secretion or KPI and cervical mucus reach the pre-ovulatory titre or values similar to that obtained in a normal menstrual cycle. The average estrone values reached just before hCG in our series was 14.5 μg whereas the average KPI for the same purpose was 71 %. The cervical mucus showed a +++ score.

In 8 cycles evaluated, estrone peak coincided with the day of the BBT dip and maximum cervical mucus (+++) response in 87.5 % cycles, but coincided with the KPI peak on the same day in only 62.5 % cycles which is similar to what is seen in normal cycles.

The KPI peak in most cases precedes the estrone peak. Probably the reason for this is, that after the hCG administration, the estrone values continue to rise as a result of synergistic action of the two gonadotropins, HMG and hCG, whereas the vaginal smear which also reflects progestational activity probably shows early changes of regression by fall of KPI due to pre-ovulatory secretion of progesterone (3). Table 1 shows the KPI and estrone patterns immediately after hCG administration.

Table 1. K. P. I. and estrone patterns immediately after hCG administration.

No. of cycles	K. P. I.		Urinary estrone	
	Fall	Rise	Fall	Rise
16*	60 %	40 %	12.5 %	87.5 %

*In one patient there was no follow up and in three cycles ovarian response to HMG was poor and hence hCG was not given.

Figure 4 shows a patient of primary amenorrhea with steep rise of KPI with HMG treatment in relation to urinary estrone. KPI was about 80 % and urinary estrone 12.5 µg, when hCG was given. Cervical mucus took six days to change from + to +++. After hCG, KPI rose to 94 % while estrone continued to rise to 32 µg. In this cycle, coitus took place on days 11, 12 and 13 and resulted in normal pregnancy.

Figure 5 shows a patient of secondary amenorrhea who responded to Clomid with ovulatory cycles for about a year, but did not conceive. Eventually she was treated with gonadotropins

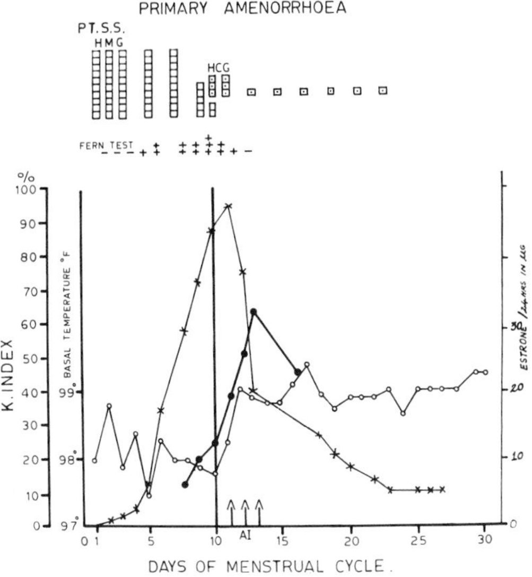

FIG 4. Shows patient S. S. a case of primary amenorrhea on gonadotropin therapy. x——x KPI; o——o BBT; ●——● estrone.

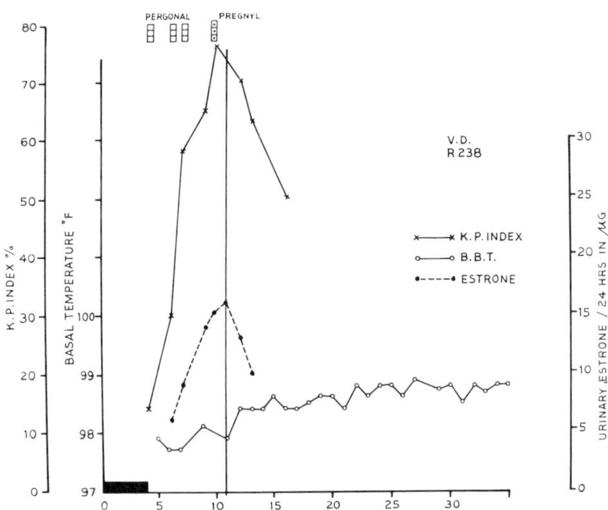

FIG 5. Shows patient V. D. a case of secondary amenorrhea on her first gonadotropin therapy resulting in pregnancy.

resulting in pregnancy in the very first cycle. HCG was given when estrone was 14 µg and KPI was 75 % and cervical mucus +++. The estrone curve again shows rise after hCG whereas KPI tends to decline.

Most investigators are not agreed on the necessity of monitoring ovarian function closely, in patients treated with Clomid or Clomid with hCG. However, if the objective is to diagnose time of ovulation as closely as possible, assessment of pre-ovulatory estrogenic activity by direct hormone assays and by end-organ effect may be necessary, thus indicating the optimum time for coitus or for administration of hCG in such cases.

Figure 6A and 6B show two cases of secondary amenorrhea treated with Clomid and hCG. HCG was given when cervical mucus reached ++ to +++ score, KPI reached 65 % in one case and 52 % in another and when urinary estrone was 14 µg in both the cases. In the former, following hCG, KPI fell whereas the estrone values continued to rise to 20 µg and ovulation appeared to have occurred on that day; thereafter the titres fell. In the latter, both KPI and estrone increased following hCG, for a day or so coinciding with the BBT dip on day 17 and then fell. This therapy resulted in successful conception.

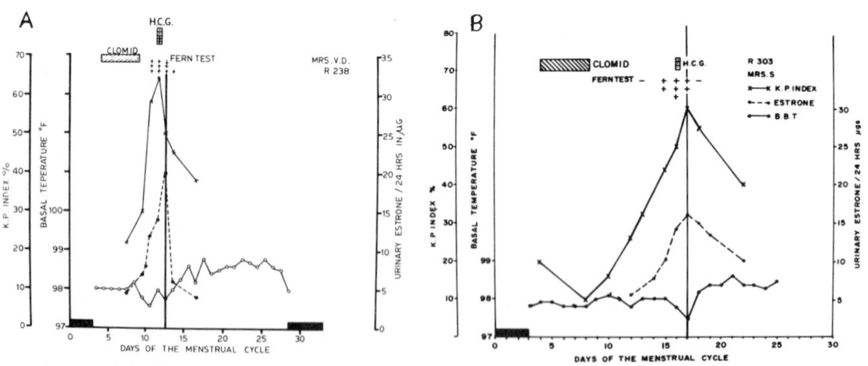

FIG 6A. Shows patient of secondary amenorrhea treated with clomid and hCG x——x KPI; o——o BBT; ●——● estrone.
FIG 6B. Shows patient S.A. a case of secondary amenorrhea treated with clomid +hCG resulting in a successful conception. The KPI peak, the estrone peak and the BBT dip seem to coincide on day 17.

Table 2. Summary of the result of clomid and gonadotropin therapy

Type of therapy	No. of patients*	No. of cycles	No. of ovulation	No. of pregnancies
HMG + hCG	5	12	11	4
Only HMG	3	3	nil	nil
Clomid + hCG	4	5	4	nil

*Two patients had more than one type of therapy.

While the pre-ovulatory phase and dosage of HMG can be fairly regulated by serial estrone assays, KPI and cervical mucus changes, the parameters for ovulation and luteal activity are assessed by biphasic shift of BBT, pregnanediol or progesterone secretion, endometrial biopsy and progestational changes in vaginal smears. Of these, the adequacy of luteal function can be best assessed by assay of progestational hormones, or the degree of regression and progestational changes in vaginal smears. Hormone assays take time, and endometrial biopsy is not usually done in each and every cycle. Vaginal smear pattern during the second half of the cycle can thus be used, to indicate whether further administration of hCG is necessary.

Though the number of patients and treated cycles are limited, the results in properly selected cases of amenorrhea appear quite satisfactory (Table 2). Mild degree of over-stimulation like pain in the lower abdomen and moderate enlargement of the ovaries were noted in 7 out of 12 cycles.

It is obvious that the objective of using these various parameters along with gonadotropin therapy is to find the correct dose and timing of HMG and hCG for an individual subject which will produce changes in endogenous ovarian hormones as close to normal ovulatory cycle as possible. Thus the chances of obtaining normal and single pregnancies are likely to improve.

ACKNOWLEDGEMENTS

Thanks are due to the Dean, T.N. Medical College and Nair Hospital for allowing the publication of this data. The assistance of Shri. K.B.O. Pillai for staining the smears and in the typing of the manuscript is gratefully acknowledged.

REFERENCES

1. Brown, J.B., Mac Naughton, C., Smith, M.A. and Smith, B. (1968). J. Endocrinology 40, 175.
2. Brown, J.B. and Beischer, N.A. (1972). Obst. Gynecol. Survey. 27, 205.
3. Johansson, E.D.B. and Gemzell, C. (1969). Acta Endo. (Kbh). 62, 89.

REGULATION OF GONADAL FUNCTION IN THE MALE BY GONADOTROPINS

H.G. Burger, H.W.G. Baker, D.M. de Kretser, B. Hudson, P. Franchimont and R.J. Pepperell

The male gonad has two major functions, androgen secretion and gamete production, both of which are under gonadotropic control. In this review of recent advances in the physiology of the gonadotropins, we describe our studies of the secretory rates of LH and FSH in normal men, and discuss both short and long-term relationships between gonadotropin and gonadal steroid levels in peripheral blood. The application to clinical problems of knowledge gained concerning the feedback control of gonadotropin secretion, both in relation to gonadal steroids and to spermatogenesis is considered.

GONADOTROPIN PRODUCTION RATES

A. Luteinizing hormone

The determination of LH secretion rate is complicated by the occurrence of episodic short-time fluctuations in the plasma concentrations of the hormone, and by uncertainty regarding the most appropriate assay standard to be used. Production rates in 10 normal men whose ages ranged from 19 to 52 years were calculated from the metabolic clearance rate (MCR) (determined by the constant infusion technique) and the mean plasma LH determined from 2 - 12 samples, usually collected at 15 min intervals over 3 hr. Plasma LH concentration was expressed in mIU per ml, using a pituitary standard which had been bio-assayed in terms of the Second International Reference Preparation of Human Menopausal Gonadotropin (2nd - IRP HMG) (1). In the assay used, 1 µg LER 907 was equivalent to 40 mIU LH. If 2nd IRP HMG was used directly as the assay standard, the results (in mIU/ml) would be 5.2 times greater. For the majority of studies highly purified iodinated hLH (LER 1533 B76 - 93) was infused, equilibrium being reached 3-6 hr after commencement of the infusion ; identical results were obtained even if unlabeled LH was used. The disappearance curves of unlabeled and iodinated LH, and of the LH component of clinical grade human pituitary gonadotropin did not differ significantly from each other. The initial immunological half-life of LH was 42.4 $\pm$ 6 min. The mean MCR for the normal men was 44.6 ml/min or 23.4 ml/min/m^2; in 10 women, 4 of whom were normal and 6 anovulatory, MCR was 30.5 ml/min, or 18.4 ml/min/m^2, the difference between men and women being statistically significant. The value for MCR in women is slightly higher than the range of 23 - 25 ml/min reported by Kohler et al. (2) and the values in men are considerably greater than those recently reported by Marshall et al. (3).

In normal men, the secretion rate of LH varies from 44.6 to 122.9 with a mean of 84.6 IU per day. This figure may be compared with a mean urinary excretion of LH in seven of these normal men of 35.0 IU per day, (equivalent to 42 % of the production rate), using radioimmunoassay of ethanolic extracts of urine and the 2nd-IRP HMG as standard. When LH (1012 IU over 8 hr) was administered to 6 women with ovulatory disturbances, a mean of 36 % of the administered dose (in terms of 2nd IRP-HMG) was found in the urine in the succeeding 24 hr.

B. Follicle Stimulating Hormone

Preliminary studies using labeled and unlabeled FSH have indicated the extreme difficulty of achieving plateau levels of the hormone; even with infusions lasting for 16 hours, the immunoprecipitable plasma radioactivity was still rising slowly. It was possible to estimate that the MCR was of the order of 6-10 ml/min which gives a calculated FSH secretion rate in normal men of approximately 25 IU/day (range 6-66). It is of interest that the ratio of LH to FSH activity in pituitary extracts (4) of 2.4 is of a similar order of magnitude to that of secretion rates - 3.3. In 3 normal men, urinary FSH excreted in 24 hr averaged 39 % of the estimated production rate, while the mean recovery of infused FSH was 24.2 % in 24 hr.

REGULATION OF TESTICULAR HORMONE SECRETION

A. Long-term studies

Examination of blood levels of gonadotropins and testosterone as a function of age indicates that during pubertal development,

LH and testosterone rise in parallel, while there is a more abrupt rise in FSH levels between stages 1 and 2 of puberty; increases in pubic hair and testicular volume also occur in parallel with this change in LH and testosterone concentration (Fig 1). The literature on the hormonal changes during puberty has been reviewed recently (6). With advancing age, there is a change in the relationship between the pituitary and the testes; a gradual decline in

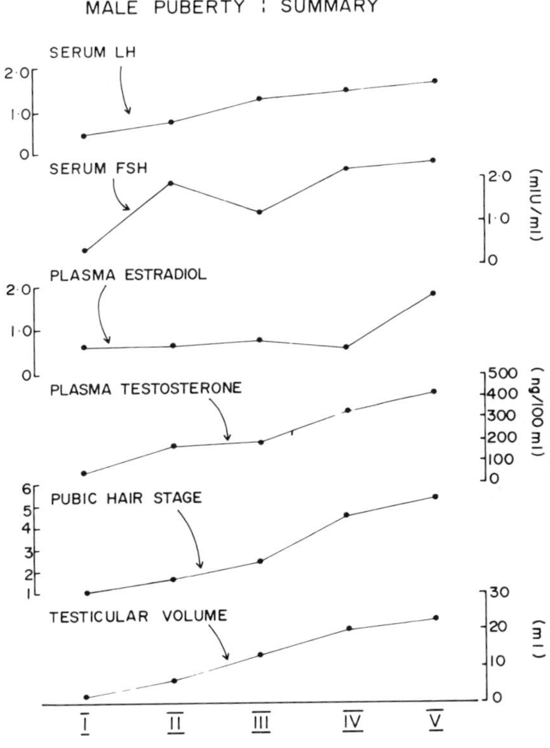

FIG 1. Changes in serum LH and FSH, plasma estradiol and testosterone, pubic hair and testicular volume from stages I - V of puberty [after Baker et al. (5)].

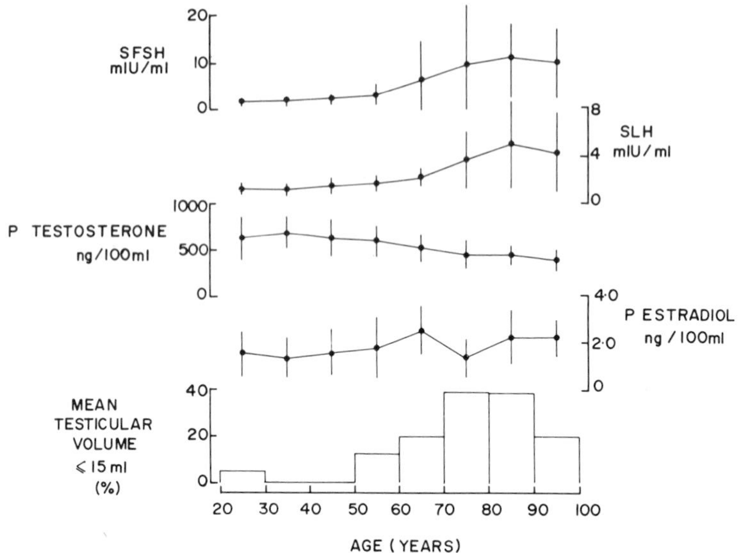

FIG 2. Changes in serum FSH and LH, plasma testosterone and estradiol and frequency of finding a mean testicular volume ≤ 15 ml in men from the third to tenth decades.

plasma testosterone levels occurs after the fourth decade, whilst LH and FSH levels rise (Fig 2); because there is an increase in sex steroid binding globulin capacity over the age of 60, free testosterone levels fall with advancing age, confirming the findings of Vermeulen et al. (7). The fact that the absolute response of testis to stimulation with hCG in old men is less than that in younger men (8) provides confirmatory evidence of a decrease in testicular function in the former; the rise in gonadotropin concentrations presumably reflects a diminution of the negative feedback effects of the testicular androgens and of a possible factor (Inhibin) produced by the germinal epithelium.

B. Short-term studies

The recent observations of short-term fluctuations in the levels of the gonadotropins (9-11) and testosterone (11-13) has posed new problems for the diagnostician and the investigator. Changes in LH may be over a 300-900 % range and several authors have indicated that there is an apparent lack of association between the LH and testosterone peaks seen during 10-15 min sampling experiments. It would thus seem relevant to examine two questions : first, to what extent does a single plasma gonadotropin level give a reliable indication of an individual's gonadotropic function and second, is there any relationship between episodes of LH secretion and testosterone levels in plasma.

C. Relationships between single and multiple gonadotropin determinations

In order to examine what correlation exists between single and multiple estimations of serum gonadotropin concentrations, blood samples were drawn at 15 min intervals for 3 hr in 15 normal men and 31 patients with oligo- or azoospermia. The mean levels of FSH and LH of the multiple samples for both these groups were compared with a "normal" range previously established for single samples from 55 normal men of a comparable age range (20-50 years); these mean values were then categorized as being high, normal or low with respect to this normal range. Of the 31 infertile men evaluated in this way, mean FSH levels were above the normal range in 10; all individual samples were also above normal, indicating that a single estimate would have been adequate for correct classification. Twenty patients had mean values in the normal range; however, in 5, individual samples fell above the upper limit of normal and in 2, individual samples were abnormally low. One patient had a mean level below the lower limit of normal, though one individual sample was above that limit. Thus, as regards the finding of a single sample with an FSH content above the normal range, 10 of 15 patients were correctly classified, but 5 patients with a normal mean FSH level could have been misclassified. For LH, mean values were high in 9, normal in 20 and low in 2. Of the 9 with elevated mean levels, individual samples were within the normal range in 6 (generally at or just below the upper limit); of the 20 classed as normal, individual values were high in 7. The two with low mean values both had individual concentrations in the normal range.

When the normal individuals were examined, 13 of 15 were in the previously assigned normal range for FSH and in one of these, some individual samples were high; 2 patients had high levels. In 12 of 15 normal men, mean LH levels were in the normal range, but in 6, high single samples were observed. In three, all samples were above the previously established normal range. It can be concluded that classification of a patient's gonadotropic status is open to error if only a single determination is made, and that caution must be exercised particularly with values at the extremes of the normal range. In the author's laboratory, a value of 6.0 mIU/ml for serum FSH in the presence of azoospermia would indicate irreversible damage to the germinal epithelium.

D. Urinary gonadotropin excretion

In order to assess whether the diagnostic accuracy of gonadotropin determinations could be improved, the daily excretion rate

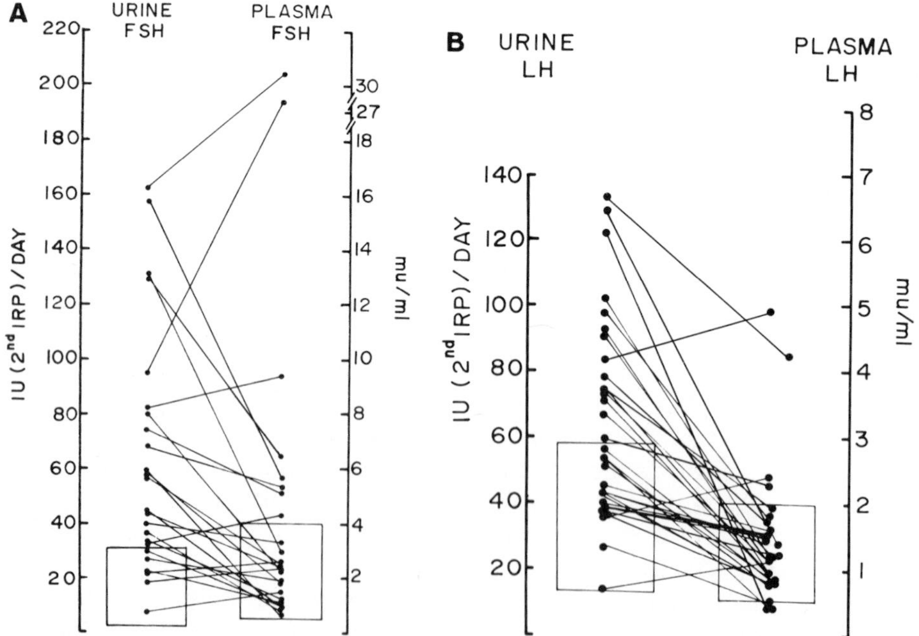

FIG 3. Comparison of serum FSH (3A) and LH (3B) (as measured on a single sample) and 24 hr urinary excretion of FSH and LH in men with testicular disorders. The normal range for each radioimmunoassay, which utilized the same anti-FSH and anti-LH serum, is shown as a box.

of both hormones has been measured in ethanolic extracts of urine from 24 oligospermic and azoospermic patients. These values were compared to the plasma gonadotropin levels (Fig 3A). Eighteen of these patients had elevated 24 hr urinary excretion rates of FSH but in only 8 of these were the plasma levels elevated. In 27 patients, the daily excretion rate of LH was measured and compared with plasma levels (Fig 3B); 4 had elevated plasma levels, but in 14 the urinary excretion rate was greater than normal. The estimation of urinary gonadotropin excretion may be of particular value during puberty, in the light of recent evidence (14) that nocturnal levels of LH were higher than those during the day at that time. It must be pointed out, however, that there may be considerable variation in the urinary excretion of gonadotropin in normal subjects, as illustrated by the findings in the normal young man shown in Fig 4.

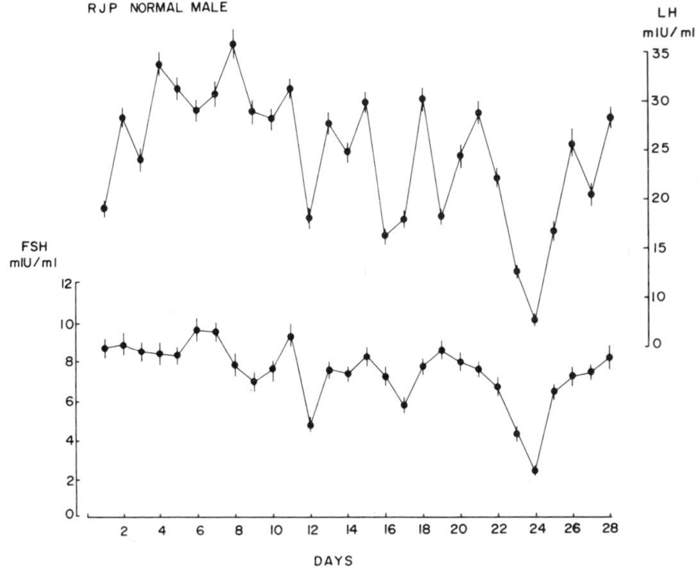

Fig 4. Daily variation in the urinary excretion of immunoreactive FSH and LH in a normal man aged 29 years. The bars indicate the error of the individual estimate ($\pm$ 1 S. D).

E. Relationship between LH and testosterone

A number of studies have suggested that there appears to be a lack of correlation between endogenous LH and testosterone levels when multiple (13) or continuous (1) sampling is undertaken. Furthermore, Marshall et al. (3) administered 1210 IU of LH to 4 normal men and observed a significant rise in 17-β hydroxy androgens in only one.

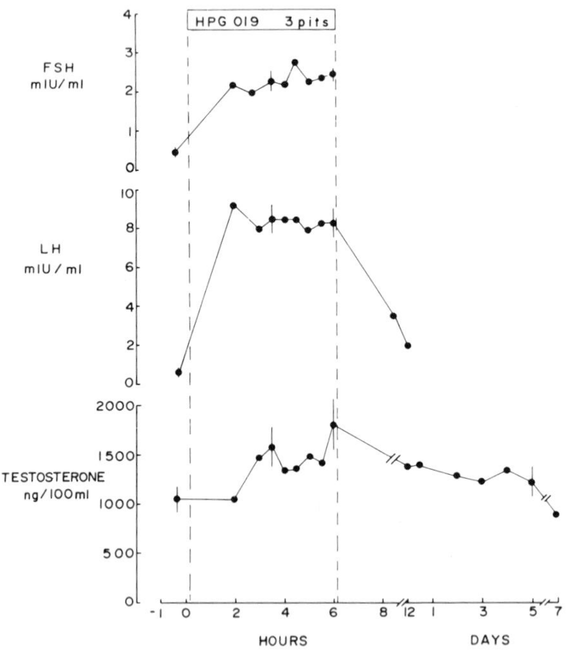

FIG 5. Responses of plasma FSH, LH and testosterone to the infusion of human pituitary gonadotropin (HPG, batch 019, Commonwealth Serum Laboratories, Melbourne) in one normal man who received the equivalent of 3 human pituitaries (total of 180 IU FSH, 360 IU LH by immunoassay; the biological potency for FSH was extremely low, whilst for LH it was equivalent to immunological potency). See Pepperell et al. (4).

Naftolin et al. (12) reported that they could find no consistent relationship between testosterone levels and the onset of LH rise in a study using multiple sampling over 8 hr, but did find that one third of LH peaks were followed by a rise in testosterone and that each elevation of the latter was preceded by an LH peak. Rises in testosterone occurred 45-80 min after LH. Studies in the authors' laboratory using the infusion of human pituitary gonadotropin (3 pituitary equivalents) showed a rise in testosterone which occurred between 2 and 3 hr after commencement of the infusion in one of two normal subjects (Fig 5) and re-analysis of data from continuous sampling studies (11) and inspection of the published data of Murray and Corker (13) suggests that the interval between a rise in LH and a rise in testosterone may be about 3-4 hr. Further studies using a sufficiently long sampling time (eg. at least 12 hr) will be required to resolve this problem.

Additional data relevant to a consideration of LH - testosterone relationships comes from an analysis of the testicular response to injection of synthetic LHRH. Numerous studies have shown that, in response to conventional iv doses of 25-100 μg LHRH, a peak response in serum LH is observed at 20-30 min. Few studies of testicular responsiveness to an abrupt LH elevation of this type have been reported. In 4 normal men, plasma FSH, LH and testosterone levels were measured from 20 min before to 4 hr following a single iv injection of 100 μg LHRH. There was a rise in testosterone approximately 3 hr after the LHRH injection in 3 of the 4. Variability of testosterone levels under basal conditions again renders interpretation of such data difficult, but the findings are consistent with a latent interval 3-4 hr between LH stimulus and testosterone response. The findings emphasise the need for studies over a longer interval to elucidate this relationship.

FEEDBACK BETWEEN TESTIS AND PITUITARY

A number of aspects of the feedback control of gonadotropin secretion have been reviewed recently by the present authors (6, 15, 16). From the viewpoint of the clinician, the practical application of knowledge gained by a study of pituitary-testicular feedback is in the ability to assess hypothalamic and pituitary function on the one hand, and testicular function, particularly in relation to delayed puberty and to disorders of fertility on the other. Certain combinations of values of FSH, LH and testosterone on single blood samples give adequate diagnostic information; thus, the finding of markedly elevated levels of FSH and LH, together with a low level of plasma testosterone provides unequivocal confirmation of the presence of severe testicular damage. On the other hand, the finding of FSH, LH and testosterone levels in the low portion of the normal range in, for example, a 16 year old boy who shows no sign of pubertal development provides neither diagnostic nor prognostic information and emphasises the need for dynamic evaluation of the pituitary - testicular relationship. This can include assessment of testicular reserve with hCG, of hypothalamic - pituitary function with clomiphene citrate and of pituitary responsiveness to LHRH.

CLINICAL APPLICATIONS

Two of the clinical problems mentioned above will be discussed briefly to illustrate the application of such investigations. In a study of retarded puberty in patients not suffering from primary gonadal disorders, Franchimont et al. (17) have suggested a classification of affected patients into two groups on the basis of their responses to clomiphene and to LHRH. In the first group of six boys aged 6-17, there was a significant rise in LH, and a less constant rise in FSH, following clomiphene administration; LHRH injection led to 8-10 fold rises in LH and 1.6 - 2.7 fold rises in FSH. In all these patients spontaneous puberty occured within two years following their investigations. In the second group, which included 6 patients with hypogonadotropic hypogonadism and anosmia and five other patients with delayed puberty aged 17 - 25 years, there was no response to clomiphene, and a minimal (less than 4-fold) or no response to LHRH. Prognosis in this group appears poor, and active treatment is indicated for their isolated deficiency of gonadotropin synthesis and/or release.

The assessment of men presenting with infertility should include investigations which can give both prognostic information and a guide to appropriate therapy. Of great importance is the recognition of the small number of patients with gonadotropin deficiency, in whom replacement therapy with hCG alone, or with FSH and LH (with hCG) is likely to restore fertility. In them, low or low-normal gonadotropin levels are usually unresponsive to clomiphene but may respond to LHRH, particularly in the presence of a hypothalamic disorder. It is also important to recognise those patients with irreversible damage to the germinal epithelium, as in seminiferous tubular hyalinization or germinal cell aplasia (the Sertoli-cell only syndrome). Here the most important single finding is a clear-cut elevation in serum FSH (Fig 6) (17, 18). Investigation of men with oligospermia and azoospermia whose testicular biopsies indicate the presence of hypospermatogenesis or of germinal cell arrest reveal the presence of FSH elevation in 20 % of the former and 50 % of the latter (17, 18) and of elevated LH levels and low testosterone concentrations in a significant number. In the majority of men with these testicular disorders administration of clomiphene is associated with normal FSH and LH responses, while responses to LHRH may be normal or even exaggerated (6).

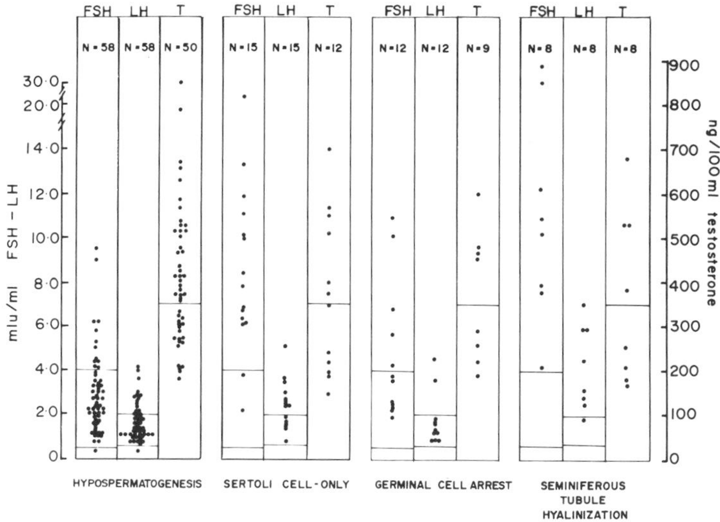

FIG 6. The levels of FSH, LH and testosterone in serum and plasma of men with testicular disorders are grouped according to the histological appearance of the biopsy. The normal ranges for FSH and LH are indicated by the horizontal lines, whilst the lower limit of normal for plasma testosterone is similarly indicated.

HCG stimulation of testosterone production, in contrast, frequently leads to a relatively poor response (16, 17), which is particularly noticeable after the second of the four daily hCG injections (3000 IU per day) used in the stimulation test. This highlights probable deficiencies in interstitial cell function in males with oligo- or azoospermia and disorders of spermatogenesis.

CONCLUSION

In this review, some aspects of the normal production rates of the gonadotropins, and the relationship of these to the urinary excretion of immunoreactive FSH and LH, have been discussed. Some of the problems still remaining in the interpretation of data on gonadotropic control of testosterone production have been mentioned, and measurements of basal levels of gonadotropins, and their responses to dynamic testing, have been related to certain clinical problems. Future studies must be directed not only to an elucidation of the basis of abnormalities in such disorders as idiopathic infertility, but to the clarification of the feedback control, specifically of FSH, an area which holds great promise in the development of potential agents to regulate male fertility.

ACKNOWLEDGEMENTS

We are grateful to Dr. L. E. Reichert for his generous gifts of purified FSH and LH and to the Australian Human Pituitary Advisory Committee for clinical grade HPG. The Hormone distribution Officer of the NIAMDD kindly provided reagents for the radioimmunoassay of FSH, and Dr. Anne Hartree provided LH for use as tracer in the LH assay. Drs. E. Keogh and M. Suthers and Sister L. Sievers kindly assisted in the collection of blood samples, and Dr. Christina Wang, Misses. G. May, L. Lindley and A. Dulmanis provided excellent technical assistance. We thank Miss. Christine Freestone for drawing the figures and Miss. Sandy Robertson for secretarial assistance.

The work was supported by grants from the National Health and Medical Research Council of Australia and the Belgian Foundation for Medical Research, and by the Allen and Hanbury's Fellowship (Dr. R. J. Pepperell).

REFERENCES

1. Alford, F.P., Baker, H.W.G., Patel, Y.C., Rennie, G.C., Youatt, G., Burger, H.G. and Hudson, B. (1973). J. Clin. Endocr. 36, 108.
2. Kohlet, P.O., Roos, G.T., and Odell, W.D. (1968). J. Clin. Invest. 47, 38.
3. Marshall, J.C., Anderson, D.C., Russell Fraser, T. and Harsoulis, P. (1973). J. Endocrinol. 56, 431.
4. Pepperell, R.J., Taft, H.P., Schiff, P., Brown, J.B., Evans, J.H., de Kretser, D.M. and Burger, H.G. (1973). The Endocrine Society of Australia, Proceedings of the 16th Annual Meeting, Abstract 34.
5. Baker, H.W.G., Court, J.M., de Kretser, D.M., Hudson, B. and Wang, C. (1973). The Endocrine Society of Australia, Proceedings of the 16th Annual Meeting, Vol. 16, Abstract 18.
6. Franchimont, P. and Burger, H. (1973). In "Human growth hormone and gonadotropins in health and disease", North Holland, Amsterdam (in press).
7. Vermeulen, A., Rubens, R., and Verdonck, L. (1972). J. Clin. Endocrinol. Metab. 34, 730.
8. Longcope, C. (1973). Steroids 21, 583.
9. Nankin, H.R. and Troen, P. (1971). J. Clin. Endocrinol. Metab. 33, 558.
10. Naftolin, F., Yen, S.S.C. and Tsai, C.C. (1972). Nature New Biol. 236, 92.
11. Alford, F.P., Baker, H.W.G., Burger, H.G., de Kretser, D.M., Hudson, B., Johns, M.W., Masterton, J.P., Patel, Y.C. and Rennie, G.C. (1973). J. Clin. Endocr. 37 (in press).
12. Naftolin, F., Judd, H.L., and Yen, S.S.C. (1973). J. Clin. Endocrinol. Metab. 36, 285.
13. Murray, M.A.F. and Corker, C.S. (1973). J. Endocrinol. 56, 157.
14. Boyer, R.M., Finkelstein, J., Roffwarg, H., Kapen, S., Weitzman, E. and Hellman, L. (1972). New Eng. J. Med. 287, 582.
15. Burger, H.G., Baker, H.W.G., Hudson, B. and Taft, H.P. (1972) In "Gonadotropins", B.B. Saxena, C.G. Beling, H.M. Gandy, (Eds). Wiley-Interscience, New York. pp 569.

16. Burger, H.G., Franchimont, P., de Kretser, D.M. and Hudson, B. (1973). Workshop Conference on Gonadotropins and Gonadal Steroids, Academic Press, New York (in press).
17. De Kretser, D.M., Burger, H.G., Fortune, D., Hudson, B., Long, A.R., Paulsen, C.A. and Taft, H.P. (1973). J. Clin. Endocrinol. Metab. 35, 392.
18. De Kretser, D.M., Burger, H.G. and Hudson, B. (1973). In Proceedings of Serono International Symposium on Male Fertility and Sterility, R. Mancini (Ed). Academic Press, (in press).

SERUM GONADOTROPIN LEVELS IN MEN WITH HYPOGONADISM : MESTEROLONE IN THE TREATMENT OF OLIGOZOOSPERMIA

G.K. Rastogi, B.N. Datta, R.J. Dash, M.K. Sinha

INTRODUCTION

Decreased gonadal function in adult men could manifest itself in the reduction of either one or both the functions of the testes, namely, spermatogenesis and the secretion of androgens. Male potency, in addition to hormonal influences, is dependent on neural and psychological factors. The present paper describes the levels of serum gonadotropins in different types of male hypogonadism. In a small group, the response of serum gonadotropins to synthetic LHRH has also been evaluated. Mesterolone (17 β -hydroxy-1 α -methyl-5 α -Androstan-3-one) therapy has been evaluated in disorders of spermatogenesis.

MATERIALS AND METHODS

Blood samples were collected in the morning from 54 eugonadal men (aged 18 to 60 years), 24 men with idiopathic azoospermia, 24 men with oligozoospermia (semen-spermatozoa count less than 40,000,000/ml on three consecutive counts), 7 men with cytogenetically proved Klinefelter's syndrome, 6 men with unexplained failure of testicular development, 12 men presenting with impotence and a group of diabetic men with and without impotence. Whenever possible, blood was collected on two consecutive days and serum stored at -20°. Men with disordered spermatogenesis had normal libido, potency and virility; testicular biopsy was obtained from a significant number of them. Mesterolone, a weak peripherally acting androgen, was administered orally, in a dose of 25 mg three times daily for 6 to 9 months to 8 men with azoo- and 14 men with oligozoospermia. Repeated semen examinations were carried out at intervals of 6 weeks. For the LHRH test, 100 µg of the peptide was injected soon after obtaining 2 basal samples. Further samples were collected after 20 and 60 min. LH and FSH were estimated by using homologous radioimmunoassays standardized in our laboratory (1), utilizing reagents gifted by the National Pituitary Agency, NIH, U.S.A. The standards used were MRC human LH 68/40 and for FSH, IRP-HMG-II, both supplied by the National Institute of Medical Research, London, England. The lower limit of detection for both LH and FSH was 2 mU/ml.

RESULTS AND COMMENTS

Figure 1 shows the serum FSH and LH levels in men with different types of hypogonadism. In 43 eugonadal men, the serum LH levels ranged from undetectable to 27 mU/ml with a mean of 9.7 ± 1 (SEM). The serum FSH concentration in 54 men ranged from undetectable to 10 mU/ml, with a mean of 3.8 ± 0.35. These values are comparable with those reported in the West utilizing similar standards (2,3,4). The mean serum LH of 11.2 ± 2 (range 2-33.6 mU/ml) in 24 oligozoospermic males was not significantly different ($p > 0.05$) from that in eugonadal men. However, the mean serum FSH concentration in this group, 11.4 ± 2 (range, undetectable to 35), was significantly higher ($p < 0.05$) than that in eugonadal men. In 24 azoospermic men, the mean LH, 13.0 ± 2.7 (range 2-49) and the mean FSH, 16.6 ± 2.2 (range 2 - 37.8), were both significantly ($p < 0.05$) higher than those in eugonadal men. These findings are slightly different from those of Franchimont et al. (2), who did not find much elevation in the serum LH levels in such patients. As is evident from Figure 2, we also found a good correlation between the histological grading of spermatogenesis (5) and the serum FSH levels, but no correlation between the stage of spermatogenesis and serum LH levels. Serum FSH levels were usually elevated when gametogenesis was arrested before spermatid formation. These findings support the views of Franchimont et al. (2) and Steinberger (6) that FSH is necessary for the meiotic division and formation of spermatids. Mesterolone at the dose administered to the azoospermics does not significantly alter the circulating gonadotropin levels (7) and failed to improve spermatogenesis. However, out of fourteen oligozoospermics, in ten, a mean increase in sperm count of 35,000,000/ml was observed. In such cases, where a decrease in mobility was present, a significant improvement was noticed after Mesterolone therapy. Although oligozoospermics with improved sperm-count and motility have been shown to effect conception (7), none of the patients in the present

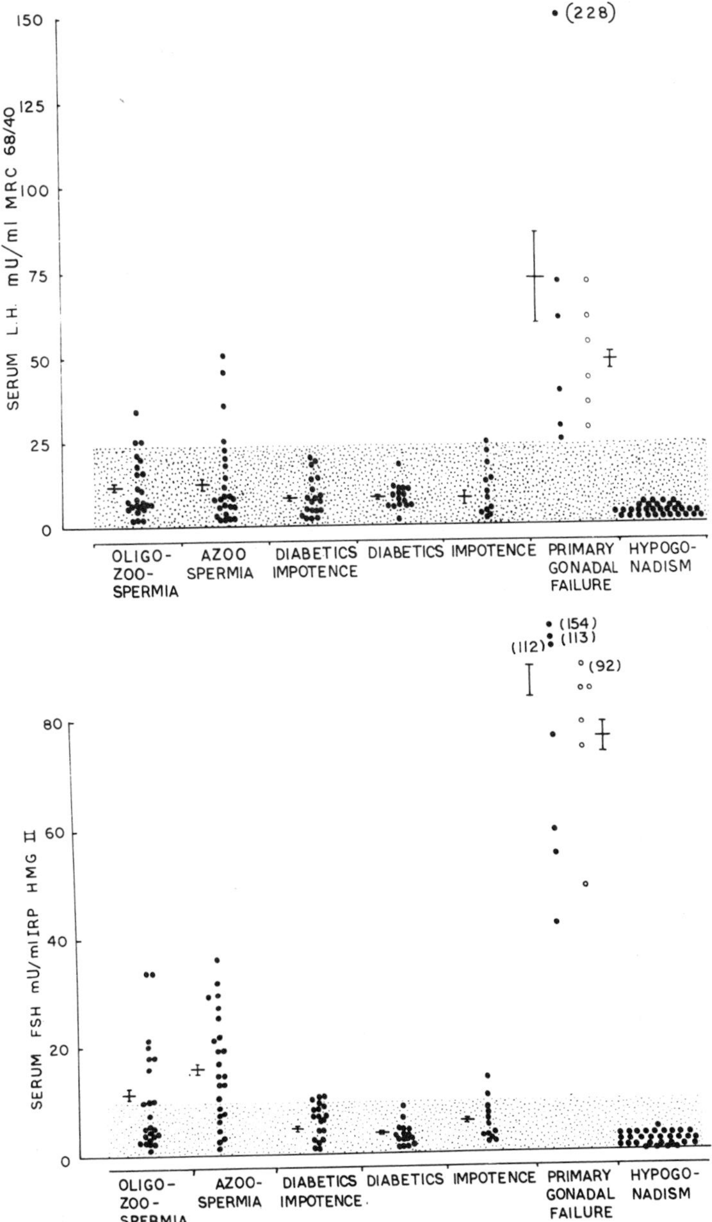

FIG 1. Serum LH and FSH levels in men with hypogonadism. The shaded area shows the range in eugonadal men.

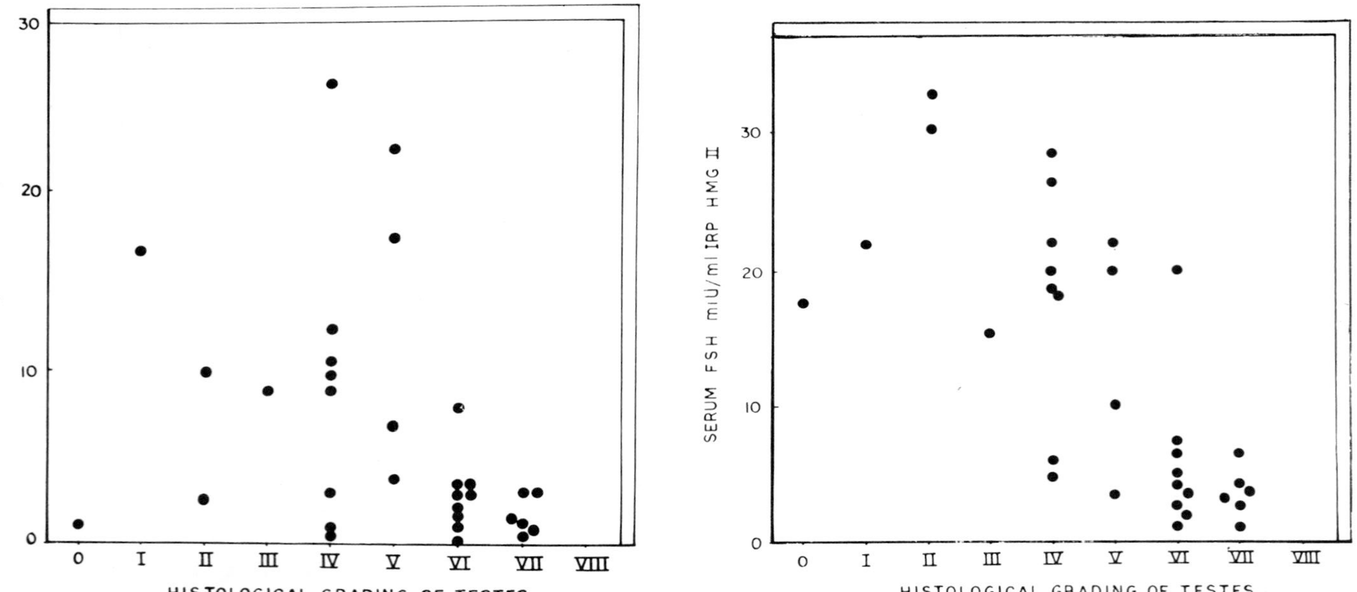

FIG 2. Relationship between stage of gametogenesis on histology in oligo and azoospermic men and serum LH and FSH levels.

study succeeded in this respect.

There was a profound elevation in serum LH and FSH levels in primary gonadal failure: Klinefelter's syndrome (n=7) mean LH 79 ± 26.6 and mean FSH 89.8 ± 14.3; primary testicular failure (n=6) mean LH 47.6 ± 6.3 and mean FSH 79.2 ± 6.2.

Hypospermatogenesis, a decreased Ketosteroid excretion and a decreased potence are frequently met with in diabetes mellitus; the causes for these are multifactorial and not dependent on endocrinologic disturbances (8). The mean serum LH and FSH levels in 16 diabetics with normal sexual potency (7.9 ± 0.8 and 3.7 ± 0.6, respectively and in 19 diabetic men with impotence (LH 8.2 ± 1.3, FSH 6.16 ± 0.7) did not differ significantly ($p > 0.05$) from those in eugonadal men or 12 non-diabetic men with

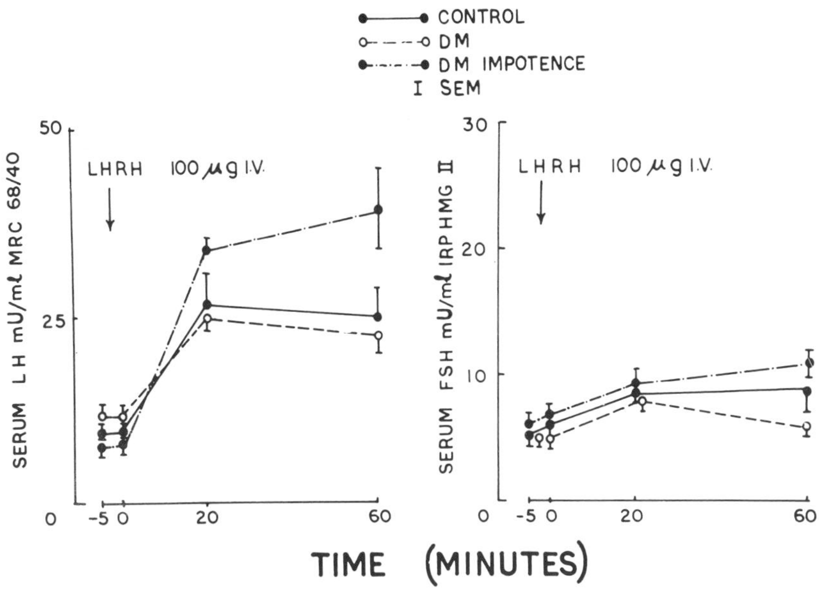

FIG 3. LH and FSH response to 100 μg synthetic LHRH in 5 eugonadal men and 5 diabetics with and 5 diabetics without impotence.

impotence (LH 10 $\pm$ 2.2, FSH 6 $\pm$ 1.1). These finds are in agreement with earlier reports. In response to LHRH, administered i v, a significant rise in both LH and FSH was evident in eugonadal men as well as diabetic men with and without impotence (Fig 3). A significant derangement of the hypothalamo-hypophysio-gonadal axis is, therefore, not likely in diabetic patients with impotence or showing deficient spermatogenesis.

REFERENCES

1. Rastogi, G.K., Dash, R.J. and Sinha, M.K. (1973). J. Ass. Phys. Ind. 21, 643.
2. Franchimont, P., Millet, D., Venderely, E., Letawe, J., Legros, J.J., and Netter, A. (1972). J. Clin. Endocr. 34, 1003.
3. Neil, J., Teterson, J.R., Midgley, A.R. Jr., and Jaffe, R.B. (1968). J. Clin. Endocr. 28, 1473.
4. Saxena, B.B., Demura, H., Gandy, H.M. and Peterson, R.E. (1968). J. Clin. Endocr. 28, 519.
5. Clerment, Y. (1963). Amer. J. Anat. 112, 35.
6. Steinberger, E. (1971). Phys. Rev. 51. 1.
7. Petry, R., Rausch-Stroomann, J.G., Hienz, H.A., Senge, T. and Mauss, J. (1968). Acta. Endocrinol. 59, 497.
8. Singhal, K.C., Rastogi, G.K., Aikat, B.K. and Chhuttani, P.N. (1969). Ind. J. Path. Bact. 12, 145.

CONCLUDING REMARKS

A. V. Nalbandov

My primary reason for rising at this time is to speak on behalf of the many foreign guests of the Symposium. We wish to take this opportunity to thank the organizer of the meeting, Dr. N.R. Moudgal, for including us among the speakers. We find that this important and exceedingly fruitful meeting has provided us with much new and meaningful information which all of us will take home with us and use in our own work in one way or another.

Accordingly, I request that all of us rise and express our appreciation to Raghu for a job well done.

Neither can I miss this opportunity to express our appreciation for the presence of the delightful, colorful, and helpful young women who brightened our work days. Equally helpful and valuable was the presence of the young men who made our stay more pleasant. To them all: our heartfelt thanks !

By applying Chinese torture methods, the Honorary President of the Symposium, Dr. C.H. Li, persuaded me to "summarize" the symposium. I finally agreed because there will be no opportunity for rebuttal on the part of any member of this audience.

Obviously, it would serve no purpose to rehash the contents of the papers the great majority of which were of high quality. Accordingly, I would like to present some random thoughts as they ran through my head as I listened. Please do not infer from the briefness of my remarks that my thoughts were few. I could easily spend the next hour or so highlighting what I consider the most outstanding contributions. However, do not fear; in deference to the general brain fatigue from which we all suffer because of the rich intellectual fare, of which we partook during this week, my remarks will be kept to no more than ten minutes.

I and my colleagues who are comparative endocrinologists, were saddened by the fact that the rat continues to be pre-eminent as the prime animal model for experimentation. This, in spite of the fact that it has been amply shown that its endocrine and reproductive systems are so specialized that they bear little or no resemblance to the systems evolved by other animals. Thus, any extrapolation from this arch endocrine artifact is hazardous,especially to man. Two examples of many will suffice. The mechanism of prolactin release is unique for the murine species as is the restricted use of prolactin as a luteotropic hormone. Untold research efforts were wasted on other mammals in which attempts were made to maintain the corpus luteum with prolactin. Equally futile were efforts to demonstrate hypothalamic differentiation by the post-natal surge of testosterone in any animal other than rats, hamsters, and perhaps rabbits. Accordingly, I would like to make a plea that serious consideration be given to the use of other experimental models to maximize the chances that the information obtained may be more easily transferable to reproductive problems besetting man. The fashion of using the term "relevance of research", e.g., its applicability, which seems to be sweeping the world will surely make it easier to obtain research support from increasingly recalcitrant granting agencies, if animal models whose reproductive patterns and endocrinology approach those of man, more closely than do those of the rat. That such models can be used has been demonstrated by scientists, who are using monkeys or domestic animals. Please do not interpret these remarks as being critical of doing "science for science's sake", but think of them as a word of caution that our tax-paying supporters may get as tired of paying for esoteric biological research as they did in the United States for space exploration. If and when this day comes, I will regret it as much as you will.

When radioimmunoassays first became available, it was shown that in most species the basel levels of FSH and LH do not change throughout the cycle until the occurrence of the ovulatory peaks of these hormones. This fact caused concern to many because it was argued that rises in hormone levels should occur in order to explain the luteotropic effect of LH and follicular growth and steroidogenesis which is usually ascribed to the gonadotropic complex. Karsch and I proposed in 1970 that this need not concern us, if we assume that in the face of unchanging hormone levels the sensitivity of the end organ may be changing. It was heartening to find that increasing attention is being directed toward the end organ and of the meaning of the concept of its "changing sensitivity". Indications are that this may turn out to depend on a change in the number and the kind of binding sites in the corpora lutea or in the follicle. Whether this will explain most of the phenomena reported at this symposium, only time will tell. I have learned over the years that glib and easy explanations frequently turn out to be over-simplified, if not totally wrong. At present these "bandwagon" phenomena include prostaglandins, cyclic AMP, binding sites, etc., which we have seen included in a variety of schemes and models presented to us.

As a nonchemist, I was tremendously impressed with the dexterity and ingenuity with which organic chemists chip away at, and otherwise mutilate and violate the integrity of FSH and LH molecules. The subunits they have produced are being avidly used by physiologists so far with conflicting results both with regard to their biological activity and their ability to be bound. Obviously the ultimate aim of the chemists is to present us with synthetic gonadotropins, but estimates as to how soon this will be accomplished vary from "very soon" to "not in our life-time".

In short, then, the intellectual content of the symposium was enormous and I will conclude with congratulating both the convener on a most well conceived symposium and the many speakers on the excellence of their data and their presentations.

Subject Index

A

Adenyl cyclase
  of chlorpromazine on LH
    stimulated, 396
  effect, of LH on ovarian, 395
  of prostaglandins on, of bovine
    corpus luteum, 378
Affinity chromatography, *see also*
  Immunosorbents
  coupling to hCG to Sepharose-4B
  problems involved in the use of,
  to purify receptor proteins, 456
Amenorrhea
  primary and secondary, 519
  use of gonadotropin therapy in the
    treatment of, 519, 524, 527
Amino acids
  composition
    of hCG, 74
    of human FSH, 37
    of human LH and subunits, 3
    of LHRF, 135
    of LH from frog and turtle, 110,
      111
  sequence
    of ovine, bovine, human, and
      porcine LH, 2, 4-6, 19
    of α and β subunits of hCG,
      82-84
Anencephaly of human fetus, effect
  on testis development, 199
Antiserum
  to FSH and LH
    characterization of, 213
    effect on, estrous cycle, 216
    follicular development in
      hamsters, 213, 216
    intraluminal water, 246
    ovulation, 241, 242
  to hCG
    immunosorbents of
      gonadotropin, 169
    preparation, and effect on
      ovulation in mice, 256, 257
    use in purification of LH and
      FSH, 170
    use in the assay of monkey
      serum LH and CG, 194
    use in studying immunopotency
      of hCG, 69, 163
    use in studying immunochemical
      properties of hCG synthe-
      sized in culture, 326-329
  to LH
    effect on LH stimulated proges-
      terone synthesis in sheep
      corpora lutea, 319, 392
    effect on progesterone secretion,
      and, pregnancy maintenance,
      263, 264
    use in studying immunological
      relatedness of LH from
      different species, 113
  to LHRH
    biological potency, preparation
      and use in radioimmuno-
      assay, 305-307
  to ovarian LH-hCG receptor, 446
  to $PGF_{2\alpha}$, effect on ovulation, 351
  to PMSG, effect on ovulation in
    mice, 258
  to prolactin
    effect on decidual cell
      response, 273
    effect on pigeon cropsac stimu-
      lation, and progesterone
      secretion, 272, 264

B

Biosynthesis
- experimental systems used in study of gonadotropin, 312, 313
- of gonadotropins, effect of LHRF on, 292, 312, 313
- of hCG, in cultivated trophoblasts, 321, 323
- of human chorionic FSH in culture, 330
- of LH, effect of testosterone propionate on, 314

C

Carbohydrate
- attachment sites, in hCG molecule, 86, 87
- composition, of human LH and its subunits, 3
  - of human FSH, 37, 46
  - of hCG, native and subunits, 85
- effect on hCG activity, 461, 471
- effect of mono- and oligosaccharides on hCG binding to its receptor, 468
- sequence, of hCG, 462
- sequential removal of, from hCG and its effect on hCG activity, 461, 471

Cell culture
- of granulosa, use in the assay of gonadotropins, 185, 191
- of luteal cells
  - effect of prostaglandins on labelled amino acid incorporation into protein, 334
  - inhibition by $PGF_{2\alpha}$ of progesterone production in, 334
  - stimulatory effect of LH on $PGF_{2\alpha}$ production, 334
  - use in studying luteotropic and luteolytic activity, 334-344

Cholesterol
- role of cytochrome P.450 in side-chain cleavage of, 403
- role of TPNH, and oxygen in side-chain cleavage of, 413
- side-chain cleavage pathway of, 403
- stoichiometry of side-chain cleavage of, 409, 410, 412

Corpora lutea
- of cycle, pregnancy and lactation, 260
- effect of lactation on, 268
- effect of LH deprival on, in hamster, 281-290
- stimulation of steroid secretion by LH in, 264
- ultrastructure of hamster, 282-285

Cyclic AMP
- binding potential and content of immature and adult rat ovary, 439
- effect of, on luteinization and progesterone secretion by granulosa cells in culture, 190
  - on alkaline phosphatase and ATPase activity of follicles, 395, 396
  - on cholesterol esterase activity in bovine corpus luteum, 384
  - on LH and FSH release, 294, 309
- effect of gonadotropins on levels in procine granulosa cell suspensions, 192
  - extraction and estimation of, 431
  - fate of endogenous, of corpora lutea, 381, 382
  - of hormones and prostaglandins on, in isolated corpora lutea and follicles, 369, 370, 395
  - increase in interstitial tissue, by LH, 501
  - of LH and FSH on, in isolated prepubertal rat ovary, 364

of LH and prostaglandins on ovarian, *in vivo* and *in vitro*, 366, 367
of LHRH on pituitary, 307, 308
of prostaglandins on pituitary, 309
role in action of LH, 376-378, 384, 385
testicular content, increase by FSH, 500, 502-509

Cytochrome P.450
presence of more than one species of, 404
purification and properties of, 404-412
role in side-chain cleavage of cholesterol, 403

E

Estrogen
effect, on intraluminal water retention, 245
on LH release, 309, 310
excretory levels of, during gonadotropin therapy, 515
relationship to ascites and ovarian enlargement, 516, 520
serum levels of, through estrous cycle of hamsters, 207-209
use of and advantages of, in planning gonadotropin therapy, 517, 518, 522, 523

Estrous cycle of hamsters
effect of FSH and LH deprivation during proestus on, 216
effect of hypophysectomy and gonadotropin therapy on, 207
follicular development during, 205, 206

F

Follicle stimulating hormone
activation of adenylate cyclase by, 486, 487
amino acid composition of, human, 37
analysis of carbohydrate moieties of, human, 37, 46
binding to membrane of seminiferous tubules, 486, 488
biological activities of native and subunits of, human, 31, 43
CD spectrum of, human, 32
component analysis of, 44
correlation of serum levels with stage of spermatogenesis, 548, 549
effect of, age of animal on ability of, to stimulate protein kinase, 488
administration of, to hypophysectomized hamsters, 207
desialylation of human, 44
LHRH on synthesis and release of, 294
effect, of neutralizing proestrus surge of, in hamsters, 216
effect, on binding of ^{125}I-hCG to granulosa cells, 412
on RNA and protein synthesis in testis, 488
on RNA polymerase activity and chromatin template activity, 491, 492
elevation of, in "Sertoli cell only" syndrome, 538, 541
fragmentation of human, 49, 50
isolation and characterization of, human pituitary, 23-26, 42-44
of subunits of human, 28, 30-39
metabolic clearance rate of, 535
methylation analysis of, 48, 49
microheterogeneity of human, 26, 42
potentiating effect of theophylline on release of, 295
role of, in follicular maturation, 248
in ovulation, 247

secretion rate in normal men and women, 532
serum levels in men during puberty, adulthood, and hypogonadism, 533, 534, 536, 537, 547, 548
serum levels of, during estrous cycle of hamster, 208, 209
stimulation of appearance of LH receptor by, 419
target cells in male, responsive to, 504, 510
unilateral ovariectomy in hamster, effect of, on serum levels, 211
Follicle stimulating hormone releasing factor
assay of, 132
effect on production of FSH from pituitary, 314
Follicular atresia
factors responsible for, 205, 210, 225
prevention of, in unilaterally ovariectomized hamsters, 210
significance of, 228, 229
Follicular development
changes in LH and FSH receptor during, 419
correlation with gonadotropin surge, 238, 239
dependence on hormones, 206, 238
effect, of FSH and LH antiserum on, in rats and hamsters, 213, 214, 238
of FSH on, in LH-deprived pregnant hamsters, 214, 215
effect of hypophysectomy on, 238
of PMSG treatment on, in hamsters, 206
of unilateral ovariectomy on, 209, 210
gonadotropin regulation of, 205, 206, 238
involvement of FSH and LH in the process of, 213
quantitative studies on, 205
role of gonadotropins in, 230
site of steroidogenesis in follicles during, 220

G

Glycosidases
effect of glycosidase inhibitors on binding of hCG to plasma membrane, 469
effect of hydrolysis of plasma membranes with, on hCG binding, 463, 464
involvement of cell surface, in hCG binding, 468
use of, in hydrolysis of hCG, 463, 464
use of, in structural investigation of human FSH, 49
Gonadotropins, *see also* LH, FSH, hCG and PMSG
binding to rat testis Leydig cell preparation, 462-473
biological activity of piscine, 122-125
biosynthesis of, 312-319
changes in, levels during puberty and adulthood, 533, 534
comparison of activities of mammalian, reptilian and piscine, using cell culture system, 188, 190
correlation of immunological and biological activity of, 161
effect of, on uterine water loss, 248
effect of a combination of, on progesterone production in cultured hamster corpora lutea, 335
effect of therapy, on estrogen excretion levels, 515

excretion of, in humans, 536
fractionation, characterization and bioassay of, of reptiles and amphibians, 104, 110
glycoprotein with dual activity from ovine pituitary and its characterization, 54-63
heterotropic activity of piscine, 126
need for, by testis and accessory organs, 199
need for, in luteal maintenance, 332
ovulation inducing activity of catfish, 122
of pituitary from reptiles and amphibians, 101
of piscine origin, 118-127
phylogenetic survey of reptilian, 114
plan of therapy, based on estrogen excretion pattern, 517, 522, 524
regulation of gonadal function in men by, 531-545
regulation of testicular hormone secretion by, 532
release from pituitary, 149
role of hypothalamus in release of, 149-154
role of, in the development of fetal testis, 199
in the development of theca interna, 220
in follicular development, 230
in function of granulosa and thecal cells, 220
secretion rate of, in humans, 537
serum levels in hypogonadal men, 539, 540, 545
serum levels on treatment with LHRH, 549
stimulation by, of $PGF_{2\alpha}$ and progestin production in luteal cell culture, 334
use of, in induction of ovulation in women, 512

Gonadotropin-releasing factor, *see also* LHRF and FSH-RF
effect of hypothalamic lesions on the release of gonadotropins, 149-150
effect of, on release of gonadotropins from pituitary, 153, 312
effect of steroids on pituitary responsiveness to LHRF, 152
involvement of cholinergic synapses in gonadotropin and prolactin release, 145
mechanism of action of, 312, 319
role of catecholamines in the release of, 154
role of cyclic nucleotides in release of gonadotropin and prolactin, 156
role of prostaglandins in mediating gonadotropin and prolactin release, 156

Granulosa
changes during ovulation, 225
changes in gonadotropin receptors during differentiation of, 416
formation of, 222
maturation of, and induction of luteinization in, 419, 421
transformation during luteinization, 227

H

Human chorionic gonadotropin
amino acid composition and sequence of α and β subunits, 74, 82-84, 461
antiserum to highly purified, 69
attachment sites of carbohydrates in, 86, 87
biological potency of, urinary, 68-71

of its subunits, 81
biological activity of tritiated, 474
biosynthesis of, in cultured trophoblasts, 321, 323
carbohydrate composition of native and subunits, 71, 72, 85, 462
effect of, and subunits on granulosa cells and luteinization in culture, 186
effect of removal of various carbohydrate components of, on biological and immunological activity, 466, 471
effect of route of administration of, on ovulation and its serum level in mice, 255
extraction, purification and analysis of, biosynthesized in culture, 321, 322
half-life of, in serum of mouse, 255
hydrolysis with specific glycosidases, 463, 464
immunopotency of urinary, 72
interaction with rat gonads, 474, 477
isoelectric focusing of molar, 95-97
isoelectric focusing of urinary, 69, 70
properties of, biosynthesized in culture, 325, 326
purification and characterization of urinary, 66, 73, 79
from hydatidiform mole, 93-99
separation of biological and immunological properties, 163-165
sialic acid content of urinary, 71, 72
of hCG synthesized in culture, 326, 328
studies on subunit recombination of urinary, 88
subunit structure of urinary, 80
uptake of ^{125}I-hCG by pseudopregnant rat ovaries and other organs, 475
Hydatidiform mole, chorionic gonadotropin from, 93
Hypogonadism
azoospermia, FSH and LH levels in men with, 535, 545
serum LH and FSH levels in men with Klinefelter's syndrome, 545, 549
use of mesterolone in therapy of oligozoospermia, 545
Hypophysectomy
ability of LH and prolactin to maintain pregnancy in hamsters following, 273, 274
effect of FSH on long-term, in hamsters, 207
effect on, estrous cycle in hamsters, 207
estrogen surge in rats, 239
follicular maturation, 238
Hypothalamus
effect of lesions on gonadotropin release, 149
effect of prostaglandins on release of LRF from, 361
localization of the gonadotropin-releasing factor in, 153
release of LRF from, 359

I

Immunosorbents
advantages of use of, 171
application of, 170
LH coated erythrocytes as, 170
preparation of, of gonadotropins, and their antibodies, 169
use of, in isolation of pituitary gonadotropins, 176
Interstitial cell stimulating hormone, *see* luteinizing hormone

Isoelectric focusing
of molar hCG, 95-97
of urinary hCG, 69, 70

L

Luteal function
effect of LH deprival on, 278
effect of prolactin antiserum on, 271, 272
relative role of LH and prolactin in, 271-278
Luteolysis
ability of LH to prevent, in hamsters, 275
changes in plasma membrane and mitochondria of hamster corpus luteum during, 289
effect of prostaglandins on, 333, 336
prostaglandins as antagonists of gonadotropin action in, 333-340
Luteinization
effect of cyclic AMP and prostaglandins on, 190, 191
effect of desialylation of hCG on, 186-188
formation of theca-lutein and granulosa lutein cells, 226, 227
of monkey granulosa cells in culture, effect of hCG and its subunits on, 186
of procine granulosa cells, effect of LH, hCG and FSH in culture on, 191
Luteinizing hormone
accessibility to tyrosyl residues of, 20, 21
amino acid, composition of hLH and its subunits, 3
of frog and reptilian, 110, 111
sequence of α and β subunits of bovine, human, porcine and ovine, 2, 4-6, 19
binding potential of ovary during pregnancy, 437, 438
CD and mass spectra of ovine, 10-13
daily excretion rate in normal and infertile men, 535
disulphide bridges of ovine, 8, 9
effect of, administration in different delay vehicles to rats on serum level, 275, 277
cyclic AMP and theophylline on release of, 295
ergot alkaloids on, level in rats, 277
intrafollicular injection of, on ovulation, 395
LHRH and its analogs on the release of, 294, 300
prostaglandins on the release of, 300, 301
effect of LH on, adenyl cyclase of luteal tissue, 394, 395
cyclic AMP in isolated rat and rabbit follicles, 369, 385
$PGF_{2\alpha}$ content of ovary, 345
ovarian cyclic AMP, 367, 368, 371
steroidogenesis, additive effects with cyclic AMP and PGE_2, 376-379
immunological relatedness of, from different species, 113
importance of sialic acid for biological activity of frog and turtle, 114
involvement in the luteotropic complex, 262
isolation from frog and turtle pituitary, 105
metabolic clearance rate of, in human, 531, 532
on the nature of interaction with its receptor, 432-435
primary structure of, subunits of ovine, 9, 16, 17

production rate in normal men and women, 531-532
purification of, receptor from luteinized rat ovaries, 444
receptor for, 419, 427
on the responsiveness to, 439
role of cyclic AMP and prostaglandins in the action of, 376
role of FSH in induction of LH receptor, 419
role of, in ovulation, 247-384
serum levels, in men during puberty and adulthood, 533, 534
during estrous cycle of hamster, 207, 208
in men with hypogonadism, 547, 548
structure comparison of bovine, human, porcine and ovine, 16, 17
structure elucidation of human and ovine, 2-8
structural homology with TSH, 18
use of cell culture system in the assay of, 186, 194, 195
variability in the primary structure of α and β subunits during evolution, 18, 19

Luteinizing hormone releasing hormone
amino acid composition of, 135
antiserum to deamidated, and its use in radioimmunoassay, 305-307
assay of, 132
biological potency of antiserum to, 306
counter-current distribution of, 130, 131
derivatization of, 134
effect of, analogs on LH release, 299, 300
effect on cyclic AMP accumulation in gonadotrophs, 297, 307, 308
effect on pituitary adenyl cyclase, 308, 309
effect on pituitary tissue culture, 313
hypothalamic content throughout estrous cycle, 307
intrinsic FSH releasing activity of, 142
isolation of, 129
mass spectrum of, 136-138
mechanism of action of, 305, 311
stimulatory effect on synthesis and release of LH and FSH from pituitary *in vivo* and *in vitro*, 292, 294, 313, 314, 317-319
structure-activity relationship of, 141
structure elucidation of, 133, 140
synthesis of, 139, 141
synthetic analogs and their activity, 140, 142
ultrastructural changes in gonadotrophs on stimulation with, 297
use of, in treatment of male infertility, 540, 549, 550

Luteotropic complex
involvement of LH and prolactin in, 262, 264, 271-278
in lactating rats, 260

M

Microheterogeneity
of human FSH, 26, 42
of molar hCG, 99
of urinary hCG, 66, 67

Monoamines
mediation through, of stimulation for release factor secretion, 357

O

Ovary
- estrogen excretory pattern as a measure of enlargement of, 516
- hyperstimulation with gonadotropins, 512, 513, 515
- gonadotropins and cyclic AMP in various compartments of rat, 364-375

Ovulation
- ability of catfish gonadotropins to induce, 122
- ability of pure LH, its β subunit and FSH to induce, 240
- action of LH and cyclic AMP on, 384, 385
- changes in theca interna, granulosa and stromal cells during, 224-226
- correlation of estrogen excretory pattern with, 519, 520
- effect of gonadotropin antisera on, 241, 242
- effect of intrafollicular injection of indomethacin, dbcAMP and cyclic AMP on, 348, 395
- effect of $PGF_{2\alpha}$ on oocyte maturation, 351
- induction of, by gonadotropins, 239, 512
- minimal time exposure to ovulating hormone, 253
- other events accompanying, 244
- ovum maturation for, 246
- preovulatory changes in prostaglandin content, 345
- on the preparedness of follicle for, 237, 238
- relative roles of FSH and LH in induction of, 237
- use of pentobarbital in studying, 243-246

P

Pregnant mare serum gonadotropin
- antiserum to, its ability on ovulation, 258
- effect on follicular development in hamster, 206
- ovulating ability of, 255

Primary structure of
- α and β subunits of ovine LH, 9, 16, 17
- variability in the, of α and β subunits during evolution, 18, 19

Progesterone
- effect of, on follicular growth, 207
- effect of, on intraluminal water dissipation, 245
- effect of ergocryptin on secretion of, 26
- effect of litter size on secretion of, and 20α-OH-P, 261
- effect of perphenazine on, 266, 267
- effect of prolactin antiserum on, 268
- secretion rhythm, during lactation, 261
- serum levels, through estrous cycle of hamster, 207, 209

Prolactin, involvement in the luteotropic complex, 264

Prolactin-inhibiting factor, synaptic transmitters involved in the release of, 154

Prostaglandins
- effect of antiserum to $PGF_{2\alpha}$ on ovulation, 351
- effect of hypothalamic PGs on release of LRF, 361
- effect of indomethacin on preovulatory elevation of, 345
- effect of LH on $PGF_{2\alpha}$ content of ovary, 345

effect of PGs on luteinization and progesterone secretion in granulosa cells in culture, 191
effect of PG-inhibitors on gonadotropin secretion, 359
effect of PGE_1 and PGE_2 on cyclic AMP in rat ovary and isolated rat corpora lutea and follicles, 367-371
effect of PG antagonist on steroidogenesis, 379
effect on ovarian arterial flow-rate, 334
effect on pituitary cyclic AMP, 309
effect on progesterone secretion, in hamster luteal cell culture, 333, 335
effect on release of LH and FSH, 300, 301, 358
failure of indomethacin to block LH-induced steroidogenesis, 350, 351
luteolytic effect of, 333
measurement of PGE and PGFs in rabbit Graafian follicles, 368
as mediators/attenuators of hormone action, 332
preovulatory changes in content of, 385, 386
rat ovarian content during estrous cycle, 345
role in LH action, 376-379
role in mediating gonadotropin and prolactin release, 156
role in ovulation
of the rabbit, 345
of rats, 358
Radioimmunoassay
at elevated temperature, 174
solid-phase method, 170, 172
Receptor
antiserum to purified rat ovarian LH, 446
assay of receptor activity, 446
changes in LH and FSH receptor during granulosa cell differentiation, 416
during pregnancy, 423
definition of, 416
effect of cyanoketone on FSH induced, stimulation of LH, 420
hCG-binding characteristics of ovarian, 450
isolation of receptor-rich pellet from corpus luteum, 417
nature of interaction of LH with its, 432-435
on the ontogenecity of LH, 438
purification and characterization of LH-hCG receptor from rat ovaries, 444-459
use of affinity chromatography in purification of, 445-447

S

Steroidogenesis
additive effect of LH and cyclic AMP on, 377-378
in bovine corpus luteum, effect of LH and cyclic AMP on, 376
changes during preovulatory period, 384
effect of 7-oxa-prostynoic acid on, 379-380
Subunits
amino acid and carbohydrate composition of human LH, 3
amino acid sequence of α and β, of ovine, bovine, human, and porcine LH, 2, 4-6, 19
of hCG, 82-84
biological activity of human FSH α and β, 31
biological activity of hCG α and β, 81

binding of LH-β to rat ovarian receptor, 435
carbohydrate composition of hCG, 85
effect of hCG subunits on luteinization in culture, 186
isolation and characterization of human FSH α and β, 28, 30-39
primary structure of α and β, of ovine LH, 9, 16, 17
recombination of, of hCG, 87, 88
use of urea in isolation of FSH, 28
variability in primary structure in α and β of ovine LH during evolution, 18, 19

T

Testis
age-dependent phosphodiesterase activity on FSH treatment, 488
blood-testis barrier, development of, 495
cell-types responsive to FSH in, 500-503
characteristics of binding of ^{125}I-hCG with receptor from, 480, 482
effect of age of tubules on responsiveness to FSH, 503
effect of cyproterone acetate on development of, 201
effect of fetal decapitation on development of, 199, 201
effect of FSH on primary spermtocyte and degeneration of spermatogonia, 492-494
FSH activation of adenylate cyclase in, 486
FSH effect on RNA and protein synthesis, and protein phosphorylation in, 488, 489
gonadotropic control of development of, 199
increase in cyclic AMP level by FSH in, 502, 503
need for the presence of fetal, 199
regulation of spermatogenesis by FSH in, 494
response of interstitial tissue to FSH, 501
responsiveness of the, in hypophysectomized rats to FSH, 505
secretion of Müllerian duct inhibiting substance by fetal, 202
secretion of testosterone by fetal, 201-202
specific binding of FSH to seminiferous tubules, 486
Testosterone
correlation of secretion, with LH secretion in men, 532, 538
secretion by fetal testis, 201-203
Theca interna
ability to synthesize estrogen, 222
changes during ovulation, 225
its formation from undifferentiated cells, in a variety of species, 220, 221
ultrastructure of, 221

U

Ultrastructure
of corpus luteum in hamster, 282-285
of a gonadotroph in culture, in the presence of LHRH, 298
of granulosa, 222, 223
of theca interna, 221
Urea
effect of, on ^{125}I-hCG binding to ovary, 477
use of, in subunit isolation of human FSH, 28

A 4
B 5
C 6
D 7
E 8
F 9
G 0
H 1
I 2
J 3